Axial Spondyloarthritis: A Clinical Approach

Axial Spondyloarthritis: A Clinical Approach

Editor: Bradley McGrath

FOSTER ACADEMICS

www.fosteracademics.com

www.fosteracademics.com

FOSTER ACADEMICS

Cataloging-in-Publication Data

Axial spondyloarthritis : a clinical approach / edited by Bradley McGrath.
p. cm.
Includes bibliographical references and index.
ISBN 978-1-64646-144-8
1. Spondyloarthropathies. 2. Spine--Diseases--Treatment. 3. Arthritis. I. McGrath, Bradley.
RC935.S67 A95 2022
616.73--dc23

Foster Academics,
118-35 Queens Blvd., Suite 400,
Forest Hills, NY 11375, USA

ISBN 978-1-64646-144-8 (Hardback)

Contents

Preface

Spondyloarthritis refers to a group of inflammatory diseases affecting the joints and enthuses. Ankylosing spondylitis is the most common of these disorders. Other disorders include psoriatic arthritis, reactive arthritis and enteropathic arthritis. Spondyloarthritis can cause tiredness, back pain, osteoporosis, psoriasis skin rash, pain or swelling in the hips, ankles, feet, knees, wrists, etc. The diagnosis of spondyloarthritis is based primarily on physical examination and medical history. An X-ray of the sacroiliac joints or an MRI may also be suggested. Pain and inflammation occurring in spondyloarthritis can be addressed with NSAIDs, while corticosteroids can be injected directly into a joint or membrane to reduce joint swelling. In cases where these drugs are insufficient to manage the symptoms, disease-modifying antirheumatic drugs may be prescribed to prevent joint damage and relieve symptoms. This book covers in detail the new frontiers in clinical management of spondyloarthritis. Different approaches, evaluations, methodologies and advanced studies on spondyloarthritis have been included herein. This book is a collective contribution of a renowned group of international experts on orthopedics and inflammatory diseases.

After months of intensive research and writing, this book is the end result of all who devoted their time and efforts in the initiation and progress of this book. It will surely be a source of reference in enhancing the required knowledge of the new developments in the area. During the course of developing this book, certain measures such as accuracy, authenticity and research focused analytical studies were given preference in order to produce a comprehensive book in the area of study.

This book would not have been possible without the efforts of the authors and the publisher. I extend my sincere thanks to them. Secondly, I express my gratitude to my family and well-wishers. And most importantly, I thank my students for constantly expressing their willingness and curiosity in enhancing their knowledge in the field, which encourages me to take up further research projects for the advancement of the area.

Editor

1

The prevalence of clinically diagnosed ankylosing spondylitis and its clinical manifestations: a nationwide register study

Sofia Exarchou[1*], Ulf Lindström[2], Johan Askling[3], Jonas K Eriksson[4], Helena Forsblad-d'Elia[2], Martin Neovius[4], Carl Turesson[1], Lars Erik Kristensen[1,5] and Lennart TH Jacobsson[2]

Abstract

Introduction: Prevalence estimates of ankylosing spondylitis vary considerably, and there are few nationwide estimates. The present study aimed to describe the national prevalence of clinically diagnosed ankylosing spondylitis in Sweden, stratified according to age, sex, geographical, and socio-economic factors, and according to subgroups with ankylosing spondylitis-related clinical manifestations and pharmacological treatment.

Methods: All individuals diagnosed with ankylosing spondylitis according to the World Health Organization International Classification of Disease codes, between 1967 and 2009, were identified from the National Patient Register. Data regarding disease manifestations, patient demographics, level of education, pharmacological treatment, and geographical region were retrieved from the National Patient Register and other national registers.

Results: A total of 11,030 cases with an ankylosing spondylitis diagnosis (alive, living in Sweden, and 16 to 64 years old in December 2009) were identified in the National Patient Register, giving a point prevalence of 0.18% in 2009. The prevalence was higher in northern Sweden, and lower in those with a higher level of education. Men had a higher prevalence of ankylosing spondylitis (0.23% versus 0.14%, $P < 0.001$), a higher frequency of anterior uveitis (25.5% versus 20.0%, $P < 0.001$) and were more likely to receive tumor necrosis factor inhibitors than women (15.6% versus 11.8% in 2009, $P < 0.001$). Women were more likely than men to have peripheral arthritis (21.7% versus 15.3%, $P < 0.001$), psoriasis (8.0% versus 6.9%, $P = 0.03$), and treatment with oral corticosteroids (14.0% versus 10.4% in 2009, $P < 0.001$).

Conclusion: This nationwide, register-based study demonstrated a prevalence of clinically diagnosed ankylosing spondylitis of 0.18%. It revealed phenotypical and treatment differences between the sexes, as well as geographical and socio-economic differences in disease prevalence.

Introduction

Ankylosing spondylitis (AS) is a chronic inflammatory disorder primarily involving the sacroiliac joints and spine. It is associated with both articular and extra-articular clinical manifestations, including peripheral arthritis, enthesitis, anterior uveitis, psoriasis, and inflammatory bowel disease. The first symptoms usually occur before the age of 30 and seldom occur after the age of 45 [1]. The chronic and often progressive nature of the disease affects individuals for most of their working lives, limiting physical function, the ability to work, and perceived quality of life [2,3]. Pharmacological treatments include non-steroidal anti-inflammatory drugs (NSAIDs), oral glucocorticoids, synthetic disease modifying anti-rheumatic drugs (sDMARDs), and tumor necrosis factor inhibitors (TNFi) [4].

Compared with rheumatoid arthritis (RA), few studies have examined the prevalence of AS. The prevalence in Europe, North America, and China is estimated at 0.03 to 1.8% [5-17]; however, estimates are lower in Japan [18] and higher in populations with a high frequency of the major risk gene, HLA-B27 [19].

The highly varying estimates in the West may reflect differences in study methodology. Studies used different

* Correspondence: sofiaexar@hotmail.com
[1]Rheumatology, Department of Clinical Sciences, Malmö, Lund University, Inga Marie Nilssons gata 32, 205 02 Malmö, Sweden
Full list of author information is available at the end of the article

sampling sources, including local health records [8,13,10], small population surveys [12,11,5,7,6,9], general epidemiological surveys [14], blood donor registers [16], and regional patient registers [15]. The population surveys performed to date also used different screening methods, including telephone interviews [5], postal surveys [6,9], and home-based interviews [7].

Accurate and contemporary prevalence estimates, including the frequency of AS-related clinical manifestations and pharmacological treatments, as well as socio-economic and geographical variations, are important for healthcare planning, and they may provide clues to possible risk factors for the disease. Furthermore, little is known about differences in disease manifestations and pharmacological treatments between the sexes at the population level. One approach to obtaining such information is to use national healthcare registers, a method that has only been used on a regional level for AS [15], but was successfully used on a national level for RA [20]. This approach is supported by the high validity of the Swedish National Patient Register (NPR) in general [21], and by our recent assessment of the validity of the International Classification of Disease (ICD) codes [22] for AS in the Swedish NPR; the ICD codes showed high validity with regard to fulfilling the established classification criteria for both AS and spondyloarthritis (SpA) [23,24].

The primary aim of the present study was to assess the total national point prevalence of clinically diagnosed AS in Sweden in December 2009, and to stratify the prevalence according to age, sex, geographical and socio-economic factors. We also stratified the prevalence according to AS-related clinical manifestations and pharmacological treatments. The secondary aim was to compare disease manifestations and pharmacological treatments between the sexes.

Methods

Setting

The data used in this nationwide, population-based study were obtained from the Swedish national healthcare registers.

Healthcare provision in Sweden is largely funded by the taxpayer and is independent of individual financial or insurance considerations. There is an upper limit to an individual's yearly costs for medical consultations and prescription medications. Patients with an inflammatory rheumatic disease such as AS are usually diagnosed at public or (less commonly) private rheumatology clinics. Such cases are rarely definitively diagnosed in a primary care setting [25].

Ethical approval for the study was granted by the Regional Ethics Committee, Karolinska Institute, Stockholm, Sweden. Patient consent was waived, as data were derived either from administrative registers that do not require informed consent or quality registers where the consent is already given at the time point of first registration.

Data sources

The NPR comprises the Inpatient Register (IPR) and the Outpatient Register (OPR). The IPR was launched in 1964, and complete national coverage (almost 100%) was achieved in 1987. The IPR contains data (medical and administrative) derived from all patients discharged from hospitals in Sweden [21]. The OPR for public specialized care was started in 2001. The national coverage of the OPR is lower (approximately 73% in 2008 and 87% in 2011) [26,27] than that of the IPR, mainly due to missing data from private caregivers. Visits to primary care facilities are not covered by the NPR. Diagnoses are registered using the Swedish version of the ICD codes [22]. The present study used the NPR to identify AS cases and AS-related clinical manifestations between 1967 and 2009. An additional table shows the ICD codes used in the present study (Additional file 1: Table S1).

The Swedish Prescribed Drug Register [28] contains information about all prescribed drugs dispensed by Swedish pharmacies since July 2005. This register was used to determine the exposure of patients with a registered diagnosis of AS to NSAIDs, oral corticosteroids, and sDMARDs during 2009. Exposure to TNFi during 2009 was based on data retrieved from the Swedish Biologics Register (the Anti-Rheumatic Therapy in Sweden Register; ARTIS) [29], which was initiated in 1999 and includes over 85% of subcutaneous and intravenous TNFi prescribed for AS [30]. An individual was considered to be "exposed" in 2009 if they had at least one prescription dispensed or, in the case of TNFi, were listed in ARTIS as receiving medication during 2009.

Demographic data were obtained from Statistics Sweden [31], which holds data on immigration, emigration, and residency, as well as data on socio-economic factors (for example, marital status and level of formal education) for all those residing in Sweden.

Vital status on 31 December 2009 was determined via the cause-of-death register [32], which provides information on the date and cause(s) of death for all residents since 1961.

All data in the Swedish national healthcare registers are accessed via a personal identification number, which provides the link between all of the registers used in the present analyses [33].

Definition of ankylosing spondylitis

All individuals with an ICD diagnosis registration of AS between 1967 and 2009 were identified from the NPR (Figure 1). The base case definition required at least one AS diagnosis to be registered in the NPR (IPR 1967 to 2009 and/or OPR 2001 to 2009) by any department at a

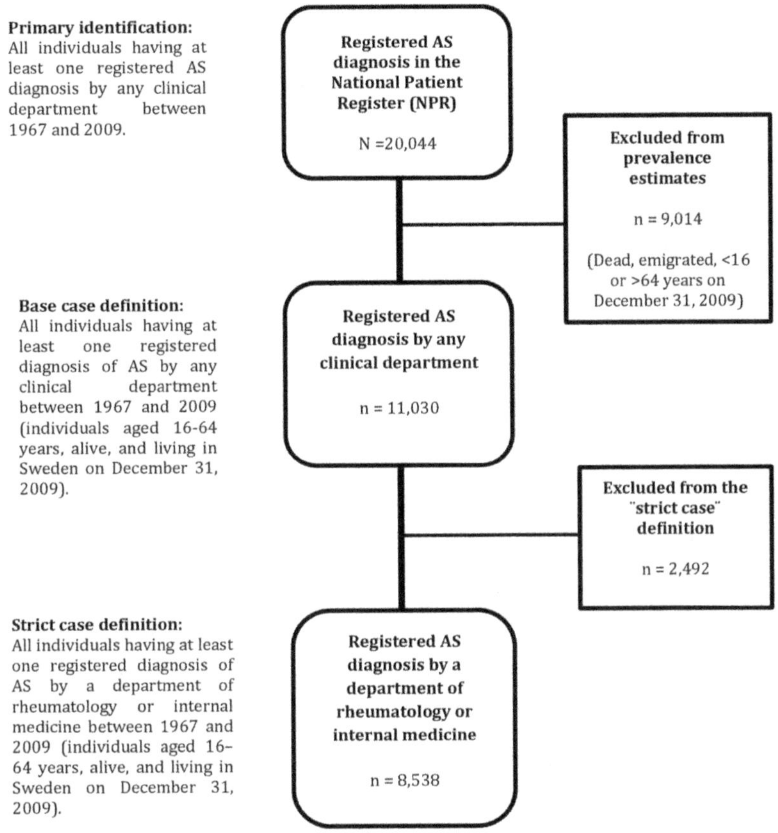

Figure 1 Flow chart showing the process of identifying patients with a registered ankylosing spondylitis (AS) diagnosis according to the World Health Organization International Classification of Disease codes in the National Patient Register between 1967 and 2009 according to the base case and strict case definition.

specialized care center. The strict case definition required at least one AS diagnosis to be registered by a department of rheumatology or internal medicine (Figure 1), a definition that we have previously found to have a high validity [23].

The case definitions used herein included individuals who had received their AS diagnosis for the first time before the age of 16, and also individuals diagnosed with juvenile idiopathic arthritis who had a subsequent diagnosis of AS. This is because these conditions were considered to be part of the same adult AS phenotype.

Results were obtained for individuals aged 16 to 64 years in 2009. The upper age limit was chosen to ensure a high case identification and at the same time minimize the flawing of the results which could be possibly caused by the inclusion of older individuals. Although >95% of patients with AS experience disease onset before the age of 45, there is a considerable delay (8 to 15 years) in obtaining a definitive diagnosis from a specialist in Sweden [23,15], meaning that a high age limit was required in order to maximize the number of cases enrolled. Moreover, since the major source used to identify AS cases, the OPR, did not start until 2001, the ability to accurately identify AS cases in older age groups with earlier disease onset, and who were exclusively diagnosed in a specialized outpatient care setting, was limited. Estimates of disease prevalence in older age groups may also be flawed due to the high mortality among AS patients [34]. Also, it may be that few AS diagnoses are made in older age groups due to either the limited impact of the disease on older people [35] or the influence of other major age-related co-morbidities on diagnosis registration patterns.

Geographical variations and level of formal education

There are six healthcare regions in Sweden: one northern, one southern, and four in between (the southeastern and western regions, and the Uppsala-Örebro and Stockholm regions). These regions were used to calculate the regional prevalence of clinically diagnosed AS and are presented in Additional file 2: Figure S1.

The level of formal education was classified into three categories (≤9 years, 10 to 12 years, and >12 years of schooling). The prevalence of clinically diagnosed AS in relation to the level of education is presented for those aged ≥30 years, the age by which the majority of the population is expected to have completed their studies.

Statistical analysis

The total point prevalence of clinically diagnosed AS was estimated on 31 December 2009 according to both the base case and strict case definitions, and after stratification according to sex and age. Despite the cumulative ascertainment of AS cases, the term "point prevalence" is used. Considering that AS is a chronic disease, individuals with a previous registered AS diagnosis, alive and living in Sweden in 2009, are assumed having an AS diagnosis on 31 December 2009 as well. The point prevalence of AS was thus calculated by taking the number of AS individuals according to each definition and dividing it by the Swedish population on 31 December 2009 with similar age. Furthermore, the prevalence was estimated for subgroups based on AS-related clinical manifestations and pharmacological treatment, by taking the number of AS individuals (according to the base case definition) having dispensed prescriptions for each pharmacological treatment during any part of 2009, or those with a registered diagnosis of AS-related disease manifestations between 1967 and 2009, and dividing it by the Swedish population on 31 December 2009 with similar age. Crude and age-/sex-standardized point prevalence estimates according to healthcare region and level of formal education were also calculated. Standardization was performed to the Swedish population aged 16 to 64 years in 2009. For comparisons between the sexes, the Chi-squared test was used for categorical variables, and the Student's *t*-test was used for normally distributed continuous variables. *P*-values <0.05 were considered statistically significant. For comparisons between geographical location and socio-economic factors, statistical significance was based on the absence of overlap between the estimated 95% confidence interval (CI). Logistic regression models adjusted for age and AS-related clinical manifestations (psoriasis, inflammatory bowel disease, anterior uveitis, and peripheral arthritis) were used to examine sex-related differences in treatment patterns. All analyses were performed using IBM SPSS Statistics for Windows, Version 20.0. Armonk, NY: IBM Corp and Microsoft Excel 2010, Microsoft Corporation, One Microsoft Way, Redmond, WA, USA.

Results

On 31 December 2009, the population of Sweden was about 9.3 million, of which 64% (5,982,237) were aged 16 to 64 years (the denominator in this study). Males accounted for 50.8%.

We identified 20,044 AS cases registered in the NPR between 1967 and 2009 (Figure 1). Of those, 11,030 were aged between 16 and 64 years, alive, and living in Sweden on 31 December 2009. Of these 11,030 individuals, 76% (n = 8,379) were registered in the OPR, 48.5% (n = 5,350) in the IPR, and 24.5% (n = 2,699) in both. Of those fulfilling the base case definition of AS, 7,041 (63.8%) were male. The mean age in 2009 was 48.3 years (standard deviation (SD) 11.3) and the mean age at the time of first AS diagnosis registration in the NPR was 38.6 years (SD 11.4) (Table 1). Of those fulfilling the base case definition, 77.4% (n = 8,538) also fulfilled the strict case definition (Figure 1).

Prevalence of clinically diagnosed ankylosing spondylitis, pharmacological treatment, and disease manifestations

The total point prevalence of clinically diagnosed AS (16 to 64 years old) on 31 December 2009, according to both base case and strict case definitions, was 0.18% (11,030/5,982,237) and 0.14% (8,538/5,982,237), respectively. Of the AS cases identified between 1967 and 2009 according to the base case definition, 68.4% had a registered visit in the NPR during the period 2005 to 2009 (7,550/11,030). The prevalence of AS according to the base case definition having any dispensed prescription for NSAIDs during 2009 was 0.10%, while the prevalence for those with any dispensed prescription for sDMARDs or TNFi during 2009, or those registered with AS-related clinical manifestations between 1967 and 2009, was considerably lower (Figure 2).

There were differences between the sexes with regard to pharmacological treatments received during 2009. Women were more often treated with oral corticosteroids than men ($P < 0.001$), whereas men were more often treated with TNFi ($P < 0.001$) (Table 1). There were also differences between the sexes regarding some AS-related clinical manifestations. Anterior uveitis was more common in men ($P < 0.001$), and peripheral arthritis and psoriasis were more common in women ($P < 0.001$ and $P = 0.03$, respectively) (Table 1). The sex-related differences with regard to treatment with TNFi (odds ratio = 1.48; 95% CI, 1.32 to 1.67; $P < 0.001$) and oral corticosteroids (odds ratio = 1.35; 95% CI, 1.20 to 1.52; $P < 0.001$) remained significant after adjustment for age and AS-related clinical manifestations (psoriasis, inflammatory bowel disease, anterior uveitis, and peripheral arthritis) in logistic regression models.

Data regarding demographics, disease manifestations, pharmacological treatment, and sex-related differences were similar regardless of whether the base case or strict case definitions of AS were used, as shown in detail in Additional file 3: Table S2.

The prevalence of clinically diagnosed AS increased linearly with age up to the age of 55 years, and then reached a plateau. For all age groups combined, the prevalence of AS was higher in men than in women (0.23% versus 0.14%; $P < 0.001$). The male-to-female ratio was highest after the age of 50; however, it was lower for younger age groups (Figure 3). The same pattern was observed for the prevalence of AS according to the strict case definition after age and sex stratification (Additional file 4: Figure S2).

Geographical location

Estimates according to healthcare region revealed that the age-/sex-standardized prevalence of clinically diagnosed

Table 1 Demographics, pharmacological treatment, and ankylosing spondylitis (AS)-related clinical manifestations in patients with an ankylosing spondylitis diagnosis in the National Patient Register (1967 to 2009) according to the base case and strict case definitions

	Base case definition				Strict case definition
	Men	Women		Total	Total
	(N = 7,041)	(N = 3,989)		(N = 11,030)	(N = 8,538)
Demographics	**Mean (SD)**		***P*-value**	**Mean (SD)**	**Mean (SD)**
Age at diagnosis registration	38.6 (11.4)	38.6 (11.3)	0.907	38.6 (11.4)	39.1 (11.0)
Age on 31 December 2009	48.6 (11.2)	47.6 (11.5)	<0.001	48.3 (11.3)	48.5 (10.9)
Pharmacological treatment during 2009†	**N (% of total)**		***P*-value†††**	**N (% of total)**	
NSAIDs	3,724 (52.9)	2,164 (54.2)	0.169	5,888 (53.4)	4,736 (55.5)
Oral corticosteroids	734 (10.4)	557 (14.0)	<0.001	1,291 (11.7)	1,078 (12.6)
sDMARDs	1,406 (20.0)	841 (21.1)	0.163	2,247 (20.4)	1,937 (22.7)
TNFi	1,100 (15.6)	471 (11.8)	<0.001	1,571 (14.2)	1,442 (16.9)
Any pharmacological treatment	4,634 (65.8)	2,653 (66.5)	0.460	7,287 (66.1)	5,974 (70.0)
AS-related clinical manifestations (1967–2009)††	**N (% of total)**		***P*-value**	**N (% of total)**	
Anterior uveitis	1,797 (25.5)	797 (20.0)	<0.001	2,594 (23.5)	2,109 (24.7)
Psoriasis	486 (6.9)	320 (8.0)	0.030	806 (7.3)	669 (7.8)
IBD	571 (8.1)	343 (8.6)	0.371	914 (8.3)	746 (8.7)
Peripheral arthritis	1,079 (15.3)	864 (21.7)	<0.001	1,943 (17.6)	1,568 (18.4)
Hip arthroplasty	527 (7.5)	319 (8.0)	0.331	846 (7.7)	658 (7.7)

Synthetic disease modifying anti-rheumatic drugs (sDMARDs): methotrexate, sulfasalazine, and leflunomide (according to Anatomical Therapeutic Chemical (ATC) codes in the prescribed drugs register). Any pharmacological treatment: non-steroidal anti-inflammatory drugs (NSAIDs), oral corticosteroids, or sDMARDs (according to ATC codes in the prescribed drugs register), or tumor necrosis factor inhibitors (TNFi) (according to the Anti-Rheumatic Therapy in Sweden Register (ARTIS)). IBD: inflammatory bowel disease (according to International Classification of Disease (ICD) codes in the National Patient Register (NPR)). Peripheral arthritis: psoriatic arthritis, reactive arthritis, polyarthritis, or any type of arthritis (according to ICD codes in the NPR). †At least one dispensed prescription during 2009 according to the Swedish prescribed drugs register or listed in ARTIS as receiving TNF-α medication during 2009. ††At least one diagnosis registered in the NPR between 1967 and 2009. †††Adjusted for age and a registered diagnosis of anterior uveitis, psoriasis, IBD, or peripheral arthritis. SD, standard deviation.

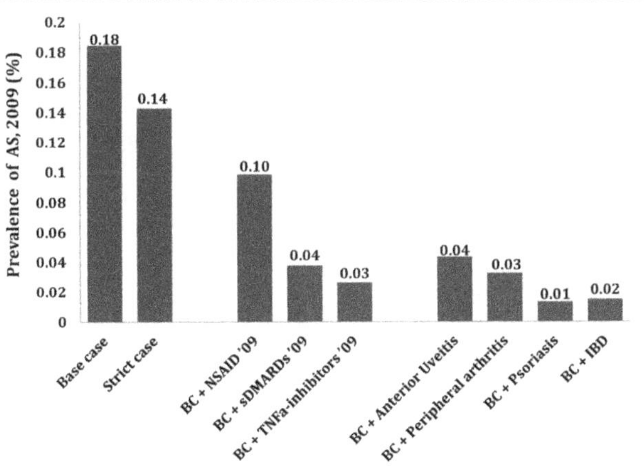

Figure 2 The point prevalence of clinically diagnosed ankylosing spondylitis (AS) in Sweden on 31 December 2009 among those aged 16 to 64 years according to the base case and strict case definitions, and the prevalence of clinically diagnosed AS in 2009 for subgroups stratified according to pharmacological treatment and disease-related clinical manifestations. Peripheral arthritis defined as psoriatic arthritis, reactive arthritis, polyarthritis, or any type of arthritis. BC, base case; IBD, inflammatory bowel disease; NSAID, non-steroidal anti-inflammatory drug; sDMARD, synthetic disease modifying anti-rheumatic drug; TNF, tumor necrosis factor.

AS was highest in the Northern Healthcare Region, which was 0.24% (95% CI, 0.23 to 0.25%), whereas that in the Southern Region was 0.16% (95% CI, 0.15 to 0.16%); however, there was no clear north–south gradient with regard to prevalence of AS across the rest of the country (Figure 4).

Level of formal education

The age-/sex-standardized prevalence of clinically diagnosed AS was lowest in the population group with >12 years of formal education (0.20%; 95% CI, 0.19 to 0.21%). A higher prevalence was observed in those with a lower level of education: ≤9 years (0.24%; 95% CI, 0.22 to 0.25%) or 10 to 12 years (0.24%; 95% CI, 0.23 to 0.24%) of schooling, as shown in Additional file 5: Figure S3. A lower prevalence of AS in the population with the highest level of education was still observed after stratification according to age in 2009 (Figure 5).

Discussion

This nationwide, register-based study revealed that the point prevalence of clinically diagnosed AS in Sweden in 2009 was 0.18%. The prevalence was lower in those with

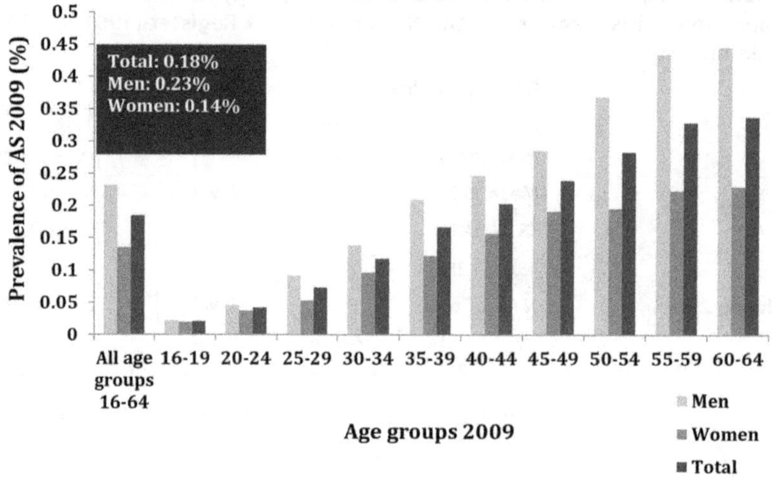

Figure 3 The age- and sex-stratified point prevalence of clinically diagnosed ankylosing spondylitis (AS) in Sweden on 31 December 2009, according to the base case definition.

the highest level of education and higher in those living in the north. Furthermore, the prevalence was higher in men than women. In addition, the frequency of anterior uveitis and treatment with TNFi was higher in men than in women. On the other hand, women had more registered diagnoses related to peripheral arthritis and psoriasis, and were more frequently treated with oral corticosteroids.

Estimates of AS prevalence vary considerably. Differences in study design and population genetics are the most likely explanations; however, geographical, environmental, and socio-economic factors may also play a role. In northern Norway, the prevalence of AS is reported to be 0.21% [13], which is very similar to our own estimates for northern Sweden. A population survey from Finland [12], which examined a representative sample of the population aged ≥30 years (The Mini-Finland Health Survey) reported a prevalence of 0.15%. Finally, a regional register-based study from southern Sweden [15] estimated the prevalence of AS in those ≥15 years old to be 0.12%, which is also consistent with the results we obtained for the southern region of Sweden when using the same age restriction and case definition criteria (data not shown).

According to the results presented herein, sex appears to play a role in AS prevalence. First, the prevalence of AS was higher in men than women across all age groups; this was expected given the results of previous studies [12,15,7]. Furthermore, a registered visit with a diagnosis of anterior uveitis was more common among men. Men were also more likely to be prescribed TNFi than women.

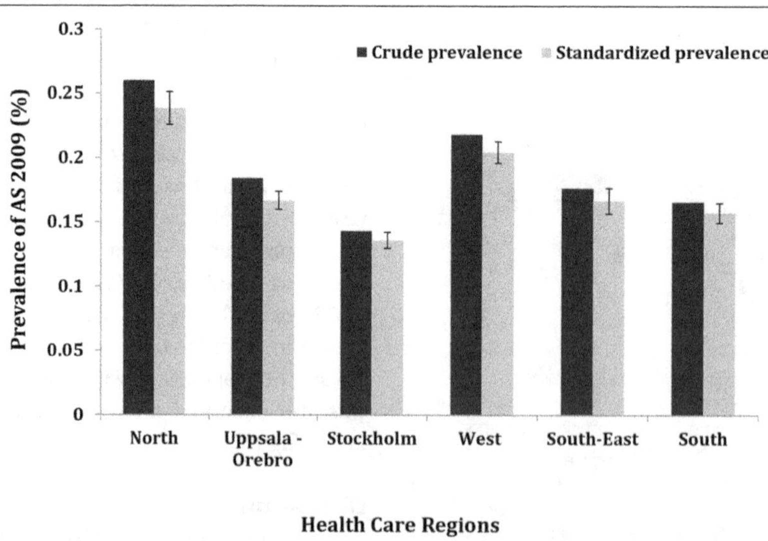

Figure 4 The point prevalence of clinically diagnosed ankylosing spondylitis (AS) in Sweden on 31 December 2009 according to the base case definition, among those aged 16 to 64 years in each healthcare region (crude and standardized according to age and sex).

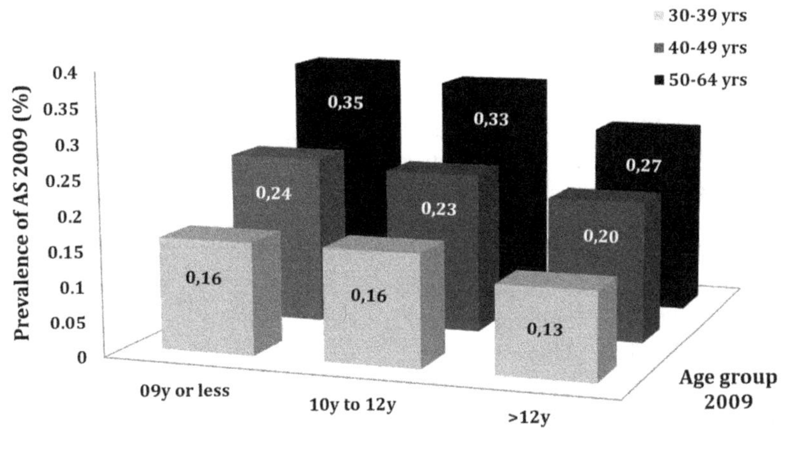

Figure 5 The point prevalence of clinically diagnosed ankylosing spondylitis (AS) in Sweden on 31 December 2009 (according to the base case definition), among those aged 30 to 64 years, stratified according to the level of formal education and age in 2009.

By contrast, a diagnosis indicating peripheral arthritis and psoriasis, and a prescription for oral corticosteroids were more common among women. These findings support the presence of sex-related phenotypic differences, which could affect treatment choices. However, the differences between the sexes with regard to pharmacological treatment remained significant, even after adjusting for such phenotypic differences.

We also found geographical and socio-economic differences in AS prevalence. Previous studies may have lacked sufficient data or the power to evaluate such differences [5,7]. The higher prevalence in northern Sweden (identified herein) and in northern Scandinavia [11,13,14] may be explained by population genetics; the prevalence of the AS-related genotype, HLA-B27, is high (24%) in the indigenous population (Sami) in these areas [11]. The frequency of HLA-B27 is lower in the non-Sami populations of northern Scandinavia (10 to 16%) and Finland (12 to 16%); however, it is still considerably higher than that in southern Europe [19]. Additionally, the present study is the first to suggest an inverse relationship between AS prevalence and the level of education. Such a relationship was also shown previously for RA [20]. It may illustrate that the (usually) early age of AS onset may affect one's ability to pursue education; however, it may also indicate that socio-economic or environmental factors may play a role in AS development. The fact that those exclusively followed in private care are not included in our study may introduce a selection bias that affects this analysis. Those with higher educational attainment (indicating higher socio-economic status) may be more likely to be treated in private clinics, and therefore are missing from our sample. However, in Sweden the majority of private healthcare providers are reimbursed by the counties for providing services covered by the same regulations and fees that apply to municipal care facilities, suggesting that the ability to contact a private rheumatologist is not strongly dependent on socio-economic status. Future studies could focus on identifying environmental factors associated with AS by linking the populations examined in the present study to other registers containing information regarding relevant early life exposure.

The present study has several strengths. First, it is the first nationwide prevalence study on clinically diagnosed AS. Previous studies were either based on regional or small national population samples, with limited generalizability. Second, in contrast to smaller regional studies, we used a uniform case ascertainment over a large geographical area, enabling us to demonstrate geographical variations in disease occurrence, which may reflect differences in genetic, environmental, and socio-economic factors. Third, the register-based approach (using AS diagnoses made by physicians) reflects the real disease burden as estimates of AS occurrence are based on clinical diagnoses, and enables the assessment of the frequency of AS-related clinical manifestations and pharmacological treatments.

The study also has a number of limitations. First, a register-based approach does not identify patients not seeking contact with a healthcare practitioner, since it only identified clinically diagnosed cases. Second, the NPR does not cover AS cases that are managed exclusively in a primary care or private setting. According to a previous study from southern Sweden, only 3% of AS patients are being followed exclusively in primary care [25], usually those with a mild disease course. In another study, the proportion of AS cases solely seeking private healthcare was estimated to be 15% [15]. Our own estimates from the biologics register show that only 4.6% of those receiving TNFi are treated exclusively privately (data not shown). Taking these factors into consideration, although we acknowledge that in particular some AS cases with mild disease or short disease duration may not be included in the present study, our underestimation of AS prevalence should be less than 10%. Finally, the validity of an AS diagnosis registered in the NPR may be questioned, as all diagnoses are based on the judgment of each individual physician and not on established classification criteria. However, we previously showed that AS diagnoses according to the strict case definition have high validity, with a positive-predictive value of 80% for fulfilling the modified New York criteria, and 89% for fulfilling any of the commonly used criteria for SpA [23]. These findings indicate that only a low percentage of patients with clinical non-radiographic axial SpA are incorrectly classified as AS in the NPR. Based on these findings, misclassification of AS diagnosis in the NPR is unlikely to have a significant impact on our results. Finally, the present study specifically addresses the prevalence of clinically diagnosed AS and not that for the whole group of axial SpA (including the non-radiographic stage). The latter is expected to be higher and thus more studies are necessary to estimate the total prevalence of axial SpA.

Conclusions

To conclude, this nationwide, register-based prevalence estimate of clinically diagnosed AS in Sweden offers a unique opportunity to improve our understanding of the real burden that AS places on the healthcare system. We identified phenotypical and pharmacological treatment differences between the sexes, and differences in disease prevalence related to geographical region and socio-economic factors, suggesting that genetic and (possibly) environmental factors may be important for the development of AS.

Additional files

Additional file 1: Table S1. Diagnostic codes indicating a diagnosis of ankylosing spondylitis (AS) and AS-related clinical manifestations according to three consecutive Swedish versions of the World Health Organization International Classification of Disease codes.

Additional file 2: Figure S1. The Swedish Healthcare regions.

Additional file 3: Table S2. Demographics, pharmacological treatments, and ankylosing spondylitis (AS)-related clinical manifestations in patients with an AS diagnosis registered in the National Patient Register (NPR) (1967 to 2009) according to the strict case definition.

Additional file 4: Figure S2. Age- and sex-stratified point prevalence of clinically diagnosed ankylosing spondylitis (AS) in Sweden on 31 December 2009, according to the strict case definition.

Additional file 5: Figure S3. The point prevalence of clinically diagnosed ankylosing spondylitis (AS) in Sweden on 31 December 2009 (according to the base case definition), among those aged 30 to 64 years, stratified according to the level of formal education (both crude and standardized according to age and sex).

Abbreviations

ARTIS: Anti-Rheumatic Therapy in Sweden Register; AS: ankylosing spondylitis; CI: confidence interval; ICD: International Classification of Disease; IPR: Inpatient Register; NPR: National Patient Register; NSAID: non-steroidal anti-inflammatory drug; OPR: Outpatient Register; RA: rheumatoid arthritis; SD: standard deviation; sDMARD: synthetic disease modifying anti-rheumatic drug; SpA: spondyloarthritis; TNFi: tumor necrosis factor inhibitors.

Competing interests

The authors declare that they have no competing interests.

Authors' contributions

SE participated in the study design, performed the data analysis, wrote the manuscript, participated in the interpretation of the results and submitted the manuscript. UL participated in the interpretation of the results and the drafting of the manuscript. JA participated in the interpretation of the results and the drafting of the manuscript. JKE contributed to the acquisition of data, participated in the interpretation of the results and the drafting of the manuscript. HFdE participated in the interpretation of the results and the drafting of the manuscript. MN participated in the interpretation of the results and the drafting of the manuscript. CT participated in the study design, the interpretation of the results and the drafting of the manuscript. LEK participated in the study design, the interpretation of the results and the drafting of the manuscript. LTHJ participated in the study design, the interpretation of the results and the drafting of the manuscript. All authors had full access to all data at all points of the manuscript planning, drafting and post-submission, and all authors have read and approved the final version of the manuscript.

Acknowledgments

The study was funded by the Oak foundation, the Swedish Rheumatism Association and the Lund University.

Author details

[1]Rheumatology, Department of Clinical Sciences, Malmö, Lund University, Inga Marie Nilssons gata 32, 205 02 Malmö, Sweden. [2]Department of Rheumatology and Inflammation Research, Sahlgrenska Academy at University of Gothenburg, Gothenburg, Sweden. [3]Clinical Epidemiology Unit & Rheumatology Unit, Department of Medicine Solna, Karolinska Institute, Stockholm, Sweden. [4]Clinical Epidemiology Unit, Department of Medicine Solna, Karolinska Institute, Stockholm, Sweden. [5]The Parker Institute, Department of Rheumatology, Bispebjerg and Frederiksberg Hospital, the Capital Region of Copenhagen, Copenhagen, Denmark.

References

1. Feldtkeller E, Bruckel J, Khan MA. Scientific contributions of ankylosing spondylitis patient advocacy groups. Curr Opin Rheumatol. 2000;12:239–47.
2. Dagfinrud H, Kjeken I, Mowinckel P, Hagen KB, Kvien TK. Impact of functional impairment in ankylosing spondylitis: impairment, activity limitation, and participation restrictions. J Rheumatol. 2005;32:516–23.
3. Kristensen LE, Petersson IF, Geborek P, Joud A, Saxne T, Jacobsson LT, et al. Sick leave in patients with ankylosing spondylitis before and after anti-TNF therapy: a population-based cohort study. Rheumatology (Oxford). 2012;51:243–9.
4. Braun J, van den Berg R, Baraliakos X, Boehm H, Burgos-Vargas R, Collantes-Estevez E, et al. 2010 update of the ASAS/EULAR recommendations for the management of ankylosing spondylitis. Ann Rheum Dis. 2011;70:896–904.
5. Saraux A, Guillemin F, Guggenbuhl P, Roux CH, Fardellone P, Le Bihan E, et al. Prevalence of spondyloarthropathies in France: 2001. Ann Rheum Dis. 2005;64:1431–5.
6. Anagnostopoulos I, Zinzaras E, Alexiou I, Papathanasiou AA, Davas E, Koutroumpas A, et al. The prevalence of rheumatic diseases in central Greece: a population survey. BMC Musculoskelet Disord. 2010;11:98.
7. Trontzas P, Andrianakos A, Miyakis S, Pantelidou K, Vafiadou E, Garantziotou V, et al. Seronegative spondyloarthropathies in Greece: a population-based study of prevalence, clinical pattern, and management. The ESORDIG study. Clin Rheumatol. 2005;24:583–9.
8. Alamanos Y, Papadopoulos NG, Voulgari PV, Karakatsanis A, Siozos C, Drosos AA. Epidemiology of ankylosing spondylitis in Northwest Greece, 1983–2002. Rheumatology (Oxford). 2004;43:615–8.

9. De Angelis R, Salaffi F, Grassi W. Prevalence of spondyloarthropathies in an Italian population sample: a regional community-based study. Scand J Rheumatol. 2007;36:14–21.
10. Hanova P, Pavelka K, Holcatova I, Pikhart H. Incidence and prevalence of psoriatic arthritis, ankylosing spondylitis, and reactive arthritis in the first descriptive population-based study in the Czech Republic. Scand J Rheumatol. 2010;39:310–7.
11. Johnsen K, Gran JT, Dale K, Husby G. The prevalence of ankylosing spondylitis among Norwegian Samis (Lapps). J Rheumatol. 1992;19:1591–4.
12. Kaipiainen-Seppanen O, Aho K, Heliovaara M. Incidence and prevalence of ankylosing spondylitis in Finland. J Rheumatol. 1997;24:496–9.
13. Bakland G, Nossent HC, Gran JT. Incidence and prevalence of ankylosing spondylitis in Northern Norway. Arthritis Rheum. 2005;53:850–5.
14. Gran JT, Husby G, Hordvik M. Prevalence of ankylosing spondylitis in males and females in a young middle-aged population of Tromso, northern Norway. Ann Rheum Dis. 1985;44:359–67.
15. Haglund E, Bremander AB, Petersson IF, Strombeck B, Bergman S, Jacobsson LT, et al. Prevalence of spondyloarthritis and its subtypes in southern Sweden. Ann Rheum Dis. 2011;70:943–8.
16. Braun J, Bollow M, Remlinger G, Eggens U, Rudwaleit M, Distler A, et al. Prevalence of spondylarthropathies in HLA-B27 positive and negative blood donors. Arthritis Rheum. 1998;41:58–67.
17. Xiang YJ, Dai SM. Prevalence of rheumatic diseases and disability in China. Rheumatol Int. 2009;29:481–90.
18. Hukuda S, Minami M, Saito T, Mitsui H, Matsui N, Komatsubara Y, et al. Spondyloarthropathies in Japan: nationwide questionnaire survey performed by the Japan Ankylosing Spondylitis Society. J Rheumatol. 2001;28:554–9.
19. Khan MA. Epidemiology of HLA-B27 and arthritis. Clin Rheumatol. 1996;15:10–2.
20. Neovius M, Simard JF, Askling J. Nationwide prevalence of rheumatoid arthritis and penetration of disease-modifying drugs in Sweden. Ann Rheum Dis. 2011;70:624–9.
21. Ludvigsson JF, Andersson E, Ekbom A, Feychting M, Kim JL, Reuterwall C, et al. External review and validation of the Swedish national inpatient register. BMC Public Health. 2011;11:450.
22. WHO International Classification of Disease codes. http://www.who.int/classifications/icd/en/.
23. Lindström U, Exarchou S, Sigurdardottir V, Sundström B, Askling J, Eriksson JK, et al. Validity of ankylosing spondylitis and undifferentiated spondyloarthritis diagnoses in the Swedish National Patient Register. Scand J Rheumatol. 2015;23:1-8. [Epub ahead of print]
24. Kristensen LE, Jakobsen AK, Askling J, Nielsson FX, Jacobsson LT. Safety of etoricoxib, celecoxib and non-selective NSAIDs in ankylosing spondylitis and other spondyloarthritis patients: a Swedish national population based cohort study. Arthritis Care Res. 2015. doi: 10.1002/acr.22555. [Epub ahead of print]
25. Jordan KP, Joud A, Bergknut C, Croft P, Edwards JJ, Peat G, et al. International comparisons of the consultation prevalence of musculoskeletal conditions using population-based healthcare data from England and Sweden. Ann Rheum Dis. 2014;73:212–8.
26. The National Board of Health and Welfare. Coding quality in the patient register - Inpatient register 2008. (Socialstyrelsen. Kodningskvalitet i patientregistret – Slutenvård 2008). 2010. (Article in Swedish) http://www.socialstyrelsen.se/publikationer2010/2010-6-27.
27. The National Board of Health and Welfare. Coding quality in the patient register - A new tool for measuring quality. (Socialstyrelsen. Kodningskvalitet i patientregistret – Ett nytt verktyg för att mäta kvalitet). 2013. (Article in Swedish) http://www.socialstyrelsen.se/publikationer2013/2013-3-10.
28. The Swedish prescribed drug register (Läkemedelsregistret) (Page in Swedish). http://www.socialstyrelsen.se/register/halsodataregister/lakemedelsregistret.
29. Askling J, Fored CM, Geborek P, Jacobsson LT, van Vollenhoven R, Feltelius N, et al. Swedish registers to examine drug safety and clinical issues in RA. Ann Rheum Dis. 2006;65:707–12.
30. Wadström H, Eriksson JK, Neovius M, Askling J, ARTIS Study Group. How good is the coverage and how accurate are data in the swedish biologics register? Scand J Rheumatol. 2015;44:22–8.
31. Statistics Sweden. http://www.scb.se/en_/.
32. The Swedish cause-of-death register (Dödsorsaksregistret) (Page in Swedish). http://www.socialstyrelsen.se/register/dodsorsaksregistret.
33. Ludvigsson JF, Otterblad-Olausson P, Pettersson BU, Ekbom A. The Swedish personal identity number: possibilities and pitfalls in healthcare and medical research. Eur J Epidemiol. 2009;24:659–67.
34. Zochling J, Braun J. Mortality in rheumatoid arthritis and ankylosing spondylitis. Clin Exp Rheumatol. 2009;27:S127–30.
35. Exarchou S, Redlund-Johnell I, Karlsson M, Mellstrom D, Ohlsson C, Turesson C, et al. The prevalence of moderate to severe radiographic sacroiliitis and the correlation with health status in elderly Swedish men - the MrOS study. BMC Musculoskelet Disord. 2013;14:352.

2

Plasma, urine and ligament tissue metabolite profiling reveals potential biomarkers of ankylosing spondylitis using NMR-based metabolic profiles

Wei Wang[1†], Gen-jin Yang[2†], Ju Zhang[3], Chen Chen[4], Zhen-yu Jia[5], Jia Li[5] and Wei-dong Xu[5*]

Abstract

Background: Ankylosing spondylitis (AS) is an autoimmune rheumatic disease mostly affecting the axial skeleton. Currently, anti-tumour necrosis factor α (anti-TNF-α) represents an effective treatment for AS that may delay the progression of the disease and alleviate the symptoms if the diagnosis can be made early. Unfortunately, effective diagnostic biomarkers for AS are still lacking; therefore, most patients with AS do not receive timely and effective treatment. The intent of this study was to determine several key metabolites as potential biomarkers of AS using metabolomic methods to facilitate the early diagnosis of AS.

Methods: First, we collected samples of plasma, urine, and ligament tissue around the hip joint from AS and control groups. The samples were examined by nuclear magnetic resonance spectrometry, and multivariate data analysis was performed to find metabolites that differed between the groups. Subsequently, according to the correlation coefficients, variable importance for the projection (VIP) and *P* values of the metabolites obtained in the multivariate data analysis, the most crucial metabolites were selected as potential biomarkers of AS. Finally, metabolic pathways involving the potential biomarkers were determined using the Kyoto Encyclopedia of Genes and Genomes (KEGG) database, and the metabolic pathway map was drawn.

Results: Forty-four patients with AS agreed to provide plasma and urine samples, and 30 provided ligament tissue samples. An equal number of volunteers were recruited for the control group. Multidimensional statistical analysis suggested significant differences between the patients with AS and control subjects, and the models exhibited good discrimination and predictive ability. A total of 20 different metabolites ultimately met the requirements for potential biomarkers. According to KEGG analysis, these marker metabolites were primarily related to fat metabolism, intestinal microbial metabolism, glucose metabolism and choline metabolism pathways, and they were also probably associated with immune regulation.

Conclusions: Our work demonstrates that the potential biomarkers that were identified appeared to have diagnostic value for AS and deserve to be further investigated. In addition, this work also suggests that the metabolomic profiling approach is a promising screening tool for the diagnosis of patients with AS.

Keywords: Ankylosing spondylitis, NMR, Biomarkers, Metabolomics

* Correspondence: wdxushanghai@sina.com
[†]Equal contributors
[5]Department of Orthopedics, Changhai Hospital, Shanghai city, People's Republic of China
Full list of author information is available at the end of the article

Background

Ankylosing spondylitis (AS) is a form of chronic inflammatory arthritis that predominantly affects the axial skeleton causing patients to experience severe stiffness and pain [1]. In addition, AS affects the peripheral joints and is exhibited by extra-articular symptoms such as inflammatory bowel disease (IBD) and uveitis [2]. Because early AS is often asymptomatic or does not show obvious pathological changes, the diagnosis of AS is not prompt. Although the significance of early intervention has been well-recognized for a long time, the diagnostic criteria for early-stage AS may be difficult to apply, leading to delay in the use of appropriate intervention [3].

Currently diagnosing AS is a clinically driven process based on the observation of clinical symptoms and structural changes on x-rays. The structural changes on x-rays are the result of the inflammatory process but do not make the inflammatory process itself known [4]. It takes several years before the changes are visible on x-rays. Diagnostic biomarkers such as rheumatoid factor or autoantibodies against citrullinated proteins are used for the early diagnosis of rheumatoid arthritis (RA) with high specificity and selectivity [5, 6]. However, potential markers for the diagnosis of AS, such as immunoglobulin G (IgG), IgA or C-reactive protein, have not achieved sufficient diagnostic sensitivity or specificity [7]. Additionally, the high association of human leucocyte antigen B27 with AS, combined with a relatively high population prevalence, does not make it a good candidate for use as a diagnostic marker alone, but it may be useful in a combined model [4].

With the advent of microarray techniques many pathological processes can be explored and monitored globally with the aid of omics-driven, high-throughput technologies [8]. Genomics, transcriptomics and proteomics have emerged as biochemical profiling tools to provide important insight into the biology of various diseases [9]. However, these profiling methods are focused only on upstream genetic and protein variations [10]. As a rapidly developing field of systems biology, metabolomics represents a new method that delineates a wide panel of metabolic parameters and thus allows a global and potentially more personalized diagnostic method to be used in combination with conventional protocols [11]. The fundamental basis for the application of clinical metabolomics is that perturbations are in biological [12]. To date, metabolic profiling has been used to identify potential biomarkers for other arthritic diseases, including RA [13], osteoarthritis [14] and gout [15].

Several research studies but not many, have used metabolomics in the study of AS. For example, Fischer et al. found that vitamin D_3 metabolites were downregulated in AS [16]. Gao et al. found that the plasma concentrations of some amino acids were abnormally changed in AS [8]. In addition, Chen et al. found that some plasma fatty acid chains in AS could be used as potential biomarkers [1]. All of the research described above used only plasma as a test sample and mass spectrometry (MS) as a detection method.

The two most powerful and most commonly used analytical methods for metabolic fingerprinting are MS and nuclear magnetic resonance (NMR) spectrometry [17]. NMR is a non-invasive and non-destructive technique that can provide complete structural analysis of a wide range of organic molecules in complex mixtures [18]. It has a series of advantages compared with MS including simple sample preparation, not requiring chromatographic separation and being inexpensive on the basis of consumables [19]. Although a growing number of NMR-based metabolomic studies are aimed at finding potential biomarkers of several diseases, such as RA [13], prostate cancer [20] and diabetes [21], there have been no reports of using an NMR method to investigate the differences of metabolites in AS. Urine and plasma are the most frequently used specimens for exploring the systematic alteration of metabolites in humans because the collection and handling of these specimens are relatively easy [22]. Furthermore, pathologic tissues have been used as samples for metabolic profiling in a growing number of studies because these tissues can provide more metabolic information directly related to these diseases [19, 20]. However, thus far, only plasma has been used as a research sample for metabolomic studies of AS, and the results may not be comprehensive.

In the present study using NMR spectroscopy, we performed metabolic profiling to observe the metabolites in plasma and urine samples of patients with AS and healthy control subjects. Furthermore, to provide complementary information on metabolites in intact tissues, ligament tissues surrounding hip joints of patients with AS who were scheduled for hip arthroplasty were collected for metabolomic analysis. The hip joint is the most easily involved peripheral joint of AS, and ossification of the ligament is the most important pathological change [23], these are the main reasons why this ligament tissue was chosen as the test sample. To the best of our knowledge, this study is the first in which NMR has been used as a detection method and in which biological samples other than plasma have been used as test samples to perform a metabolomic study of AS to identify more suitable potential biomarkers.

Methods

Patients

Volunteers were recruited mainly from among patients with AS who were admitted to the rheumatology and immunology clinic of our hospital (Changhai Hospital, Shanghai, China) to participate in plasma and urine analyses in this study between June 2014 and June 2015. Volunteers were also recruited for the sample analysis of ligament tissues surrounding hip joints of patients with AS who were scheduled for hip arthroplasty in the department of orthopaedics of our hospital between June 2013 and June 2015. The inclusion criteria for recruitment were as follows: aged >18 years with an independent right to sign a consent form and with a diagnosis of AS (1984 New York modified criteria) [24]. The exclusion criteria were as follows: patients with other systemic diseases (hypertension, diabetes and the comorbidities of AS), patients with a history of taking medication within the last week (e.g., treated with anti-tumour necrosis factor α [anti-TNF-α], taking disease-modifying antirheumatic drugs or non-steroidal anti-inflammatory drugs), and patients who had breakfast in the morning before they came to the outpatient clinic (for plasma and urine samples). Additionally, age- and sex-matched volunteers were recruited from among the healthy population for routine physical examinations in our hospital as control subjects for plasma and urine sample analysis, and their exclusion criteria were the same as those for the AS group. Volunteers were also recruited from among patients admitted to the emergency department of our hospital for the surgical treatment of femoral neck fracture (FNF) as control subjects for ligament tissue sample analysis (no other underlying diseases were allowed for these patients to be included). All procedures performed in this study involving human participants were carried out in accordance with the 1964 Helsinki declaration and its later amendments or comparable ethical standards. This clinical study was approved by the ethics committee of Changhai Hospital (CHEC2013-176).

Sample collection and processing

Urine and plasma samples were collected from all of the fasting volunteers in the morning. Blood samples were first placed in heparin anti-coagulation tubes at room temperature and then centrifuged at 4 °C (5000 rpm for 10 minutes) [25]. Next the supernatant plasma was divided into aliquots of 300 μl in epoxy epoxide (EP) tubes and stored at −80 °C for later detection and analysis. Urine samples were collected and then centrifuged at 4 °C within 30 minutes (6000 rpm for 15 minutes). After that step, the supernatant was divided into aliquots of 540 μl in EP tubes and stored at −80 °C for later detection and analysis [26].

Samples of ligament tissue surrounding the hip joints were collected from the volunteers during hip surgery. In the operating theatre, the ligament tissue was cut into small pieces of 1 cm^3 each, aliquoted in cryogenic tubes and then stored in a liquid nitrogen tank [23]. The liquid nitrogen tank was brought to the laboratory, and the tissue was immediately homogenized into powder using an electric tissue homogenizer (60 Hz for 40 seconds). The powder was removed into an EP tube and weighed. Then, extract solution (2.85 ml/g distilled water + 4 ml/g methanol and chloroform) was added. Samples were vortexed for 15 seconds three times and kept on ice in between. Last, samples were centrifuged at 4 °C (10,000 × *g* for 10 minutes). Three hundred microliters of each supernatant (polar extracts) and subnatant (non-polar extracts) were removed into two EP tubes. Dried products of the supernatant and subnatant were obtained using freeze-drying treatment and a nitrogen blowing instrument, respectively, and they were stored at −80 °C for detection and analysis [27].

Sample preparation and spectroscopy

The plasma samples were prepared for NMR analysis by mixing 300 μl of plasma with 300 μl of PBS (1.5 M NaH_2PO_4/K_2HPO_4 pH 7.4, 10 % vol/vol D_2O) containing 0.6 mg of 3-trimethylsilyl-2,2,3,3-d_4-propionate (TMSP) as a chemical shift reference ($\delta = 0.00$ ppm). Urine samples (540 μl mixed with 60 μl of PBS) and tissue extracts (mixed with 600 μl of PBS) were processed similarly. All of the samples were then centrifuged at 4 °C (12,000 rpm for 10 minutes), and the supernatants were pipetted into 5-mm NMR tubes for NMR analysis [27].

The proton NMR spectra of the plasma, urine and tissue extract samples were recorded at 300 K on a Bruker Avance II 600-MHz spectrometer (Bruker BioSpin, Rheinstetten, Germany) operating at a ^1H frequency of 600.13 MHz and equipped with a broadband observe probe.

Standard water-suppressed one-dimensional spectra of urine and tissue extracts were acquired using the first increment of the gradient-selected nuclear Overhauser effect spectroscopy pulse sequence (recycle delay-90 degrees-t_1-90 degrees-t_m-90 degrees-acquire data) with a recycle delay of 2 seconds, a t_1 of 3 microseconds, a mixing time (t_m) of 100 milliseconds and a 90-degree pulse length of 13.70 microseconds. A total of 128 transients were acquired in 49,187 data points using a spectral width of 9590 Hz and an acquisition time of 2.56 seconds. For plasma, a water-presaturated Carr-Purcell-Meiboom-Gill pulse sequence (recycle delay-90 degrees-(τ-180 degrees-τ)$_n$-acquisition) was employed to attenuate the NMR signals from macromolecules. A spin-spin relaxation delay ($2n\tau$) of 76.8 milliseconds and a spin-echo delay τ of 400 microseconds were used. Typically, the 90-degree pulse was set to 13.7 microseconds, and 32 transients were collected in 49,178 data points for each spectrum using a spectral width of 9590 Hz. Other acquisition parameters were the same as described above [28]. After the Fourier transformation, phase correction and baseline correction were performed using the TopSpin version 3.0 software package

(Bruker BioSpin). The ^{1}H chemical shifts were referenced to the TMSP peak at $\delta = 0.00$.

Multivariate data analysis

Multivariate statistical analysis can take internal relationships and mutual influence between the variables into account; therefore, the use of multivariate statistical analysis was more reasonable than univariate statistical analysis with respect to the data source, with many objectively existing variables and mutual influences. Multivariate statistical analysis, including principal component analysis (PCA), partial least squares discriminant analysis (PLS-DA) and orthogonal projection to latent structures discriminant analysis (OPLS-DA), was performed to globally understand the metabolic changes of AS.

PCA was performed using the SIMCA-P version 11.5 software package (Umetrics AB Umea, Sweden). PCA is an unsupervised analytical pattern recognition tool that provides an overview of complex data through examination of the covariance structure. The multivariate data can be displayed in a few principal components as a set of 'scores' that highlight general trends and outliers [29].

PLS-DA and OPLS-DA were performed using a unit variance scaled approach based on the SIMCA-P version 11.5 software package (Umetrics AB). PLS-DA is a supervised regression method used to maximize the covariance between the predictor space and the response space. It can predict responses in the population using the predictor matrix. OPLS-DA was performed with the NMR data to facilitate interpretation of the loading. The model coefficients were back-calculated from the coefficients incorporating the weight of the variables and plotted with color-coded coefficients to enhance the interpretability of the model [29]. The color-coded correlation coefficients indicate the significance of the metabolite contribution in predicting the response. Two parameters, R^2Y and Q^2, were used for evaluation of the models. R^2Y explains the latent variables of the sums of squares of all x and y values. Q^2 reflects the cumulative cross-validated percentage of the total variation that can be predicted by the current latent variables. High coefficient values of R^2Y and Q^2Y (>0.5 is acceptable) showed good discrimination and predictive ability [8]. In the PLS-DA models, we used permutation tests (200 times) to observe whether there was overfitting, while the permutation test was evaluated by using cross-validation, with R^2 and Q^2 as correlation coefficients of the cross-validation. It is generally believed that the intercept of the Q^2 regression line on the y-axis (permutation plot) being 0 or less than 0 indicates a reliable and effective model, without overfitting [30].

Potential biomarker selection and metabolic pathway analysis

On the basis of parameters obtained from the multivariate analysis, we selected the metabolites whose absolute correlation coefficient values greater than the cut-off value or variable importance for projection (VIP) (value >1.0 and $P < 0.05$) as potential biomarkers for AS [10, 29, 30]. Then, the related metabolic pathways in which these potential biomarkers are involved were identified through a Kyoto Encyclopedia of Genes and Genomes (KEGG) database retrieval, and the metabolic pathway map was plotted.

Statistical methods

IBM SPSS version 20.0 software (IBM Armonk, NY, USA) was used for statistical analysis. The mean values for age, body mass index (BMI), disease duration, Bath Ankylosing Spondylitis Disease Activity Index score (BASDAI) and Bath Ankylosing Spondylitis Functional Index score (BASFI) were reported with their SDs. A P value ≤0.05 was considered to be statistically significant.

Results

Clinical population

Upon our invitation, 44 patients with AS and 44 healthy individuals as the control group consented to participate in the study of plasma and urine samples, and another 30 patients with AS and 30 patients with FNF consented to participate in the study of tissue samples. All of the participants met our inclusion or exclusion criteria, and 5 patients with AS (6.3 %) with hypertension, diabetes mellitus and AS comorbidities (iritis, ulcerative colitis and otitis media) were excluded. The clinical information of the patients and control subjects is summarized in Table 1. As listed in the table, the age, sex and BMI of the control group basically matched those of the AS group.

^{1}H NMR spectra of samples

Figure 1 shows typical ^{1}H NMR spectra of the plasma urine and tissue samples taken from randomly selected participants in the AS and control groups. The urine, plasma and polar tissue extract samples contained mainly a series of amino acids, glucose and lipids, while the non-polar tissue extract samples contained the minimum metabolites, dominated mainly by triglycerides (TG).

Multivariate data analysis of NMR data

Figure 2 shows the PCA score plots for the three sample types (urine plasma and tissue). The difference in the PCA score plots of tissue samples between the AS group and the control group was the most significant difference. The PCA score plots of plasma samples revealed incomplete but clear discrimination between patients with AS and healthy control subjects. For the urine samples, the PCA model was not able to completely distinguish

Table 1 Participant characteristics at the time of sampling

Characteristics	Urine and plasma samples			Ligament tissue samples		
	Patients with AS	HC	*P* value[a]	patients with AS	Patients with FNF	*P* value[a]
Number of participants	44	44	–	30	30	–
Age, years, mean ± SD	31.8 ± 10.9	33.8 ± 9.7	0.350	40.6 ± 12.8	46.6 ± 11.6	0.065
Range	18–59	18–57	–	20–71	31–72	–
18–29	15	12	–	6	2	–
30–49	21	22	–	14	13	–
50–79	8	10	–	10	15	–
Sex, *n* (%)			1.000			0.037
Female	6 (13.6 %)	6 (13.6 %)	–	4 (13.3 %)	11 (36.7 %)	–
Male	38 (86.4 %)	38 (86.4 %)	–	26 (86.7 %)	19 (63.3 %)	–
BMI, kg/m^2, mean ± SD	21.8 ± 2.4	22.5 ± 2.9	0.226	22.8 ± 2.0	23.7 ± 1.5	0.062
<18.5	13	12	–	9	7	–
18.5–25	25	23	–	14	15	–
>25	6	9	–	7	8	–
Disease duration, years, mean ± SD	6.8 ± 3.5	–	–	14.2 ± 4.8	–	–
<5	25	–	–	0	–	–
5–10	18	–	–	11	–	–
>10	1	–	–	19	–	–
BASDAI score	3.2 ± 1.8	–	–	5.8 ± 1.1	–	–
0–3	20	–	–	0	–	–
3–6	23	–	–	18	–	–
6–10	1	–	–	12	–	–
BASFI score	3.9 ± 2.1	–	–	5.5 ± 0.9	–	–
0–3	20	–	–	0	–	–
3–6	22	–	–	19	–	–
6–10	2	–	–	11	–	–
Treatment duration, years, mean ± SD	2.8 ± 1.5	–	–	8.4 ± 3.6	–	–
0	32	–	–	0	–	–
1–10	11	–	–	19	–	–
11–20	1	–	–	9	–	–
>20	0	–	–	2	–	–

Abbreviations: AS Ankylosing spondylitis, *FNF* Femoral neck fractures, *BMI* Body mass index, *BASDAI* Bath Ankylosing Spondylitis Disease Activity Index, *BASFI* Bath Ankylosing Spondylitis Functional Index, HC Healthy control subjects

[a]Calculated using Student's *t* test for continuous variables and chi-square test for categorical variables between patients with AS and healthy control subjects

between the patients with AS and healthy control subjects. Therefore, we focused mainly on supervised analysis results for the urine samples

The PLS-DA result is presented in Fig. 3. For these three types of samples, the score plots highlighted two clusters corresponding to the AS and control groups. In the PLS-DA model, the parameters of R^2Y and Q^2 were, respectively, 0.894 and 0.832 (plasma), 0.767 and 0.469 (urine), and 0.921 and 0.860 (tissue extracts). These results revealed the good discrimination and predictive ability of this model. Although the Q^2 value of urine samples was slightly lower, it was acceptable considering the many uncontrollable factors in human studies. Model cross-validation through permutation tests (200 times) generated intercepts of R^2 and Q^2 (respectively, 0.599 and −0.029 for plasma, 0.617 and −0.027 for urine, and 0.385 and −0.047 for tissue). The low values of the intercepts indicate that the model was not over-fitted.

The OPLS-DA analytical results and the correlation coefficient loading plots are shown in Fig. 4. The parameters of R^2Y and Q^2 were respectively, 0.894 and 0.833 (plasma), 0.767 and 0.422 (urine), and 0.921 and 0.857 (tissue extracts), which also revealed the

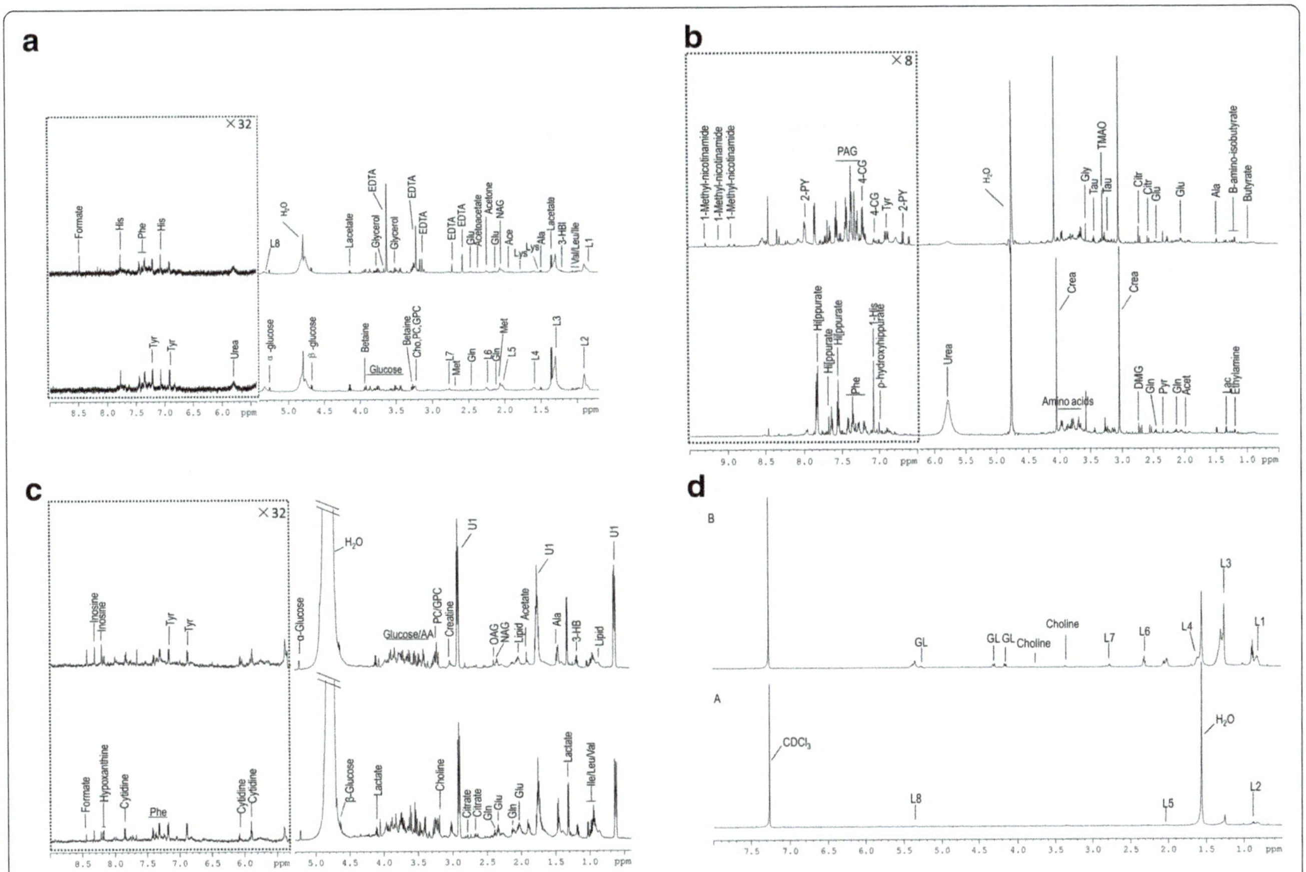

Fig. 1 Representative 600-MHz ^{1}H NMR spectra of (**a**) plasma, (**b**) urine and (**c**) polar tissue extract and (**d**) non-polar extract metabolites obtained from the AS group (*upper layer*) and control subjects (*lower layer*). *Phe* Phenylalanine, *His* Histidine, *Glu* Glutamate, *Ace* Acetate, *Lys* Lysine, *Ala* Alanine, *Val* Valine, *Leu* Leucine, *Ile* Isoleucine, *Tyr* Tyrosine, *Met* Methionine, *Gln* Glutamine, *PC* Phosphorylcholine, *GPC* Glycerophosphocholine, *OAG* O-acetyl glycoprotein, *Lac* Lactate, *Pyr* Pyruvate, *Citr* Citrate, *Gly* Glycine, *4-CG* 4-Cresol glucuronide, *GL* Glyceryl of lipids, *3-HB* 3-Hydroxybutyrate, *NAG* N-acetyl glycoprotein, *NMR* Nuclear magnetic resonance, *TG* triglycerides, *PAG* phenylacetylglycine, *2-PY* 2-Pyridone-3-carboxamide, *L1*:$C\boldsymbol{H}_3(CH_2)_n$-, *L2* $C\boldsymbol{H}_3CH_2CH_2C$=, *L3* -$(C\boldsymbol{H}_2)_n$-, *L4* $C\boldsymbol{H}_2CH_2CO$, *L5* -$C\boldsymbol{H}_2C$ = C-, *L6* $C\boldsymbol{H}_2CO$, *L7* C = $CC\boldsymbol{H}_2C$ = C, *L8* -C**H**-, *EDTA* Ethylenediaminetetraacetic acid, *AS* Ankylosing spondylitis

good discrimination and predictive ability of this model. In addition, based on our results from the correlation coefficient loading plots, correlation coefficient cut-off values for potential markers of plasma, urine and tissue samples were set at 0.294, 0.294 and 0.355, respectively.

Potential biomarkers and pathway analysis

On the basis of correlation coefficients, VIP values and *P* values of the metabolites obtained from the multivariate analysis, we selected 20 metabolites from plasma ($n = 13$), urine ($n = 7$) and tissue ($n = 2$) as potential biomarkers for AS (Table 2). The box-and-whisker plots of these potential

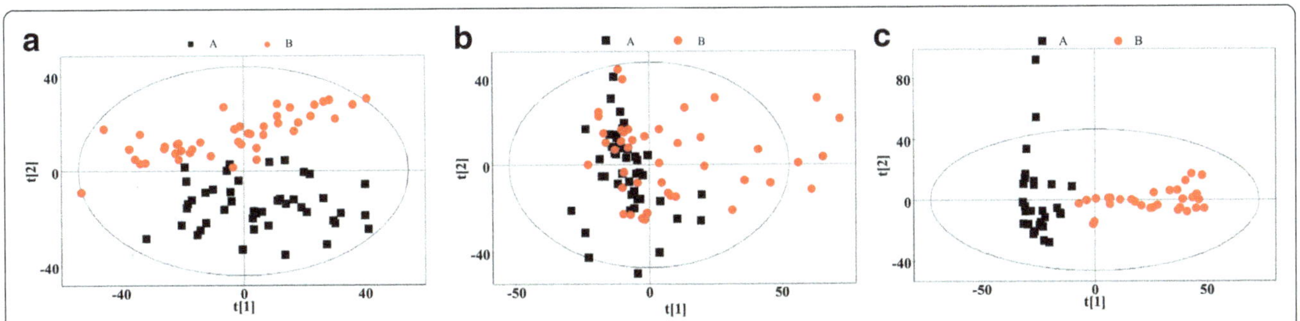

Fig. 2 Principal component analysis (PCA) score plots based on the 1H NMR spectra of (**a**) plasma, (**b**) urine and (**c**) tissue metabolites obtained from the ankylosing spondylitis patients (AS, red circles) and healthy controls (HC, black squares). PC1 and PC2 explained (A-plasma) 34.5 % and 13.6 %, (B-urine) 31.5 % and 13.4 %, (C-tissue)48.2 % and 22.7 % of the variables, respectively

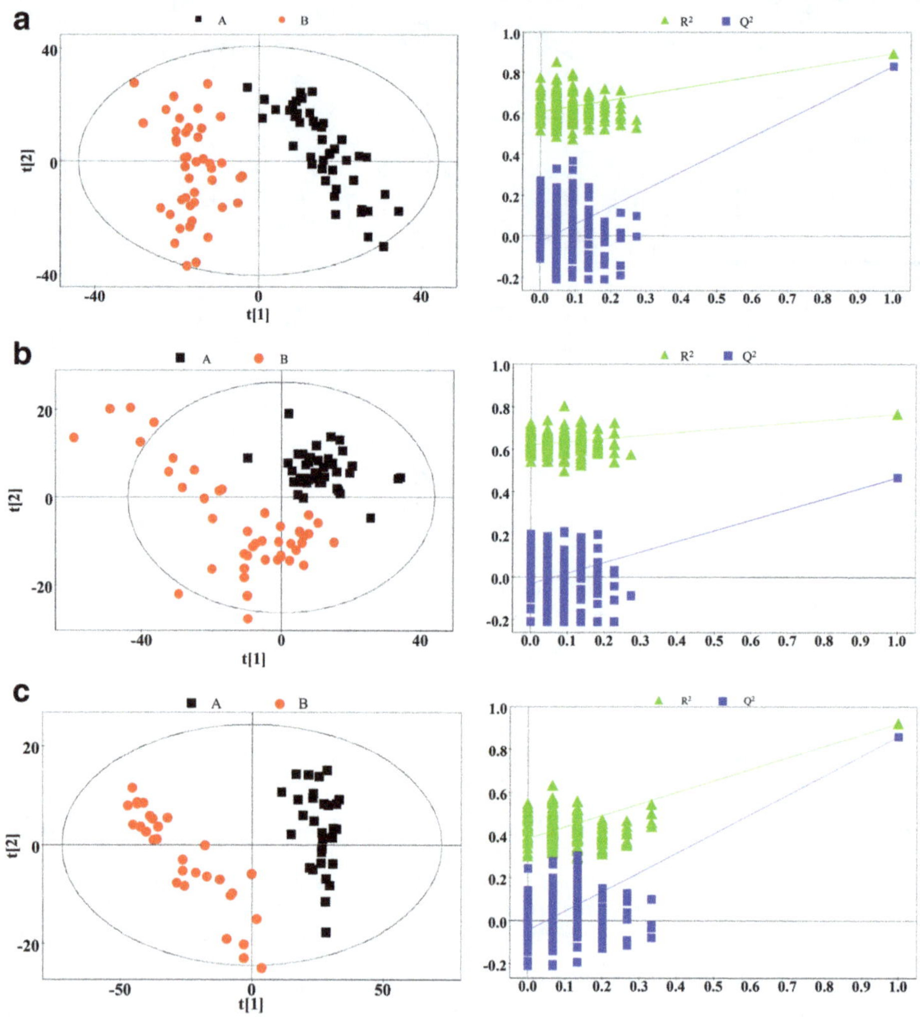

Fig. 3 Partial least squares discriminant analysis (PLS-DA) score plots (*left panel*) and statistical validation of the corresponding PLS-DA model by permutation analysis (*right panel*) based on the ^{1}H nuclear magnetic resonance spectra of (**a**) plasma, (**b**) urine and (**c**) tissue metabolites obtained from the patients with ankylosing spondylitis (*red circles*) and from the healthy control subjects and patients with femoral neck fracture (*black squares*). Principal component 1 (PC1) and PC2 explained (**a**) 42.1 % and 16.0 %, (**b**) 39.4 % and 11.3 %, and (**c**) 51.6 % and 18.7 % of the variables, respectively

biomarkers also suggested the presence of significant intergroup differences (Fig. 5). On this basis, by KEGG pathway database retrieval, we found that these metabolites were associated mainly with metabolic pathways such as fat metabolism, intestinal microbial metabolism, glucose metabolism and choline metabolism, as well as probably with immune regulation. Finally, we combined these results to draw a metabolic pathway map (Fig. 6) to show a more intuitive correlation between these metabolites.

Discussion

The diagnosis of AS is not prompt owing to the lack of effective diagnostic biomarkers. With effective and potentially disease-modifying treatments such as TNF inhibitors becoming widely available [31], the diagnostic delay becomes the critical rate-limiting factor for the mobility and quality of life of patients with AS. As an effective tool, metabolomics has been playing a great role in studies aimed at finding diagnostic biomarkers for various types of cancer [32]. In recent years, few studies have been reported on the metabolomics of AS [1, 2, 16], and the common point is that MS and only plasma samples are used in these studies. In the present study, for the first time to our knowledge, we used NMR along with plasma, urine and ligament tissues as samples in metabolomic investigations in an effort to define more meaningful potential diagnostic biomarkers for AS.

All metabolites with significant changes could be candidates for AS biomarkers (i.e. potential biomarkers). Nevertheless, no single biomarker can characterize AS, and fluctuating metabolic changes in amino acids are not specific biomarkers of any disease [29]. Thus, a panel of markers rather than a single compound may be promising tools for making an accurate diagnosis of AS

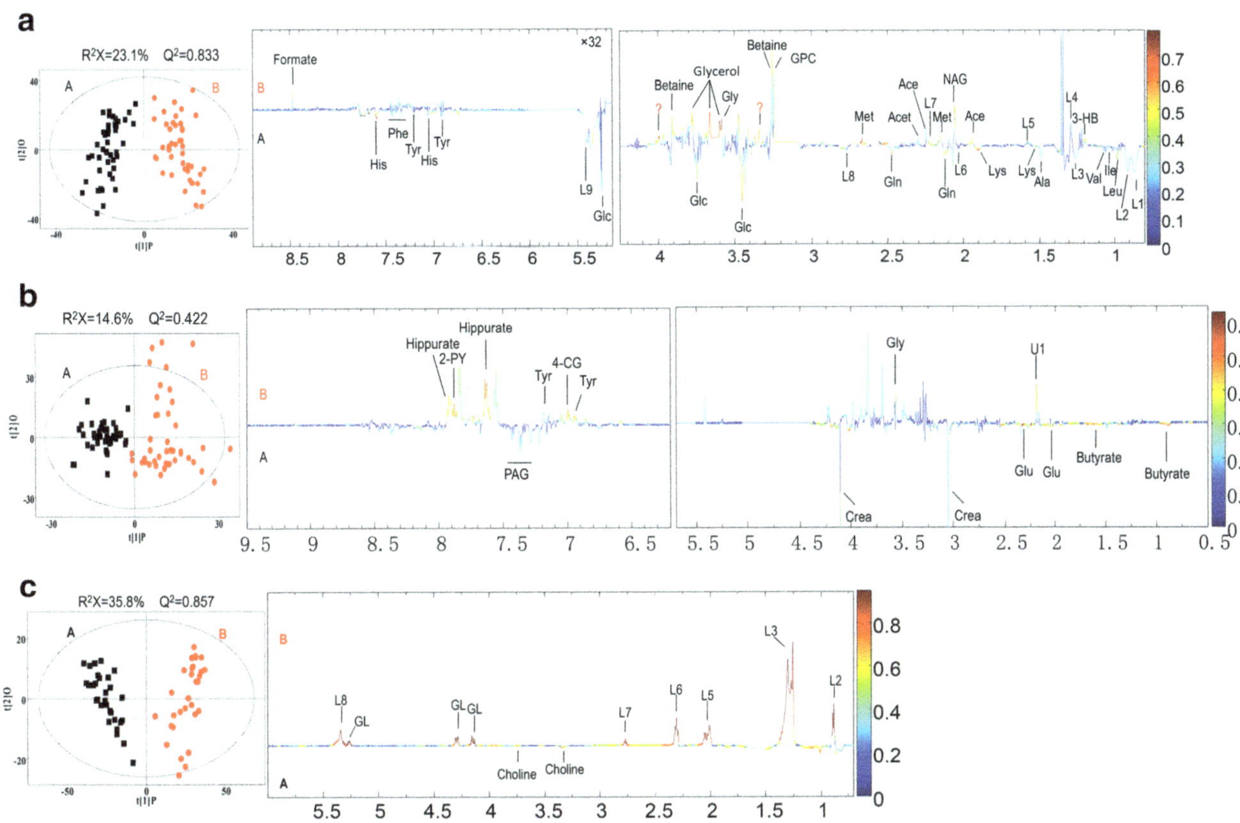

Fig. 4 Orthogonal projection to latent structures discriminant analysis score plots (*left panel*) and the corresponding coefficient loading plots (*right panel*) based on the ^{1}H nuclear magnetic resonance spectra of (**a**) plasma, (**b**) urine and (**c**) tissue metabolites obtained from the patients with ankylosing spondylitis (*red circles*) and from the healthy control subjects and patients with femoral neck fracture (*black squares*). *2-PY* 2-Pyridone-3-carboxamide, *4-CG* 4-Cresol glucuronide, *Ace* Acetate, *Ala* Alanine, *Crea* Creatinine, *GL* Glycerol of lipids, *Gln* Glutamine, *Glu* Glutamate, *Gly* Glycine, *GPC* Glycerophosphocholine, *His* Histidine, *Ile* Isoleucine, *L1* $\boldsymbol{CH_3}(CH_2)n$., *L2* $\boldsymbol{CH_3}CH_2CH_2C$=, *L3* -($\boldsymbol{CH_2}$)n-, *L4* $\boldsymbol{CH_2}CH_2CO$, *L5* -$\boldsymbol{CH_2}$C = C-, *L6* $\boldsymbol{CH_2}$CO, *L7* C = C$\boldsymbol{CH_2}$C = C, *L8* -$\boldsymbol{CH}$ = $\boldsymbol{CH}$-, *Lac* Lactate, *Leu* Leucine, *Lys* Lysine, *Met* Methionine, *NAG* N-acetyl glycoprotein, *PAG* Phenylacetylglycine, *Phe* Phenylalanine, *Pyr* Pyruvate, *Tyr* Tyrosine, *Val* Valine

[12]. On the basis of these detection methods and multivariate data analysis, we selected 20 different metabolites as potential biomarkers for AS.

The TG content was significantly decreased in the plasma of patients with AS while its metabolite level in plasma (glycerol) was significantly increased. More importantly, three metabolites of the β-oxidation of its downstream fatty acids—namely, acetoacetate, acetone and 3-hydroxybutyrate (3-HB)—were significantly increased in the plasma of patients with AS. In addition, two branched-chain amino acids (leucine and valine) were decreased in AS plasma. Branched-chain amino acids have long been thought to be closely related to fat metabolism, especially for leucine. It has been confirmed in relevant reports that lack of leucine can promote the metabolism of peripheral fats and energy [33]. Additionally, 2-pyridone-3-carboxamide (2-PY) is increased in AS urine, which is reported to be related to fat metabolism as well [34]. All of the above results suggest that the fat metabolic pathways may be active in AS. In addition, we have also reported in previous studies that the expression levels of some β-oxidation-related enzymes were up-regulated in AS, that is the active status of fat metabolism may be related to the pathogenesis of AS [23]. Moreover, Ottaviani et al. reported that BMI tends to increase during the course of AS treatment [35], implying that BMI values are partly related to the severity of AS. Syrbe et al. also reported that the serum levels of some adipokines (resistin and visfatin) were up-regulated in patients with AS, while serum resistin levels are related to markers of inflammation [36]. Gao et al. found that plasma levels of glycerol were increased in AS. Similarly, they suggested that the increased glycerol levels may result from the large in vivo fat consumption in patients with AS [8]. Therefore, we concluded that the fat metabolism in AS may be very active and that TG, glycerol, acetoacetate, acetone, 3-HB, leucine, valine and 2-PY are the key metabolites reflecting these abnormalities. It is worth noting that TG content in the AS ligament tissue increased dramatically instead (Fig. 5). We think this may be an

Table 2 Summary of potential biomarkers of ankylosing spondylitis by plasma, urine and tissue metabolomic analysis

Metabolite	Sample type	Status[a]	Chemical shift	Correlation coefficient (AS vs HC)[b]	VIP value[b]	FC[c]	*P* value[d]
Leucine	Plasma	↓	0.96 (d), 0.97 (d), 1.72 (m), 1.72 (m), 3.73 (t)	−0.452	0.698	0.932	0.045
Valine	Plasma	↓	1.00 (d), 1.05 (d), 2.28 (m), 3.62 (d)	−0.302	1.090	0.86	<0.001
3-HB	Plasma	↑	1.20 (d), 2.32 (dd), 2.42 (dd), 4.16 (m)	0.422	1.328	1.254	<0.001
Alanine	Plasma	↓	1.48 (d), 3.77 (q)	−0.332	1.664	0.770	<0.001
NAG	Plasma	↑	2.05 (s)	0.570	0.065	1.207	<0.001
Methionine	Plasma	↑	2.14 (s), 2.16 (m), 2.65 (t), 3.87 (t)	0.597	1.701	1.325	<0.001
TG (L1, L2, L3, L5, L7, L8)	Plasma	↓	0.86 (t), 0.88 (t), 1.27 (m), 2.01 (m), 2.76 (m), 5.30 (m)	−0.400	0.977	0.814–1.077	<0.05
Acetone	Plasma	↑	2.23 (s)	0.298	1.358	1.415	<0.001
Acetoacetate	Plasma	↑	2.29 (s)	2.294	0.884	1.249	<0.001
Betaine	Plasma	↑	3.26 (s), 3.91 (s)	0.334	0.287	1.038	0.030
Glycerol	Plasma	↑	3.65 (dd), 3.56 (dd), 3.77 (m)	0.328	1.400	1.207	<0.001
Glucose	Plasma	↓	3.42 (dd), 3.54 (dd), 3.71 (dd), 3.78 (m), 3.84 (m), 5.26 (d)	−0.317	0.559	0.909	0.013
Glutamate	Plasma	↓	2.07 (m), 2.35 (m), 3.75 (m)	−0.374	1.300	0.789	<0.001
Butyrate	Urine	↓	0.90 (t), 1.56 (m), 2.16 (t)	−0.447	1.533	0.896	0.003
Creatinine	Urine	↓	3.04 (s), 3.93 (s)	−0.331	1.330	0.814	0.018
Glycine	Urine	↑	3.56 (s)	3.392	1.088	1.298	0.009
Hippurate	Urine	↑	7.84 (d), 7.64 (t), 7.56 (dd)	0.421	0.772	1.320	0.017
PAG	Urine	↓	8.03 (d), 7.36 (m), 7.37 (m), 7.43 (m)	−0.306	1.213	0.895	0.028
Glutamate	Urine	↓	2.07 (m), 2.35 (m), 3.75 (m)	−0.429	1.541	0.919	0.002
2-PY	Urine	↑	7.83 (dd), 8.55 (d)	0.461	0.700	1.182	0.049
TG (L2, L3, L5, L6, L7, L8)	Tissue	↑	0.88 (t), 1.27 (m), 2.01 (m), 2.30 (m), 2.76 (m), 5.33 (m)	0.946	1.060	2.490–7.039	<0.001
Choline	Tissue	↓	4.14 (m), 4.29 (m), 5.26 (m)	−0.680	0.718	0.242	<0.001

Abbreviations: AS Ankylosing spondylitis, *VIP* Variable importance for projection, *FC* Fold change, *3-HB* 3-Hydroxybutyrate, *NAG* N-acetyl glycoprotein, *TG* Triglycerides, *PAG* Phenylacetylglycine, *2-PY* 2-Pyridone-3-carboxamide, *L1* $C\boldsymbol{H}_3(CH_2)_n$-, *L2* $C\boldsymbol{H}_3CH_2CH_2C$=, *L3* -$(C\boldsymbol{H}_2)_n$-, *L5* -$C\boldsymbol{H}_2C$ = C-, *L6* $C\boldsymbol{H}_2CO$, *L7* C = $CC\boldsymbol{H}_2C$ = C, *L8* -C***H*** = C***H***-

[a]Relative concentrations compared with healthy control subjects: ↑ = up-regulated; ↓ = down-regulated

[b]Correlation coefficient and VIP value were obtained from orthogonal projection to latent structures discriminant analysis

[c]Fold change between patients with AS and healthy control subjects

[d]*P* value determined using Student's *t* test

ectopic fat deposition phenomenon. It has been found in some studies that patients with fat deposition in local tissue often also have an increased level of inflammatory cytokines (such as TNF-α and interleukin 6) [37, 38], which is consistent with the chronic inflammatory environment in patients with AS.

IBD has been considered one of the most extra-articular symptoms of AS [39] and the pathogenesis of IBD is closely related to intestinal microorganisms [40]. Four of the potential biomarkers we detected are closely related to intestinal microbial metabolism. The levels of glycine and hippurate were significantly increased in AS urine. Hippurate is produced in the gut by microorganisms using glycine and benzoic acid as building blocks [41]. It is normally found in urine, and an increased level of hippurate indicates disorder of the gut microbiota [42]. In addition, an increased hippurate level in the urine has been associated with leanness [43], which is also consistent with our results related to abnormal fat metabolism. Phenylacetylglycine (PAG) and butyrate are also decreased in AS urine. Butyrate has been considered to regulate the intestinal flora balance, and the addition of low doses of butyrate to the diet has a certain therapeutic effect on ulcerative colitis [44]. On one hand, a decreased level of PAG in the urine may also be associated with intestinal flora metabolism disorder [45]. On the other hand, previous studies have found that sulphate-reducing bacteria were increased in the faeces of patients with AS, and such bacteria were suggested to be correlated with the pathogenic mechanism of IBD [46]. In addition, some authors believe that the intestinal microbial composition in patients with AS is changed compared with that in healthy individuals [47, 48], and *Dialister* has been suggested as the potential marker of AS [48]. Therefore, the evidence described above suggests that the changes of butyrate, hippurate, glycine

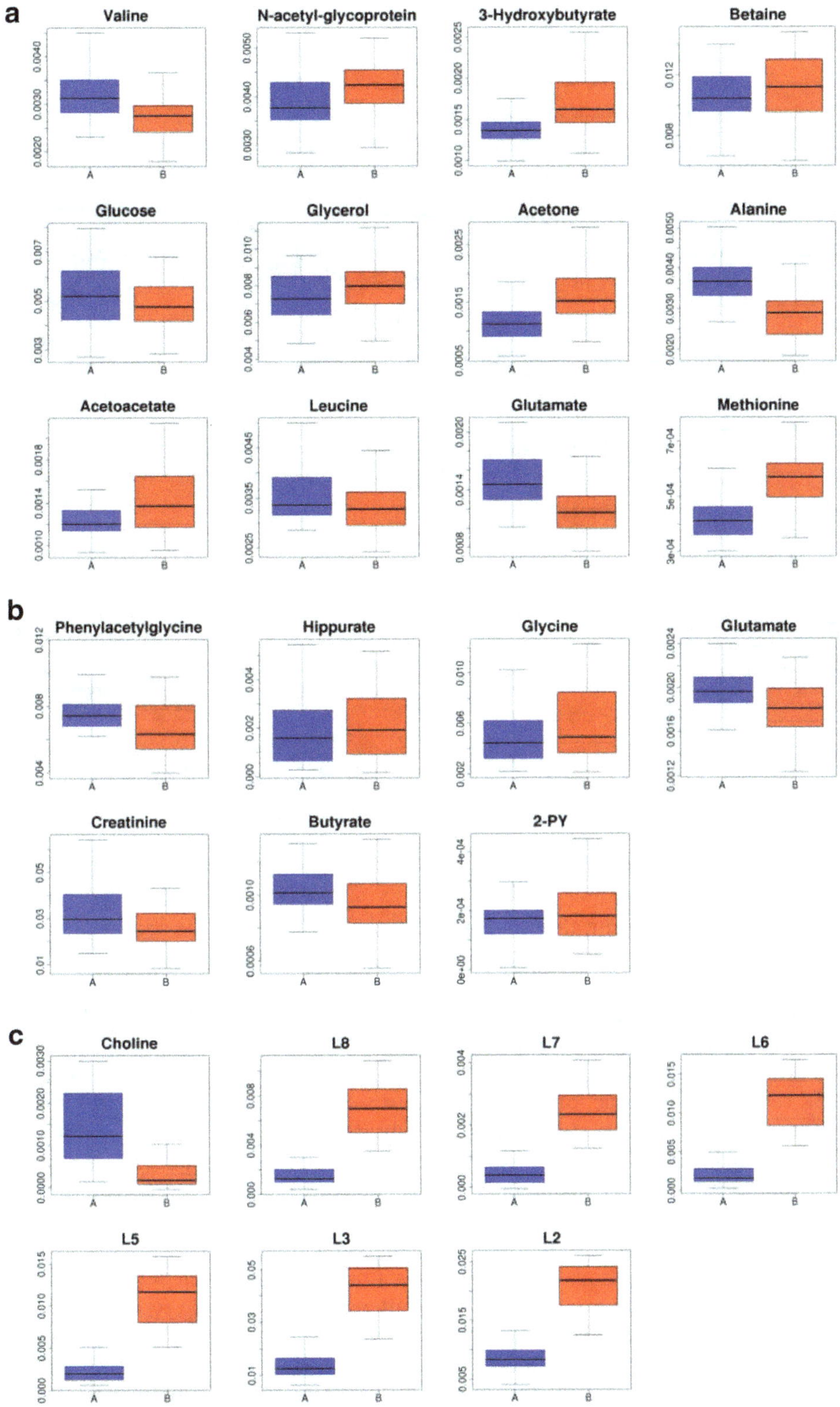

Fig. 5 Box-and-whisker plots showing the relative levels of selected potential biomarkers for AS in (**a**) plasma, **b**) urine and **c**) tissue. *Horizontal line* in the middle portion of the boxes represents the median; *bottom* and *top boundaries of boxes* represent the lower and upper quartiles, respectively; and whiskers represent the 5th and 95th percentiles. *AS* Ankylosing spondylitis, *HC* Healthy control subjects, *FNF* Femoral neck fracture, *2-PY* 2-Pyridone-3-carboxamide, *L2* $C\boldsymbol{H}_3CH_2CH_2C{=}$, *L3* $-(C\boldsymbol{H}_2)_n-$, *L5* $-C\boldsymbol{H}_2C=C-$, *L6* $C\boldsymbol{H}_2CO$, *L7* $C=CC\boldsymbol{H}_2C=C$, *L8* $-C\boldsymbol{H}=C\boldsymbol{H}-$

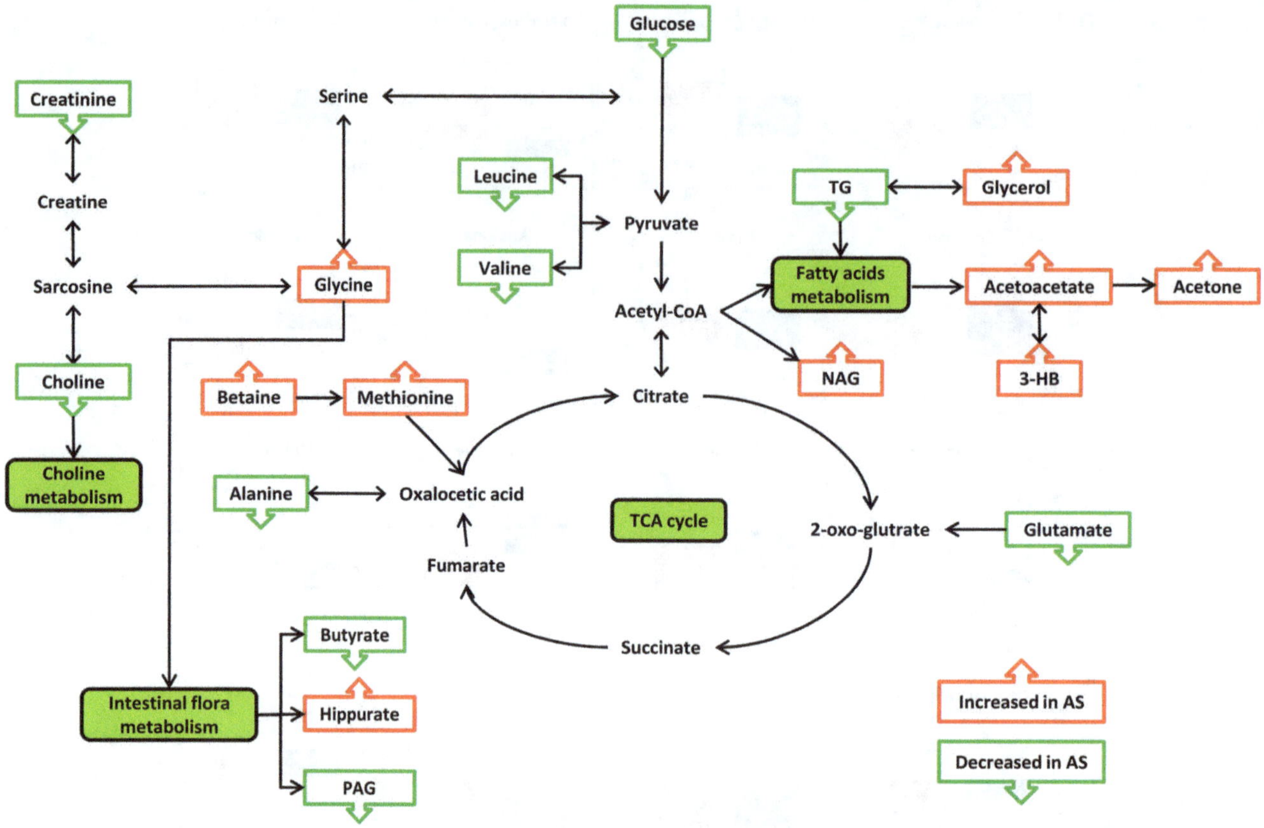

Fig. 6 Altered metabolic pathways for the most relevant distinguishing metabolites (potential biomarkers) between the patients with AS and the healthy control subjects and patients with femoral neck fracture. *Green boxes* indicate metabolites that were up-regulated in AS, while *red boxes* indicate metabolites that were down-regulated. *AS* Ankylosing spondylitis, *3-HB* 3-Hydroxybutyrate, *NAG* N-acetyl glycoprotein, *TG* Triglycerides, *PAG* Phenylacetylglycine, *CoA* Coenzyme A, *TCA* Tricarboxylic acid

and PAG levels in the urine may indicate that they are the key metabolites of the abnormal intestinal microbial metabolism in AS.

In our previous research we reported that insulin receptor (INSR) may be a key upstream protein that leads to an unusually active fat metabolism [12] and that over-expressed INSR can enhance the action of insulin and disrupt glucose metabolism. In this study, plasma glucose was decreased, which might be a result of the over-expression of INSR. In addition, as two important precursors of gluconeogenesis, alanine and glutamate were significantly decreased in AS plasma (glutamate was reduced in urine, too), which may also be the reason for the decline in the glucose concentration.

We also found abnormal choline metabolism in AS. Choline was decreased significantly in the ligaments of patients with AS. Choline has an affinity for fat and can promote the transport of fat out of the liver in the form of phospholipids through the blood or it can improve the use of fatty acids themselves in the liver to prevent the abnormal deposition of fat in some organs or tissues [49]. Therefore, the ectopic fat deposition phenomenon in the ligament may be related to the significant decrease in choline. Furthermore, as a precursor of choline, the urinary creatinine level in patients with AS was decreased. A decreased level of urinary creatinine is commonly found in chronic kidney disease, and AS is occasionally complicated with renal disease [50]. Therefore, the decreased urinary creatinine may be a manifestation of AS complicated with extra-articular symptoms.

AS is a typical autoimmune disease and its pathogenesis is closely related to immune system disorder. We found that plasma levels of betaine, methionine and N-acetyl glycoprotein (NAG) were noticeably increased. Methionine is a precursor of methionine enkephalin (MENK), and the latter is involved in the regulation of immune response in addition to affecting cell proliferation. Effects of MENK on the immune system are observed mainly in immune stimulation at lower concentrations [51]. Thus, an elevated plasma level of methionine may reflect reduced synthesis of MENK, which further results in an aggressive autoimmune reaction leading to AS. Because betaine is a precursor of methionine [52], the elevation of both betaine and methionine in AS may be inter-related, and plasma NAG elevation may also suggest an immune system disorder in AS because NAG can acetylate glycoproteins, which are important for white blood cell recognition [53].

In general, the metabolomic profiles we have obtained are promising. With good discrimination and predictive ability in multivariate analysis models, the profiles could aid in making decisions on a more invasive diagnostic procedure. However, some limitations of this research need to be noted. First, the sample was limited in size, and the results should be validated with a larger number of patients with AS in the future. Second, the disease activity in patients with AS was not evaluated, and further work is required to address the relationship between potential biomarkers and disease activity. Third, some comorbidities of AS may affect the patient's own metabolic status, although we excluded this category of patients in advance. However, considering the possible existence of bias, we still need to pay attention to this problem when interpreting the results. Fourth, the medication history of the patients, which may also influence the results of metabolic profiling, was not interpreted in our results.

Conclusions

In this study, NMR along with three sample types—urine, plasma and ligament tissue—were used for the first time in a metabolomic study of AS to obtain more comprehensive metabolomic profiles and later select potential biomarkers that may help decrease the delay in the diagnosis of AS. Disorders of four metabolic pathways as well as immune function may exist in patients with AS, and 20 differential metabolites that play critical roles in these metabolic pathways or physiological functions can be considered as potential biomarkers for AS. Further validation studies are needed to confirm these results before this method can be transferred from bench to bedside.

Abbreviations

2-PY: 2-Pyridone-3-carboxamide; 3-HB: 3-Hydroxybutyrate; 4-CG: 4-Cresol glucuronide; Ace: Acetate; Ala: Alanine; AS: Ankylosing spondylitis; BASDAI: Bath Ankylosing Spondylitis Disease Activity Index; BASFI: Bath Ankylosing Spondylitis Functional Index; BMI: Body mass index; Citr: Citrate; CoA: Coenzyme A; EDTA: Ethylenediaminetetraacetic acid; EP: Epoxy epoxide; FC: Fold change; FNF: Femoral neck fracture; GL: Glycerol of lipids; Gln: Glutamine; Glu: Glutamate; Gly: Glycine; GPC: Glycerophosphocholine; HC: Healthy control subjects; His: Histidine; IBD: Inflammatory bowel disease; Ig: Immunoglobulin; Ile: Isoleucine; INSR: Insulin receptor; KEGG: Kyoto Encyclopedia of Genes and Genomes; L1: $CH_3(CH_2)n$.; L2: $CH_3CH_2CH_2C$=; L3: -$(CH_2)n$-; L4: CH_2CH_2CO; L5: -CH_2C = C-; L6: CH_2CO; L7: C = CCH_2C = C; L8: -CH = CH-.; Lac: Lactate; Leu: Leucine; Lys: Lysine; MENK: Methionine encephalin; Met: Methionine; MS: Mass spectrometry; NAG: N-acetyl glycoprotein; NMR: Nuclear magnetic resonance; OAG: O-acetyl glycoprotein; OPLS-DA: Orthogonal projection to latent structures discriminant analysis; PAG: Phenylacetylglycine; PC: Phosphorylcholine; PCA: Principal component analysis; Phe: Phenylalanine; PLS-DA: Partial least squares discriminant analysis; Pyr: Pyruvate; RA: Rheumatoid arthritis; TCA: Tricarboxylic acid; TG: Triglycerides; t_m: Mixing time; TMSP: 3-Trimethylsilyl-2,2,3,3-d_4-propionate; TNF-α: Tumour necrosis factor α; Tyr: Tyrosine; Val: Valine; VIP: Variable importance for projection;

Acknowledgements

We appreciate the cooperation of all the patients who volunteered and the staff at the outpatient centre and inpatient department. We also express our sincere gratitude to the rheumatologist (Dong-bao Zhao) who helped to get the samples. We acknowledge Suzhou Bionovogene for providing help with performing ^{1}H NMR-based metabolic analysis using the NMR imaging equipment.

Funding

No funding.

Authors' contributions

WW carried out the sample processing, analysis and interpretation of data, participated in the NMR detection, and drafted the manuscript. GY carried out the NMR detection, participated in the analysis and interpretation of data, and revised the manuscript. JZ carried out the acquisition of urine samples, performed the statistical analysis, and helped to revise the manuscript. CC carried out the acquisition of plasma samples and interpretation of data, and also helped to revise the manuscript. ZJ carried out the acquisition of tissue samples and interpretation of data, and also helped to revise the manuscript. JL participated in the design of the study, performed the statistical analysis, and helped to revise the manuscript. WX conceived of the study, participated in its design and coordination, and helped to draft the manuscript. All authors read and approved the final manuscript.

Competing interests

The authors declare that they have no competing interests.

Author details

[1]Department of Orthopedics, Chengdu Military General Hospital, Chengdu city, People's Republic of China. [2]School of Pharmacy, Second Military Medical University, Shanghai city, People's Republic of China. [3]Department of Rheumatology, Changhai Hospital, Shanghai city, People's Republic of China. [4]Physical Examination Center, Changhai Hospital, Shanghai city, People's Republic of China. [5]Department of Orthopedics, Changhai Hospital, Shanghai city, People's Republic of China.

References

1. Chen R, Han S, Dong D, Wang Y, Liu Q, Xie W, et al. Serum fatty acid profiles and potential biomarkers of ankylosing spondylitis determined by gas chromatography-mass spectrometry and multivariate statistical analysis. Biomed Chromatogr. 2015;29(4):604–11.
2. Sundström B, Johansson G, Kokkonen H, Cederholm T, Wållberg-Jonsson S. Plasma phospholipid fatty acid content is related to disease activity in ankylosing spondylitis. J Rheumatol. 2012;39(2):327–33.
3. Harrison BJ, Symmons DP, Barrett EM, Silman AJ. The performance of the 1987 ARA classification criteria for rheumatoid arthritis in a population based cohort of patients with early inflammatory polyarthritis. J Rheumatol. 1998;25(12):2324–30.
4. de Vlam K. Soluble and tissue biomarkers in ankylosing spondylitis. Best Pract Res Clin Rheumatol. 2010;24:671–82.
5. Braun J, Sieper J. Classification criteria for rheumatoid arthritis and ankylosing spondylitis. Clin Exp Rheumatol. 2009;27(4 Suppl 55):S68–73.
6. Tilleman K, Van Steendam K, Cantaert T, De Keyser F, Elewaut D, Deforce D. Synovial detection and autoantibody reactivity of processed citrullinated isoforms of vimentin in inflammatory arthritides. Rheumatology. 2008;47:597–604.
7. Chandra PE, Sokolove J, Hipp BG, Lindstrom TM, Elder JT, Reveille JD, et al. Novel multiplex technology for diagnostic characterization of rheumatoid arthritis. Arthritis Res Ther. 2011;13:R102.
8. Gao P, Lu C, Zhang F, Sang P, Yang D, Li X, et al. Integrated GC-MS and LC-MS plasma metabonomics analysis of ankylosing spondylitis. Analyst. 2008; 133(9):1113–284.

9. Chan EC, Koh PK, Mal M, Cheah PY, Eu KW, Backshall A, et al. Metabolic profiling of human colorectal cancer using high-resolution magic angle spinning nuclear magnetic resonance (HR-MAS NMR) spectroscopy and gas chromatography mass spectrometry (GC/MS). J Proteome Res. 2009;8:352–61.
10. Chen T, Xie G, Wang X, Fan J, Qiu Y, Zheng X, et al. Serum and urine metabolite profiling reveals potential biomarkers of human hepatocellular carcinoma [published erratum appears in Mol Cell Proteomics. 2011;10(7): A110.004945]. Mol Cell Proteomics. 2011;10(7):M110.004945.
11. Suzuki N. Mass spectrometry-based quantitative analysis and biomarker discovery. J Pharm Soc Jpn. 2011;131(9):1305–9.
12. Jiang M, Chen T, Feng H, Zhang Y, Li L, Zhao A, et al. Serum metabolic signatures of four types of human arthritis. J Proteome Res. 2013;12:3769–79.
13. Lauridsen MB, Bliddal H, Christensen R, Danneskiold-Samsøe B, Bennett R, Keun H, et al. ^{1}H NMR spectroscopy-based interventional metabolic phenotyping: a cohort study of rheumatoid arthritis patients. J Proteome Res. 2010;9(9):4545–53.
14. Lu C, Zha Q, Chang A, He Y, Lu A. Pattern differentiation in Traditional Chinese Medicine can help define specific indications for biomedical therapy in the treatment of rheumatoid arthritis. J Altern Complement Med. 2009;15(9):1021–5.
15. Hügle T, Kovacs H, Heijnen IA, Daikeler T, Baisch U, Hicks JM, et al. Synovial fluid metabolomics in different forms of arthritis assessed by nuclear magnetic resonance spectroscopy. Clin Exp Rheumatol. 2012;30(2):240-5.
16. Liu J, Zhu P, Peng J, Li K, Du J, Gu J, et al. Identification of disease-associated proteins by proteomic approach in ankylosing spondylitis. Biochem Biophys Res Commun. 2007;357:531–6.
17. Gowda GA, Zhang S, Gu H, Asiago V, Shanaiah N, Raftery D. Metabolomics-based methods for early disease diagnostics. Expert Rev Mol Diagn. 2008;8:617–33.
18. Cao Z, Wu LP, Li YX, Guo YB, Chen YW, Wu RH. Change of choline compounds in sodium selenite-induced apoptosis of rats used as quantitative analysis by in vitro 9.4T MR spectroscopy. World J Gastroenterol. 2008;14:3891–6.
19. Viant MR, Lyeth BG, Miller MG, Berman RF. An NMR metabolomic investigation of early metabolic disturbances following traumatic brain injury in a mammalian model. NMR Biomed. 2005;18:507–16.
20. Cheng LL, Burns MA, Taylor JL, He W, Halpern EF, McDougal WS, et al. Metabolic characterization of human prostate cancer with tissue magnetic resonance spectroscopy. Cancer Res. 2005;65:3030–4.
21. Sharma K, Karl B, Mathew AV, Gangoiti JA, Wassel CL, Saito R, et al. Metabolomics reveals signature of mitochondrial dysfunction in diabetic kidney disease. J Am Soc Nephrol. 2013;24:1901–12.
22. Cao H, Huang H, Xu W, Chen D, Yu J, Li J, et al. Fecal metabolome profiling of liver cirrhosis and hepatocellular carcinoma patients by ultra performance liquid chromatography–mass spectrometry. Anal Chim Acta. 2011;691:68–75.
23. Xu WD, Yang XY, Li DH, Zheng KD, Qiu PC, Zhang W, et al. Up-regulation of fatty acid oxidation in the ligament as a contributing factor of ankylosing spondylitis: a comparative proteomic study. J Proteomics. 2015;113:57–72.
24. Rudwaleit M, Braun J, Sieper J. ASAS classification criteria for axial spondyloarthritis [in German]. Z Rheumatol. 2009;68(7):591–3.
25. Teahan O, Gamble S, Holmes E, Waxman J, Nicholson JK, Bevan C, et al. Impact of analytical bias in metabonomic studies of human blood serum and plasma. Anal Chem. 2006;78:4307–18.
26. Culeddu N, Chessa M, Porcu MC, Fresu P, Tonolo G, Virgilio G, et al. NMR-based metabolomic study of type 1 diabetes. Metabolomics. 2012;8:1162–9.
27. Lin CY, Wu H, Tjeerdema RS, Viant MR. Evaluation of metabolite extraction strategies from tissue samples using NMR metabolomics. Metabolomics. 2007; 3(1):55–67.
28. Liu G, Yang G, Fang T, Cai Y, Wu C, Wang J, et al. NMR-based metabolomic studies reveal changes in biochemical profile of urine and plasma from rats fed with sweet potato fiber or sweet potato residue. RSC Adv. 2014;4:23749–58.
29. Lin Z, Jin H, Guo X, Yang Z, Zhao L, Tang S, et al. Distinguishing pancreatic cancer from chronic pancreatitis and healthy individuals by ^{1}H nuclear magnetic resonance-based metabonomic profiles. Clin Biochem. 2012;45:1064–9.
30. Umetrics AB. User's guide to SIMCA-P, SIMCA-P+ version 11.5. Umea, Sweden: Umetrics AB; 2005.
31. van der Heijde D, Sieper J, Maksymowych WP, Dougados M, Burgos-Vargas R, Landewé R, et al. 2010 Update of the international ASAS recommendations for the use of anti-TNF agents in patients with axial spondyloarthritis. Ann Rheum Dis. 2011;70:905–8.
32. Jung J, Jung Y, Bang EJ, Cho SI, Jang YJ, Kwak JM, et al. Noninvasive diagnosis and evaluation of curative surgery for gastric cancer by using NMR-based metabolomic profiling. Ann Surg Oncol. 2014;21 Suppl 4:S736–42.
33. Xia T, Cheng Y, Zhang Q, Xiao F, Liu B, Chen S, et al. S6K1 in the central nervous system regulates energy expenditure via MC4R/CRH pathways in response to deprivation of an essential amino acid. Diabetes. 2012;61(10):2461–71.
34. Delaney J, Hodson MP, Thakkar H, Connor SC, Sweatman BC, Kenny SP, et al. Tryptophan-NAD$^+$ pathway metabolites as putative biomarkers and predictors of peroxisome proliferation. Arch Toxicol. 2005;79(4):208–23.
35. Ottaviani S, Allanore Y, Tubach F, Forien M, Gardette A, Pasquet B, et al. Body mass index influences the response to infliximab in ankylosing spondylitis. Arthritis Res Ther. 2012;14:R115.
36. Syrbe U, Callhoff J, Conrad K, Poddubnyy D, Haibel H, Junker S, et al. Serum adipokine levels in patients with ankylosing spondylitis and their relationship to clinical parameters and radiographic spinal progression. Arthritis Rheumatol. 2015;67(3):678–85.
37. Marra F, Bertolani C. Adipokines in liver diseases. Hepatology. 2009;50:957–69.
38. Grunfeld C, Feingold KR. The metabolic effects of tumor necrosis factor and other cytokines. Biotherapy. 1991;3:143–58.
39. Bae JM, Choo JY, Kim KJ, Park KS. Association of inflammatory bowel disease with ankylosing spondylitis and rheumatoid arthritis: a nationwide population-based study. Mod Rheumatol. 2016;26:1-6.
40. Orel R, Kamhi TT. Intestinal microbiota, probiotics and prebiotics in inflammatory bowel disease. World J Gastroenterol. 2014;20(33):11505–24.
41. Nicholson JK, Holmes E, Wilson ID. Gut microorganisms, mammalian metabolism and personalized health care. Nat Rev Microbiol. 2005;3(5):431–8.
42. Yang Y, Wang L, Wang S, Huang R, Zheng L, Liang S, et al. An integrated metabonomic approach to studying metabolic profiles in rat models with insulin resistance induced by high fructose. Mol Biosyst. 2014;10:1803–11.
43. Waldram A, Holmes E, Wang Y, Rantalainen M, Wilson ID, Tuohy KM, et al. Top-down systems biology modeling of host metabotype-microbiome associations in obese rodents. J Proteome Res. 2009;8(5):2361–75.
44. Roediger WE, Nance S. Selective reduction of fatty acid oxidation in colonocytes: correlation with ulcerative colitis. Lipids. 1990;25(10):646–52.
45. Gooda Sahib Jambocus N, Saari N, Ismail A, Khatib A, Mahomoodally MF, Abdul Hamid A. An investigation into the antiobesity effects of *Morinda citrifolia* L. leaf extract in high fat diet induced obese rats using a ^{1}H NMR metabolomics approach. J Diabetes Res. 2016;2016:2391592.
46. Stebbings S, Munro K, Simon MA, Tannock G, Highton J, Harmsen H, et al. Comparison of the faecal microflora of patients with ankylosing spondylitis and controls using molecular methods of analysis. Rheumatology (Oxford). 2002;41(12):1395–401.
47. Costello ME, Ciccia F, Willner D, Warrington N, Robinson PC, Gardiner B, et al. Brief report: intestinal dysbiosis in ankylosing spondylitis. Arthritis Rheumatol. 2015;67(3):686–91.
48. Tito RY, Cypers H, Joossens M, Varkas G, Van Praet L, Glorieus E, et al. Dialister as microbial marker of disease activity in spondyloarthritis. Arthritis Rheumatol. doi:10.1002/art.39802.
49. Buchman AL, Dubin MD, Moukarzel AA, Jenden DJ, Roch M, Rice KM, et al. Choline deficiency: a cause of hepatic steatosis during parenteral nutrition that can be reversed with intravenous choline supplementation. Hepatology. 1995;22:1399–403.
50. Korkmaz C, Ozcan A, Akcar N. Increased frequency of ultrasonographic findings suggestive of renal stones in patients with ankylosing spondylitis. Clin Exp Rheumatol. 2005;23(3):389–92.
51. Liu XH, Huang DA, Yang FY, Hao YS, Du GG, Li PF, et al. A new cytokine: the possible effect pathway of methionine enkephalin. World J Gastroenterol. 2003;9(1):169–73.
52. Xie G, Lu L, Qiu Y, Ni Q, Zhang W, Gao YT, et al. Plasma metabolite biomarkers for the detection of pancreatic cancer. J Proteome Res. 2015;14(2):1195–202.
53. Zhang L, Jin H, Guo X, Yang Z, Zhao L, Tang S, et al. Distinguishing pancreatic cancer from chronic pancreatitis and healthy individuals by ^{1}H nuclear magnetic resonance-based metabonomic profiles. Clin Biochem. 2012;45(13-14):1064–9.

3

Work productivity is associated with disease activity and functional ability in Italian patients with early axial spondyloarthritis: an observational study from the SPACE cohort

Manouk de Hooge†, Roberta Ramonda*†, Mariagrazia Lorenzin, Paola Frallonardo, Leonardo Punzi, Augusta Ortolan and Andrea Doria

Abstract

Background: Spondyloarthritis often affects young people, typically in their working years. The aim of our study was to investigate work productivity and its relationship with disease activity and physical functioning in Italian patients with axial spondyloarthritis (axSpA) with chronic back pain (CBP) for ≥3 months and ≤2 years, and onset < 45 years of age.

Methods: Baseline absenteeism, presenteeism, work productivity loss (assessed by the Work Productivity and Activity Impairment questionnaire (WPAI)), and disease activity (assessed by the Bath Ankylosing Spondylitis Disease Activity Index (BASDAI)/Ankylosing Spondylitis Disease Activity Score (ASDAS)) and functional ability (assessed by the Bath Ankylosing Spondylitis Disease Functional Index (BASFI)) of patients with axSpA (rheumatologist's diagnosis) included in the Italian section of the Spondyloarthritis Caught Early (SPACE) cohort were collected. Multivariate linear regression analysis was used to evaluate the associations between work productivity and disease activity/physical functioning.

Results: Absenteeism in 51 patients with axSpA was low (8.3 %). A decrease in work productivity was related to an increase in disease activity. Disease activity was strongly correlated with absenteeism ($p < 0.01$), presenteeism ($p < 0.01$) and work productivity loss ($p < 0.001$). In addition, decreased work productivity was related to a decrease in functional ability. Physical functioning was correlated with absenteeism ($p < 0.001$), presenteeism ($p < 0.05$) and work productivity loss ($p < 0.001$).

Conclusions: Impairment of work productivity was correlated with disease activity and physical functioning in Italian patients with axSpA with CBP for ≥3 months and ≤2 years, with onset <45 years of age.

Keywords: Spondyloarthritis, Work, Back pain, Disease activity

Background

Spondyloarthritis (SpA) are a group of chronic inflammatory rheumatic diseases that share several clinical characteristics. They can be subdivided into axial SpA (axSpA) or peripheral SpA depending on the predominant musculoskeletal site involved [1]. Patients with axSpA can be further subdivided into two groups: patients with radiographic evidence of sacroiliitis (ankylosing spondylitis, AS) or without radiographic sacroiliitis (non-radiographic axSpA, nr-axSpA). Patients with axSpA often suffer from impaired function, activity limitations and decreased health-related quality of life (HRQoL) [2–4]. AxSpA usually occurs during young adulthood, before the third decade [5]; thus, function impairment and activity limitations can have important socioeconomic consequences because they affect patients who have just started working. The work participation of axSpA patients with longstanding disease has previously been reported in several studies, which showed correlation between decreased work productivity and increased disease-related sick leave [6–8]. Limitations in physical functioning are also strongly associated with

* Correspondence: roberta.ramonda@unipd.it
†Equal contributors
Rheumatology Unit, Department of Medicine –DIMED, University of Padova, Via Giustiniani 2, 35128 Padova, Italy

work restrictions in patients with axSpA [2, 6]. Besides limitations in work productivity when performing paid work, patients with axSpA also seem to be limited in performing daily activities such as taking care of the family, studying or housekeeping [6].

A study focusing on three European countries (Netherlands, Belgium and France) showed that the work status and productivity of patients with AS differ among these countries [9], decreasing the generalizability of the correlation between work productivity and disease activity or physical functioning in patients with axSpA as identified in previous studies. The prevalence of axSpA in Italy is 1.06 % [10] and the prevalence of nr-axSpA is estimated to be 0.35 % [11]. Few data on work productivity in Italian patients with axSpA are available [12]; it is therefore important to get a clear picture on how this disease impacts the work productivity. The aim of our study was to investigate work productivity and its relationship with disease activity and physical functioning in Italian patients with short-term chronic back pain (CBP) who participated in the Italian section of the Spondyloarthritis Caught Early (SPACE) cohort. In particular presenteism, absenteeism, and work productivity loss (WPL) were considered. Presenteism represents the reduced work productivity due to disease; absenteeism is the percentage of hours missed due to disease; WPL gives an indication of the total work impairment due to disease.

Methods

Patients

Patients who were at least 16 years old, suffering from CBP (≥3 months, ≤2 years, onset < 45 years of age) of unknown origin and referred to a rheumatologist were included in the Italian section of the SPACE cohort. This is an ongoing observational cohort study, which was originally launched at the Leiden University Medical Centre (LUMC) in January 2009.

In March 2012 the SpA study group of the Rheumatology Unit at the University of Padua opened an Italian branch of the SPACE cohort. Eligible patients underwent physical examination, laboratory tests, radiographic imaging and magnetic resonance imaging (MRI) of the sacroiliac joints and spine according to a standardized protocol. In addition, patients completed questionnaires on disease activity, physical functioning, pain and impairment due to the disease, and work productivity. The SPACE cohort has been extensively described in a previous publication [13]. An experienced rheumatologist diagnosed axSpA. Only baseline data were used in these analyses. At this time point, all patients were treated with non-steroidal anti-inflammatory drugs. No patients were treated with synthetic or biological disease modifying anti-rheumatic drugs.

Questionnaires

The Work Productivity and Activity Impairment (WPAI) questionnaire is validated to assess the impact of a disease (here axSpA) on work productivity and on other daily activities [14, 15]. The Italian version of the WPAI was used to obtain the data in our study (from http://www.reillyassociates.net/WPAI_Translations.html) [16]. By using six items, the questionnaire measures: (Question (Q)1) patients' employment status; (Q2) number of hours missed at work due to axSpA; (Q3) number of hours missed at work due to due to other reasons; (Q4) number of hours worked effectively according to the patient's own judgment; (Q5) degree of disease influence on work productivity, according to the patient; and (Q6) degree of disease influence on activities not related to work, according to the patient [13].

The WPAI questionnaire allows the calculation of absenteeism, presenteeism and work productivity loss (WPL). Presenteeism represents the reduced work productivity due to disease, which is rated on a 0–100 % numeric scale, and is calculated as the degree of disease influence on work productivity/10 (question (Q)5). Absenteeism is the percentage of hours missed due to disease (and not due to other reasons) and is calculated as follows the number of hours missed at work due to axSpA (Q2)/(number of hours missed at work due to axSpA (Q2) + number of hours worked effectively (Q4)) [14]. The WPL gives an indication on the total work impairment due to disease and is derived from presenteeism and absenteeism as follows: absenteeism + ((1-Absenteism) × (Presenteeism)). All scores are to be multiplied by 100 to be expressed as percentages. The higher the presenteeism, absenteeism or WPL scores, the greater the work impairment is due to disease.

It has to be underlined that as patients could do both paid work and other daily activities, they reported separately on the WPAI items for paid work (in the form of employee or self-employment) and/or daily activities (in the form of domestic work, studying, voluntary work or taking care of family members). The disease activity and physical functioning of patients were assessed with self-reported questionnaires: the Bath Ankylosing Spondylitis Disease Activity Index (BASDAI), the Bath Ankylosing Spondylitis Functional Index (BASFI) and the Ankylosing Spondylitis disease activity score (ASDAS), which combines items from the BASDAI, patient global assessment and serum C-reactive protein (CRP) [17]. Four ASDAS categories were defined: inactive disease (ASDAS <1.3), moderate disease activity (ASDAS ≥1.3 and <2.1), high disease activity (ASDAS ≥2.1 and ≤3.5) and very high disease activity (ASDAS >3.5) [18]. BASDAI and BASFI continuous scores were converted into dichotomous scores. BASDAI <4 indicated low disease activity and BASDAI ≥4 indicated high disease activity [17]. As there is no BASFI score for impaired and unimpaired physical functioning, we arbitrarily choose a BASFI score ≥2.5 to indicate impaired physical functioning.

Statistical analyses

Patient characteristics were reported by descriptive statistics. The Mann-Whitney test was used to evaluate the association between work productivity and disease activity (evaluated by BASDAI) and physical functioning. The Kruskal-Wallis test was used to evaluate the relationship between work productivity and the four ASDAS states. Multivariate linear regression analyses were performed to evaluate the association of BASDAI, ASDAS and BASFI continuous scores with presenteeism, absenteeism and WPL, adjusted for age, gender, HLA-B27 positivity and duration of CBP. SPSS 21 was used to perform statistical analysis.

Results

Out of 51 patients enrolled in the study, 100 % fulfilled the ASAS criteria for axSpA; 4 (7.8 %) were diagnosed as having AS and 47 (92.2 %) as having nr-axSpA. Mean age at CBP onset was 29.7 (SD ± 8.7) years, 21 patients (41.2 %) were men and 16 patients (31.4 %) were HLA-B27 positive. All 51 patients had at least two features of SpA and the maximum disease activity and physical functioning scores were 9.1 (BASDAI), 4.2 (ASDAS) and 8.9 (BASFI). Other patient characteristics, including work status and mean scores for disease activity and physical functioning, are reported in Table 1. A detailed description of patient characteristics has been published before [19].

Table 1 Baseline characteristics of Italian patients with axSpA included in the SPACE cohort (n = 51)

Characteristic	Value
Age of onset back pain, mean (± SD)	29.7 (± 8.7)
Male, *n*	21 (41.2 %)
Marital state	
- Married	15 (45.1 %)
- Unmarried (with partner)	13 (25.5 %)
- Unmarried (without partner)	23 (29.4 %)
Education level	
- Only primary school	3 (5.9 %)
- Secondary education	28 (54.9 %)
- University education	20 (39.2 %)
Duration (months) back pain, mean (± SD)	12.9 (± 5.9)
Work status	
- Employed, *n*	28 (54.9 %)
- Self employed, *n*	7 (13.7 %)
- Domestic work, *n*	8 (15.7 %)
- Studying, *n*	11 (21.6 %)
- Voluntary work, *n*	2 (3.9 %)
- Care taking of family members, *n*	3 (5.9 %)
ASDAS, mean (± SD)	2.3 (± 1.0)
BASDAI, mean (± SD)	4.5 (± 2.6)
BASFI, mean (± SD)	1.7 (± 2.1)

axSpA axial spondyloarthritis, *SPACE* Spondyloarthritis Caught Early, *ASDAS* Ankylosing Spondylitis Disease Activity Score, *BASDAI* Bath Ankylosing Spondylitis Disease Activity Index, *BASFI* Bath Ankylosing Spondylitis Functional Index

Work productivity

When looking at all 51 patients, they worked 36.4 (±13.9) hours and missed 4.2 (± 8.4) hours per week due to axSpA, presenteeism was 28.6 %, absenteeism 8.3 % and WPL 33.7 %. Table 2 shows the hours worked and missed due to axSpA, presenteeism, absenteeism and WPL of patients with paid jobs (employed and self-employed) or performing voluntary work, domestic work, care of family and/or studying. There were 35 patients (68.6 %) in paid work; 6 of them combined paid work with voluntary work (n = 1), domestic work (n = 1), care of the family (n = 2), studying (n = 1) or a combination (n = 1). Patients spent less time (27.6 hours) in daily activities compared to income-earning jobs (35.7 hours). There was no difference between patients involved in paid work and other daily activities in the number of missed hours/week due to the disease. However, while patients in paid work missed <4 hours/week, patients doing domestic work missed >6 hours/week. Patients with paid work had greater productivity loss due to disease (presenteeism = 32.6 % vs 18.6 %, $p = 0.031$). Absenteeism was in general relatively low in this cohort (7.9 % in income-earning patients and 8.3 % in patients performing other activities).

Relationship between work productivity and disease activity or physical functioning

We identified decrease in work productivity alongside increased disease activity (ASDAS). Hours missed at work ($p = 0.087$), absenteeism ($p = 0.050$), presenteeism ($p = 0.205$) and WPL ($p = 0.012$) increased with the progressive increase in disease activity (ASDAS). Patients with very high disease activity (ASDAS ≥3.5) worked on average 10 hours less than patients with inactive disease (ASDAS ≤1.3) ($p = 0.122$). Presenteeism ($p = 0.049$) and WPL ($p = 0.007$) were significantly increased in patients with BASDAI ≥4 compared to patients with BASDAI <4 (Table 2).

Although the number of hours worked were similar ($p = 0.737$), hours missed at work ($p = 0.021$), the degree on disease influence on daily activities (Q6; $p = 0.020$), absenteeism ($p = 0.014$), presenteeism ($p = 0.010$) and WPL ($p = 0.000$) were significantly higher in patients

Table 2 Work productivity of patients with axSpA according to work status, disease activity (ASDAS/BASDAI), functional ability (BASFI)

	Hours worked per week mean (± SD)	Hours missed per week due to axSpA mean (± SD)	Hours missed per week due to other reasons mean (± SD)	Activity impairment due to axSpA% mean (± SD)	Absenteeism mean% (± SD)	Presenteeism mean% (± SD)	WPL mean% (± SD)
Work status							
Paid work	35.7 (± 12.9)	3.4 (± 6.8)	2.1 (± 3.5)	4.1 (± 2.8)	7.9 (± 14.0)	32.6 (± 31.2)*	36.6 (± 30.0)
- Employed	33.8 (± 9.4)	3.6 (± 7.4)	2.4 (± 3.8)	4.2 (± 2.9)			
- Self employed	43.6 (± 21.4)	2.6 (± 3.3)	1.0 (± 1.7)	3.4 (± 2.4)			
Other daily activities	27.6 (± 12.4)	4.3 (± 9.4)	0.6 (± 1.5)	4.6 (± 3.5)	8.3 (± 13.9)	18.6 (± 28.8)*	25.6 (± 28.5)
- Domestic work	29.1 (± 10.9)	6.4 (± 13.8)	0.8 (± 2.1)	6.1 (± 3.7)			
- Studying	29.0 (± 13.0)	3.7 (± 6.7)	0.4 (± 0.9)	3.6 (± 3.4)			
- Voluntary work	6.0 (0)	-	3.0 (0)	0.5 (± 0.7)			
- Taking care of family members	14.7 (± 9.5)	1.0 (± 1.7)	-	4.3 (± 2.9)			
ASDAS score (disease activity)							
< 1.3 (inactive)	41.4 (± 9.6)	0.8 (± 2.1)	2.8 (± 4.7)	2.6 (± 2.8)	1.7 (± 4.0)*	14.5 (± 21.1)	15.3 (± 22.2)*
1.3–2.1 (moderate)	33.5 (± 18.9)	3.0 (± 6.4)	1.7 (± 3.1)	2.9 (± 2.7)*	5.7 (± 10.0)*	20.9 (± 25.1)	26.3 (± 23.0)*
2.1 – 3.5 (high)	36.9 (± 13.5)	3.3 (± 5.4)	1.2 (± 2.2)	5.2 (± 2.6)*	7.3 (± 10.9)*	32.2 (± 31.2)	36.9 (± 30.1)*
≥ 3.5 (very high)	31.2 (± 10.2)	16.0 (± 16.7)	-	7.0 (± 3.7)	29.2 (± 24.6)*	55.0 (± 44.6)	68.3 (± 28.8)*
BASDAI score (disease activity)							
< 4 (low)	37.6 (± 14.9)	2.3 (± 5.0)	1.9 (± 3.7)	2.5 (± 2.5)***	4.4 (± 8.3)	17.4 (± 24.0)*	20.5 (± 24.4)*
≥ 4 (high)	35.5 (± 13.1)	5.8 (± 10.2)	1.2 (± 2.3)	5.8 (± 2.8)***	11.5 (± 17.0)	37.9 (± 34.1)*	44.5 (± 30.9)*
BASFI score (physical function)							
< 2.5 (low)	35.9 (± 13.5)	2.2 (± 4.4)*	1.8 (± 3.3)	3.6 (± 2.9)***	4.8 (± 8.5)*	21.3 (± 26.2)**	24.8 (± 26.3)**
≥ 2.5 (high)	38.2 (± 15.3)	10.8 (± 13.8)*	0.7 (± 2.0)	6.9 (± 2.6)***	19.6 (± 21.8)*	52.5 (± 36.2)**	62.5 (± 24.7)**

axSpA axial spondyloarthritis, *ASDAS* Ankylosing Spondylitis Disease Activity Score, *BASDAI* Bath Ankylosing Spondylitis Disease Activity Index, *BASFI* Bath Ankylosing Spondylitis Functional Index; $*p < 0.05$; $**p < 0.01$; $***p < 0.001$

with low BASFI scores (<2.5) compared to patients with high BASFI scores (≥2.5).

Table 3 shows that the associations between work productivity and disease activity and physical functioning were statistically significant on linear regression analyses. Results were adjusted for age, gender, HLA-B27 positivity, duration of CBP. There was no interaction between marital status or educational level and work productivity or BASDAI/ASDAS.

Table 3 Relationship between work productivity and disease activity and functional ability in patients with early axSpA

	R^2	ß-estimated	95 % CI
Absenteeism			
ASDAS	0.30	6.08	2.8–10.8
BASDAI	0.29	2.65	1.1–4.3
BASFI	0.51	4.32	2.9–5.8
Presenteeism			
ASDAS	0.28	16.04	7.1–25.0
BASDAI	0.25	5.80	2.2–9.4
BASFI	0.16	4.62	0.4–8.9
Work productivity loss			
ASDAS	0.36	18.86	10.8–27.0
BASDAI	0.34	7.12	3.9–10.4
BASFI	0.29	7.31	3.6–11.1

Data are adjusted for age, gender, human leucocyte antigen (HLA)-B27 positivity and duration of chronic back pain. *axSp*, axial spondyloarthritis, *ASDAS* Ankylosing Spondylitis disease activity score, *BASDAI* Bath Ankylosing Spondylitis Disease Activity Index, *BASFI* Bath Ankylosing Spondylitis Functional Index, *CI* confidence interval

Discussion

In this study we found work productivity impairment to be correlated to both disease activity and physical functioning in Italian patients with axSpA with CBP ≥3 months and ≤2 years, with onset < 45 years of age. In addition, absenteeism was very low compared to that in patients in other countries.

In our study, patients with axSpA with income-earning jobs worked 2.2 hours/week less than the general Italian population with income-earning jobs, who work 36 hours/week (as reported on http://dati.istat.it (June 2015)). We identified 7.9 % absenteeism in patients with paid work, which is similar to the sick leave in the general Italian population (8.4 %). However, the rate of sick leave in our patients with axSpA is much lower than reported in other studies. A Dutch study in patients with early SpA (with <5 years disease duration) reported a rate of 28 % for sick leave in the Amsterdam area [20], a rate almost 7 times higher than in the general population in Amsterdam and 3.5 times higher compared to our data. This difference may be due to the higher average age and the longer disease duration in these Dutch patients with respect to our patients. Moreover, 74 % of Dutch patients had a defined diagnosis of AS, while our patients had nr-axSpA in 92.2 % of cases.

Sick leave rates reported in the literature largely vary between several countries with 47 % in Belgium, 48 % in France and 52 % in the Netherlands, while the sick leave rate was reported as 28 % in Sweden and 16 % in the UK [9, 21, 22]. It has to be pointed out that the great majority of these studies were focused on patients with longstanding AS. In this severely affected patient group, the sick leave rate was expected to be higher due to the proven effect of AS on work productivity [23]. Like absenteeism, presenteeism seems to be lower in our patients compared to other studies. The few available data on presenteeism show rates of 41 % in patients with early SpA and 45 % in patients with AS of 10–18 years disease duration, while we identified a presenteeism rate of 32.6 % in patients with early axSpA [23]. This indicates that Italian patients with early axSpA have reduced work productivity, but the disease does not lead to more sick leave, compared to the general Italian population.

Several studies show correlation between WPL and increased disease activity and decreased physical functioning [9, 24]. In addition, Haglund et al. found BASDAI and BASFI not only to be correlated with presenteeism but also with activity impairment going beyond patients' paid work [25]. Although those studies focused on patients with longstanding AS, the results of our study were similar, supporting the idea that disease activity more than disease duration can impact on work ability and productivity.

This study was based on a small sample size. Even though the number of patients was relatively small the authors found the results to be of importance, as there are no available data on this matter in Italy. In the future, a longitudinal study could be conducted to more intensively investigate the course of disease activity and its relationship with work productivity. Another limitation of our study was the use of self-report questionnaires to determine disease activity, physical functioning and work productivity.

Self-report questionnaires tend to give a biased view, which can lead to either underestimation or overestimation of the findings. Nevertheless, the validity of these questionnaires was tested and considered good [17]. Therefore validated, standardized questionnaires are often used in these studies and are the preferred tool to assess disease outcome. The strength of our study was the absence of bias due to non-responders, as all 51 patients reported back.

Conclusions

In conclusion, our analyses showed that absenteeism and presenteeism rates were lower in Italian patients with axSpA with ≤2 years disease duration compared to the rates in other European countries. In addition, in these Italian patients with early axSpA, work productivity correlated with disease activity and physical functioning, as previously was found in in several European studies of patients with longstanding AS.

Abbreviations

AS: ankylosing spondylitis; ASDAS: Ankylosing Spondylitis Disease Activity Score; axSpA: axial spondyloarthritis; BASDAI: Bath Ankylosing Spondylitis Disease Activity Index; BASFI: Bath Ankylosing Spondylitis Functional Index; CBP: chronic back pain; CRP: C-reactive protein; HLA-B27: human leukocyte antigen-B27; LUMC: Leiden University Medical Centre; MRI: magnetic resonance imaging; nr-axSpA: non-radiographic axial spondyloarthritis; SpA: spondyloarthritis; SPACE: Spondyloarthritis Caught Early; WPAI: work productivity and activity impairment; WPL: work productivity loss

Acknowledgement

The authors wish to thank Linda Inverso Moretto, English mother language, for assisting in editing the English version of this manuscript.

Funding

The study was not supported by any specific grant.

Authors' contributions

MDH designed the study, analyzed and interpreted data, drafted the manuscript and revised it. RR designed the study, analyzed and interpreted data and revised the manuscript. ML participated in the acquisition of data, analyzed and interpreted data and revised the manuscript. PF and LP participated in the analysis and interpretation of data and critically revised the manuscript. AO participated in the acquisition of data, analyzed and interpreted data, helped draft the manuscript and revised it. AD gave substantial contribution to the interpretation of data and revised the manuscript. All of the authors gave final approval of this version.

Competing interests

The authors declare that they have no competing interests.

References

1. Rudwaleit M, van der Heijde D, Landewé R, Listing J, Akkoc N, Brandt J, et al. The development of Assessment of SpondyloArthritis international Society classification criteria for axial spondyloarthritis (part II): validation and final selection. Ann Rheum Dis. 2009;68:777–83.

2. Dagfinrud H, Kjeken I, Mowinckel P, Hagen KB, Kvien TK. Impact of functional impairment in ankylosing spondylitis: impairment, activity limitation, and participation restrictions. J Rheumatol. 2005;32:516–23.
3. Singh JA, Strand V. Spondyloarthritis is associated with poor function and physical health-related quality of life. J Rheumatol. 2009;36:1012–20.
4. Van Echteld I, Cieza A, Boonen A, Stucki G, Zochling J, Braun J, et al. Identification of the most common problems by patients with ankylosing spondylitis using the international classification of functioning, disability and health. J Rheumatol. 2006;33:2475–83.
5. Sieper J, Rudwaleit M, Khan MA, Braun J. Concepts and epidemiology of spondyloarthritis. Best Pract Res Clin Rheumatol. 2006;20:401–17.
6. Boonen A, Brinkhuizen T, Landewé R, van der Heijde D, Severens JL. Impact of ankylosing spondylitis on sick leave, presenteeism and unpaid productivity, and estimation of the societal cost. Ann Rheum Dis. 2010;69:1123–8.
7. Strömbeck B, Jacobsson LTH, Bremander A, Englund M, Heide A, Turkiewicz A, et al. Patients with ankylosing spondylitis have increased sick leave–a registry-based case-control study over 7 yrs. Rheumatology (Oxford). 2009;48:289–92.
8. Forejtová Š, Mann H, Štolfa J, Vedral K, Fenclová I, Némethová D, et al. Factors influencing health status and disability of patients with ankylosing spondylitis in the Czech Republic. Clin Rheumatol. 2008;27:1005–13.
9. Boonen A, van der Heijde D, Landewé R, Spoorenberg A, Schouten H, Rutten-van Mölken M, et al. Work status and productivity costs due to ankylosing spondylitis: comparison of three European countries. Ann Rheum Dis. 2002;61:429–37.
10. De Angelis R, Salaffi F, Grassi W. Prevalence of spondyloarthropathies in an Italian population sample: a regional community-based study. Scand J Rheumatol. 2007;36:14–21.
11. Strand V, Rao SA, Shillington AC, Cifaldi MA, McGuire M, Ruderman EM. Prevalence of axial spondyloarthritis in United States rheumatology practices: assessment of Spondyloarthritis International Society criteria versus rheumatology expert clinical diagnosis. Arthritis Care Res (Hoboken). 2013;65(8):1299–306.
12. Ramonda R, Marchesoni A, Carletto A, Bianchi G, Cutolo M, Ferraccioli G, ATLANTIS study group, et al. Patient-reported impact of spondyloarthritis on work disability and working life: the ATLANTIS survey. Arthritis Res Ther. 2016;18:78.
13. Van den Berg R, de Hooge M, van Gaalen F, Reijnierse M, Huizinga T, van der Heijde D. Percentage of patients with spondyloarthritis in patients referred because of chronic back pain and performance of classification criteria: Experience from the spondyloarthritis caught early (SPACE) cohort. Rheumatology (Oxford). 2013;52:1492–9.
14. Reilly MC, Gooch KL, Wong RL, Kupper H, van der Heijde D. Validity, reliability and responsiveness of the Work Productivity and Activity Impairment Questionnaire in ankylosing spondylitis. Rheumatology (Oxford). 2010;49:812–9.
15. Martindale J, Shukla R, Goodacre J. The impact of ankylosing spondylitis/axial spondyloarthritis on work productivity. Best Pract Res Clin Rheumatol. 2015;29:512–23.
16. WPAI. Calculation work productivity loss. Available from: http://www.reillyassociates.net/WPAI_Scoring.html. Accessed 7 Sept 2015.
17. Zochling J. Measures of symptoms and disease status in ankylosing spondylitis: Ankylosing Spondylitis Disease Activity Score (ASDAS), Ankylosing Spondylitis Quality of Life Scale (ASQoL), Bath Ankylosing Spondylitis Disease Activity Index (BASDAI), Bath Ankylosing Sp. Arthritis Care Res (Hoboken). 2011;63(Suppl):S47–58.
18. Machado P, Landewé R, Lie E, Kvien TK, Braun J, Baker D, et al. Ankylosing Spondylitis Disease Activity Score (ASDAS): defining cut-off values for disease activity states and improvement scores. Ann Rheum Dis. 2011;70:47–53.
19. Lorenzin M, Ortolan A, Frallonardo P, Vio S, Lacognata C, Oliviero F, et al. Spine and sacroiliac joints on magnetic resonance imaging in patients with early axial spondyloarthritis: prevalence of lesions and association with clinical and disease activity indices from the Italian group of the SPACE study. Reumatismo. 2016;68:72–82.
20. Van der Weijden MA, Boonen A, van der Horst-Bruinsma IE. Problems in work participation and resource use should not be underestimated in patients with early spondyloarthritis. J Rheumatol. 2014;41:2413–20.
21. Haglund E, Bremander A, Bergman S, Jacobsson LT, Petersson IF. Work productivity in a population-based cohort of patients with spondyloarthritis. Rheumatology (Oxford). 2013;52:1708–14.
22. Healey EL, Haywood KL, Jordan KP, Garratt A, Packham JC. Impact of ankylosing spondylitis on work in patients across the UK. Scand J Rheumatol. 2011;40:34–40.
23. Boonen A, Chorus A, Miedema H, van der Heijde D, Landewé R, Schouten H, et al. Withdrawal from labour force due to work disability in patients with ankylosing spondylitis. Ann Rheum Dis. 2001;60:1033–9.
24. Ward MM, Kuzis S. Risk factors for work disability in patients with ankylosing spondylitis. J Rheumatol. 2001;28:315–21.
25. Haglund E, Petersson IF, Bremander A, Bergman S. Predictors of Presenteeism and Activity Impairment Outside Work in Patients with Spondyloarthritis. J Occup Rehabil. 2015;25:288–95.

4

A longitudinal study of fecal calprotectin and the development of inflammatory bowel disease in ankylosing spondylitis

Eva Klingberg[1*], Hans Strid[2,3], Arne Ståhl[4], Anna Deminger[1], Hans Carlsten[1], Lena Öhman[4,5] and Helena Forsblad-d'Elia[1,6]

Abstract

Background: Patients with ankylosing spondylitis (AS) are at increased risk of developing inflammatory bowel disease (IBD). We aimed to determine the variation in fecal calprotectin in AS over 5 years in relation to disease activity and medication and also to study the incidence of and predictors for development of IBD.

Methods: Fecal calprotectin was assessed at baseline ($n = 204$) and at 5-year follow-up ($n = 164$). The patients answered questionnaires and underwent clinical evaluations. At baseline and at 5-year follow-up, ileocolonoscopy was performed in patients with fecal calprotectin ≥500 mg/kg and ≥200 mg/kg, respectively. The medical records were checked for diagnoses of IBD during the follow-up period.

Results: Fecal calprotectin >50 mg/kg was found in two-thirds of the patients at both study visits. In 80% of the patients, fecal calprotectin changed by <200 mg/kg between the two measuring points. Baseline fecal calprotectin was positively correlated with Ankylosing Spondylitis Disease Activity Score based on C-reactive protein, Bath Ankylosing Spondylitis Disease Activity Index, Bath Ankylosing Spondylitis Functional Index, C-reactive protein, erythrocyte sedimentation rate, and fecal calprotectin at 5-year follow-up. The use of nonsteroidal anti-inflammatory drugs (NSAIDs) was associated with higher fecal calprotectin, and 3-week cessation of NSAIDs resulted in a drop of a median 116 mg/kg in fecal calprotectin. The use of tumor necrosis factor (TNF) blockers was associated with lower fecal calprotectin at both visits, but the users of TNF receptor fusion proteins had significantly higher fecal calprotectin than users of anti-TNF antibodies at 5-year follow-up. The 5-year incidence of Crohn's disease (CD) was 1.5% and was predicted by high fecal calprotectin.

Conclusions: Fecal calprotectin was elevated in a majority of the patients and was associated with disease activity and medication at both visits. CD developed in 1.5% of the patients with AS, and a high fecal calprotectin was the main predictor thereof. The results support a link between inflammation in the gut and the musculoskeletal system in AS. We propose that fecal calprotectin may be a potential biomarker to identify patients with AS at risk of developing IBD.

Keywords: Ankylosing spondylitis, Spondylarthritis, Inflammatory bowel disease, Fecal calprotectin, Crohn's disease, Ulcerative colitis, Intestinal inflammation

* Correspondence: eva.klingberg@vgregion.se
[1]Department of Rheumatology and Inflammation Research, Sahlgrenska Academy at the University of Gothenburg, Guldhedsgatan 10A, S-413 46 Gothenburg, Sweden
Full list of author information is available at the end of the article

Background

Ankylosing spondylitis (AS), Crohn's disease (CD), and ulcerative colitis (UC) are inflammatory diseases that have many common features. Several risk genes are shared between the spondylarthritides and inflammatory bowel disease (IBD), and the diseases can show coinheritance [1–4]. Patients with IBD can develop peripheral arthritis (10–20%), sacroiliitis (10–20%), and anterior uveitis (0.5–3%) [5–9]. Studies have revealed the presence of endoscopic and histologic gut inflammation in 40–60% of patients with AS and in 46% of patients with early spondylarthritis (SpA) [10–13]. The subclinical gut inflammation in AS is often localized to the colon or the distal ileum. Histologically, the inflammation has been divided into an acute form and a chronic form, the latter resembling CD and conferring an increased risk for subsequent development of IBD [14–16]. Approximately 5–10% of patients with SpA eventually develop IBD, with CD being more common than UC [17, 18]. There is a lack of knowledge about what predicts the development of IBD in AS, however, and clinical studies on the subject are rare [19].

Fecal calprotectin is an unspecific marker for gut inflammation. Calprotectin belongs to the family of calcium-binding calgranulins (or S100 proteins) and consists of heterodimers of the two proteins S100A8 and S100A9. Calprotectin is an abundant protein in the neutrophils, constituting up to 40–60% of the cytosolic protein content, and it is also found in gut epithelial cells, monocytes, and macrophages. The level of calprotectin in feces is proportional to the level of neutrophil inflammation in the gut [20]. Fecal calprotectin is clinically used to discriminate IBD from irritable bowel syndrome and correlates well with clinical, endoscopic, and histologic measures of disease activity in IBD [21, 22]. Fecal calprotectin is also increased in enteropathy caused by nonsteroidal anti-inflammatory drugs (NSAIDs) [23].

We have previously investigated the levels of fecal calprotectin in a cohort of 204 patients with AS. We found that 68% of the patients had elevated levels (>50 mg/kg) and that fecal calprotectin was associated with higher disease activity but not with gastrointestinal symptoms [24]. The same patients were then invited to be reexamined at a 5-year follow-up examination.

The aims of this 5-year prospective study on AS were (1) to investigate the intraindividual variations in fecal calprotectin over time in relation to disease activity, disease manifestations, and medication; (2) to study the 5-year incidence of IBD; and (3) to identify predictors for the development of IBD.

Methods

Patients

All patients fulfilling the modified New York criteria for AS who were registered at the rheumatology clinics at Sahlgrenska University Hospital and the hospitals of Borås and Alingsås were invited to participate in the study in 2009, hereafter called *baseline* [24, 25]. Exclusion criteria were diagnosed IBD, psoriasis, dementia, pregnancy, and difficulties in understanding the Swedish language. Altogether, 204 patients were included at baseline and 164 (80%) patients were reexamined at the 5-year follow-up in 2014. All patients gave their written informed consent. The study was approved by the regional ethics committee in Gothenburg and was carried out in accordance with the Helsinki declaration. A flowchart of the enrollment of the patients and the study procedures is shown in Fig. 1. The patients underwent the same assessments at both visits, including physical examinations and responding to questionnaires. Blood and stool samples were collected. The medical records of all the included patients at baseline were checked for ileocolonoscopies, episodes of gut inflammation, or diagnoses of IBD.

Questionnaires

The Ankylosing Spondylitis Disease Activity Score based on C-reactive protein ($ASDAS_{CRP}$), Bath Ankylosing Spondylitis Disease Activity Index (BASDAI), Bath Ankylosing Spondylitis Patient Global Score, and Bath Ankylosing Spondylitis Functional Index (BASFI) were used to assess disease activity and physical function. Back mobility was measured for the calculation of Bath Ankylosing Spondylitis Metrology Index (BASMI) [26].

Stool samples

Stool samples were collected by the patients and sent to the laboratory, where the samples were immediately frozen. After thawing of the samples, fecal calprotectin was analyzed using an enzyme-linked immunosorbent assay (ELISA) kit (Bühlmann Laboratories AG, Schönenbuch, Switzerland). The same ELISA kit and procedures were used at baseline and at 5-year follow-up. In the general population, fecal calprotectin is <50 mg/kg, according to the manufacturer of the kit.

Blood samples

Blood samples were analyzed for hemoglobin, erythrocyte sedimentation rate (ESR), and C-reactive protein (CRP) using standard laboratory techniques. Serum calprotectin was analyzed at baseline by ELISA (PhiCal; Immundiagnostik AG, Bensheim, Germany) following the manufacturer's instructions. According to the manufacturer, the normal range for serum calprotectin is 500–3000 ng/ml.

Ileocolonoscopy

At baseline, all patients with fecal calprotectin ≥500 mg/kg were asked to send in a new stool sample. NSAID use was not stopped. If their fecal calprotectin remained ≥500 mg/kg, the patients were advised to undergo a clinical routine

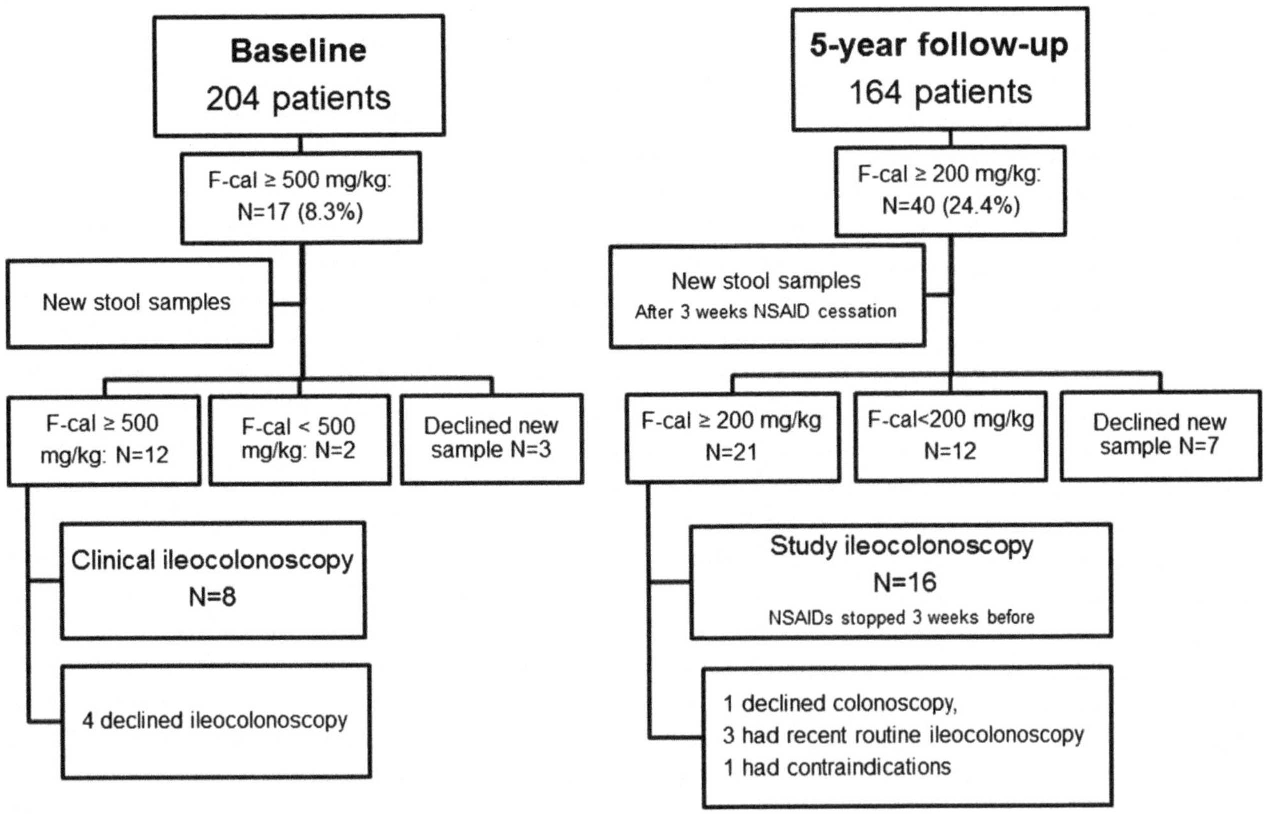

Fig. 1 Flowchart of the study procedures. Ileocolonoscopies were performed at different thresholds of fecal calprotectin at baseline and 5-year follow-up. *F-cal* Fecal calprotectin, *NSAID* Nonsteroidal anti-inflammatory drug

ileocolonoscopy (Fig. 1). At 5-year follow-up, all patients with fecal calprotectin ≥200 mg/kg were asked to send in another stool sample after pausing NSAID medication for 3 weeks. If their fecal calprotectin remained >200 mg/kg when retested, the patients were referred for ileocolonoscopy. Before the ileocolonoscopy, NSAIDs were again paused for 3 weeks. At 5-year follow-up, all ileocolonoscopies were performed by one endoscopist (HS) and followed the same procedure.

Data analyses

Data from all patients who participated at baseline (n = 204) were analyzed with the aim of determining the 5-year incidence of IBD and the predictors thereof. For all other data analyses, only the patients who participated both at baseline and at 5-year follow-up (n = 164) were included.

Statistical analyses

Statistical analyses were performed using IBM SPSS Statistics 23 software (IBM, Armonk, NY, USA). Descriptive statistics are presented as median and IQR. In comparisons between groups, the Mann-Whitney U test was used for continuous variables, and the chi-square test or Fisher's exact test was used for categorical variables. The Wilcoxon signed-rank test was used for repeated measurements. Correlations were calculated using Spearman's correlation (r_s). Owing to its skewed distribution, fecal calprotectin was log-transformed and used as an outcome in linear regression with a stepwise model. All tests were two-tailed, and $p \leq 0.05$ was considered statistically significant.

Results

Characteristics of the study population

In total, 164 patients, comprising 45% women and 55% men, completed the study and were examined at the two study visits (baseline and 5-year follow-up). The characteristics of the study population are provided in Table 1.

Intraindividual variation in fecal calprotectin between baseline and 5-year follow-up

Fecal calprotectin was elevated (>50 mg/kg) in 70.7% (116 of 164) of the patients at baseline and in 63.4% (104 of 164) of the patients at 5-year follow-up. The levels of fecal calprotectin did not differ between baseline and follow-up (p = 0.660) (Table 1).

The change in fecal calprotectin between baseline and the 5-year follow-up was ≤50 mg/ml in 48% of the patients, 51–100 mg/kg in 16%, and 101–200 mg/kg in 16%. The median change between baseline and 5-year follow-up for calprotectin was 1.5 (IQR −52.7 to 52.7) mg/kg. The intraindividual

Table 1 Characteristics of the 164 patients with ankylosing spondylitis at baseline and 5-year follow-up

	Baseline	5-Year follow-up	*p* Value
Sex, female/male	74 (45)/90 (55)		
Age, years	49.5 (41–62)	54.5 (46–67)	<0.001
Years since onset of AS symptoms	22 (13–34)	27 (18–39)	<0.001
Years since AS diagnosis	12 (5–23)	17 (10–28)	<0.001
HLA-B27-positive	141 (86)		
Fecal calprotectin, mg/kg	86 (45–222)	82 (35–190)	0.660
Fecal calprotectin level			
≤ 50 mg/kg	48 (29.3)	60 (36.6)	0.660
51–199 mg/kg	69 (42.1)	64 (39.0)	
200–499 mg/kg	32 (19.5)	29 (17.7)	
500–999 mg/kg	13 (7.9)	8 (4.9)	
>1000 mg/kg	2 (1.2)	3 (1.8)	
Serum calprotectin, ng/ml	645 (282–705)	No data	N/A
CRP, mg/L	2 (1–6)	3 (1–6)	0.434
ESR, mm/h	11 (7–18)	8 (4–14)	<0.001
$ASDAS_{CRP}$ score	2.2 (1.6–3.0)	2.1 (1.3–2.7)	<0.001
BASDAI score	3.1 (1.6–5.2)	3.2 (1.8–5.2)	0.713
BAS-G score	2.7 (1.2–5.7)	2.8 (1.4–5.9)	0.187
BASFI score	2.3 (1.0–3.8)	2.3 (1.0-4.1)	0.443
BASMI score	2.8 (2.0–4.0)	3.4 (2.4–4.6)	<0.001
Current smoker	15 (9.1)	11(6.7)	0.388
NSAIDs	128 (78)	125 (76)	0.868
Daily use	73 (45)	66 (40)	
As needed	55 (34)	59 (36)	
TNF blockers	33 (20)	39 (24)	0.238
Infliximab	24 (15)	21 (13)	0.664
Adalimumab	4 (2)	8 (5)	0.289
Golimumab	0 (0)	4 (2)	N/A
Etanercept	5 (3)	6 (4)	1.000
DMARDs			
Methotrexate	35 (21)	29 (18)	0.189
Sulfasalazine	16 (10)	8 (5)	0.004
Regular occurrence of gastrointestinal symptoms			
Loose stools	70 (43)	66 (40)	0.401
Mucus in diarrhea	25 (15)	34 (21)	0.405
Blood in stools	22 (13)	21 (13)	1.000
Blood in diarrhea	8 (5)	9 (5)	1.000
Abdominal pain	24 (15)	33 (20)	0.210
Obstipation	54 (33)	41 (25)	0.008
Reflux symptoms	65 (40)	62 (38)	0.391
Epigastric pain	47 (29)	46 (28)	1.000

Abbreviations: AS Ankylosing spondylitis, *CRP* C-reactive protein, *DMARD* Disease-modifying antirheumatic drug, *ESR* Erythrocyte sedimentation rate, $ASDAS_{CRP}$ Ankylosing Spondylitis Disease Activity Score based on C-reactive protein, *BASDAI* Bath Ankylosing Spondylitis Disease Activity Index, *BAS-G* Bath Ankylosing Spondylitis Patient Global Score, *BASFI* Bath Ankylosing Spondylitis Functional Index, *BASMI* Bath Ankylosing Spondylitis Metrology Index, *NSAID* nonsteroidal anti--inflammatory drug, *TNF* tumor necrosis factor

Data are presented as median and [interquartile range] or number (%)

correlation coefficient for fecal calprotectin at baseline and follow-up was $r_S = 0.512$ ($p < 0.001$) (Fig. 2a).

Fecal calprotectin correlates with disease activity and physical function

At both visits, fecal calprotectin was positively and significantly correlated with parameters reflecting higher disease activity and poorer function at the same visit, such as CRP, ESR, $ASDAS_{CRP}$, BASDAI, BASFI, and BASMI. In addition, fecal calprotectin at baseline was positively associated with higher levels of CRP, ESR, $ASDAS_{CRP}$, and BASFI at 5-year follow-up (Table 2).

The patients who were smoking at baseline (9%) had, in comparison with nonsmokers, significantly higher fecal calprotectin at 5-year follow-up (median [IQR] 107 [43–402] vs. 85 [45–221] mg/kg, $p = 0.026$). Baseline serum calprotectin was also positively correlated with fecal calprotectin, both at baseline ($r_S = 0.252$, $p = 0.001$) and at 5-year follow-up ($r_S = 0.170$, $p = 0.030$).

Fecal calprotectin and medication

The medications used at baseline and 5-year follow-up are listed in Table 1. Fecal calprotectin was significantly higher in NSAID users than in nonusers at both study visits (baseline median [IQR] 105 [45–262] vs. 68 [44–93] mg/kg, $p = 0.032$; 5-year follow-up 93 [44–215] vs. 40 [23–120] mg/kg, $p = 0.011$) (Fig. 3a). The users of anti-tumor necrosis factor (anti-TNF) antibodies (infliximab, adalimumab, golimumab) had significantly lower fecal calprotectin than patients without TNF blocker therapy at both visits (baseline 43 [17–84] vs. 99 [54–256] mg/kg, $p = 0.004$; 5-year follow-up 48 [26–135] vs. 89 [40–210] mg/kg, $p = 0.022$), whereas no such difference was found between users of TNF receptor fusion proteins (etanercept) and nonusers of TNF blockers. At 5-year follow-up, the patients treated with TNF receptor fusion proteins had significantly higher fecal calprotectin than the patients treated with anti-TNF antibodies (200 [93–555] vs. 48 [26–135] mg/kg; $p = 0.016$) (Fig. 3b). Comedication with methotrexate and a TNF blocker was common. Methotrexate was mostly taken in low doses (5–15 mg weekly). At 5-year follow-up, the use of methotrexate among patients on anti-TNF antibodies was not significantly different from the use in patients taking etanercept (18 of 33 [54.5%] vs. 2 of 6 [33%]; $p = 0.407$ by Fisher's exact test).

Although the patients treated with TNF blockers had a significantly lower frequency of NSAID intake than the patients without TNF blockers, the significant differences in fecal calprotectin between users and nonusers of disease-modifying antirheumatic drugs and/or TNF blockers remained after adjustment for NSAID use. Linear regression analysis was performed with log-transformed fecal calprotectin at 5-year follow-up as an outcome measure, and the following baseline values were used as covariates: sex, age, serum calprotectin, fecal calprotectin, CRP, $ASDAS_{CRP}$, BASFI, smoking, and use of NSAIDs and anti-TNF antibodies/TNF receptor fusion proteins. Only fecal calprotectin at baseline ($\beta = 0.001$, SE $= 0.000$, 95% CI 0.0008–0.0015, $p < 0.001$) and smoking at

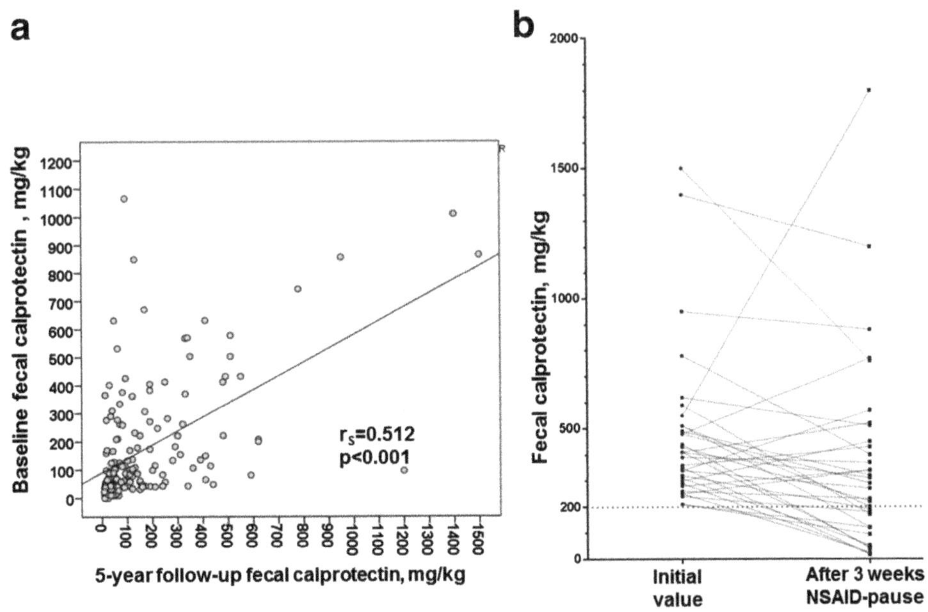

Fig. 2 **a** Scatterplot of fecal calprotectin at baseline and 5-year follow-up in 164 patients with ankylosing spondylitis (AS). **b** Fecal calprotectin before and after a 3-week pause of nonsteroidal anti-inflammatory drug (NSAID) use at 5-year follow-up in 33 patients with AS

Table 2 Spearman's correlations between fecal calprotectin and parameters reflecting disease activity and physical function at baseline and 5-year follow-up

	CRP		ESR		$ASDAS_{CRP}$		BASDAI		BASFI		BASMI	
	Baseline	5-year follow-up	Baseline	5-year follow-up	Baseline	5-year follow-up	Baseline	5-year follow-up	Baseline	5-year follow-up	Baseline	5-year follow-up
FC Baseline	0.280	0.209	0.222	0.169	0.260	0.240	0.190	N.S.	0.166	0.166	N.S.	N.S.
p-value	< 0.001	$p = 0.007$	$p = 0.004$	$p = 0.031$	$p = 0.001$	$p = 0.002$	$p = 0.016$		$p = 0.034$	$p = 0.034$		
FC 5-year	N.S.	0.219	N.S.	0.172	N.S.	0.207	N.S.	N.S.	N.S.	0.154	N.S.	0.207
p-value		$p = 0.005$		$p = 0.027$		$p = 0.008$				$p = 0.048$		$p = 0.008$

Abbreviations: CRP C-reactive protein, *ESR* Erythrocyte sedimentation rate, *$ASDAS_{CRP}$* Ankylosing Spondylitis Disease Activity Score based on C-reactive protein, *BASDAI* Bath Ankylosing Spondylitis Disease Activity Index, *BASFI* Bath Ankylosing Spondylitis Functional Index, *BASMI* Bath Ankylosing Spondylitis Metrology Index, *FC* fecal calprotectin

baseline (B = 0.241, SE = 0.121, 95% CI 0.002–0.479, $p = 0.048$) remained independently associated with higher fecal calprotectin at 5-year follow-up ($R^2 = 0.247$).

Gastrointestinal symptoms

A high frequency of gastrointestinal symptoms (diarrhea, presence of blood or mucus in stools, obstipation, abdominal pain, tenesmus, reflux symptoms, and epigastric pain) was reported by the participants both at baseline and at 5-year follow-up (Table 1). There were no significant associations between the levels of fecal calprotectin and gastrointestinal symptoms at any of the time points, however.

Fecal calprotectin before and after of 3-week NSAID pause

At 5-year follow-up, the patients who had fecal calprotectin ≥200 mg/kg ($n = 40$ [24%]) were asked to send in a new stool sample after pausing NSAID use for 3 weeks, which a total of 33 patients did. After the 3-week NSAID pause, fecal calprotectin dropped by 116 (−20 to 289) mg/kg from a range of 410 (295–510) mg/kg to 290 (120–480) mg/kg ($p = 0.005$) (Fig. 2b).

Development of gut inflammation during 5 years of follow-up

Ileocolonoscopies were performed in 8 patients at baseline and in 16 patients at 5-year follow-up (Fig. 1). The findings from the ileocolonoscopies are summarized in Table 3. Altogether, 10 (41.7%) of the 24 patients who underwent ileocolonoscopy had inflammatory changes in the gut biopsies. In addition, five patients (20.8%) had only macroscopic changes.

At 5-year follow-up, 3 patients (1.5%) were diagnosed with CD (corresponding to an annual incidence of 294 new cases per 100,000 person-years), and 1 patient (0.5%) was diagnosed with lymphocytic colitis. No cases of UC

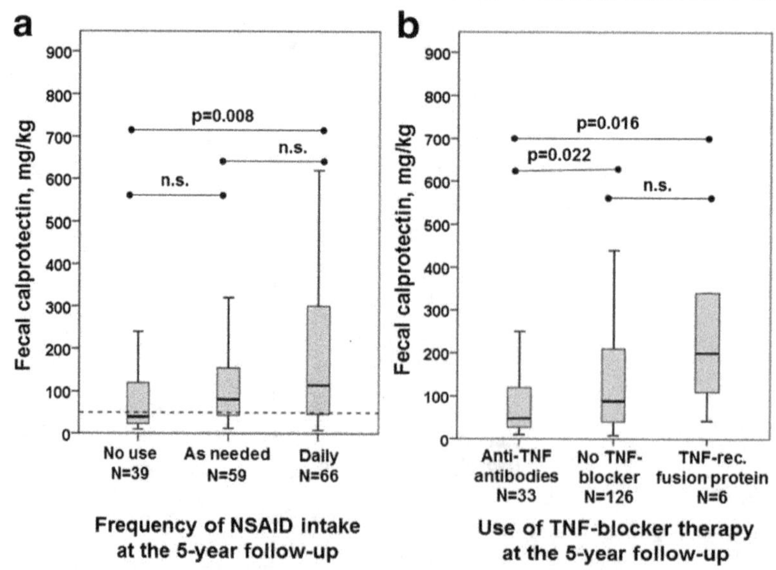

Fig. 3 **a** Box plot showing the association between fecal calprotectin and frequency of NSAID intake at 5-year follow-up. **b** Box plot showing the distribution of fecal calprotectin among patients on anti-TNF antibodies (infliximab, adalimumab, golimumab) vs. no TNF blocker therapy vs. TNF receptor fusion proteins (etanercept) at 5-year follow-up. Values are median (*horizontal lines*), IQR (*boxes*), and total range (*whiskers*). *NSAID* Nonsteroidal anti-inflammatory drug, *TNF* Tumor necrosis factor

Table 3 Development of gut inflammation in 204 patients with ankylosing spondylitis between baseline and 5-year follow-up

Type of inflammation	Baseline	5-Year follow-up	Total
Diagnosis of Crohn's disease	1	2	3
Diagnosis of ulcerative colitis	0	0	0
Diagnosis of lymphocytic colitis	1	0	1
Subclinical findings in the distal ileum			5
Macroscopic changes: aphthous ulcerations		1	
Microscopic changes: chronic inflammation		1	
Both macroscopic and microscopic changes	2	1	
Subclinical findings in the colon			6
Macroscopic changes: ulcerations	3	1	
Microscopic changes: chronic inflammation		1	
Both macroscopic and microscopic changes		1	
Total			15

were found. Additionally, five patients (2.5%) demonstrated characteristics of subclinical CD with aphthous ulcerations and/or chronic inflammation in the distal ileum, and another six patients (2.9%) had ulcerations and/or chronic inflammation in the colon. In total, 15 patients (7.4%) demonstrated characteristics of inflammation in the large or small intestine during the 5-year follow-up period.

Predictors for development of CD

At baseline, the patients who developed CD had, in comparison with the other patients, higher fecal calprotectin (570 [271–570] mg/kg vs. 85 [43–230]; $p = 0.014$) and more often reported having diarrhea containing mucus (3 of 3 vs. 30 of 201; $p = 0.004$). No significant associations were found between the development of CD and the other baseline parameters. A receiver operating characteristic (ROC) curve was created with baseline fecal calprotectin as the test variable and development of CD as the categorical state variable. The area under the curve was 0.913 (95% CI 0.805–1.000; $p = 0.014$). Using a threshold for baseline fecal calprotectin of 266 mg/kg, based on this ROC curve, the sensitivity for development of CD was 100% and the specificity was 78.7%.

Discussion

In this longitudinal 5-year study of a well-characterized cohort of patients with AS, we followed the intraindividual variation in fecal calprotectin in relation to disease activity and medication, and we determined the incidence and predictors for IBD. Fecal calprotectin was elevated (>50 mg/kg) in approximately two-thirds of the patients at both the baseline and 5-year follow-up visits. The intraindividual variation was moderate; in 80% of the patients, fecal calprotectin changed <200 mg/kg between the two measurement time points. Smoking and elevated fecal calprotectin at baseline were the strongest predictors for high fecal calprotectin at 5-year follow-up. Of the 204 patients included at baseline, 1.5% were diagnosed with CD and 0.5% with lymphocytic colitis at 5-year follow-up. High fecal calprotectin and presence of mucus in diarrhea at baseline were the main predictors of development of CD in this cohort.

Our results indicate that gut inflammation in AS is associated with higher disease activity in rheumatic disease. Increased fecal calprotectin at baseline was associated with higher $ASDAS_{CRP}$, BASDAI, BASFI, CRP, and ESR at 5-year follow-up. Early prospective studies showed a link between active gut inflammation and persistence of joint and spine inflammation as well as more chronic radiographic changes in the sacroiliac joint and spine [18, 27]. Researchers in two cross-sectional studies reported higher fecal calprotectin in AS than in healthy control subjects [28, 29]. One of the studies showed a positive correlation between fecal calprotectin and BASDAI, BASFI, ESR, and CRP [29]. In studies with the Belgian Inflammatory Arthritis and spoNdylitis cohorT (GIANT) of early SpA, the presence of histological gut inflammation was associated with higher BASDAI and higher BASMI and was also linked to a greater degree of bone marrow edema in the sacroiliac joints visualized by magnetic resonance imaging [13, 30]. The longitudinal results of our study support they hypothesis that inflammation in the gut and the musculoskeletal system may be linked. If gut inflammation is the cause or the consequence of locomotor disease is unknown, however, and fecal calprotectin is only a surrogate measure for gut inflammation.

In a recent report based on the GIANT cohort, fecal calprotectin, serum calprotectin, and CRP were also significantly higher in patients with microscopic gut inflammation [31]. We found that serum calprotectin at baseline was positively correlated with fecal calprotectin, both at baseline and at 5-year follow-up, but serum calprotectin was not a significant predictor for the development of CD.

In the present study, the use of anti-TNF antibodies was associated with lower fecal calprotectin, whereas use of TNF receptor fusion proteins was associated with higher levels of fecal calprotectin, at 5-year follow-up. Infliximab and adalimumab, but not etanercept, are efficacious in the treatment of CD and UC [32]. Similarly, in earlier studies, more flares and onset of IBD were observed in patients with AS treated with etanercept than in patients treated with infliximab [33, 34].

The 5-year incidence of CD in the present study was 1.5%, which corresponds to an annual incidence of 294 new cases per 100,000 person-years. This can be compared with the highest reported annual incidence of CD in the general population of 12.7 per 100,000 person years in Europe and 20.2 per 100,000 person-years in North America [35]. Mielants et al. reported an incidence of IBD of 5% in a cohort of 217 patients with SpA or AS during a median follow-up of 5.5 years [19]. Similarly to our study, CD was more common than UC in their study. In contrast to our study, ileocolonoscopy was performed on all patients at inclusion, and 49 patients underwent a second endoscopy. Because patients with fecal calprotectin <200 mg/kg were not examined with endoscopy in our study, cases with IBD despite lower fecal calprotectin may have been missed. Moreover, the earlier studies were performed in the "prebiologic era," which may have affected the results. Furthermore, a few patients with persistently elevated fecal calprotectin declined ileocolonoscopy.

In our study, elevated fecal calprotectin and presence of mucus in diarrhea at baseline were the only significant predictors of the development of CD. The low number of new cases of CD ($n = 3$) may have affected the robustness of the results and the possibility of finding other significant predictors.

The high use of NSAIDs among patients with AS is a problem when studying gut inflammation. NSAID-induced enteropathy is difficult to distinguish from AS-associated gut inflammation and is associated with increased fecal calprotectin [23]. In the present study, NSAID use was stopped for 3 weeks before retesting fecal calprotectin and before ileocolonoscopies, which resulted in a drop of a median of 116 mg/kg in fecal calprotectin. We found that 3-week cessation of NSAID use before testing fecal calprotectin was a reasonable course of action and acceptable for most patients.

The strengths of the present study are its prospective design with two measurement time points, the relatively large and well-characterized cohort, and cessation of NSAIDs before ileocolonoscopy at follow-up. The study's weaknesses are that ileocolonoscopy was not performed in all patients, which may have resulted in a lower incidence of IBD. The ileocolonoscopies were also performed at different thresholds of fecal calprotectin at baseline and 5-year follow-up (Fig. 1).

Conclusions

Fecal calprotectin was elevated in two-thirds of the patients with AS and was positively associated with parameters reflecting higher disease activity and poorer physical function at both study visits. Use of NSAIDs and TNF receptor fusions proteins was associated with higher levels of fecal calprotectin, whereas use of anti-TNF antibodies was associated with lower levels of fecal calprotectin. Further studies are needed to prove whether anti-TNF treatment has an effect on subclinical gut inflammation in AS and whether it can prevent the development of IBD. The 5-year incidence of CD was 1.5%, and elevated fecal calprotectin at baseline was the strongest predictor of the development of IBD. On the basis of these results, we propose that fecal calprotectin may be a potential biomarker to identify patients with AS at risk of developing IBD. Thus, fecal calprotectin quantification should be considered, especially in patients with high disease activity and gastrointestinal symptoms. If possible, NSAIDs should be stopped temporarily before measuring fecal calprotectin to reduce the confounding effect of NSAID enteropathy on the measurement.

Abbreviations

AS: Ankylosing spondylitis; ASDAS: Ankylosing Spondylitis Disease Activity Score; $ASDAS_{CRP}$: Ankylosing Spondylitis Disease Activity Score based on C-reactive protein; BASDAI: Bath Ankylosing Spondylitis Disease Activity Index; BASFI: Bath Ankylosing Spondylitis Functional Index; BAS-G: Bath Ankylosing Spondylitis Patient Global Score; BASMI: Bath Ankylosing Spondylitis Metrology Index; CD: Crohn's disease; CRP: C-reactive protein; DMARD: Disease-modifying antirheumatic drug; ELISA: Enzyme-linked immunosorbent assay; ESR: Erythrocyte sedimentation rate; GIANT: Belgian Inflammatory Arthritis and spoNdylitis cohorT; IBD: Inflammatory bowel disease; NSAID: Nonsteroidal anti-inflammatory drug; ROC: Receiver operator characteristic; SpA: Spondylarthritis; TNF: Tumor necrosis factor; UC: Ulcerative colitis

Acknowledgements

We thank all the patients who participated in the study.

Funding

This work was supported by grants from the Health and Medical Care Executive Board of the Västra Götaland, Rune and Ulla Amlövs Foundation for Rheumatology Research, Göteborg Association against Rheumatism, the Swedish Association Against Rheumatism, the Medical Society of Göteborg, and the Region Västra Götaland (agreement concerning research and education of doctors), Controlling Chronic Inflammatory Diseases with Combined Efforts (COMBINE), the Margareta Rheuma Research Foundation, and the Swedish Society of Medicine.

Authors' contributions

EK participated in the design of the study, examined the patients, collected data, performed statistical analyses, and drafted the manuscript. HS participated in the design of the study, performed the ileocolonoscopies, and participated in the collection and interpretation of data. AS was responsible for the fecal analyses and interpretation of data. AD participated in the design of the study, examined the patients, and collected data. HC participated in the design of the study and the interpretation of data. LÖ participated in the design of the study and the collection and interpretation of data. HFd'E supervised the study and was responsible for study design and interpretation of data. All authors critically reviewed the manuscript, approved the final version to be published, and agreed to be accountable for all aspects of the work.

Competing interests

The authors declare that they have no financial or nonfinancial competing interests.

Author details
[1]Department of Rheumatology and Inflammation Research, Sahlgrenska Academy at the University of Gothenburg, Guldhedsgatan 10A, S-413 46 Gothenburg, Sweden. [2]Department of Internal Medicine, Södra Älvsborgs Sjukhus, Borås, Sweden. [3]Department of Internal Medicine and Clinical Nutrition, Sahlgrenska Academy at the University of Gothenburg, Gothenburg, Sweden. [4]Department of Microbiology and Immunology, Sahlgrenska Academy at the University of Gothenburg, Gothenburg, Sweden. [5]Sweden School of Health and Education, University of Skövde, Skövde, Sweden. [6]Rheumatology Unit, Department of Public Health and Clinical Medicine, Umeå University, Umeå, Sweden.

References

1. Reveille JD. Genetics of spondyloarthritis—beyond the MHC. Nat Rev Rheumatol. 2012;8(5):296–304.
2. Jacques P, Van Praet L, Carron P, Van den Bosch F, Elewaut D. Pathophysiology and role of the gastrointestinal system in spondyloarthritides. Rheum Dis Clin North Am. 2012;38(3):569–82.
3. Thjodleifsson B, Geirsson AJ, Bjornsson S, Bjarnason I. A common genetic background for inflammatory bowel disease and ankylosing spondylitis: a genealogic study in Iceland. Arthritis Rheum. 2007;56(8):2633–9.
4. Bjarnason I, Helgason KO, Geirsson AJ, Sigthorsson G, Reynisdottir I, Gudbjartsson D, et al. Subclinical intestinal inflammation and sacroiliac changes in relatives of patients with ankylosing spondylitis. Gastroenterology. 2003;125(6):1598–605.
5. Orchard TR, Wordsworth BP, Jewell DP. Peripheral arthropathies in inflammatory bowel disease: their articular distribution and natural history. Gut. 1998;42(3):387–91.
6. Orchard TR, Holt H, Bradbury L, Hammersma J, McNally E, Jewell DP, et al. The prevalence, clinical features and association of HLA-B27 in sacroiliitis associated with established Crohn's disease. Aliment Pharmacol Ther. 2009;29(2):193–7.
7. de Vlam K, Mielants H, Cuvelier C, De Keyser F, Veys EM, De Vos M. Spondyloarthropathy is underestimated in inflammatory bowel disease: prevalence and HLA association. J Rheumatol. 2000;27(12):2860–5.
8. Baeten D, De Keyser F, Mielants H, Veys EM. Ankylosing spondylitis and bowel disease. Best Pract Res. 2002;16(4):537–49.
9. Vavricka SR, Schoepfer A, Scharl M, Lakatos PL, Navarini A, Rogler G. Extraintestinal manifestations of inflammatory bowel disease. Inflamm Bowel Dis. 2015;21(8):1982–92.
10. Lee YH, Ji JD, Kim JS, Bak YT, Lee CH, Kim CH, et al. Ileocolonoscopic and histologic studies of Korean patients with ankylosing spondylitis. Scand J Rheumatol. 1997;26(6):473–6.
11. Mielants H, Veys EM, Cuvelier C, de Vos M. Ileocolonoscopic findings in seronegative spondylarthropathies. Br J Rheumatol. 1988;27 Suppl 2:95–105.
12. Leirisalo-Repo M, Turunen U, Stenman S, Helenius P, Seppala K. High frequency of silent inflammatory bowel disease in spondylarthropathy. Arthritis Rheum. 1994;37(1):23–31.
13. Van Praet L, Van den Bosch FE, Jacques P, Carron P, Jans L, Colman R, et al. Microscopic gut inflammation in axial spondyloarthritis: a multiparametric predictive model. Ann Rheum Dis. 2013;72(3):414–7.
14. Cuvelier C, Barbatis C, Mielants H, De Vos M, Roels H, Veys E. Histopathology of intestinal inflammation related to reactive arthritis. Gut. 1987;28(4):394–401.
15. Mielants H, Veys EM, Cuvelier C, De Vos M, Goemaere S, De Clercq L, et al. The evolution of spondyloarthropathies in relation to gut histology. II. Histological aspects. J Rheumatol. 1995;22(12):2273–8.
16. Van Praet L, Jacques P, Van den Bosch F, Elewaut D. The transition of acute to chronic bowel inflammation in spondyloarthritis. Nat Rev Rheumatol. 2012;8(5):288–95.
17. Stolwijk C, van Tubergen A, Castillo-Ortiz JD, Boonen A. Prevalence of extra-articular manifestations in patients with ankylosing spondylitis: a systematic review and meta-analysis. Ann Rheum Dis. 2015;74(1):65–73.
18. De Vos M, Mielants H, Cuvelier C, Elewaut A, Veys E. Long-term evolution of gut inflammation in patients with spondyloarthropathy. Gastroenterology. 1996;110(6):1696–703.
19. Mielants H, Veys EM, De Vos M, Cuvelier C, Goemaere S, De Clercq L, et al. The evolution of spondyloarthropathies in relation to gut histology. I. Clinical aspects. J Rheumatol. 1995;22(12):2266–72.
20. Tibble J, Teahon K, Thjodleifsson B, Roseth A, Sigthorsson G, Bridger S, et al. A simple method for assessing intestinal inflammation in Crohn's disease. Gut. 2000;47(4):506–13.
21. Foell D, Wittkowski H, Roth J. Monitoring disease activity by stool analyses: from occult blood to molecular markers of intestinal inflammation and damage. Gut. 2009;58(6):859–68.
22. Gisbert JP, McNicholl AG. Questions and answers on the role of faecal calprotectin as a biological marker in inflammatory bowel disease. Dig Liver Dis. 2009;41(1):56–66.
23. Higuchi K, Umegaki E, Watanabe T, Yoda Y, Morita E, Murano M, et al. Present status and strategy of NSAIDs-induced small bowel injury. J Gastroenterol. 2009;44(9):879–88.
24. Klingberg E, Carlsten H, Hilme E, Hedberg M, Forsblad-d'Elia H. Calprotectin in ankylosing spondylitis – frequently elevated in feces, but normal in serum. Scand J Gastroenterol. 2012;47(4):435–44.
25. van der Linden S, Valkenburg HA, Cats A. Evaluation of diagnostic criteria for ankylosing spondylitis: a proposal for modification of the New York criteria. Arthritis Rheum. 1984;27(4):361–8.
26. Sieper J, Rudwaleit M, Baraliakos X, Brandt J, Braun J, Burgos-Vargas R, et al. The Assessment of SpondyloArthritis international Society (ASAS) handbook: a guide to assess spondyloarthritis. Ann Rheum Dis. 2009;68 Suppl 2:ii1–44.
27. Mielants H, Veys EM, Cuvelier C, De Vos M, Goemaere S, De Clercq L, et al. The evolution of spondyloarthropathies in relation to gut histology. III. Relation between gut and joint. J Rheumatol. 1995;22(12):2279–84.
28. Matzkies FG, Targan SR, Berel D, Landers CJ, Reveille JD, McGovern DP, et al. Markers of intestinal inflammation in patients with ankylosing spondylitis: a pilot study. Arthritis Res Ther. 2012;14(6):R261.
29. Duran A, Kobak S, Sen N, Aktakka S, Atabay T, Orman M. Fecal calprotectin is associated with disease activity in patients with ankylosing spondylitis. Bosn J Basic Med Sci. 2016;16(1):71–4.
30. Van Praet L, Jans L, Carron P, Jacques P, Glorieus E, Colman R, et al. Degree of bone marrow oedema in sacroiliac joints of patients with axial spondyloarthritis is linked to gut inflammation and male sex: results from the GIANT cohort. Ann Rheum Dis. 2014;73(6):1186–9.
31. Cypers H, Varkas G, Beeckman S, Debusschere K, Vogl T, Roth J, et al. Elevated calprotectin levels reveal bowel inflammation in spondyloarthritis. Ann Rheum Dis. 2016;75(7):1357–62.
32. Sandborn WJ, Hanauer SB, Katz S, Safdi M, Wolf DG, Baerg RD, et al. Etanercept for active Crohn's disease: a randomized, double-blind, placebo-controlled trial. Gastroenterology. 2001;121(5):1088–94.
33. Braun J, Baraliakos X, Listing J, Davis J, van der Heijde D, Haibel H, et al. Differences in the incidence of flares or new onset of inflammatory bowel diseases in patients with ankylosing spondylitis exposed to therapy with anti-tumor necrosis factor alpha agents. Arthritis Rheum. 2007;57(4):639–47.
34. Toussirot E, Houvenagel E, Goeb V, Fouache D, Martin A, Le Dantec P, et al. Development of inflammatory bowel disease during anti-TNF-alpha therapy for inflammatory rheumatic disease: a nationwide series. Joint Bone Spine. 2012;79(5):457–63.
35. Ye Y, Pang Z, Chen W, Ju S, Zhou C. The epidemiology and risk factors of inflammatory bowel disease. Int J Clin Exp Med. 2015;8(12):22529–42.

5

Incorporating assessment of the cervical facet joints in the modified Stoke ankylosing spondylitis spine score is of additional value in the evaluation of spinal radiographic outcome in ankylosing spondylitis

Fiona Maas[1*], Suzanne Arends[1,2], Elisabeth Brouwer[1], Hendrika Bootsma[1], Reinhard Bos[2], Freke R. Wink[2] and Anneke Spoorenberg[1,2]

Abstract

Background: To aim was to investigate the additional value of incorporating the de Vlam cervical facet joint score in the modified ankylosing spondylitis (AS) spine score (mSASSS) for the evaluation of spinal radiographic outcome in AS.

Method: Baseline and 4-year radiographs from 98 consecutive patients from the Groningen Leeuwarden AS (GLAS) cohort, who had AS treated with TNF-α inhibitors, were scored by two readers; the vertebral bodies were assessed according to the mSASSS (0–72) and cervical facet joints (C2–C7) were assessed according to the method of de Vlam (0–15). The combined AS spine score (CASSS) was calculated as the sum of both total scores (range 0–87) and compared with the original mSASSS according to three aspects of the Outcome Measures in Rheumatology Clinical Trials (OMERACT) filter: feasibility, discrimination, and truth.

Results: Feasibility: the CASSS was calculated in 91% of the patients. No additional radiographs were necessary and the assessment took only a few extra minutes. Discrimination: both scoring methods had excellent inter-observer reliability (intra-class correlation coefficient (ICC) status scores >0.99, progression scores 0.92). Incorporating the cervical facet joints did not result in an increase in measurement error. The CASSS detected more patients with definite damage (61% vs. 57%) and definite progression (55% vs. 48%). Truth: higher CASSS scores at baseline and higher progression scores were seen in 41 (46%) and 22 (25%) patients, respectively. Cervical rotation correlated better with cervical CASSS than with cervical mSASSS (Spearman's rho = 0.68 vs. 0.59).

Conclusions: The CASSS is a relevant and easy modification of the mSASSS. It captures more patients with AS who have spinal radiographic damage and progression, which is of great additional value in the evaluation of radiographic outcome in this heterogeneous and overall slowly progressing disease.

Keywords: Ankylosing spondylitis, Spinal damage, Outcome measure, Radiography, OMERACT

* Correspondence: f.maas@umcg.nl
[1]Rheumatology and Clinical Immunology, University Medical Center Groningen, University of Groningen, P.O. Box 30.0019700 RB Groningen, The Netherlands
Full list of author information is available at the end of the article

Background

Evaluation of structural damage is essential for the diagnosis and monitoring of ankylosing spondylitis (AS). The primary locations of interest are the sacroiliac joints and the spine. Changes in the sacroiliac joints are especially important for diagnosis, whereas changes in the spine are more sensitive for monitoring disease outcome [1]. Many sites in the spine can be evaluated including the vertebral bodies, vertebral margins and ligaments, intervertebral spaces, and the facet joints [1].

Until now, the modified Stoke AS spine score (mSASSS) is found to be the best and most widely used scoring method to assess evidence of spinal damage on conventional radiographs in randomized controlled trials (RCTs) and cohort studies [2]. This scoring method includes the anterior elements of the cervical and lumbar spine. Despite good reliability of the scoring method, the mSASSS has only moderate sensitivity to change [3]. In our previous analysis in 210 patients with AS treated with TNF-α, the smallest detectable change (SDC) for 2-year progression rates was larger than the mean progression at the group level (2.3 vs. 1.6, respectively) [4]. SDC refers to the change in scores that can be detected without measurement error [5]. This indicates that the mean observed progression at the group level might be a result of measurement error instead of representing "real" progression. For progression over a time period ≥4 years, the SDC was smaller than the mean progression suggesting that at least 4 years of follow up is needed for sufficient discriminatory power of the mSASSS to detect changes.

The change in radiographic evidence of damage is an important subject of interest in monitoring the effects of treatment on spinal radiographic progression in clinical studies. However, this is hampered by the nature of AS, a slowly and very heterogeneously progressing disease [6, 7]. Therefore, researchers have attempted previously to improve the performance of the mSASSS by incorporating more spinal elements into the scoring method. Including anterior elements of the lower part of thoracic spine (T10–T12) in the mSASSS has resulted in higher status and progression scores and a larger proportion of patients identified with (new) syndesmophytes compared to the original mSASSS [8]. However, in a longitudinal study including 809 radiographs from 195 patients with AS, in most cases the three additional thoracic vertebrae were not visible on lateral radiographs of the lumbar spine (in 64% of the radiographs), which is an important limitation to feasibility [9].

Besides the anterior elements of the vertebral bodies as scored in the mSASSS, the facet joints or zygapophyseal joints are frequently affected in AS [10–12] The presence of facet joint damage is associated with longer disease duration, greater disease activity, and most importantly, with worse spinal mobility [10, 12]. Longitudinal studies on the course of spinal mobility showed that the majority of patients with AS develop moderate to severe impairment of spinal mobility. Patients with severe spinal restrictions had severe spinal deformity [13, 14]. Due to the anatomy of the facet joints, damage to these joints results in reduced cervical rotation [12]. Reduced cervical rotation hampers patients in all kinds of daily activities. Therefore, inclusion of the facet joints in a radiographic scoring method seems clinically relevant.

The presence and development of radiographic evidence of damage in the facet joints is not always concurrent with damage or radiographic progression of the anterior elements of the spine [10, 12]. In our recent study in 99 patients with AS treated with TNF-α inhibitors, we found that the majority of patients who developed new ankylosis of the cervical facet joints did not develop new syndesmophytes in the cervical spine [12]. These findings indicate that evaluation of the cervical facet joints in addition to the anterior elements of the spine could improve construct validity and possibly also the sensitivity of the mSASSS to change.

Radiographic damage of facet joints can be scored with the method of de Vlam et al. [10] In particular, the cervical facet joints are easy to score on lateral radiographs [10, 15], which is in contrast with scoring the lumbar facet joints. For this, three-quarter-oblique lumbar spine radiographs are needed. However, the reproducibility of oblique radiographic assessment might be limited [16]. Most important, the cervical facet joints can be scored more reliably than the lumbar facet joints [10].

The aim of the present study was to investigate the additional value of incorporating the de Vlam cervical facet joint score in the mSASSS for the evaluation of spinal radiographic outcome in AS. In order to investigate the applicability of a new scoring method, the Outcome Measures in Rheumatology Clinical Trials (OMERACT) filter has been proposed, which includes three aspects: feasibility, discrimination, and truth [17, 18]. The combined AS spine score (CASSS), a composite scoring method, was compared with the original mSASSS according to these three aspects of the OMERACT filter.

Methods

The present analysis was performed in 98 consecutive patients from the Groningen Leeuwarden AS (GLAS) cohort study, who had AS and for whom lateral-projection radiographs of the cervical and lumbar spine were available at baseline and after 4 years of follow up. All patients were treated with TNF-α inhibitors because of persistent high disease activity despite conventional treatment. As described previously, the GLAS cohort is a large ongoing, prospective, longitudinal, observational,

Dutch cohort study in which patients are followed according to a fixed protocol and treated according to the national and international guidelines [4, 12]. Patients were 18 years or older, and fulfilled the modified New York criteria for AS and the assessment of spondyloarthritis (ASAS) criteria for starting TNF-α blocking therapy [19].

The GLAS cohort was approved by the local ethics committees of the Medical Center Leeuwarden (MCL) and the University Medical Center Groningen (UMCG), and all patients gave written informed consent according to the Declaration of Helsinki.

Radiological assessments

Lateral radiographs of the cervical and lumbar spine were scored independently by two trained readers (FM and RC). The anterior corners of the vertebrae (lower C2 to upper T1) were scored according to the mSASSS (range 0–72): 0 = normal, 1 = erosion, sclerosis, and/or squaring, 2 = non-bridging syndesmophyte, and 3 = bridging syndesmophyte [2, 3]. In addition, the cervical facet joints (C2–C3 to C6–C7) were scored according to the method of de Vlam et al.: 0 = normal, 1 = joint space narrowing or erosion, 2 = partial blurring or ankylosis, and 3 = complete blurring or ankylosis (range 0–15) [10, 12]. Abnormalities related to degenerative changes, defined as a reduction in intervertebral disk space height and horizontal bone spurs (>45°) at the facet joints and/or vertebral bodies [20], were not taken into account and therefore not scored. All patient identifying information and the performance dates were removed from the radiographs in order to blind readers to patient characteristics and time sequence. Scoring radiographic progression with unknown time sequence was used to diminish reader bias, as all patients were treated with TNF-α inhibitors.

For both scoring methods, a total score was calculated based on the average of the total scores of both readers. A third reader (AS) independently reassessed the radiographs in case of discrepancy in the total scores above the 95% limits of agreement or when there was discrepancy in the presence of non-bridging or bridging syndesmophytes and the presence of partial or complete ankylosis of the facet joints. The score of the primary reader closest to the third reader was used.

A composite score of the mSASSS and the total facet joint score was calculated by summing the total scores of both scoring methods. This combination score was named the combined AS spine score (CASSS) and had a scoring range of 0–87. For the mSASSS, the presence or development of definite damage was defined as the presence or development of ≥1 non-bridging or bridging syndesmophyte. In the CASSS, the presence or development of definite damage was defined as the presence or development of (partial) ankylosis in ≥1 facet joints or the presence or development of ≥1 non-bridging or bridging syndesmophytes [12].

OMERACT filter

The OMERACT filter consists of three aspects in order to judge the applicability of measurement instruments: feasibility, discrimination, and truth [17, 18]. The CASSS was compared with the original mSASSS as the gold standard according to these three aspects of the OMERACT filter.

Feasibility

The feasibility aspect of the OMERACT filter focuses on the question: "Can the measure be applied easily, given constraints of time, money, and interpretability?" To answer this question, information was given about required radiographs, the time needed for scoring, and the ability to score and obtain total scores for both the mSASSS and CASSS.

Discrimination

The discrimination aspect of the OMERACT filter addresses the question: "Does the measure discriminate between situations of interest?" These situations can relate to states at one time point or change in states over time. The discrimination aspect captures reliability and sensitivity to change. Inter-observer reliability for the mSASSS and the CASSSS status and progression scores was analyzed using the ICC (two-way mixed effects model, single measures, absolute agreement). Bland and Altman plots were constructed and the SDCwas calculated as:

$$1.96 * SD_{\Delta(\text{Progression score})/(\sqrt{2}*\sqrt{k})}$$

in which k represents the number of readings) [4], to explore systemic error and measurement error. Cohen's kappa and the percentage of absolute agreement were used to explore the inter-observer reliability of measuring the presence or development of definite damage according to both scoring methods. ICCs and kappas of 0.00–0.20 were interpreted as poor, of 0.20–0.40 as fair, of 0.40–0.60 as moderate, of 0.60–0.80 as good, and of 0.80–1.00 as excellent [21].

For sensitivity to change, the mean and median mSASSS and CASSSS status and progression scores were reported and the standardized response mean (SRM: the average of the progression scores divided by SD of the progression scores) was calculated. An SRM <0.5 was interpreted as small, 0.5–0.8 as moderate, and >0.8 as large [22]. In addition, the percentage of patients with maximal scores at baseline (ceiling effect) (and thus, not able to be identified with progression according to the scoring methods), and the percentage of patients with progression >0, with progression ≥ the SDC, and with definite progression during 4 years of follow-up were reported.

Truth

The truth aspect of the OMERACT filter focuses on the questions: "Is the measure truthful, does it measure what is intended? Is the result unbiased and relevant?" Information about the relevance of scoring the cervical facet joints was investigated by examining the absolute differences in status and progression scores of the CASSS compared to the mSASSS using the Wilcoxon signed-rank test. The CASSS and mSASSS had a common element of construct validity because they both included the anterior elements of the spine. The construct validity of incorporating assessment of the cervical facet joints in the mSASSS was evaluated by comparing the damage and progression of damage in the cervical facet joints to the vertebral bodies scored in the mSASSS.

Correlation between the mSASSS and the total facet joint score was investigated using Spearman's correlation coefficient. In addition, the correlation between the mSASSS or the CASSS and spinal mobility measures (cervical rotation, occiput-to-wall distance, lateral spinal flexion, modified Schober test, and chest expansion), physical function (Bath AS functional index (BASFI)), and quality of life (AS quality of life (ASQoL) questionnaire) was investigated using Spearman's correlation coefficients. Correlation of 0.00–0.20 was interpreted as very weak, 0.20–0.40 as weak, 0.40–0.60 as moderate, 0.60–0.80 as strong and 0.80–1.00 as very strong [21]. Data on cervical rotation were only available at 4 years in the GLAS cohort. [12] Therefore, correlation between scores and this measurement was investigated at 4 years instead of at baseline.

Additional statistical analysis

Descriptive statistics were used; results were expressed as number of patients (%), mean ± SD or median (IQR) for categorical, normally distributed and non-normally distributed data, respectively. The chi-square or Fisher's exact test, independent samples *t* test, and Mann-Whitney *U* test were used as appropriate to compare groups. A *p* value ≤0.05 was considered statistically significant. Statistical analysis was performed using IBM SPSS Statistics 22 (SPSS, Chicago, IL, USA).

Results

Study population

The baseline characteristics of the 98 patients with AS for whom spinal radiographs were available are described in Table 1. Patients had high disease activity at baseline, which reduced rapidly after start of TNF-α blocking therapy and stabilized during follow up (mean Bath ankylosing spondylitis disease activity index (BASDAI) was 3.0 ± 2.1, mean ankylosing spondylitis disease activity score (ASDAS) 2.0 ± 0.9, and median C-reactive protein (CRP) 3 (IQR 2–7) at 4 years). Baseline characteristics such as male gender, age, symptom duration, and human leukocyte antigen (HLA)-B27 status were comparable to other AS cohorts.

Table 1 Baseline characteristics of the AS study population

	All patients n = 98	Patients with available CASSS n = 89
Male gender	74 (76)	66 (74)
Age (years)	41.8 ± 11.2	41.0 ± 11.1
Symptom duration (years)	16 (7–24)	16 (7–24)
Time since diagnosis (years)	7 (2–15)	7 (2–16)
HLA-B27+	82 (84)	74 (83)
BMI (kg/m^2)	26.1 ± 3.5	25.4 ± 3.0
Current smoker	30 (37)	28 (38)
Total smoking duration (years)	12 (0–25)	12 (0–24)
History of IBD	9 (9)	9 (10)
History of uveitis	27 (28)	25 (28)
History of psoriasis	11 (11)	11 (12)
Peripheral arthritis	21 (21)	18 (20)
NSAID use	79 (85)	72 (85)
DMARD use	23 (23)	23 (26)
BASDAI (0–10)	5.9 ± 1.6	5.8 ± 1.7
$ASDAS_{CRP}$	3.8 ± 0.8	3.8 ± 0.8
CRP (mg/L)	15 (7–25)	15 (7–25)
Occiput-to-wall distance (cm)	5.0 (0.0–11.1)	4.5 (0.0–10.0)
Lateral spinal flexion (cm)	7.9 (5.0–11.5)	8.1 (5.5–11.7)
Modified Schober test (cm)	3.0 (1.2–4.0)	4.5 (0.0–10.0)
Chest expansion (cm)	3.0 (2.0–4.0)	3.0 (2.0–4.0)
BASFI (0–10)	5.6 (3.7–7.1)	5.5 (3.6–7.1)
ASQoL (0–18)	10 (7–13)	9 (7–12)

Values are presented as number of patients (%), mean ± SD, or median (IQR). Total smoking duration: current and past smoking. Peripheral arthritis: presence of ≥1 swollen joints (range 0–44). *AS* ankylosing spondylitis, *CASSS* combined AS spine score, *HLA* human leukocyte antigen, *BMI* body mass index, *NSAID* non-steroidal anti-inflammatory drug, *DMARD* disease-modifying antirheumatic drug, *BASDAI* bath AS disease activity index, *ASDAS* AS disease activity score, *GDA* global disease activity, *CRP*, C-reactive protein, *BASFI* bath AS functional index, *ASQoL* AS quality of life questionnaire

Feasibility

CASSS was assessed on the same cervical radiographs as used for the mSASSS and the assessment took only a few extra minutes. Total scores for the mSASSS were calculable in 94 (96%) patients and total scores for CASSS were calculable in 89 (91%) patients; >3 vertebral edges and ≥1 facet joint were not visible in 2 patients, >3 vertebral edges were not visible in 2 patients, and ≥1 facet joint was not visible in 5 patients. Facet joints at the levels of lower C6 to upper T1 and/or C6–C7 were not visible in these patients.

For further comparison, we used 89 patients with AS for whom radiographic data were available for both the mSASSS and CASSS in all analyses. The baseline characteristics of these patients are shown in Table 1. The nine patients without CASSS data were significantly older, had higher body mass index (BMI), worse spinal mobility, and worse quality of life.

Discrimination

Reliability

Inter-observer reliability was excellent and was similar for the mSASSS and CASSS with ICCs >0.99 for status scores and 0.92 for progression scores. Bland and Altman plots revealed no systematic error in either scoring method (Fig. 1).

For mSASSS, Cohen's kappa was 0.86 for the presence of definite damage and 0.87 for the development of definite damage, with percentages of absolute agreement of 93% for both definite damage and definite progression. For CASSS, the reliability and absolute agreement was even better; Cohen's kappa was 0.98 for the presence of definite damage and 0.89 for the development of definite damage, with percentages of absolute agreement of 99% and 94%, respectively.

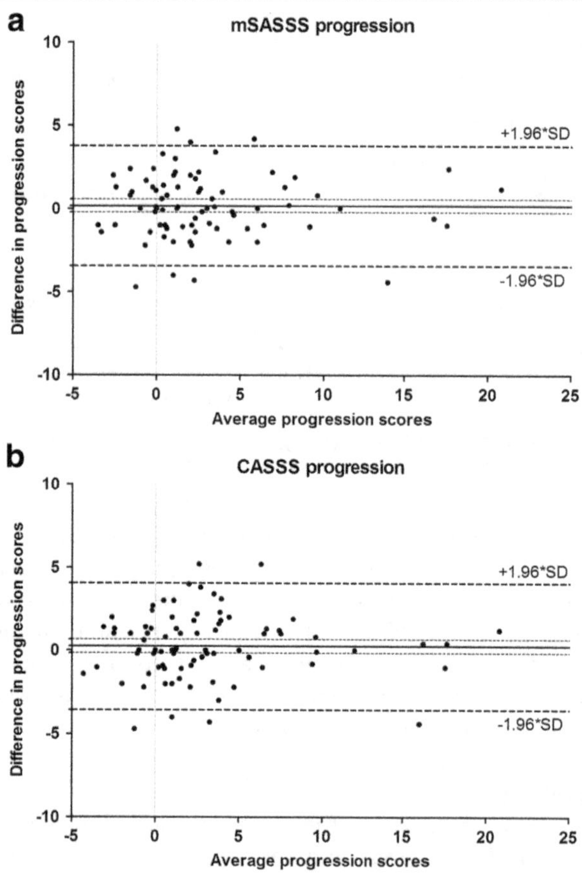

Fig. 1 Bland and Altman plots show differences between readers in progression scores in assessed using the modified Stoke ankylosing spondylitis spine score (*mSASSS*) (**a**) and the combined ankylosing spondylitis spine score (*CASSS*) (**b**), plotted against the average scores of both readers and the 95% limits of agreement (+/− 1.96*SD)

Sensitivity to change

At the group level, mean status scores at baseline were 19.3 ± 18.7 for the mSASSS and 21.8 ± 21.3 for the CASSS, showing large variation in radiographic damage according to both methods. Mean progression scores over 4 years of follow up were 2.7 ± 4.6 and 3.0 ± 4.8, respectively. The SDC using the mSASSS or the CASSS was smaller than the mean 4-year progression rate (Table 2). The SRM was 0.59 for the mSASSS and 0.63 for the CASSS (Table 2).

At the individual patient level, the CASSS resulted in more patients identified with definite damage at baseline (61% vs. 57%), fewer patients with the maximum score (1% vs. 3%), and more patients with definite progression during follow up (55% vs. 48%) (Table 2).

Truth

In comparison to the mSASSS, scoring radiographic damage using the CASSS resulted in 41 patients (46%) with higher baseline scores and 22 (25%) with higher progression scores (Fig. 2). Ten patients (11%) had lower progression scores as a result of scoring with unknown time sequence. Differences in scores were seen over the whole spectrum of the mSASSS, both in patients without damage and in patients with very advanced disease according to the mSASSS. No fan-out pattern was observed.

There was moderate correlation between the cervical facet joint score and the mSASSS (Spearman's rho = 0.49). There was weak correlation between change in score for the cervical facet joints over 4 years and change in the mSASSS (Spearman's rho = 0.16).

For radiographic damage assessed using either the mSASSS or the CASSS, there was strong correlation with the occiput-to-wall distance and with lateral spinal flexion; there was moderate correlation with the modified Schober test; and there was weak correlation with chest expansion and with the BASFI. There was no correlation between damage identified by either the mSASSS or the CASSS and the ASQoL (Table 3). Cervical rotation at 4 years was somewhat better correlated with the CASSS than with the mSASSS (Table 3).

Additional analysis using only the cervical mSASSS (range 0–36) and the cervical CASSS (range 0–51) showed that the cervical CASSS was more strongly

Table 2 Status and progression scores and proportion of patients with damage and progression according to the mSASSS and the composite CASSS

	mSASSS (range 0–72)	CASSS (range 0–87)
Status scores		
Observed range	0–72	0–87
Mean ± SD	19.3 ± 18.7	21.8 ± 21.3
Median (IQR)	11.3 (5.1–29.9)	13.5 (5.4–36.6)
Definite damage	51 (57)	54 (61)
Maximum score	3 (3)	1 (1)
Progression scores		
Observed range	−3.5–20.8	−4.3–20.8
Mean ± SD	2.7 ± 4.6	3.0 ± 4.8
Median (IQR)	1.2 (0.0–3.6)	1.6 (0.0–4.2)
SDC	1.8	1.9
SRM	0.59	0.63
Progression >0	64 (72)	64 (72)
Progression ≥ SDC	40 (45)	41 (46)
Definite progression	43 (48)	49 (55)

Values are presented as mean ± SD, median (IQR), or number of patients (%). *mSASSS* modified stoke ankylosing spondylitis spine score, *CASSS* combined ankylosing spondylitis spine score, *SDC* smallest detectable change, *SRM* standardized response mean

correlated with cervical rotation (Spearman's rho = 0.68) than the cervical mSASSS (Spearman's rho = 0.59).

Discussion

This is the first study investigating the additional value of cervical facet joints in the evaluation of spinal radiographic outcome in patients with AS, a slowly progressive disease in which both the anterior and posterior elements of the spine are affected [1, 7]. The composite scoring method CASSS, which combines the assessment of damage at the cervical facet joints (according to de Vlam) with the assessment of damage at the anterior corners of the cervical and lumbar vertebral bodies (the mSASSS), was compared with the original mSASSS using the three aspects of the OMERACT filter: feasibility, discrimination, and truth [17, 18].

The feasibility of the CASSS was very good; no extra radiographs were needed, it took only a few extra minutes to perform the CASSS, and the cervical facet joints were clearly visible in >90% of the patients. The lumbar facet joints were not included in the new scoring method because previous studies have shown that lumbar facet joints are more difficult to score than cervical facet joints. A study in 73 patients with psoriatic arthritis (PsA) showed that lumbar facet joints could be scored on lateral and anterior-posterior radiographs in 73–82% of the patients whereas cervical facet joints could be scored in 93–95% of the patients [15]. In the study of de Vlam et al., the

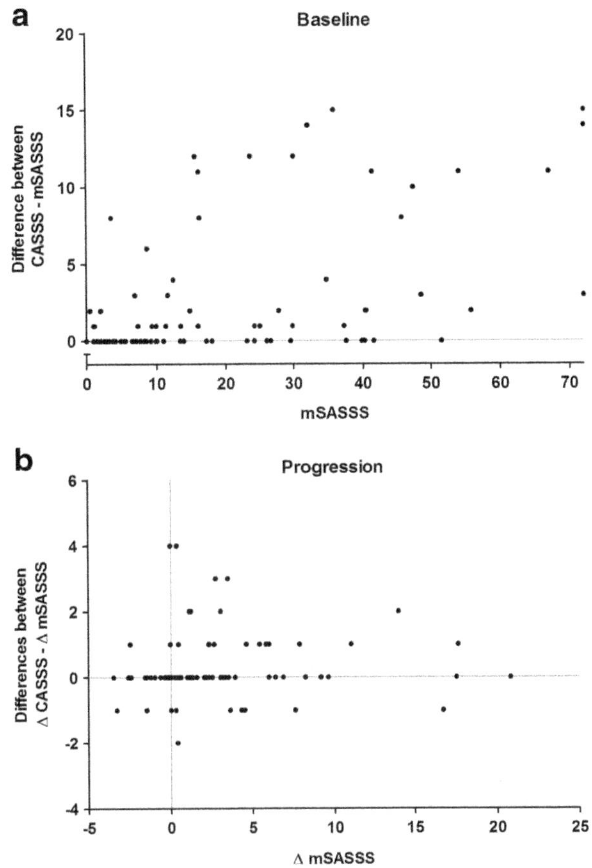

Fig. 2 Differences in status and progression scores when comparing the composite score (combined ankylosing spondylitis spine score (*CASSS*)) (range 0–87) with modified Stoke ankylosing spondylitis spine score (*mSASSS*) (range 0–72). *X-axis* mSASSS status scores at baseline (**a**) and progression scores during 4 years of follow-up (**b**). *Y-axis*: differences between mSASSS and CASSS status and progression scores

Table 3 Correlation between radiographic damage assessed using the mSASSS and CASSS and spinal mobility, physical function, and quality of life at baseline

	mSASSS	CASSS
Cervical rotation[a]	−0.56**	−0.63**
Occiput-to-wall distance	0.64**	0.67**
Lateral spinal flexion	−0.62**	−0.61**
Modified Schober test	−0.44**	−0.45**
Chest expansion	−0.33**	−0.35**
BASFI	0.24*	0.26*
ASQoL	0.03	−0.01

Correlation is expressed as Spearman's rho. [a]Analysis performed with 4 years of data. *mSASSS* modified stoke ankylosing spondylitis spine score, *CASSS* combined ankylosing spondylitis spine score, *BASFI* Bath ankylosing spondylitis functional index, *ASQoL* ankylosing spondylitis quality of life questionnaire. *Statistically significant correlation $p \leq 0.05$. **Statistically significant correlation $p \leq 0.01$

inter-observer and intra-observer reliability was only poor to moderate for scoring individual lumbar facet joints on oblique radiographs (weighted kappa for the stages ranged between 0.19 and 0.52), but there was moderate to good reliability for scoring individual cervical facet joints on lateral projection radiographs (weighted kappa ranged between 0.55 and 0.66) [10].

As spinal radiographic progression in AS is a slow and very heterogeneous process, a reliable scoring method is needed with low measurement error and good discriminatory properties to detect changes over time. In our study the inter-observer reliability was excellent for both the mSASSS and the CASSS, with comparable SDCs (1.8 and 1.9, respectively). This implies that, although it involves scoring additional sites, the CASSS could be used without an increase in measurement error. The SDCs were smaller than the mean mSASSS and CASSS progression rates over 4 years and therefore "real" changes could be assessed during 4 years of follow up using either scoring method.

The most important benefit of the CASSS over the mSASSS is that the CASSS had better discriminatory properties and better construct validity than the mSASSS. The composite scoring method detected more patients with definite damage at baseline (61% vs. 57%). Seven percent of the patients with evidence of definite progression during 4 years of follow up according to the CASSS did not have progression according to the mSASSS. In addition, almost half of all patients had higher status scores and 25% had higher progression scores according to the CASSS. Differences in scores were found over the whole spectrum of the mSASSS. This confirms that not only the vertebral bodies but also the facet joints are frequently involved in AS, even if no damage or progression is observed or when patients have very advanced disease according to the original mSASSS [10–12].

There was weak correlation between disease progression in the facet joints and progression in the vertebral bodies. This suggests that the damage does not develop in the facet joints synchronically with the most typical AS-related damage, i.e., the development of syndesmophytes. It has been thought that damage in the facet joints is not specific to AS as these joints are also affected by degenerative changes [23]. The most characteristic degenerative changes in the facet joints are osteophyte formation (more horizontally oriented, >45°), joint space narrowing, sclerosis, and joint irregularity [20]. In patients with degenerative disc disease who are candidates for lumbar spine surgery, facet joint osteoarthritis was not observed in the absence of disc degeneration [24]. It is thought that degenerative changes begin in the disc, followed by changes in the facet joints [20, 24]. Therefore, the whole structure at each vertebral level was evaluated in the present study in order to distinguish between AS-specific changes and degenerative changes.

In a USA population based study from 1970, cervical osteoarthritis (not specifically facet joint osteoarthritis) was very rare before the age of 45 years (prevalence <2%). The prevalence of cervical osteoarthritis was 19% in adults aged 45–64 years, and in adults aged 65 years or older it was 56–57% [25]. The hallmark radiographically demonstrated characteristic of AS is ankylosis of the vertebral column. In our study partial or complete facet joint ankylosis was already evident in 19% of the patients aged <45 years. In patients aged 45–64 years, 34% had partial or complete facet joint ankylosis and 33% of patients aged 65 years or older had ankylosis. Incident partial or complete ankylosis was evident within 4 years of follow up in 14% of our patients with AS; half of these patients were younger than 45 years. This shows that AS-related cervical facet joint involvement begins at a relatively young age in comparison to osteoarthritis.

In our previous analysis we demonstrated that facet joint damage is associated with longer symptom duration, higher disease activity (ASDAS and CRP), worse spinal mobility (occiput-to-wall distance), and presence of extra-articular manifestations (inflammatory bowel disease (IBD), uveitis, and psoriasis) [12]. These findings, in combination with the strong correlation between CASSS and cervical rotation, occiput-to-wall distance, and lateral spinal flexion, as found in the present study, highlight the fact that damage in the cervical facet joints is common in AS, and is also evident at a younger age. Incorporating cervical facet joint scores is therefore of clinical relevance and improves the construct validity of the assessment of spinal radiographic damage in AS.

Previously, researchers in the field of PsA also developed a composite scoring method, the psoriatic arthritis spondylitis radiology index (PASRI). This scoring method combines the mSASSS of at the level of lower T12 to upper S1 and lower C2 to upper C6, the cervical facet joints (presence or absence of ankylosis), and the sacroiliac joints (SI) score (modified New York criteria) [13]. Although intra-observer and inter-observer reliability are excellent for the PASRI (range 0–72) in AS [26], it is very difficult to reliably score status and progression of disease at the SI joints in AS [27]. Besides this, the most important advantage of the CASSS over the PASRI is that the original mSASSS remains intact and, therefore, it is possible to obtain separate data on the mSASSS and the cervical facet joints. In this way, the original mSASSS scores in new studies can easily be compared with scores from former studies using only the mSASSS.

Our study was the first to investigate radiographic evidence of progression of disease at the cervical facet joints in patients with AS who had active disease and had started treatment with TNF-α inhibitors. The results may not be generalizable to all patients with axial spondyloarthritis (SpA). As potent biologic agents such as TNF-α inhibitors are available for the treatment of active disease in AS, it is unethical to withhold this treatment long-term in patients with active disease. Therefore, it was not possible to compare radiographic evidence of progression at the cervical facet joints in patients with and without TNF-α inhibitors in order to evaluate the effect of treatment. Further validation of the CASSS is needed in patients with axial SpA at different stages of disease duration, disease activity, and treatment strategies, and in long-term follow up. Data on radiographic evidence of progression at the vertebral bodies (mSASSS) show that at >4 years of follow up at least are needed to show radiographic evidence of diminishing progression during treatment with TNF-α inhibitors in this disease of overall slow progression [4, 28].

The assessment was performed with unknown time sequence to diminish possible reader bias due to knowledge of the applied therapy. However, it caused some negative progression scores (in 11 patients according to the CASSS and in 19 patients according to the mSASSS). Excessive bone formation in AS is an irreversible process, and therefore, negative progression is a result of measurement error. Reading radiographs in chronological time order is more sensitive to detect changes but less appropriate with respect to reader bias when the applied treatment regimens are known [29]. Future studies should determine the discrimination and truth aspects of the CASSS scored in chronological time order when radiographs from patients receiving conventional and biological treatment are randomized.

Conclusions

The CASSS seems a promising scoring method to evaluate spinal radiographic outcome in AS. In our prospective observational cohort study we demonstrated that standardized scoring of the cervical facet joints in addition to the mSASSS is a feasible and reliable modification that provides better construct validity than the original mSASSS. Furthermore, the composite CASSS captures more patients with radiographic evidence of spinal disease progression, which is very valuable in this heterogeneous and overall slowly progressing disease.

Key messages

- Incorporation of the cervical facet joints in the mSASSS is feasible, reliable and relevant for the assessment of spinal radiographic outcome in AS
- The combined AS spine score (CASSS) captured more patients with AS with damage and progression and correlated better with cervical rotation than mSASSS
- The original mSASSS and the cervical facet joint score of de Vlam can easily be extracted from the CASSS

Abbreviations

AS: Ankylosing spondylitis; ASAS: Assessment of spondyloarthritis; ASDAS: Ankylosing spondylitis disease activity score; ASQoL: AS quality of life questionnaire; BASDAI: Bath ankylosing spondylitis disease activity index; BASFI: Bath ankylosing spondylitis functional index; BMI: Body mass index; C: Cervical; CASSS: combined ankylosing spondylitis spine score; CRP: C-reactive protein; DMARD: Disease-modifying antirheumatic drug; GDA: Global disease activity; GLAS: Groningen Leeuwarden ankylosing spondylitis; HLA: Human leukocyte antigen; ICC: Intra-class correlation coefficient; IQR: Interquartile range; L: lumbar; MCL: Medical Center Leeuwarden; mSASSS: modified Stoke ankylosing spondylitis spine score; NSAID: Non-steroidal anti-inflammatory drug; OMERACT: Outcome Measures in Rheumatology Clinical Trials; PsA: Psoriatic arthritis; RCT: Randomized controlled trial; SD: Standard deviation; SDC: Smallest detectable change; SI: sacroiliac; SpA: Spondyloarthritis; SRM: Standardized response mean; T: Thoracic; TNF-α: Tumor necrosis factor-alpha; UMCG: University Medical Center Groningen

Acknowledgements

The authors would like to thank all patients who participated in the GLAS cohort. Furthermore, the authors wish to acknowledge Mrs. R.N. Chaudhry for her contribution to radiographic data collection and scoring, Dr. P.M. Houtman, Mrs. W. Gerlofs, Mrs. S. Katerbarg, Mrs. A. Krol, Mrs. R. Rumph, and Mrs. B. Burmania for their contribution to clinical data collection.

Funding

The GLAS cohort was supported by an unrestricted grant from Pfizer pharmaceuticals. Pfizer had no role in the design, conduct, interpretation, or publication of this study.

Authors' contributions

FM had full access to all of the data in the study and takes responsibility for the integrity of the data and the accuracy of the data analysis. FM performed the reading of radiographs, the statistical analysis and interpretation of data, and drafted the manuscript. SA participated in the design of the study, contributed to the statistical analysis and interpretation of data, and critically revised the manuscript. EB participated in the design of the study, performed the acquisition of data, and critically revised the manuscript. HB participated in the design of the study and critically revised the manuscript. RB and FW contributed to the acquisition of clinical data and critically revised the manuscript. AS participated in the design of the study, performed the acquisition of data, contributed to the statistical analysis and interpretation of data, and critically revised the manuscript. All authors read and approved the final manuscript.

Competing interests

F. Maas: none declared; S. Arends: grant/research support from Pfizer; E. Brouwer: grant/research support from Pfizer; H. Bootsma: none declared; R. Bos: none declared; F.R. Wink: consultant for Abbvie; A. Spoorenberg: grant/research support from Abbvie, Pfizer, UCB and consultant for Abbvie, Pfizer, MSD, UCB, and Novartis.

Author details

[1]Rheumatology and Clinical Immunology, University Medical Center Groningen, University of Groningen, P.O. Box 30.0019700 RB Groningen, The Netherlands. [2]Rheumatology, Medical Center Leeuwarden, Leeuwarden, The Netherlands.

References

1. Braun J, Golder W, Bollow M, Sieper J, van der Heijde D. Imaging and scoring in ankylosing spondylitis. Clin Exp Rheumatol. 2002;20(6 Suppl 28): S178–84.
2. Wanders AJ, Landewé RB, Spoorenberg A, Dougados M, van der Linden S, Mielants H, van der Tempel H, van der Heijde DM. What is the most appropriate radiologic scoring method for ankylosing spondylitis? A comparison of the available methods based on the Outcome Measures in Rheumatology Clinical Trials filter. Arthritis Rheum. 2004;50(8):2622–32.
3. Spoorenberg A, de Vlam K, van der Linden S, Dougados M, Mielants H, van de Tempel H, van der Heijde D. Radiological scoring methods in ankylosing spondylitis. Reliability and change over 1 and 2 years. J Rheumatol. 2004; 31(1):125–32.
4. Maas F, Arends S, Brouwer E, Essers I, van der Veer E, Efde M, van Ooijen PM, Wolf R, Veeger NJGM, Bootsma H, Wink FR, Spoorenberg. Reduction in spinal radiographic progression in ankylosing spondylitis patients receiving prolonged treatment with TNF-α inhibitors. Arthritis Care Res (Hoboken). 2016. doi: 10.1002/acr.23097. [Epub ahead of print]
5. Bruynesteyn K, Boers M, Kostense P, van der Linden S, van der Heijde D. Deciding on progression of joint damage in paired films of individual patients: smallest detectable difference or change. Ann Rheum Dis. 2005; 64(2):179–82.
6. Baraliakos X, Listing J, von der Recke A, Braun J. The natural course of radiographic progression in ankylosing spondylitis–evidence for major individual variations in a large proportion of patients. J Rheumatol. 2009; 36(5):997–1002.
7. Ramiro S, Stolwijk C, van Tubergen A, van der Heijde D, Dougados M, van den Bosch F, Landewé R. Evolution of radiographic damage in ankylosing spondylitis: a 12 year prospective follow-up of the OASIS study. Ann Rheum Dis. 2015;74(1):52–9.
8. Baraliakos X, Listing J, Rudwaleit M, Sieper J, Braun J. Development of a radiographic scoring tool for ankylosing spondylitis only based on bone formation: addition of the thoracic spine improves sensitivity to change. Arthritis Rheum. 2009;61(6):764–71.
9. Ramiro S, van Tubergen A, Stolwijk C, Landewé R, van de Bosch F, Dougados M, van der Heijde D. Scoring radiographic progression in ankylosing spondylitis: should we use the modified Stoke Ankylosing Spondylitis Spine Score (mSASSS) or the Radiographic Ankylosing Spondylitis Spinal Score (RASSS)? Arthritis Res Ther. 2013;15(1):R14.
10. de Vlam K, Mielants H, Veys EM. Involvement of the zygapophyseal joint in ankylosing spondylitis: relation to the bridging syndesmophyte. J Rheumatol. 1999;26(8):1738–45.
11. Lee JY, Kim JI, Park JY, Choe JY, Kim CG, Chung SH, Lee DK, Chang HK. Cervical spine involvement in longstanding ankylosing spondylitis. Clin Exp Rheumatol. 2005;23(3):331–8.
12. Maas F, Spoorenberg A, Brouwer E, van der Veer E, Bootsma H, Bos R, Wink FR, Arends S. Radiographic damage and progression of the cervical spine in ankylosing spondylitis patients treated with TNF-α inhibitors: facet joints versus vertebral bodies. Semin Arthritis Rheum 2016. doi: 10.1016/j.semarthrit.2016.11.003. [Epub ahead of print]
13. Carette S, Graham D, Little H, Rubenstein J, Rosen P. The natural disease course of ankylosing spondylitis. Arthritis Rheum. 1983;26(2):186–90.
14. Ramiro S, Landewé RB, van der Heijde D, Stolwijk C, Dougados M, van den Bosch F, van Tubergen A. Hierarchy of impairment of spinal mobility measures in ankylosing spondylitis: twelve-year data. Arthritis Care Res (Hoboken). 2015;67(11):1571–7.
15. Lubrano E, Marchesoni A, Olivieri I, D'Angelo S, Spadaro A, Parsons WJ, Cauli A, Salvarani C, Mathieu A, Porter G, Helliwell PS. Psoriatic arthritis spondylitis radiology index: a modified index for radiologic assessment of axial involvement in psoriatic arthritis. J Rheumatol. 2009;36(5):1006–11.
16. Pathria M, Sartoris DJ, Resnick D. Osteoarthritis of the facet joints: accuracy of oblique radiographic assessment. Radiology. 1987;164(1):227–30.
17. Boers M, Brooks P, Strand CV, Tugwell P. The OMERACT filter for outcome measures in rheumatology. J Rheumatol. 1998;25(2):198–9.
18. Boers M, Kirwan JR, Tugwell P, Beaton D, Bingham III CO, Conaghan PG, D'Agostion MA, de Wit M, Gossec L, March L, Simon LS, Singh JA, Strand V, Wells G. The OMERACT handbook. Published by OMERACT. Available at: http://www.omeract.org/. Updated May 5, 2016.
19. Braun J, Davis J, Dougados M, Sieper J, van der Linden S, van der Heijde D, Working Group ASAS. First update of the international ASAS consensus statement for the use of anti-TNF agents in patients with ankylosing spondylitis. Ann Rheum Dis. 2006;65:316–20.
20. Gellhorn AC, Katz JN, Suri P. Osteoarthritis of the spine: the facet joints. Nat Rev Rheumatol. 2013;9:216–24.
21. Landis JR, Koch GG. The measurement of observer agreement for categorical data. Biometrics. 1977;33:159–74.
22. Husted JA, Gladman DD, Cook RJ, Farewell VT. Responsiveness of health status instruments to changes in articular status and perceived health in patients with psoriatic arthritis. J Rheumatol. 1998;25(11):2146–55.
23. Berven S, Tay BB, Colman W, Hu SS. The lumbar zygapophyseal (facet) joints: a role in the pathogenesis of spinal pain syndromes and degenerative spondylolisthesis. Semin Neurol. 2002;22:187–96.
24. Fujiwara A, Tamai K, Yamato M, An HS, Yoshida H, Saotome K, Kurihashi A. The relationship between facet joint osteoarthritis and disc degeneration of the lumbar spine: an MRI study. Eur Spine J. 1999;8(5):396–401.
25. Dodge HJ, Mikkelsen WM, Duff IF. Age-sex specific prevalence of radiographic abnormalities of the joints of the hands, wrists and cervical spine of adult residents of the Tecumseh, Michigan, Community Health Study area, 1962-1965. J Chronic Dis. 1970;23(3):151–9.
26. Biagioni BJ, Gladman DD, Cook RJ, Eder L, Wakhlu A, Shen H, Chandran V. Reliability of radiographic scoring methods in axial psoriatic arthritis. Arthritis Care Res (Hoboken). 2014;66(9):1417–22.
27. Sepriano A, Rudwaleit M, Sieper J, van den Berg R, Landewé R, van der Heijde D. Five-year follow-up of radiographic sacroiliitis: progression as well as improvement? Ann Rheum Dis. 2016;75(6):1262–3.
28. Haroon N, Inman RD, Learch TJ, Weisman MH, Lee M, Rahbar MH, Ward MM, Reveille JD, Gensler LS. The impact of tumor necrosis factor α inhibitors on radiographic progression in ankylosing spondylitis. Arthritis Rheum. 2013; 65(10):2645–54.
29. van Tuyl LH, van der Heijde D, Knol DL, Boers M. Chronological reading of radiographs in rheumatoid arthritis increases efficiency and does not lead to bias. Ann Rheum Dis. 2014;73:391–5.

6

Monosodium urate crystal deposition associated with the progress of radiographic grade at the sacroiliac joint in axial SpA: a dual-energy CT study

Junqing Zhu[1], Aiwu Li[2], Ertao Jia[2], Yi Zhou[3], Juan Xu[2], Shixian Chen[2], Yinger Huang[2], Xiang Xiao[4] and Juan Li[2,1*]

Abstract

Background: Previous studies have revealed that ankylosing spondylitis (AS), as the progenitor of axial spondyloarthritis (AxSpA), has been characterized by the insidiously progressive nature of sacroiliitis and spondylitis. Dual-energy computed tomography (DECT) has recently been used to analyse the deposition of monosodium urate (MSU) crystals with higher sensitivity and specificity. However, it remains unclear whether the existence of the MSU crystal deposition detected by DECT at the sacroiliac joint in patients with AxSpA also is associated with the existing structural damage. Here, we performed this study to show the DECT MSU crystal deposits in AxSpA patients without coexisting gout and to ascertain the relationship between the MSU crystal deposition and the structural joint damage of sacroiliac joints.

Methods: One hundred and eighty-six AxSpA patients without coexisting gout were recruited. The plain radiographs of the sacroiliac joint were obtained, along with the DECT scans at the pelvis and the clinical variables. All statistics based on the left or right sacroiliac joint damage grading (0–4) were calculated independently. Bivariate analysis and ordinal logistic regression was performed between the clinical features and radiographic grades at the sacroiliac joint.

Results: At the pelvis, large quantities of MSU crystal deposition were found in patients with AxSpA. The average MSU crystal volume at the left sacroiliac joint, the right sacroiliac joint, and the pelvis were 0.902 ± 1.345, 1.074 ± 1.878, and 5.272 ± 9.044 cm^3, values which were correlated with serum uric acid concentrations ($r = 0.727, 0.740, 0.896$; $p < 0.001$). In bivariate analysis, wide clinical variables were associated with the changes in sacroiliac joint damage. Further, the AxSpA duration, BASFI score, and the volume of MSU crystal at both sides of sacroiliac joint were associated with the progress of radiographic grade at the sacroiliac joints in the ordinal logistic models (left AOR = 1.180, 3.800, 1.920; right AOR = 1.190, 3.034, 1.418; $p < 0.01$).

Conclusions: Large quantities of MSU crystal deposition detected by DECT were found at the pelvis in AxSpA patients without coexisting gout. In addition to AxSpA duration and BASFI score, the MSU crystal deposition at the sacroiliac joint is associated with the progress of radiographic grade at sacroiliac joints in those patients.

Keywords: Axial Spondyloarthritis (AxSpA), Ankylosing spondylitis (AS), Dual-energy computed tomography (DECT), Monosodium urate (MSU) crystal, Sacroiliac joint

* Correspondence: lj40038@126.com
[2]Department of Internal Medicine of Traditional Chinese Medicine, College of Traditional Chinese Medicine, Southern Medical University, Guangzhou, Guangdong 510510, China
[1]Department of Rheumatology, Nanfang Hospital, Southern Medical University, Guangzhou, Guangdong 510515, China
Full list of author information is available at the end of the article

Background

The term spondyloarthritis (SpA) encompasses a group of diseases including axial SpA (AxSpA) and peripheral SpA, classifications which have been proposed by the Assessment of SpondyloArthritis International Society (ASAS) [1, 2]. It is estimated that SpA, with an incidence between 0.5 and 10.6 per 100,000 people per year, affects approximately 0.4–1.9% of the population across the globe [3]. In addition to what is now known as nonradiographic AxSpA (nr-AxSpA), ankylosing spondylitis (AS) has been characterized by the insidiously progressive nature of sacroiliitis and spondylitis, which leads to a significant reduction in quality of life and an increased mortality rate [4]. Although the aetiology and pathogenesis of AxSpA has not yet been fully elucidated, the current view is that it involves both inflammatory erosive osteopenia and unusual bony overgrowth [5, 6]. Precisely because the primal mechanism in autoimmune disorders is the loss of tolerance to self-proteins by environment-gene interactions, the coexistence of different rheumatic diseases is common. For example, AS grouped under the term AxSpA occurs in patients with rheumatoid arthritis (RA) [7, 8], gouty arthritis [9], multiple sclerosis [10, 11], and systemic lupus erythematosus [12].

There are few epidemiological publications regarding the coexistence of AxSpA and gout, but the study has revealed that AS concurrent with gout is more common than previously believed [9]. Although AxSpA and gout are two distinct rheumatic diseases, they share a few clinical characteristics, including inflammatory joint pain and excellent response to non-steroidal anti-inflammatory drugs (NSAIDs). AxSpA usually leads to structural damage and functional limitation, exemplified in patients with AS [13]. At the same time, structural joint damage is also frequently observed in patients with advanced gout as a result of monosodium urate (MSU) crystal deposition [14–16]. Therefore, in patients with coexisting AS and gout, it is hard to discriminate whether the inflammatory joint pain and structural joint damage are due to AS disease activity, the MSU crystal deposition, or both.

Dual-energy computed tomography (DECT) has been used to analyse the deposition of MSU crystal with high sensitivity (100%) and specificity (89%) [17]. The sensitivity and specificity of DECT for gout were only 0.87 and 0.84 [18], because the deposition of MSU crystal is a necessary but not a sufficient condition. Besides, DECT MSU crystal deposition was observed in both multiple joints and soft tissues in patients with asymptomatic hyperuricaemia, and was associated with increasingly severe coronary calcification [19, 20]. In addition, our study found a large quantity of MSU crystal deposition with DECT in AxSpA patients without coexisting gout, according to the 1977 American Rheumatism Association classification criteria [21]. However, whether the existence of MSU crystal deposition in those patients has contributed to the structural joint damage is still unclear.

The purpose of our study was to show the DECT MSU crystal deposits at the pelvis in AxSpA patients without coexisting gout, and further to analyse whether the MSU crystal deposition at the sacroiliac joint is associated with the structural joint damage of the sacroiliac joint in those patients.

Methods

One hundred and eighty-six patients with AxSpA were recruited from rheumatology clinics at Nanfang Hospital in China during the period of October 2012 to July 2015. All participants had AxSpA described by the ASAS classification criteria [1, 2] and had not been diagnosed with gout, according to the 1977 American Rheumatism Association classification criteria [21].

The plain radiographs of the sacroiliac joint, a DECT scan of pelvis, and the clinical variables were obtained at a follow-up appointment. In brief, each sacroiliac joint on a plain radiograph was graded on a scale of 0–4 according to the modified New York criteria [22]. DECT scans were performed on a dual-source X-ray tube 128 detector row scanner (Somatom Definition Flash, Siemens Healthcare, Erlangen, Germany). All scans were performed using the same image protocol: acquisition at 128 mm × 0.6 mm and pitch of 0.7. The two X-ray tubes are operated simultaneously at 80 kV and 140 kV. The image reconstructions were done using proprietary software (Siemens Multimodality Workplace, Software version MMWP Syngo CT 2010A, Siemens Healthcare, Erlangen, Germany), with a 512 × 512 matrix, to 0.75-mm slices, with a 0.5-mm increment. The parameter ratio for urate was set at 1.28. Two readers, blinded to the clinical variables and plain radiographic scores, evaluated the DECT scans for the presence and volumes of MSU crystal, independently. MSU crystal was considered present at each site only if reported by both readers and the average volume of MSU crystal was calculated [23].

The clinical variables, including age, gender, AxSpA disease duration, HLA-B27 positivity, erythrocyte sedimentation rate (ESR, mm/h), C-reactive protein (CRP, mg/l), total back pain (10-cm visual analogue scale, VAS), patient's global assessment (PGA) of disease activity (10-cm VAS), pain and swelling of peripheral arthritis (10-cm VAS), duration of morning stiffness (10-cm VAS), use of non-steroidal anti-inflammatory drugs (NSAIDs), use of disease-modifying anti-rheumatic drugs (DMARDs), use of biologic DMARDs, serum uric acid (μmol/L), MSU crystal positivity, and volume of MSU crystal (cm^3) were all assessed. In addition, the Ankylosing Spondylitis Disease Activity Score (ASDAS) [24] and the grading for disease activity [25] were calculated as previous study. The Bath Ankylosing Spondylitis Functional Index (BASFI) scores were calculated according to the average scores of ten questions [26].

All statistics based on the left or right sacroiliac joint damage grading were calculated independently with IBM SPSS (Version 20.0, IBM Corp., Armonk, NY, USA). Measurement data were presented as mean ± standard deviation (mean ± SD) or with a 95% confidence interval (CI), while count data were presented as numbers (n). One-way analysis of variance (ANOVA) was used to evaluate the statistical differences among groups. The non-normal distribution measurement data were tested with the Kruskal-Wallis rank-sum test. To count data, Pearson's chi-square (x^2) and Fisher's exact test were used for the comparison. Interobserver reproducibility for the volume of MSU crystals by two readers was assessed by the intraclass correlation coefficient (ICC) and limits of agreement by Bland-Altman analysis [27]. The ICC values, 95%CI, and the p values were reported. Spearman's correlation analysis was performed to evaluate the association between serum uric acid and the average volume of MSU crystal. Spearman's rank correlation coefficient (r) and p values were reported. Bivariate analysis was performed between the clinical features and radiographic grades. The odds ratios (OR) and its 95%CI were reported. In addition, the ordinal logistic regression was used to identify the effect of each potential factor adjusted for others. Variables with $p < 0.05$ in bivariate analysis were included in the ordinal logistic models. The adjusted odds ratios (AOR) 95%CI were reported. A test of parallel lines was also performed to evaluate the appropriateness of the ordinal logistic model. A $p < 0.05$ was considered statistically significant. All p values were two-tailed.

Results

Clinical characteristics of the patients with AxSpA

The 186 patients' clinical features are shown in Table 1. Patients were predominantly young males and were HLA-B27 positive. Mean disease duration was 4.3 years, mean ESR was 25.1 mm/h, and mean serum uric acid was 362.7 μmol/L. The median ASDAS scores and BASFI scores were 2.7 ± 1.1 and 4.3 ± 1.1. Seventeen and fifty-seven patients had never used NSAIDs or biologic DMARDs. Seventeen patients had used DMARDs for less than 3 months. Large quantities of MSU crystal deposition detected by DECT were found at the pelvis in AxSpA patients without coexisting gout. The positive rates of MSU crystal at the sacroiliac joint, hip joint, and pubic symphysis were 111 (29.8%), 75 (40.3%), and 63 (33.9%). The average volumes of MSU crystal at the sacroiliac joint and pelvis were 0.29 ± 0.99 and 4.37 ± 8.46 cm^3.

The statistically significant results were found among the radiographic grade group at the left or right sacroiliac joints for disease duration, ESR, CRP, total back pain, PGA of disease activity, duration of morning stiffness, ASDAS scores, BASFI scores, use of NSAIDs/DMARDs/biologic DMARDs, as well as the presence and volume of MSU crystal on the left and right sacroiliac joints ($p < 0.05$) (Table 1).

Reproducibility of DECT MSU crystal volume measurement and correlation between the average MSU crystal volume and serum uric acid

Of the patients who showed the presence of MSU crystal deposition, 57 showed deposition at the left sacroiliac joint, 54 at the right sacroiliac joint, and 154 at the pelvis. The interobserver reproducibility analysis is shown in Table 2. ICCs for MSU crystal volume measurements at the sacroiliac joint and pelvis were all greater than 0.99 ($p < 0.001$). Bland-Altman plots illustrating the interobserver limits of agreement for MSU crystal volume measurements are shown in Fig. 1. The average MSU crystal volume measurements at the left sacroiliac joint, the right sacroiliac joint, and the pelvis were 0.902 ± 1.345, 1.074 ± 1.878, and 5.272 ± 9.044 cm^3. For further analysis, the serum uric acid concentration was correlated with the volumes of MSU crystal at the left sacroiliac joint ($r = 0.727$, $p < 0.001$), the right sacroiliac joint ($r = 0.740$, $p < 0.001$), and the pelvis ($r = 0.896$, $p < 0.001$) (Table 2).

Comparison of MSU crystal deposition and serum uric acid in patients grouped by ASDAS scores

According to the ASDAS scores, all patients were divided into four groups (Table 3). The presence of MSU crystal deposition at the left and right sacroiliac joints showed statistical differences among groups ($x^2 = 11.451$, 43.684; $p = 0.010$, <0.001). However, there was no statistical difference among groups at the hip joint and pubic symphysis for the presence of MSU crystal deposition ($x^2 = 0.676$, 0.549; $p = 0.879$, 0.908). Statistical differences were found in regards to the volumes of MSU crystal at the left sacroiliac joint ($Z = 9.198$, $p = 0.027$), the right sacroiliac joint ($Z = 34.607$, $p < 0.001$), and the pelvis ($Z = 10.517$; $p = 0.015$). In addition the ANOVA tests revealed that the serum uric acid concentration was statistically different among groups ($F = 6.322$, $p < 0.001$).

Unadjusted associations of clinical features with the grade of sacroiliac joint damage

In bivariate analysis (Table 4), wide clinical variables were associated with the changes in sacroiliac joint damage based on the radiographic grade at the left sacroiliac joint. The OR scores were 1.189 (95%CI 1.103–1.283) for disease duration, 1.024 (95%CI 1.011–1.037) for ESR,

Table 1 Characteristics of the patients with AxSpA included in the study

	Total	Based on the left sacroiliac joint damage					*p* value	Based on the right sacroiliac joint damage					*p* value
		0 grade	1 grade	2 grade	3 grade	4 grade		0 grade	1 grade	2 grade	3 grade	4 grade	
Number of cases (n)	186	4	8	73	72	29	NA	4	10	74	72	26	NA
Age (years)	26.4 ± 8.7	25.3 ± 5.4	29.4 ± 10.7	24.9 ± 8.7	27. 6 ± 8.3	26.5 ± 9.2	0.138	25.3 ± 5.4	25.7 ± 9.4	25.0 ± 8.6	27.9 ± 8.5	26.7 ± 9.4	0.133
Male/female (n)	143/43	3/1	6/2	55/18	54/18	25/4	0.763	3/1	7/3	57/17	53/19	23/3	0.564
AxSpA duration (years)	4.3 ± 4.0	0.8 ± 0.3	4.4 ± 2.5	3.1 ± 3.1	4.8 ± 3.7	6.9 ± 5.6	<0.001	0.8 ± 0.3	4.5 ± 2.9	2.8 ± 2.2	5.1 ± 4.3	7.0 ± 5.5	<0.001
HLA-B27 (+/-) (n)	164/22	3/1	6/2	68/8	65/7	25/4	0.725	3/1	9/1	64/10	66/6	22/4	0.741
ESR (mm/h)	25.1 ± 22.1	9.5 ± 10.6	10.1 ± 8.9	20.2 ± 16.5	29.1 ± 24.8	33.7 ± 25.7	0.002	9.5 ± 10.6	23.8 ± 20.1	19.2 ± 17.2	28.3 ± 23.9	35.8 ± 26.3	0.007
CRP (mg/l)	14.3 ± 17.5	1.0 ± 0.5	3.1 ± 2.4	9.2 ± 13.1	16. 6 ± 17.2	26.0 ± 23.4	<0.001	1.0 ± 0.5	9.4 ± 15.6	9.9 ± 14.3	15.1 ± 15.9	28.1 ± 23.8	<0.001
Total back pain[#]	4.9 ± 2.8	1.3 ± 0.5	1.9 ± 1.4	4.5 ± 2.6	5.4 ± 2.6	6.3 ± 2.8	<0.001	1.3 ± 0.5	3.6 ± 3.2	4.5 ± 2.6	5.2 ± 2.6	6.6 ± 2.8	<0.001
PGA of disease activity[#]	5.6 ± 3.0	2.5 ± 1.9	2.5 ± 1.8	5.3 ± 2.8	5.9 ± 2.9	7.0 ± 2.9	<0.001	2.5 ± 1.9	4.4 ± 3.7	5.1 ± 2.8	5.9 ± 2.7	7.3 ± 3.0	0.002
Pain and swelling of peripheral arthritis[#]	0.2 ± 0.5	NA	0.3 ± 0.4	0.2 ± 0.4	0.3 ± 0.5	0.4 ± 0.6	0.249	NA	0.2 ± 0.4	0.2 ± 0.4	0.3 ± 0.5	0.4 ± 0.6	0.227
Duration of morning stiffness[#]	5.4 ± 2.8	2.8 ± 1.0	2.0 ± 1.3	5.1 ± 2.7	5.8 ± 2.6	6.4 ± 2.9	<0.001	2.8 ± 1.0	4.0 ± 3.6	4.9 ± 2.6	5.8 ± 2.5	6.7 ± 2.9	0.003
ASDAS (scores)	2.7 ± 1.1	1.0 ± 0.2	1.4 ± 0.4	2.4 ± 1.3	3.0 ± 1.3	3.5 ± 1.5	<0.001	1.0 ± 0.2	2.1 ± 1.6	2.4 ± 1.3	2.9 ± 1.3	3.6 ± 1.6	<0.001
BASFI (scores)	4.3 ± 1.1	1.9 ± 0.8	2.5 ± 0.9	4.0 ± 1.0	4.6 ± 0.7	4.9 ± 0.8	<0.001	1.9 ± 0.8	3.1 ± 1.5	4.1 ± 1.0	4.5 ± 0.8	4.9 ± 0.8	<0.001
Use of NSAIDs (ever/never) (n)	169/17	0/4	8/0	68/5	67/5	26/3	<0.001	0/4	10/0	70/4	66/6	23/3	<0.001
Use of DMARDs (≥3/<3 months) (n)	169/17	1/3	6/2	69/4	68/4	25/4	0.005	1/3	8/2	70/4	67/5	23/3	0.010
Ever use of biologic DMARDs (n)													
> 12 months	28	0	4	18	4	2	<0.001	0	5	15	6	2	<0.001
≤ 12 months	42	1	3	21	15	2		1	3	24	12	2	
≤ 6 months	59	2	1	16	30	10		2	0	18	32	7	
Never	57	1	0	18	23	15		1	2	17	22	15	
Serum uric acid (μmol/L)	362.7 ± 107.9	284.0 ± 95.3	345.1 ± 77.0	361.9 ± 105.5	366.0 ± 117.7	372.2 ± 97.8	0.593	284.0 ± 95.3	325.6 ± 103.5	362.3 ± 101.9	372.4 ± 118.8	363.3 ± 94.6	0.499
MSU crystallization (+/-) (n)													
Sacroiliac joint	111/261[$]	0/4	0/8	14/59	29/43	14/15	<0.001	0/4	1/9	13/61	28/44	12/44	0.002
Hip joint	75/111	1/3	4/4	33/40	28/44	9/20	0.632	1/3	6/4	32/42	29/43	7/19	0.369
Pubic symphysis	63/123	0/4	3/5	25/48	28/44	7/22	0.244	0/4	4/6	25/49	29/43	5/21	0.112
Volume of MSU crystallization (cm^3)													
Sacroiliac joint	0.29 ± 0.99[$]	NA	NA	0.10 ± 0.30	0.31 ± 0.69	0.75 ± 1.72	0.001	NA	0.01 ± 0.01	0.10 ± 0.32	0.41 ± 1.19	0.83 ± 2.11	0.005
Total volume at pelvis	4.37 ± 8.46	0.02 ± 0.03	0.63 ± 0.99	4.36 ± 8.01	4.92 ± 10.03	4.62 ± 6.72	0.077	0.02 ± 0.03	2.15 ± 4.16	4.00 ± 7.73	5.51 ± 10.37	3.78 ± 5.91	0.118

Values are given as the numbers or the mean ± standard deviation (Mean±SD);
AxSpA axial spondyloarthritis, *n* numbers, *+/-* positive/negative, *ESR* erythrocyte sedimentation rate, *CRP* C-reactive protein, *PGA* patient's global assessment, *ASDAS* Ankylosing Spondylitis Disease Activity Score, *BASFI* Bath Ankylosing Spondylitis Functional Index, *NSAIDs* non-steroidal anti-inflammatory drugs, *DMARDs* disease-modifying anti-rheumatic drugs, *MSU* monosodium urate, *NA* not available
[#]All assessed on a visual analogue scale (0–10 cm)
[$]The sum of the data from the left and right sacroiliac joint

Table 2 The interreader reproducibility analysis of MSU crystal volume and its correlation with the serum uric acid

Joint	Reader	Volume of MSU crystallization (cm^3)		Intraclass correlation coefficient			Correlation with serum uric acid[#]	
		Mean ± SD	95% CI	*ICC*	95% CI	*p*	*r*	*p*
Left sacroiliac joint (n = 57)	Reader 1	0.900 ± 1.351	0.541–1.258	0.999	0.998-0.999	<0.001	NA	NA
	Reader 2	0.904 ± 1.340	0.549–1.260				NA	NA
	Average	0.902 ± 1.345	0.545–1.259	NA	NA	NA	0.727	<0.001
Right sacroiliac joint (n = 54)	Reader 1	1.078 ± 1.878	0.578–1.619	1.000	0.999-1.000	<0.001	NA	NA
	Reader 2	1.071 ± 1.878	0.5700–1.612				NA	NA
	Average	1.074 ± 1.878	0.574–1.616	NA	NA	NA	0.740	<0.001
Pelvis (n = 154)	Reader 1	5.237 ± 8.942	3.813–6.660	0.999	0.999-0.999	<0.001	NA	NA
	Reader 2	5.307 ± 9.150	3.850–6.764				NA	NA
	Average	5.272 ± 9.044	3.832–6.712	NA	NA	NA	0.896	<0.001

Values are given as the mean ± standard deviation (mean ± SD)
MSU monosodium urate, *ICC* intraclass correlation coefficient values, *95% CI* 95% confidence interval, r, Spearman rank correlation coefficient, *NA* not available
[#]Spearman correlation analysis between serum uric acid and the average volume of MSU crystals

1.045 (95%CI 1.027–1.063) for CRP, 1.298 (95%CI 1.169–1.440) for total back pain, 1.214 (95%CI 1.104–1.335) for PGA of disease activity, 1.849 (95%CI 1.051–3.254) for pain and swelling of peripheral arthritis, 1.242 (95%CI 1.122–1.376) for duration of morning stiffness, 1.716 (95%CI 1.397–2.107) for ASDAS scores, 3.188 (95%CI 2.330–4.364) for BASFI scores, 0.143 (95%CI 0.057–0.357) for use of biologic DMARDs more than 12 months, and 0.274 (95%CI 0.127–0.592) for use of biologic DMARDs more than 6 months. Positive associations were also observed between changes in left sacroiliac joint damage and the presence and volume of MSU crystal on the left sacroiliac joint (OR = 3.368, 1.990; 95%CI 1.841–6.160, 1.308–3.028). However, the changes in left sacroiliac joint damage were not significantly associated with age, gender (male), HLA-B27-positive status, any use of NSAIDs, use of DMARDs more than 3 months, serum uric acid, MSU crystal on the hip joint and pubic symphysis, and volume of MSU crystal on the pelvis. The same trend results were obtained in bivariate analysis for the changes in sacroiliac joint damage at the right sacroiliac joint.

Adjusted associations of clinical features with the grade of sacroiliac joint damage

In the ordinal logistic models, variables with $p < 0.05$ in bivariate analysis were included (complex model 1 and 3, Table 5). For the radiographic grade at the left sacroiliac joint, the adjusted factors were AxSpA duration, total back pain, BASFI score, and the volume of MSU crystal at the left sacroiliac joint (AOR = 1.187, 1.428, 3.837, 2.018; 95%CI 1.089–1.294, 1.040–1.962, 2.263–6.506, 1.144–3.560; $p < 0.001$, $p = 0.028$, $p < 0.001$, $p = 0.015$). The same adjusted factors were obtained at the right sacroiliac joint, except the variable of total back pain. The AOR values were 1.188, 3.092, and 1.387 (95%CI 1.090–1.295, 1.896–5.044, 1.022–1.882; $p < 0.001$, $p < 0.001$, $p = 0.036$) for the variables of AxSpA duration, BASFI score, and the volume of MSU crystal at the right sacroiliac joint.

In addition, the simplified models (simplified model 2 and 4, Table 5), which excluded the repeated variables of the ASDAS score and presence of MSU crystal deposition, were also performed. The AxSpA duration, BASFI score, and the volume of MSU crystal at the left sacroiliac joint (AOR = 1.180, 3.800, 1.920; 95%CI 1.086–1.283, 2.250–6.417, 1.209–3.049; $p < 0.001$, $p < 0.001$, $p = 0.006$) were associated with the progress of radiographic grade at the left sacroiliac joint after being adjusted for other potential factors, while the duration of morning stiffness was a protective factor (AOR = 0.682, 95%CI 0.494–0.942, $p = 0.020$). In the simplified ordinal logistic model at the right sacroiliac joint, AxSpA duration, BASFI score, and the volume of MSU crystal at the right sacroiliac joint were the main factors when others factors were adjusted (AOR = 1.190, 3.034, 1.418; 95%CI 1.096–1.293, 1.870–4.922, 1.075–1.870; $p < 0.001$, $p < 0.001$, $p = 0.014$).

The test for parallel lines was not significant in the complex model 1, simplified model 2, and simplified model 4 ($x^2 = 34.904$, 13.028, 40.234; $p = 0.773$, 1.000, 0.288), which suggests that the models are appropriate. However, the parameter estimation is less stable for complex model 2 ($x^2 = 59.877$, $p = 0.036$).

The MSU crystal at the sacroiliac joint with radiographic sacroiliac joint damage in four separate patients with AxSpA

Examples of corresponding radiographic and DECT images of affected sacroiliac joints are shown in Fig. 2. Four male patients (patient 1–4), aged 36, 44, 23, and 27 years old, had serum uric acid levels of 407 μmol/L,

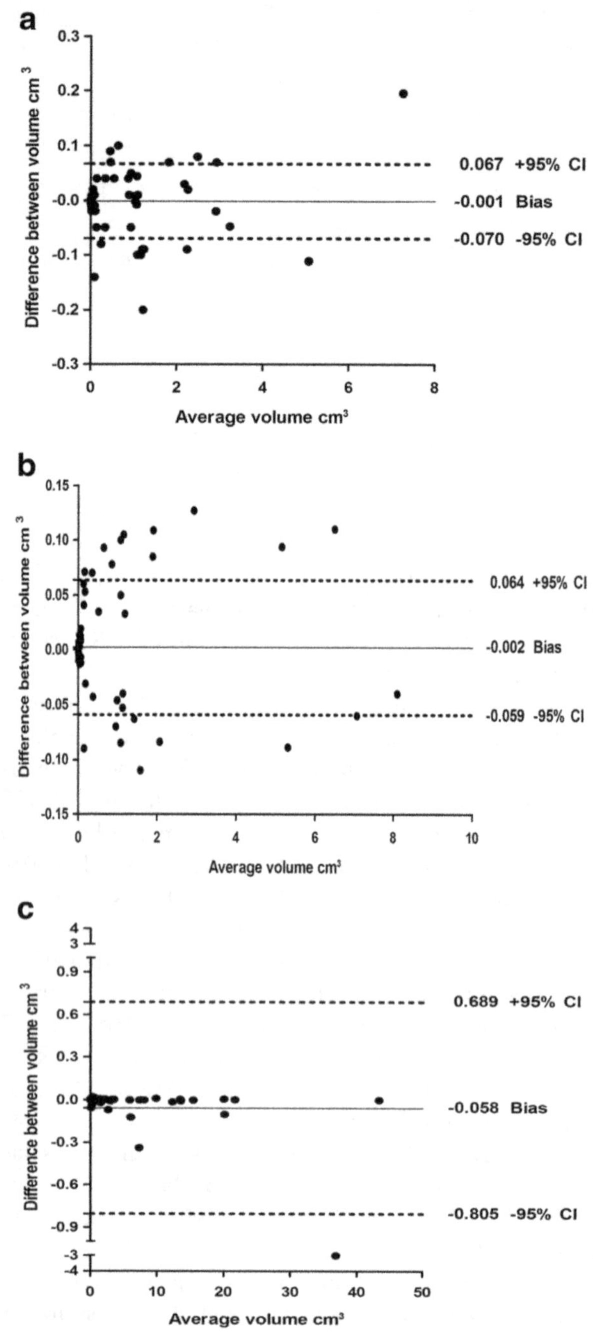

Fig. 1 Bland-Altman plots for interobserver reproducibility analysis. **a** The dual-energy computed tomography (DECT) monosodium urate (MSU) crystal volume at the *left* sacroiliac joint. **b** The DECT MSU crystal volume at the *right* sacroiliac joint. **c** The DECT MSU crystal volume at the pelvis. *Solid line* shows bias and *dashed lines* show the 95% limits of agreement

370 μmol/L, 572 μmol/L, and 464 μmol/L, respectively. As seen in Fig. 2a, four AxSpA patients were graded with a scale of 0, 0, II, III at the left sacroiliac joint and 0, I, II, III at the right sacroiliac joint, respectively, on plain radiographs. A large quantity of MSU crystal deposition was found at the sacroiliac joint or the surrounding area (Fig. 2b). The close relationship between MSU crystal deposition and radiographic structural damage (erosion, joint space narrowing, and new bone formation features) is shown at the sacroiliac joints of patients 2–4 (Fig. 2c-d).

Discussion

The umbrella of AxSpA encompasses both nr-AxSpA and classic AS by ASAS [1, 2]. However, the range of diagnoses for AxSpA may cause difficulty among a large population with back pain, especially with sacroiliitis in gout or crystal deposition diseases [28]. First, the publication of classification criteria for AxSpA has produced some false-positive and false-negative cases, due to the way that the aforementioned diseases may mimic AxSpA in clinical manifestations. Second, the coexistence of AxSpA with other rheumatic diseases is common. For example, with an increasing mean age of AS onset and a decreasing mean age of gout onset [29, 30] AS coexisting with gout is more common [9]. Finally, at a certain stage of disease duration in AxSpA patients without the gout history, the deposition of MSU crystal may only be transient, which is hard to detect with traditional radiology methods, but has a positive impact on disease progression.

Fortunately, the recently developed DECT imaging method has provided higher sensitivity and specificity for MSU crystal deposition in patients with symptomatic gout and asymptomatic hyperuricaemia [19]. Therefore, a DECT finding of MSU crystal deposition has been included in the 2015 American College of Rheumatology and the European League Against Rheumatism (ACR/EULAR) gout classification criteria [31]. Although a subclinical MSU crystal deposition by DECT is insufficient for a diagnosis of gout, those depositions are, in fact, widespread in the body of patients or even normal individuals. A previous study reported that 20% of hyperuricaemic RA patients show DECT MSU crystal depositions, which are significantly associated with seronegativity [32]. Moreover, MSU crystal deposition was also observed in multiple joints and soft tissues of the body in patients with asymptomatic hyperuricaemia and was associated with increasing severity of coronary calcification [19, 20]. Indeed, we have found a few cases of MSU crystal deposition depicted in green with DECT at painful joints or skeleton regions not only in patients with asymptomatic hyperuricemia, but also in patients with iliac condensing ostitis, reactive arthritis, osteoarthritis, rheumatoid arthritis, and AxSpA in our clinical practice, when patients were considered for other causes of inflammatory activity. It may be meaningful that the MSU crystal deposited at those joints or skeleton regions. Those depositions may be involved in the process

Table 3 Comparison of MSU crystal deposits at different regions and serum uric acid in patients grouped by ASDAS scores

	ASDAS scores				x^2/Z/F	p
	ASDAS < 1.3 (n = 38)	1.3 ≤ ASDAS < 2.1 (n = 38)	2.1 ≤ ASDAS ≤ 3.5 (n = 50)	ASDAS > 3.5 (n = 60)		
MSU crystallization (+/-) (n)#						
Left sacroiliac joint	8/30	6/32	16/34	27/33	11.451	0.010
Right sacroiliac joint	3/35	4/34	11/39	36/24	43.684	<0.001
Hip joint	15/23	16/22	22/28	22/38	0.676	0.879
Pubic symphysis	11/27	13/25	18/32	21/39	0.549	0.908
Volume of MSU crystallization (cm^3)$						
Left sacroiliac joint	0.21 ± 0.62	0.14 ± 0.47	0.49 ± 1.34	0.23 ± 0.57	9.198	0.027
Right sacroiliac joint	0.04 ± 0.18	0.13 ± 0.52	0.35 ± 1.09	0.57 ± 1.62	34.607	<0.001
Total volume at pelvis	2.41 ± 6.51	2.69 ± 5.04	7.40 ± 11.49	4.13 ± 7.77	10.517	0.015
Serum uric acid (μmol/L)&	321.0 ± 100.4	326.2 ± 104.2	397.9 ± 109.4	382.9 ± 99.8	6.322	<0.001

Values are given as the numbers or the mean ± standard deviation (Mean±SD)
ASDAS Ankylosing Spondylitis Disease Activity Score, *MSU* monosodium urate
#Pearson chi-square (x^2) test
$Kruskal-Wallis rank-sum test
&One-way analysis of variance (ANOVA)

of inflammation and bone destruction in primary diseases. In this study we reported that a large amount of MSU crystal deposition detected with DECT was in pelvic, hip joint, and sacroiliac joint regions in AxSpA patients without gout. Those findings indicated that it might be easy to ignore these regions in patients with AxSpA when it coexists with MSU crystal deposition, which may play an important role in the occurrence or development of the disease.

As is commonly known, hyperuricaemia and MSU crystal deposition are the central risk factors for development of gout. Three stages of MSU crystal deposition have been proposed: reduced urate solubility, MSU nucleation, and MSU crystal growth [33]. But there is no inevitable corresponding relationship between hyperuricaemia, MSU crystal deposition, and gout. For example, a recent study has shown that imaging evidence of MSU crystal deposition appears only in 24% of asymptomatic patients [23]. In addition, our study also found MSU crystal deposits in AxSpA patients without gout history. Further analysis revealed that serum uric acid concentration was correlated with the volume of MSU crystal at the sacroiliac joints and the pelvis. Therefore, there are more details to be discovered in future research. On the one hand, it is still unclear why MSU crystal deposition forms in some joints, soft tissues, or skeleton regions of individuals with or without gout. There must be some factors in the microenvironment of the specific location that promote the deposition of MSU crystal. Examples are temperature, pH level, concentration of ions, and proteins all of which may also be influenced by interactions with each other [33]. On the other hand, it is currently not known whether the deposition of MSU crystal at different positions makes sense in the course of the disease. Indeed, some studies have indicated that silent deposition of MSU crystal in asymptomatic hyperuricemia patients is associated with more severe coronary calcification [20]. Interestingly, we also found that, in patients with AxSpA, the presence and volumes of MSU crystal at the sacroiliac joints were statistically different when grouped by radiographic grade, but not at the hip joint, pubic symphysis, or pelvis.

Previous studies have shown that smoking status, alcohol use, HLAB27 positivity, CRP, poor responsiveness to NSAIDs, and inflammation at magnetic resonance imaging (MRI) of the sacroiliac joint could predict the radiographic sacroiliitis progression in patients with AxSpA [34–36]. In this study, similar results were found, namely that disease duration, ESR, CRP, total back pain, PGA of disease activity, pain and swelling of peripheral arthritis, duration of morning stiffness, ASDAS scores, BASFI scores, and any use of biologic DMARDs were associated with the grade of sacroiliac joint damage in patients with AxSpA by bivariate analysis, apart from the presence and volumes of MSU crystal at the sacroiliac joint. Further, the ordinal logistic regression analysis also shows that the disease duration, BASFI scores, and volume of MSU crystal at the sacroiliac joint are associated with the structural joint damage of sacroiliac joints in patients with AxSpA when other potential factors have been adjusted.

Those results suggest that more attention should be paid to AxSpA patients with no response to antirheumatic therapy, especially in those with coexisting MSU crystal deposition. Additionally, it suggest that there might be some common pathogenesis or

Table 4 Bivariate analysis between the grade of sacroiliac joint damage and clinical features#

Characteristics	Based on the left sacroiliac joint damage			Based on the right sacroiliac joint damage		
	Unadjusted *OR*	*95% CI*	*p* value	Unadjusted *OR*	*95% CI*	*p* value
Age, per year	1.016	0.985–1.047	0.324	1.025	0.994–1.057	0.121
Male, vs female	1.303	0.692–2.454	0.412	1.281	0.680--2.412	0.444
AxSpA duration, per year	1.189	1.103–1.283	<0.001	1.195	1.108–1.289	<0.001
HLA-B27 positive, vs negative	1.248	0.546–2.850	0.599	1.197	0.524–2.732	0.670
ESR, per mm/h	1.024	1.011–1.037	<0.001	1.023	1.010–1.036	<0.001
CRP, per mg/l	1.045	1.027–1.063	<0.001	1.041	1.024–1.059	<0.001
Total back pain, per score	1.298	1.169–1.440	<0.001	1.263	1.139–1.399	<0.001
PGA of disease activity, per score	1.214	1.104–1.335	<0.001	1.221	1.110–1.343	<0.001
Pain and swelling of peripheral arthritis, per score	1.849	1.051–3.254	0.033	1.950	1.105–3.441	0.021
Duration of morning stiffness, per score	1.242	1.122–1.376	<0.001	1.234	1.115–1.367	<0.001
ASDAS, per score	1.716	1.397–2.107	<0.001	1.671	1.362–2.048	<0.001
BASFI, per score	3.188	2.330–4.364	<0.001	2.811	2.081–3.797	<0.001
Ever use of NSAIDs, vs never	1.893	0.740–4.842	0.183	1.372	0.543–3.471	0.504
Use of DMARDs ≥3 months, vs <3 months	1.922	0.751–4.922	0.173	1.967	0.769–5.034	0.158
Ever use of biologic DMARDs, vs never						
≥ 12 months	0.143	0.057–0.357	<0.001	0.182	0.074–0.444	<0.001
≤ 12 months	0.274	0.127–0.592	0.001	0.244	0.113–0.531	<0.001
≤ 6 months	0.795	0.404–1.567	0.508	0.757	0.383–1.493	0.421
Never	NA	NA	NA	NA	NA	NA
Serum uric acid, per μmol/L	1.001	0.999–1.004	0.358	1.001	0.999–1.004	0.276
MSU crystallization positive, vs negative						
Left sacroiliac joint	3.368	1.841–6.160	<0.001	NA	NA	NA
Right sacroiliac joint	NA	NA	NA	3.225	1.749–5.946	<0.001
Hip joint	0.715	0.415–1.232	0.227	0.674	0.390–1.163	0.156
Pubic symphysis	0.971	0.554–1.703	0.919	0.928	0.529–1.628	0.795
Volume of MSU crystallization, per cm^3						
Left sacroiliac joint	1.990	1.308–3.028	0.001	NA	NA	NA
Right sacroiliac joint	NA	NA	NA	1.470	1.125–1.922	0.005
Total volume at pelvis	1.015	0.983–1.047	0.370	1.015	0.983–1.047	0.367

AxSpA axial spondyloarthritis, *ESR* erythrocyte sedimentation rate, *CRP* C-reactive protein, *PGA* patient's global assessment, *ASDAS* Ankylosing Spondylitis Disease Activity Score, *BASFI* Bath Ankylosing Spondylitis Functional Index, *NSAIDs* non-steroidal anti-inflammatory drugs, *DMARDs* disease-modifying anti-rheumatic drugs, *MSU* monosodium urate, *OR* odds ratios, *95% CI* 95% confidence interval, *NA* not available

#Including clinical variables and the DECT scans results

interacting mechanisms between AxSpA and MSU crystal deposition, which ultimately results in damage to the sacroiliac joint. On the one hand, the structural damage mentioned above occurs through alteration of physiological bone turnover with excessive osteoclast activation, which was abnormally regulated by the receptor activator of nuclear factor-κB (RANK), RANK ligand (RANKL), and the osteoprotegerin (OPG) signaling pathway [37, 38]. Although new bone formation evolving into ankylosis is an important feature of AxSpA, the process of inflammation and subsequent bone erosion also occurs synchronously [39]. Meanwhile, bone erosion was also recognized at some interface of MSU crystal deposition, which erodes the bone and cartilage to cause significant structural damage [23]. On the other hand, a large amount of common inflammatory and proinflammatory factors have been involved in the promotion of bone damage, such as tumour necrosis factor alpha, interleukin (IL)-1, IL-6 [40, 41]. Accordingly, our observation that volumes of MSU crystal at the sacroiliac joints are associated with the progress of radiographic grade at sacroiliac joints is consistent with the current understanding of the pathogenesis, but the exact interacting mechanism needs further investigation.

Table 5 The ordinal logistic regression analysis of clinical features # independently associated with the grade of sacroiliac joint damage

Characteristics	Based on the left sacroiliac joint damage						Based on the right sacroiliac joint damage					
	Complex model 1			Simplified model 2			Complex model 3			Simplified model 4		
	AOR	*95% CI*	*p* value	*AOR*	*95% CI*	*p* value	*AOR*	*95% CI*	*p* value	*AOR*	*95% CI*	*p* value
AxSpA duration, per year	1.187	1.089–1.294	0.000	1.180	1.086–1.283	0.000	1.188	1.090–1.295	0.000	1.190	1.096–1.293	0.000
ESR, per mm/h	1.003	0.981–1.025	0.794	1.003	0.982–1.025	0.755	1.001	0.981–1.022	0.905	1.003	0.982–1.024	0.781
CRP, per mg/l	1.038	0.999–1.079	0.058	1.018	0.991–1.046	0.194	1.025	0.987–1.065	0.196	1.008	0.981–1.036	0.576
Total back pain, per score	1.428	1.040–1.962	0.028	1.246	0.975–1.591	0.078	1.315	0.959–1.803	0.089	1.166	0.916–1.484	0.212
PGA of disease activity, per score	1.040	0.784–1.380	0.786	0.975	0.746–1.275	0.856	1.023	0.780–1.342	0.868	0.970	0.751–1.252	0.815
Pain and swelling of peripheral arthritis, per score	1.517	0.795–2.897	0.207	1.356	0.725–2.534	0.341	1.858	0.978–3.532	0.059	1.657	0.890–3.084	0.111
Duration of morning stiffness, per score	0.723	0.519–1.008	0.056	0.682	0.494–0.942	0.020	0.836	0.607–1.150	0.271	0.792	0.581–1.079	0.139
ASDAS, per score	0.492	0.179–1.354	0.170	NA	NA	NA	0.526	0.194–1.429	0.208	NA	NA	NA
BASFI, per score	3.837	2.263–6.506	0.000	3.800	2.250–6.417	0.000	3.092	1.896–5.044	0.000	3.034	1.870–4.922	0.000
Ever use of biologic DMARDs, vs never												
≥ 12 months	1.051	0.308–3.581	0.937	1.144	0.337–3.885	0.829	1.425	0.417–4.872	0.572	1.414	0.421–4.754	0.575
≤ 12 months	0.961	0.333–2.778	0.942	1.098	0.385–3.132	0.861	0.971	0.329–2.866	0.958	1.020	0.357–2.916	0.971
≤ 6 months	1.999	0.806–4.962	0.135	1.830	0.745–4.495	0.188	2.461	0.976–6.204	0.056	2.128	0.869–5.211	0.099
Never	NA	NA	NA	NA	NA	NA	NA	NA	NA	NA	NA	NA
MSU crystallization positive, vs negative												
Left sacroiliac joint	0.895	0.391–2.049	0.794	NA	NA	NA	NA	NA	NA	NA	NA	NA
Right sacroiliac joint	NA	NA	NA	NA	NA	NA	1.291	0.542–3.075	0.565	NA	NA	NA
Volume of MSU crystallization, per cm^3												
Left sacroiliac joint	2.018	1.144–3.560	0.015	1.920	1.209–3.049	0.006	NA	NA	NA	NA	NA	NA
Right sacroiliac joint	NA	NA	NA	NA	NA	NA	1.387	1.022–1.882	0.036	1.418	1.075–1.870	0.014

Complex model 1 and 3, variables with $p < 0.05$ in bivariate analysis were included based on the radiographic grade at each sacroiliac joint; simplified model 2 and 4, the models with the repeated variables of the ASDAS score and MSU crystals deposits positive were excluded

AxSpA axial spondyloarthritis, *ESR* erythrocyte sedimentation rate, *CRP* C-reactive protein, *PGA* patient's global assessment, *ASDAS* Ankylosing Spondylitis Disease Activity Score, *BASFI* Bath Ankylosing Spondylitis Functional Index, *DMARDs* disease-modifying anti-rheumatic drugs, *MSU* monosodium urate, *AOR* adjusted odds ratios, *95% CI* 95% confidence interval, *NA* not available

[#]Including clinical variables and the DECT scans results

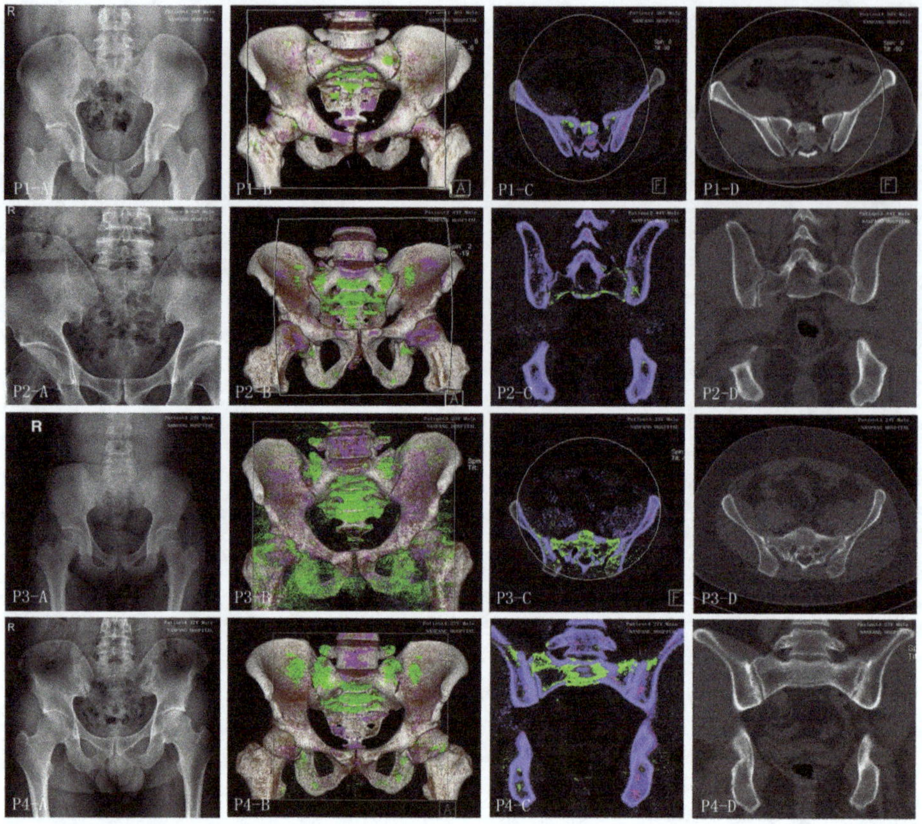

Fig. 2 Four axial spondyloarthritis (AxSpA) patients with monosodium urate (MSU) crystal and radiographic structural damage at the sacroiliac joint. For each set of images, panel **a** shows the sacroiliac joint on plain radiographs, panel **b** shows the three-dimensional reconstruction dual-energy computed tomography (DECT) images, panel **c** shows the corresponding coronal (patient 2 and 4) or axial (patient 1 and 3) DECT images, and panel **d** shows the corresponding level of computed tomography (CT) images. A large quantity of MSU crystal deposition shown as *green* was found at the sacroiliac joint or the surrounding area in the DECT images. Four male patients (patient 1–4), aged 36, 44, 23, and 27 years old, had serum uric acid levels of 407 μmol/L, 370 μmol/L, 572 μmol/L, and 464 μmol/L, respectively. They were graded with a scale of 0, 0, II, III at the *left* sacroiliac joint and 0, I, II, III at the *right* sacroiliac joint, respectively, on plain radiographs

There are several limitations of this study. First, the disease category for AxSpA includes classic AS and nr-AxSpA [1, 2]. A subgroup analysis has not been performed, due to the limited sample size. Second, structural damage grading at the sacroiliac joint was estimated by plain radiograph, according to the modified New York criteria [22]. The radiological scoring methods with CT [42, 43], which has higher density resolution and repeatability, should be applied in the structural damage assessment. Third, this study is a cross-sectional analysis. Further prospective studies would be valuable to confirm the precise contribution of MSU crystal deposition to the structural damage of the sacroiliac joints in patients with AxSpA.

Conclusions

In summary, the present study reveals that large quantities of MSU crystal deposition detected by DECT have been found in AxSpA patients without coexisting gout. In addition, it provides further evidence that the MSU crystal deposition at the sacroiliac joint in those patients has been associated with the progress of radiographic grade at sacroiliac joints, apart from AxSpA duration and BASFI score.

Abbreviations

ACR/EULAR: American College of Rheumatology and the European League Against Rheumatism; AS: ankylosing spondylitis; ASAS: Assessment of SpondyloArthritis International Society; ASDAS: Ankylosing Spondylitis Disease Activity Score; AxSpA: Axial spondyloarthritis; BASFI: Bath Ankylosing Spondylitis Functional Index; CRP: C-reactive protein; DECT: Dual-energy computed tomography; DMARDs: Disease-modifying anti-rheumatic drugs; ESR: Erythrocyte sedimentation rate; MRI: Magnetic resonance imaging; MSU: Monosodium urate; NSAIDs: Non-steroidal anti-inflammatory drugs; PGA: Patient's global assessment; SpA: Spondyloarthritis; VAS: visual analogue scale

Acknowledgements

Not applicable.

Funding
This work was supported by the President Foundation of Nanfang Hospital, Southern Medical University (No. 2016C024) and the Natural Science Foundation of China (No. 81573730). The funders had no role in study design, data collection and analysis, decision to publish, or preparation of the manuscript.

Authors' contributions
JZ designed the study, performed the statistical analyses, drafted the manuscript, and revised the manuscript. AL participated in the design of the study, helped to carry out the statistical analyses and revised the manuscript. YZ participated in the statistical analyses, finished the compiling of tables and plotting of graphs, and revised the manuscript. JX collected the clinical variables and helped with the compiling of tables. SC helped to collect the clinical variables and carry out the statistical analyses. YH helped to collect the clinical variables and produce the graphs. EJ and XX performed the plain radiographic scores as well as the DECT scan assessment for the presence and volumes of MSU crystal. JL conceived of the study, participated in the design, helped to draft the manuscript, and was accountable for all aspects of the work. All authors read and approved the final manuscript.

Competing interests
The authors declare that they have no competing interests.

Author details
[1]Department of Rheumatology, Nanfang Hospital, Southern Medical University, Guangzhou, Guangdong 510515, China. [2]Department of Internal Medicine of Traditional Chinese Medicine, College of Traditional Chinese Medicine, Southern Medical University, Guangzhou, Guangdong 510510, China. [3]Department of Obstetrics, Guangdong Women and Children Hospital, Guangzhou, Guangdong 511400, China. [4]Department of Radiology, Nanfang Hospital, Southern Medical University, Guangzhou, Guangdong 510515, China.

References

1. Rudwaleit M, van der Heijde D, Landewe R, Listing J, Akkoc N, Brandt J, Braun J, Chou CT, Collantes-Estevez E, Dougados M, Huang F, Gu J, Khan MA, Kirazli Y, Maksymowych WP, Mielants H, Sorensen IJ, Ozgocmen S, Roussou E, Valle-Onate R, Weber U, Wei J, Sieper J. The development of Assessment of SpondyloArthritis international Society classification criteria for axial spondyloarthritis (part II): validation and final selection. Ann Rheum Dis. 2009;68:777–83.
2. Rudwaleit M, Landewe R, van der Heijde D, Listing J, Brandt J, Braun J, Burgos-Vargas R, Collantes-Estevez E, Davis J, Dijkmans B, Dougados M, Emery P, van der Horst-Bruinsma IE, Inman R, Khan MA, Leirisalo-Repo M, van der Linden S, Maksymowych WP, Mielants H, Olivieri I, Sturrock R, de Vlam K, Sieper J. The development of Assessment of SpondyloArthritis international Society classification criteria for axial spondyloarthritis (part I): classification of paper patients by expert opinion including uncertainty appraisal. Ann Rheum Dis. 2009;68:770–6.
3. Bakland G, Nossent HC. Epidemiology of spondyloarthritis: A review. Curr Rheumatol Rep. 2013;15:351.
4. Exarchou S, Lie E, Lindstrom U, Askling J, Forsblad-d'Elia H, Turesson C, Kristensen LE, Jacobsson LT. Mortality in ankylosing spondylitis: results from a nationwide population-based study. Ann Rheum Dis. 2016;75:1466–72.
5. Smith JA. Update on ankylosing spondylitis: current concepts in pathogenesis. Curr Allergy Asthma Rep. 2015;15:489.
6. Itulescu TC, Alexandrescu C, Voinea LM. Ocular involvement in spondylarthritis–new mechanisms, new therapies. Oftalmologia. 2014;58:27–35.
7. Dundar U, Cevik H, Demirdal US, Toktas H. Use of rituximab to treat a patient with coexistence of rheumatoid arthritis and ankylosing spondylitis: 18 months follow-up. Int J Rheum Dis. 2014. doi:10.1111/1756-185X.12303.
8. Borman P, Ayhan F, Okumus M. Coexistence of rheumatoid arthritis and ankylosing spondylitis. Clin Rheumatol. 2011;30:1517–8.
9. Ho HH, Yu KH, Chen JY, Lin JL, Wu YJ, Luo SF, Liou LB. Coexisting ankylosing spondylitis and gouty arthritis. Clin Rheumatol. 2007;26:1655–61.
10. Lourbopoulos A, Ioannidis P, Boura E, Antoniadis D, Karacostas D, Grigoriadis N. Coexistence of multiple sclerosis and ankylosing spondylitis: report of two cases. Eur Neurol. 2013;70:149–54.
11. Borman P, Tuncay F, Koybasi M, Ergun U, Inan L. Coexistence of ankylosing spondylitis and multiple sclerosis. Acta Neurol Belg. 2011;111:340–3.
12. Singh S, Sonkar GK, Singh U. Coexistence of ankylosing spondylitis and systemic lupus erythematosus. J Chin Med Assoc. 2010;73:260–1.
13. Gran JT. An epidemiological survey of the signs and symptoms of ankylosing spondylitis. Clin Rheumatol. 1985;4:161–9.
14. Abraham Z, Gluck Z. Acute gout of the right sacroiliac joint. J Dermatol. 1997;24:781–3.
15. Kwan BY, Osman S, Barra L. Spinal gout in a young patient with involvement of thoracic, lumbar and sacroiliac regions. Joint Bone Spine. 2013;80:667–8.
16. Konatalapalli RM, Demarco PJ, Jelinek JS, Murphey M, Gibson M, Jennings B, Weinstein A. Gout in the axial skeleton. J Rheumatol. 2009;36:609–13.
17. Glazebrook KN, Guimaraes LS, Murthy NS, Black DF, Bongartz T, Manek NJ, Leng S, Fletcher JG, McCollough CH. Identification of intraarticular and periarticular uric acid crystals with dual-energy CT: initial evaluation. Radiology. 2011;261:516–24.
18. Ogdie A, Taylor WJ, Weatherall M, Fransen J, Jansen TL, Neogi T, Schumacher HR, Dalbeth N. Imaging modalities for the classification of gout: systematic literature review and meta-analysis. Ann Rheum Dis. 2015; 74:1868–74.
19. Dalbeth N, House ME, Aati O, Tan P, Franklin C, Horne A, Gamble GD, Stamp LK, Doyle AJ, McQueen FM. Urate crystal deposition in asymptomatic hyperuricaemia and symptomatic gout: a dual energy CT study. Ann Rheum Dis. 2015;74:908–11.
20. Andres M, Quintanilla MA, Sivera F, Sanchez-Paya J, Pascual E, Vela P, Ruiz-Nodar JM. Silent monosodium urate crystals deposits associate with severe coronary calcification in asymptomatic hyperuricemia: "an exploratory study". Arthritis Rheumatol. 2016;68:1531–9.
21. Wallace SL, Robinson H, Masi AT, Decker JL, McCarty DJ, Yu TF. Preliminary criteria for the classification of the acute arthritis of primary gout. Arthritis Rheum. 1977;20:895–900.
22. van der Linden S, Valkenburg HA, Cats A. Evaluation of diagnostic criteria for ankylosing spondylitis. A proposal for modification of the New York criteria. Arthritis Rheum. 1984;27:361–8.
23. Dalbeth N, Aati O, Kalluru R, Gamble GD, Horne A, Doyle AJ, McQueen FM. Relationship between structural joint damage and urate deposition in gout: a plain radiography and dual-energy CT study. Ann Rheum Dis. 2015;74: 1030–6.
24. van der Heijde D, Lie E, Kvien TK, Sieper J, Van den Bosch F, Listing J, Braun J, Landewe R. ASDAS, a highly discriminatory ASAS-endorsed disease activity score in patients with ankylosing spondylitis. Ann Rheum Dis. 2009; 68:1811–8.
25. Machado P, Landewe R, Lie E, Kvien TK, Braun J, Baker D, van der Heijde D. Ankylosing Spondylitis Disease Activity Score (ASDAS): defining cut-off values for disease activity states and improvement scores. Ann Rheum Dis. 2011;70:47–53.
26. Calin A, Garrett S, Whitelock H, Kennedy LG, O'Hea J, Mallorie P, Jenkinson T. A new approach to defining functional ability in ankylosing spondylitis: the development of the Bath Ankylosing Spondylitis Functional Index. J Rheumatol. 1994;21:2281–5.
27. Rajan A, Aati O, Kalluru R, Gamble GD, Horne A, Doyle AJ, McQueen FM, Dalbeth N. Lack of change in urate deposition by dual-energy computed tomography among clinically stable patients with long-standing tophaceous gout: a prospective longitudinal study. Arthritis Res Ther. 2013; 15:R160.
28. Braun J, Baraliakos X, Kiltz U, Heldmann F, Sieper J. Classification and diagnosis of axial spondyloarthritis–what is the clinically relevant difference? J Rheumatol. 2015;42:31–8.
29. Yu KH, Luo SF. Younger age of onset of gout in Taiwan. Rheumatology (Oxford). 2003;42:166–70.
30. Will R, Calin A, Kirwan J. Increasing age at presentation for patients with ankylosing spondylitis. Ann Rheum Dis. 1992;51:340–2.
31 Neogi T, Jansen TLTA, Dalbeth N, Fransen J, Schumacher HR, Berendsen D, Brown M, Choi H, Edwards NL, Janssens HJEM, Lioté F, Naden RP, Nuki G, Ogdie A, Perez-Ruiz F, Saag K, Singh JA, Sundy JS, Tausche A, Vaquez-

Mellado J, Yarows SA, Taylor WJ. 2015 Gout classification criteria: an American College of Rheumatology/European League Against Rheumatism collaborative initiative. Ann Rheum Dis. 2015;74:1789–98.
32 Petsch C, Araujo EG, Englbrecht M, Bayat S, Cavallaro A, Hueber AJ, Lell M, Schett G, Manger B, Rech J. Prevalence of monosodium urate deposits in a population of rheumatoid arthritis patients with hyperuricemia. Semin Arthritis Rheum. 2016;45:663–8.
33 Chhana A, Lee G, Dalbeth N. Factors influencing the crystallization of monosodium urate: a systematic literature review. BMC Musculoskelet Disord. 2015;16:296.
34 Dougados M, Demattei C, van den Berg R, Hoang VV, Thevenin F, Reijnierse M, Loeuille D, Feydy A, Claudepierre P, van der Heijde D. Rate and predisposing factors of sacroiliac radiographic progression after a 2 years follow-up period in recent onset spondyloarthritis. Arthritis Rheumatol. 2016;68:1904–13.
35 Poddubnyy D, Rudwaleit M, Haibel H, Listing J, Marker-Hermann E, Zeidler H, Braun J, Sieper J. Rates and predictors of radiographic sacroiliitis progression over 2 years in patients with axial spondyloarthritis. Ann Rheum Dis. 2011;70:1369–74.
36 Blachier M, Canoui-Poitrine F, Dougados M, Lethuaut A, Fautrel B, Ferkal S, Le Corvoisier P, Farrenq V, Poulain C, Ghaleh B, Bastuji-Garin S, Claudepierre P. Factors associated with radiographic lesions in early axial spondyloarthritis. Results from the DESIR cohort. Rheumatology (Oxford). 2013;52:1686–93.
37 Chhana A, Callon KE, Pool B, Naot D, Watson M, Gamble GD, McQueen FM, Cornish J, Dalbeth N. Monosodium urate monohydrate crystals inhibit osteoblast viability and function: implications for development of bone erosion in gout. Ann Rheum Dis. 2011;70:1684–91.
38 McGonagle D, Wakefield RJ, Tan AL, D'Agostino MA, Toumi H, Hayashi K, Emery P, Benjamin M. Distinct topography of erosion and new bone formation in achilles tendon enthesitis: implications for understanding the link between inflammation and bone formation in spondylarthritis. Arthritis Rheum. 2008;58:2694–9.
39 Jacques P, Lambrecht S, Verheugen E, Pauwels E, Kollias G, Armaka M, Verhoye M, Van der Linden A, Achten R, Lories RJ, Elewaut D. Proof of concept: enthesitis and new bone formation in spondyloarthritis are driven by mechanical strain and stromal cells. Ann Rheum Dis. 2014;73:437–45.
40 Punzi L, Scanu A, Ramonda R, Oliviero F. Gout as autoinflammatory disease: new mechanisms for more appropriated treatment targets. Autoimmun Rev. 2012;12:66–71.
41 Hreggvidsdottir HS, Noordenbos T, Baeten DL. Inflammatory pathways in spondyloarthritis. Mol Immunol. 2014;57:28–37.
42 Ozgocmen S, Ardicoglu O, Kaya A. The relationship of clinical and laboratory measurements to two different radiological scoring methods in ankylosing spondylitis. J Back Musculoskelet Rehabil. 2000;15:37–40.
43 Taylor HG, Wardle T, Beswick EJ, Dawes PT. The relationship of clinical and laboratory measurements to radiological change in ankylosing spondylitis. Br J Rheumatol. 1991;30:330–5.

7

MRI evidence of structural changes in the sacroiliac joints of patients with non-radiographic axial spondyloarthritis even in the absence of MRI inflammation

Walter P. Maksymowych[1*], Stephanie Wichuk[1], Maxime Dougados[2], Heather Jones[3], Annette Szumski[4], Jack F. Bukowski[3], Lisa Marshall[3] and Robert G. Lambert[5]

Abstract

Background: Studies have shown that structural lesions may be present in patients with non-radiographic axial spondyloarthritis (nr-axSpA). However, the relevance of structural lesions in these patients is unclear, particularly without signs of inflammation on magnetic resonance imaging (MRI). We assessed the presence of structural lesions at baseline on MRI in the sacroiliac joints (SIJ) of patients with nr-axSpA with and without SIJ inflammation on MRI.

Methods: Bone marrow edema (BME) was assessed on short tau inversion recovery (STIR) scans from 185 patients with nr-axSpA, by two independent readers at baseline using the Spondyloarthritis Research Consortium of Canada (SPARCC) score. Structural lesions were evaluated on T1 weighted spin echo scans, with readers blinded to STIR scans, using the SPARCC MRI SIJ structural score. Disease characteristics and structural lesions were compared in patients with SIJ BME (score ≥2) and without SIJ BME (score <2).

Results: Both SIJ BME and structural lesions scores were available for 183 patients; 128/183 (69.9%) patients had SIJ BME scores ≥2 and 55/183 (30.1%) had scores <2. Frequencies of MRI structural lesions in patients with vs without SIJ BME were: erosions (45.3% vs 10.9%, $P < 0.001$), backfill (20.3% vs 0%, $P < 0.001$), fat metaplasia (10.9% vs 1.8%, $P = 0.04$), and ankylosis (2.3% vs 1.8%, $P =$ ns). Significantly more patients with both SIJ BME and structural lesions were male and/or HLA-B27 positive than patients with only SIJ BME. Mean (SD) spinal scores (23 discovertebral units) were significantly higher in patients with SIJ structural lesions than without: 6.5 (11.5) vs 3.3 (5.1), respectively, $P = 0.01$.

Conclusions: In patients with nr-axSpA, SIJ structural lesions, particularly erosions, may be present on MRI when radiographs are normal or inconclusive, even in patients negative for MRI SIJ inflammation. They may reflect more severe disease with greater spinal inflammation.

Keywords: Non-radiographic axial spondyloarthritis, Magnetic resonance imaging, Sacroiliac joint, Structural lesion

* Correspondence: Walter.Maksymowych@ualberta.ca
[1]Department of Medicine, University of Alberta, 568 Heritage Medical Research Building, Edmonton, AB T6G 2S2, Canada
Full list of author information is available at the end of the article

Background

Treatment of axial spondyloarthritis (axSpA) is increasingly aimed at intervention early in the disease course before radiographic sacroiliitis has appeared and when response to treatment is greatest. Thus, magnetic resonance imaging (MRI) is an important tool for the diagnosis of SpA because it can identify inflammation prior to the detection of radiographic changes [1–5].

The Assessment of SpondyloArthritis international Society (ASAS) classification system for axSpA is based on whether patients meet clinical criteria or imaging criteria [6–8]. Patients who meet the ASAS criteria for axSpA and do not meet the modified New York criteria for radiographic sacroiliitis are considered to have non-radiographic axSpA (nr-axSpA). According to the ASAS classification criteria, bone marrow edema (BME)/osteitis on MRI is a requirement for patients with nr-axSpA who meet the criteria via the MRI arm [8]. However, this may also occur nonspecifically, and some patients with nr-axSpA do not have MRI evidence of inflammation [1, 2].

Recent studies have described several structural lesions on MRI in the sacroiliac joints (SIJ) [9–11]. Erosion is considered present when there is a breach in the cortical bone of either the iliac or sacral bones, which appears dark on both T1 weighted spin echo (T1WSE) and short tau inversion recovery (STIR) sequences, together with loss of the bright signal from adjacent marrow matrix on T1WSE MRI [12]. The T1WSE MRI sequence may also reveal a lesion in bone marrow adjacent to subchondral bone characterized by a homogeneous increase in marrow signal, indicative of accumulation of lipid, and a distinct border [10]. The histopathologic nature of this lesion remains unclear; while it may reflect adipose tissue, it may also reflect lipid accumulation in various cell types, which can occur during the course of differentiation into different phenotypes. Because it has now been shown that this lesion indicates tissue transformation following resolution of BME, it has been termed fat metaplasia [9, 13]. Recent work has shown that similar tissue develops at sites of erosion following resolution of inflammation; this has been termed "backfill" [9]. Standardized definitions for these diverse lesions have recently been developed and validated together with a semi-quantitative scoring method that assesses each individual lesion [10].

Although limited studies have demonstrated that structural lesions may already be evident in non-radiographic SpA defined according to physician expert opinion [1, 2], the majority of these patients had concomitant BME. Thus, it is unclear to what degree these diverse lesions are relevant in patients classified according to ASAS criteria, particularly in the absence of MRI inflammation, such as patients who meet the clinical but not the imaging arm of the criteria. We therefore aimed to assess the relative frequency of structural and inflammatory lesions as seen on MRI in the SIJ of patients with nr-axSpA. We also compared the disease characteristics and severity in patients with and without MRI SIJ structural lesions, anticipating that these lesions might reflect a more severe phenotype of disease.

Methods

Details of the EMBARK study (ClinicalTrials.gov identifier: NCT01258738), a phase IIIb, 104-week clinical study, have been published previously [14, 15]. Briefly, patients had axSpA per the ASAS classification criteria, were aged 18–49 years, had symptoms for >3 months and <5 years, Bath Ankylosing Spondylitis Disease Activity Index (BASDAI) score ≥4, and had an inadequate response to ≥2 nonsteroidal anti-inflammatory drugs (NSAIDs). Patients were excluded if they met the modified New York criteria for radiographic axSpA or if they had ever received a tumor necrosis factor (TNF) inhibitor for a condition other than inflammatory bowel disease. Patients met either the ASAS imaging criteria (sacroiliitis on imaging and ≥1 SpA feature) or the clinical criteria (human leukocyte antigen (HLA)-B27 positive and ≥2 other SpA features). Patients were randomized to double-blind etanercept 50 mg/week or placebo for 12 weeks, and then all patients were switched to etanercept for the remainder of the study [14]. For this report, both treatment arms were pooled and only baseline data are presented.

The study was conducted in accordance with the International Conference on Harmonisation guidelines for Good Clinical Practice and the ethical principles of the Declaration of Helsinki. Written informed consent was obtained from all patients prior to enrollment. The institutional review board or independent ethics committee at each participating center reviewed and approved all consent forms and the study protocol (see "Acknowledgments" for details).

This was a post-hoc cross-sectional analysis of patients with baseline lesion scores. The primary analysis was assessment of the presence of structural lesions on MRI in patients with SIJ BME (score ≥2) versus without SIJ BME (score <2). Sensitivity analysis was performed by evaluating the presence of structural lesions in patients who were ASAS MRI positive versus negative.

Evaluation of BME of the SIJ and spine

Two independent central readers, blinded to treatment and patient characteristics, assessed STIR scans of the SIJ and spine for BME using the Spondyloarthritis Research Consortium of Canada (SPARCC) scores [16–18]. For all assessments, the mean score of the two readers was used [14]. An adjudicator reviewed MRI scans with pre-specified reader discrepancies, and in these cases, the mean of all three readers' scores was used. The pre-specified reader discrepancies are provided in Additional file 1: Table S1. Spinal BME was evaluated using the 23-discovertebral unit (DVU) score, which ranges from 0 to 414. This scoring system assesses all 23 vertebral units of the spine from vertebrae C2/3 to L5/S1 [18]. A score ≥2 for SIJ BME was considered positive MRI evidence of inflammation, as reported previously [19]. This cutoff has been validated in the literature [20].

Evaluation of structural lesions

Two different readers (who developed the SPARCC scoring method), scored structural lesions using the SPARCC MRI SIJ structural score (SSS), which assesses fat metaplasia, erosion, backfill, and ankylosis on T1WSE MRI [10]. The readers were independent and blinded to patient characteristics, treatment, and the corresponding STIR scan. Figure 1 shows an example of erosion at baseline on T1WSE MRI in a case that was negative on STIR MRI.

The two readers scored the presence of lesions dichotomously (yes/no) in SIJ quadrants for erosion and fat metaplasia and in SIJ halves for backfill and ankylosis using a data entry system based on a diagram of the SIJ [10]. Five consecutive semi-coronal slices were evaluated beginning with the transitional slice and scrolling anteriorly. The transitional slice was defined as the first cartilaginous slice with a visible section of the ligamentous joint when assessed anteriorly to posteriorly [10]. Erosion and fat metaplasia each received a score of 0–8 per slice for five slices, for a total score of 0–40. Backfill and ankylosis each received a score of 0–4 per slice for five slices, for a total score of 0–20. A SPARCC SSS >0 was required from both readers for identification of a structural lesion of erosion, backfill, fat metaplasia, or ankylosis.

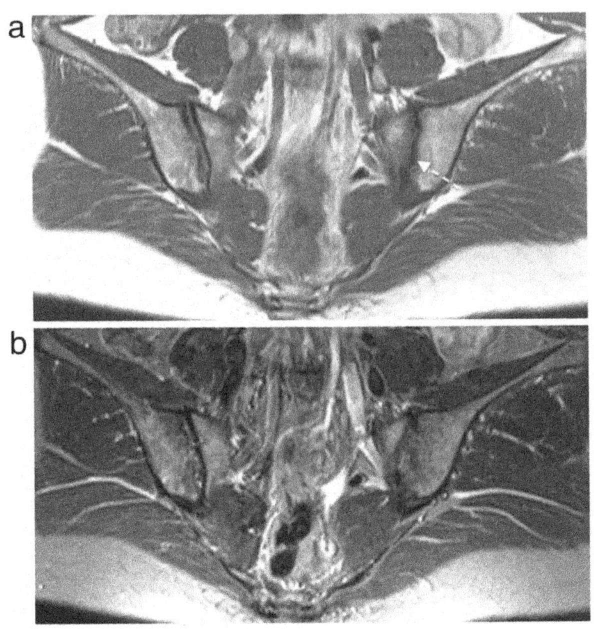

Fig. 1 Erosion of the left iliac bone on T1 weighted spin echo magnetic resonance imaging (MRI) (**a**) and in the absence of inflammation on short tau inversion recovery MRI (**b**)

Structural lesions seen on T1WSE MRI: standardized definitions

This study used standardized definitions of structural lesions of the SIJ on MRI, which were developed by the Canada-Denmark MRI Working Group and then extended in a subsequent report to include backfill [9, 10, 12]. These definitions are provided below. See Additional file 2 for images of the lesion types on T1WSE MRI.

- Erosion: on T1WSE is the full-thickness loss of the dark appearance of iliac or sacral cortical bone at its anticipated location as well as loss of the normal bright appearance of adjacent bone marrow.
- Backfill: on T1WSE is the complete loss of iliac or sacral cortical bone at its anticipated location as well as increased signal clearly demarcated from adjacent normal marrow by dark signal with irregular contour reflecting sclerosis at the border of the eroded bone.
- Fat metaplasia: increased signal on T1WSE sequences. To be scored in the SPARCC SSS method, there must be homogeneous signal across the lesion, and it must extend >1 cm in depth from the joint surface.
- Ankylosis: bone marrow signal on T1WSE between the sacral and iliac bone marrow with a full-thickness loss of the dark appearance of the iliac and sacral cortical bone.

Statistical analysis

Proportions of patients with lesions scored >0 (i.e. with any lesions or specific lesions) were determined according to the presence or absence of SIJ BME (primary strata) and according to ASAS MRI positive and negative status (secondary strata); differences in proportions were tested using Cochran-Mantel-Haenszel (CMH) tests. The presence of SIJ BME and structural lesions was evaluated according to the radiographic grade of sacroiliitis using CMH tests. Differences in demographics and baseline disease characteristics, including 23-DVU spinal score, were analyzed by presence or absence of any SSS lesions (>0 or =0) overall and separately by presence or absence of SIJ BME (≥2 or <2). Each type of structural lesion was evaluated in this manner as well. These analyses were performed using analysis of variance, the chi-square test, or the Wilcoxon-Mann-Whitney test.

Cumulative probability plots were derived to compare the SSS lesion scores of specific structural lesions according to the presence or absence of SIJ BME. These data were also analyzed using simple descriptive statistics with one-way analysis of variance and the Wilcoxon-Mann-Whitney test to test for differences in SIJ BME subgroups. Inter-observer intra-class correlation coefficients (ICC) were determined for structural lesion scores to evaluate scoring consistency between the two MRI readers. Additionally, the proportion of patients with individual lesion scores >0 was compared between two different definitions: scores from both readers were >0, and the score from at least one reader was >0. Spearman correlation was tested to analyze the relationship between continuous spinal inflammation, i.e. the 23-DVU spinal score, and continuous patient characteristics, i.e. age and symptom duration, and between continuous spinal inflammation and continuous structural lesions. Multivariate stepwise regression analysis was used to determine whether age, gender, symptom duration, presence/absence of SIJ BME, or presence of specific structural lesions was significantly associated with the 23-DVU spinal score.

Results

Patients

MRI scans at baseline were available for 185 patients. The mean (standard deviation (SD)) age was 32.0 (7.8) years; 60.5% were male, and the mean (SD) duration of disease symptoms was 2.4 (1.8) years. A total of 133/182 (71.9%) patients were HLA-B27 positive and 152/185 (82.2%) met the ASAS MRI imaging criteria.

A total of 77/185 (41.6%) patients had ≥1 structural lesion on MRI comprising erosion (65/185, 35.1%), backfill (26/185, 14.1%), fat metaplasia (15/185, 8.1%), and ankylosis (4/185, 2.2%). SIJ BME data were available for 183 patients; 128/183 (69.9%) patients had SIJ BME and 55/183 (30.1%) did not. Of the patients with SIJ BME, 69/128 (53.9%) had a structural lesion on MRI, compared with 7/55 (12.7%) patients without SIJ BME ($P < 0.001$). Relative frequencies of MRI structural lesions in patients with versus without SIJ BME were: erosion (58/128, 45.3% vs 6/55, 10.9%; $P < 0.001$), backfill (26/128, 20.3% vs 0/55, 0%; $P < 0.001$), fat metaplasia (14/128, 10.9% vs 1/55, 1.8%; $P = 0.04$), and ankylosis (3/128, 2.3% vs 1/55, 1.8%; P = nonsignificant (ns)) (Fig. 2).

Of the patients who were ASAS MRI positive, 69/152 (45.4%) had a structural lesion on MRI, compared with 8/33 (24.2%) who were ASAS MRI negative ($P = 0.03$). For ASAS MRI positive versus negative patients, relative frequencies of structural lesions were: erosion (58/152, 38.2% vs 7/33, 21.2%; P = ns), backfill (23/152, 15.1% vs

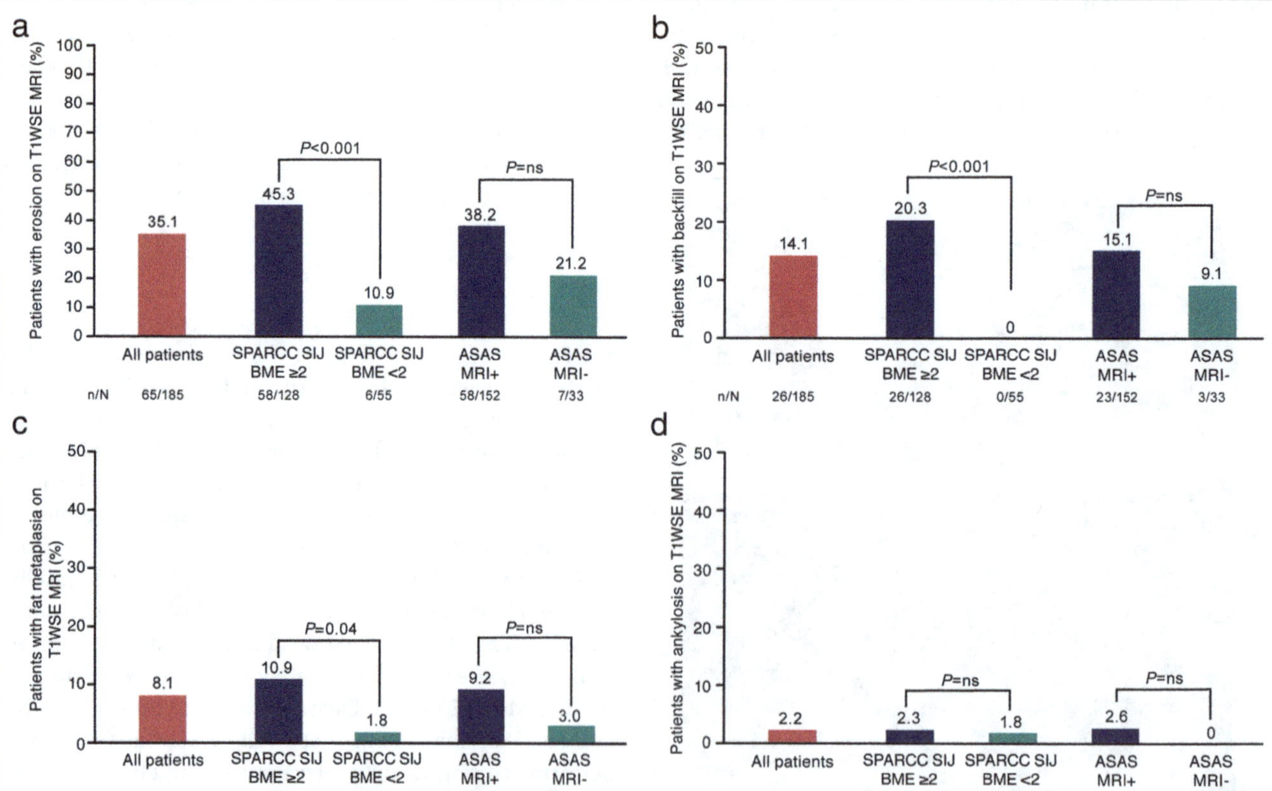

Fig. 2 Proportion of patients with erosion (**a**), backfill (**b**), fat metaplasia (**c**), and ankylosis (**d**) on T1 weighted spin echo (*T1WSE*) magnetic resonance imaging (*MRI*). *ns* nonsignificant, *SPARCC* Spondyloarthritis Research Consortium of Canada, *SIJ*, sacroiliac joint, *BME* bone marrow edema, *ASAS* Assessment of SpondyloArthritis international Society

3/33, 9.1%; P = ns), fat metaplasia (14/152, 9.2% vs 1/33, 3.0%; P = ns), and ankylosis (4/152, 2.6% vs 0/33, 0%; P = ns) (Fig. 2).

A comparison of the demographics and baseline disease characteristics between patients with the presence (SSS >0) or absence (SSS = 0) of any structural lesion according to those with and without SIJ BME is provided in Table 1. The percentage of male patients was significantly higher in the group with both SIJ BME and structural lesions (82.6% male) than in the group with only SIJ BME (47.5%, P < 0.001). Additionally, age was significantly lower in the group with both SIJ BME and structural lesions (30.3 years) compared to the group with only SIJ BME (33.5 years, P = 0.01). Symptom duration was similar across the groups. More patients were HLA-B27-positive who had both SIJ BME and structural lesions (87.0%) than those with only SIJ BME (62.7%, P = 0.002). Mean BASDAI and mean BASFI were significantly higher in the group with SIJ BME and no structural lesions (6.4 cm and 4.6 cm, respectively) than in the group with both SIJ BME and structural lesions (5.7 cm and 3.7 cm, P = 0.03 and 0.04, respectively). For the patients without SIJ BME, the small sample size of only seven patients in the SSS >0 category precluded interpretation of this subgroup.

When characterized according to the presence or absence of structural lesions in the SIJ, mean (SD) 23-DVU spinal scores were higher overall in those patients with structural lesions in the SIJ: 6.5 (11.5) vs 3.3 (5.1), respectively, P = 0.01. Similar differences in demographic and baseline disease characteristics were also observed when comparisons were made according to the presence or absence of individual structural lesions, with more male patients, higher B27 positivity, and greater spinal inflammation, especially in patients with erosion or backfill (Table 2).

The cumulative probability plots demonstrate visually that the structural lesions of erosion, backfill, and fat metaplasia occurred to a greater extent in patients with than without SIJ BME (Fig. 3), which is confirmed by the significant differences in these SIJ BME subgroups in the Wilcoxon-Mann-Whitney tests (see Additional file 1: Table S2). For ankylosis, there was little difference between the patients with and without SIJ BME. The mean (SD) and median (Q1, Q3) SPARCC SSS

Table 1 Demographics and baseline disease characteristics according to the presence or absence of SIJ inflammation and structural lesions

	SPARCC SIJ BME ≥2 (N = 128)			SPARCC SIJ BME <2 (N = 55)			Total (N = 183)		
	SSS >0 n = 69	SSS = 0 n = 59	P value	SSS >0 n = 7	SSS = 0 n = 48	P value	SSS >0 n = 76	SSS = 0 n = 107	P value
Age, years*	30.3 (6.8)	33.5 (7.7)	0.01	33.9 (11.9)	32.6 (8.5)	0.73	30.6 (7.3)	33.1 (8.0)	0.04
Male, n (%)†	57 (82.6)	28 (47.5)	<0.001	3 (42.9)	22 (45.8)	1.0	60 (79.0)	50 (46.7)	<0.001
BMI, kg/m²*	24.5 (3.6)	25.2 (4.6)	0.34	25.3 (5.6)	25.4 (5.2)	0.96	24.6 (3.8)	25.3 (4.9)	0.29
Symptom duration, years*	2.5 (2.2)	2.7 (1.4)	0.47	2.6 (1.5)	1.9 (1.4)	0.22	2.5 (2.2)	2.4 (1.4)	0.64
HLA-B27 positive, n (%)‡	60 (87.0)	37 (62.7)	0.002	6 (85.7)	29 (60.4)	0.40	66 (86.8)	66 (61.7)	<0.001
Anterior uveitis, n (%)‡	7 (10.1)	6 (10.2)	1.0	0	1 (2.1)	1.0	7 (9.2)	7 (6.5)	0.58
IBD, n (%)‡	0	0	1.0	0	1 (2.1)	1.0	0	1 (0.9)	1.0
PsO, n (%)‡	8 (11.6)	10 (17.0)	0.45	0	5 (10.4)	1.0	8 (10.5)	15 (14.0)	0.51
PsO family history, n (%)‡	4 (5.8)	1 (1.7)	0.38	0	3 (6.3)	1.0	4 (5.3)	4 (3.7)	0.72
ASDAS-CRP	3.1 (1.1)	3.1 (0.9)	0.98	2.3 (1.2)	2.8 (0.8)	0.11	3.0 (1.1)	3.0 (0.9)	0.85
CRP, mg/l	7.7 (9.6)	7.6 (14.7)	0.96	5.3 (9.3)	5.0 (7.0)	0.93	7.5 (9.6)	6.4 (11.9)	0.53
BASDAI, 0–10	5.7 (2.0)	6.4 (1.6)	0.03	4.5 (2.3)	6.0 (1.6)	0.03	5.6 (2.0)	6.2 (1.6)	0.02
BASFI, 0–10 cm VAS	3.7 (2.5)	4.6 (2.6)	0.04	3.0 (1.4)	3.9 (2.2)	0.30	3.6 (2.5)	4.3 (2.4)	0.07
BASMI, 0–10	1.0 (1.2)	1.4 (1.5)	0.14	1.2 (0.9)	1.4 (1.4)	0.72	1.1 (1.2)	1.4 (1.4)	0.10
SPARCC spine score, 23-DVU, 0–414	6.9 (11.9)	4.0 (5.8)	0.10	2.5 (3.9)	2.5 (3.9)	0.99	6.5 (11.5)	3.3 (5.1)	0.01
SPARCC spine score, 23-DVU 0–414, median§	2.0	1.5	0.39	1.0	0.8	0.85	2.0	1.5	0.12

Values are mean (standard deviation) unless stated otherwise. P values are from one-way analysis of variance (ANOVA) with treatment as factor, unless stated otherwise. *ASDAS-CRP* Ankylosing Spondylitis Disease Activity Score based on C-reactive protein, *BASDAI* Bath Ankylosing Spondylitis Disease Activity Index, *BASFI* Bath Ankylosing Spondylitis Functional Index, *BASMI* Bath Ankylosing Spondylitis Metrology Index, *BME* bone marrow edema, *BMI* body mass index, *CRP* C-reactive protein, *DVU* discovertebral units, *HLA* human leukocyte antigen, *IBD* inflammatory bowel disease, *PsO* psoriasis, *SIJ* sacroiliac joint, *SSS* SIJ structural score, *VAS* visual analog scale

*P values calculated using one-way ANOVA comparing means between groups

†P values from the chi-square test

‡P values from Fisher's exact test (two-tailed)

§ P value from the Wilcoxon-Mann-Whitney test

Table 2 Demographics and baseline disease characteristics according to baseline SIJ inflammation and structural lesions

	SPARCC SIJ BME	Erosion		Backfill		Fat metaplasia		Ankylosis	
	≥2 *n* = 128	>0 *n* = 58	0 *n* = 70	>0 *n* = 26	0 *n* = 102	>0 *n* = 14	0 *n* = 114	>0 *n* = 3	0 *n* = 125
	<2 *n* = 55	>0 *n* = 6	0 *n* = 49	>0 *n* = 0	0 *n* = 55	>0 *n* = 1	0 *n* = 54	>0 *n* = 1	0 *n* = 54
Age, years	≥2	30.0 (6.1)	33.2 (8.0)	28.9 (6.9)	32.5 (7.3)	32.3 (7.6)	31.7 (7.3)	26.3 (1.2)	31.9 (7.4)
	<2	35.3 (12.4)	32.4 (8.4)	—	32.7 (8.8)	40.0	32.6 (8.9)	25.0	32.9 (8.9)
Male, *n* (%)	≥2	51 (87.9)	34 (48.6)	21 (80.8)	64 (62.8)	12 (85.7)	73 (64.0)	3 (100)	82 (65.6)
	<2	3 (50.0)	22 (44.9)	—	25 (45.5)	1 (100)	24 (44.4)	0	25 (46.3)
BMI, kg/m^2	≥2	24.6 (3.5)	25.1 (4.5)	24.7 (3.8)	24.9 (4.2)	25.1 (3.1)	24.8 (4.2)	25.9 (4.9)	24.8 (4.1)
	<2	26.7 (4.8)	25.3 (5.3)	—	25.4 (5.2)	30.1	25.4 (5.3)	17.3	25.6 (5.2)
Symptom duration, years	≥2	2.5 (2.3)	2.7 (1.5)	3.0 (2.9)	2.5 (1.5)	3.2 (1.7)	2.5 (1.9)	4.0 (1.2)	2.5 (1.9)
	<2	2.4 (1.5)	2.0 (1.4)	—	2.0 (1.4)	0.3	2.0 (1.4)	4.0	2.0 (1.4)
HLA-B27 positive, *n* (%)	≥2	50 (86.2)	47 (67.1)	25 (96.2)	72 (70.6)	12 (85.7)	85 (74.6)	3 (100)	94 (75.2)
	<2	5 (83.3)	30 (61.2)	—	35 (63.6)	1 (100)	34 (63.0)	1 (100)	34 (63.0)
Anterior uveitis, *n* (%)	≥2	5 (8.6)	8 (11.4)	1 (3.9)	12 (11.8)	2 (14.3)	11 (9.7)	1 (33.3)	12 (9.6)
	<2	0	1 (2.0)	—	1 (1.8)	0	1 (1.9)	0	1 (1.9)
IBD, *n* (%)	≥2	0	0	0	0	0	0	0	0
	<2	0	1 (2.0)	—	1 (1.8)	0	1 (1.9)	0	1 (1.9)
PsO, *n* (%)	≥2	6 (10.3)	12 (17.1)	2 (7.7)	16 (15.7)	3 (21.4)	15 (13.2)	0	18 (14.4)
	<2	0	5 (10.2)	—	5 (9.1)	0	3 (5.6)	0	5 (9.3)
PsO family history, *n* (%)	≥2	4 (6.9)	1 (1.4)	0	5 (4.9)	1 (7.1)	4 (3.5)	0	5 (4.0)
	<2	0	3 (6.1)	—	3 (5.5)	0	3 (5.6)	0	3 (5.6)
ASDAS-CRP	≥2	3.0 (1.1)	3.1 (0.9)	3.2 (1.1)	3.0 (1.0)	2.7 (0.7)	3.1 (1.0)	3.1 (0.1)	3.1 (1.0)
	<2	2.4 (1.3)	2.8 (0.8)	—	2.8 (0.9)	0.7	2.8 (0.8)	1.8	2.8 (0.9)
CRP, mg/l	≥2	7.6 (9.7)	7.7 (13.9)	8.6 (9.5)	7.4 (12.8)	4.0 (4.1)	8.1 (12.8)	2.8 (2.2)	7.7 (12.3)
	<2	5.8 (10.0)	4.9 (7.0)	—	5.0 (7.2)	1.3	5.1 (7.3)	2.2	5.1 (7.3)
BASDAI, 0–10	≥2	5.6 (2.0)	6.4 (1.7)	5.9 (2.3)	6.1 (1.7)	5.4 (1.9)	6.1 (1.8)	6.8 (1.2)	6.0 (1.9)
	<2	4.7 (2.5)	5.9 (1.6)	—	5.8 (1.7)	0.4	5.9 (1.6)	3.5	5.8 (1.7)
BASFI, 0–10 cm VAS	≥2	3.6 (2.6)	4.5 (2.5)	3.7 (2.8)	4.2 (2.5)	3.6 (2.0)	4.2 (2.6)	4.5 (0.7)	4.1 (2.6)
	<2	3.0 (1.6)	3.9 (2.2)	—	3.8 (2.1)	0.5	3.8 (2.1)	2.9	3.8 (2.2)
BASMI, 0–10	≥2	1.1 (1.3)	1.3 (1.4)	1.1 (1.5)	1.2 (1.3)	0.9 (1.1)	1.3 (1.4)	1.3 (2.2)	1.2 (1.3)
	<2	1.2 (1.0)	1.4 (1.3)	—	1.3 (1.3)	0	1.4 (1.3)	1.3	1.3 (1.3)
SPARCC spine score, 23-DVU, 0–414	≥2	7.5 (12.8)	4.0 (5.7)	9.1 (16.1)	4.6 (7.1)	5.6 (7.7)	5.5 (9.9)	11.7 (14.9)	5.4 (9.6)
	<2	2.8 (4.2)	2.5 (3.9)	—	2.5 (3.9)	3.5	2.5 (3.9)	1.0	2.5 (3.9)

Values are mean (standard deviation) unless stated otherwise. *ASDAS-CRP* Ankylosing Spondylitis Disease Activity Score based on C-reactive protein, *BASDAI* Bath Ankylosing Spondylitis Disease Activity Index, *BASFI* Bath Ankylosing Spondylitis Functional Index, *BASMI* Bath Ankylosing Spondylitis Metrology Index, *BME* bone marrow edema, *BMI* body mass index, *CRP* C-reactive protein, *DVU* discovertebral units, *HLA* human leukocyte antigen, *IBD* inflammatory bowel disease, *PsO* psoriasis, *SIJ* sacroiliac joint, *SPARCC* Spondyloarthritis Research Consortium of Canada, *VAS* visual analog scale

values for the individual structural lesions according to the presence or absence of SIJ BME are provided in Additional file 1: Table S2.

MRI structural lesions and SIJ BME according to radiographic grade

An analysis of the presence of SIJ BME and structural lesions according to radiographic grade did not identify a linear relationship between these measurements. However, the frequency of MRI structural lesions was greatest in those patients with radiographic unilateral grade 1 and contralateral grade 2 changes in the SIJ (Table 3).

A univariate analysis of the relationship between 23-DVU spinal score and select dichotomous patient characteristics, including structural lesions, determined that male patients and patients with SIJ BME had significantly higher 23-DVU spinal scores (see Additional file 1: Table S3). According to Spearman correlation, 23-DVU spinal score did not correlate with age, symptom duration, or individual structural lesions when evaluated as continuous risk factors (Spearman correlation −0.006 to 0.128). Multivariate

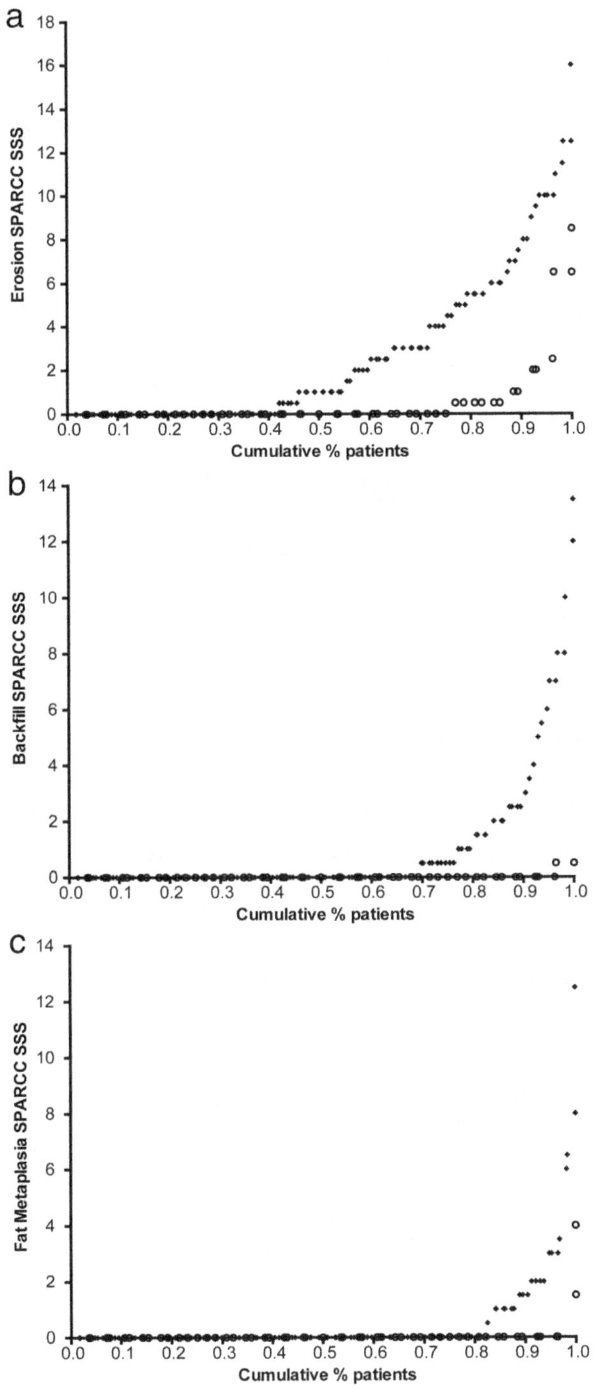

Fig. 3 Cumulative probability plots for structural lesions according to Spondyloarthritis Research Consortium of Canada (*SPARCC*) sacroiliac joint (*SIJ*) score (≥2 vs <2): erosion (**a**), backfill (**b**), and fat metaplasia (**c**)

stepwise regression analysis indicated that male sex and the presence of backfill are the best set of significant factors associated with 23-DVU spinal score; parameter estimates (SE): male sex: 2.8 (1.2), $P = 0.02$; backfill: 4.4 (1.7), $P = 0.01$.

Additional file 1: Table S4 presents the proportion of patients with individual lesion scores >0, according to two different definitions: at least one reader scored >0, and both readers scored >0. The table demonstrates that, as expected, the number of patients with structural lesions was somewhat higher using the first definition. The inter-observer ICC for structural lesions shows that, overall, there was little variation in the interpretations of the two readers (see Additional file 1: Table S5).

Discussion

The results of this study demonstrate that structural lesions on MRI, particularly erosions, may occur in nr-axSpA when radiographs are normal or inconclusive, and even in the absence of SIJ BME on MRI. Additionally, mean 23-DVU spinal scores were higher in patients with SIJ structural lesions than without. On analysis of the patient demographics, in the group with SIJ BME, most patients with SIJ structural lesions were male and most were HLA-B27 positive. These data support the concept that nr-axSpA is an early stage of axSpA and that structural lesions in the SIJ are associated with a more severe phenotype characterized by more active spinal inflammation.

Prospective analysis will be necessary to determine whether assessment of these MRI structural lesions is of prognostic significance for the development of spinal ankylosis, which has much greater clinical significance than in the SIJ. Resolution of inflammation in erosions becomes evident on T1-weighted MRI scans by the appearance of a new lesion that fills the cavity in excavated bone [21]. This tissue is called "backfill" and is brighter than normal marrow on T1-weighted MRI. With further tissue remodeling, ankylosis may then develop at the site of backfill [9], at which point the backfill is no longer evident, as bright marrow traverses the joint space from the iliac to the sacral bones. Similar tissue that is brighter than normal marrow on T1-weighted MRI may be observed in subchondral bone marrow, especially following resolution of BME, and has been termed fat metaplasia [10]. It has been proposed that this tissue in subchondral bone and at erosions may reflect a reparative phenotype associated with an increased propensity toward ankylosis. A preliminary report suggests that the presence of fat metaplasia in the SIJ predicts development of spinal ankylosis [22], which would support this hypothesis.

In addition, the presence of structural lesions in the SIJ may reflect a more severe disease phenotype with progression to involve the spine, as recorded in our data by the higher 23-DVU spinal scores. It has been suggested that there is a window of opportunity for disease modification with anti-inflammatory agents by

Table 3 MRI inflammatory and structural lesions according to radiographic grading of sacroiliitis

Radiographic grade	MRI inflammation	MRI structural lesion				
	SPARCC SIJ BME ≥ 2	SSS > 0	Erosion > 0	Fat Metaplasia > 0	Backfill > 0	Ankylosis > 0
Bilateral grade 0	23/37 (62.2)	11/38 (28.9)	10/38 (26.3)	2/38 (5.3)	3/38 (7.9)	0/38 (0)
Unilateral grade 1	25/40 (62.5)	10/41 (24.4)	10/41 (24.4)	2/41 (4.9)	2/41 (4.9)	0/41 (0)
Unilateral grade 2	6/6 (100)	2/6 (33.3)	1/6 (16.7)	0/6 (0)	2/6 (33.3)	0/6 (0)
Bilateral grade 1	28/41 (68.3)	15/41 (36.6)	9/41 (22.0)	0/41 (0)	5/41 (12.2)	2/41 (4.9)
Unilateral grade 1 and contralateral grade 2	46/59 (78.0)	39/59 (66.1)	35/59 (59.3)	11/59 (18.6)	14/59 (23.7)	2/59 (3.4)
P value*	0.16	<0.001	<0.001	0.008	0.03	0.45

Values are *n/N* (%). *BME* bone marrow edema, *MRI* magnetic resonance imaging, *SIJ* sacroiliac joint, *SPARCC* Spondyloarthritis Research Consortium of Canada, *SSS* sacroiliac joint structural score
*Cochran-Mantel-Haenszel test *P* value for general association

treating acute inflammatory lesions before bone formation pathways are triggered in more complex inflammatory lesions [23]. Consequently, the presence of structural lesions in the SIJ may help select patients for intervention with anti-TNF agents early in the disease course.

The analysis comparing SIJ BME and structural lesions with radiographic grade did not identify a linear relationship between these measurements, although the highest frequency of MRI structural lesions was observed in those cases with radiographic grade 1 and contralateral grade 2. MRI SIJ structural lesions occurred frequently in patients with normal SIJs on radiographs, reflecting the greater sensitivity of MRI over radiography for identification of structural lesions as well as inflammation.

There are several limitations to this study. One is the interpretation of the T1WSE MRI scans. The results of the inter-observer ICC analysis for the readings suggest that the scores provided by each reader were very similar. However, due to the complexities of scoring erosions and backfill on T1WSE MRI scans, it is necessary to use caution when interpreting the results. Erosion may be difficult to discern on T1WSE MRI because it requires loss of dark signal signifying a breach of cortical bone. Backfill is a heterogeneous lesion on T1WSE MRI, which requires both irregular dark signal signifying sclerotic bone together with bright signal medial to this signifying fat metaplasia. It is important to be clear that the study was not designed to draw conclusions on the diagnostic utility of structural lesions, because the population was selected for active disease and there were no controls. Further validation using computed tomography would be helpful for the understanding of both lesions.

Conclusions

This study demonstrated that in patients with nr-axSpA, structural lesions, particularly erosions, may be present on MRI of the SIJ when radiographs are normal or inconclusive. Although structural lesions were more likely in patients with MRI SIJ BME, they were also present in the absence of MRI SIJ BME. Patients with structural lesions are more likely to be male, HLA-B27 positive, and have higher 23-DVU spinal scores. Prospective data are necessary to understand the prognostic implications associated with these lesions and the impact of treatment.

Additional files

Additional file 1: Table S1. Pre-specified cases adjudicated by a blinded third reader. **Table S2.** SPARCC SSS for lesions, according to SIJ BME. **Table S3.** Univariate analysis of relationship between spinal inflammation and select patient characteristics at baseline. **Table S4.** Proportion of patients with SPARCC SSS lesions >0, according to two different definitions. **Table S5.** Inter-observer intra-class correlation coefficients for structural lesions.

Additional file 2: Lesions seen on T1 weighted spin echo MRI.

Abbreviations

ASAS: Assessment of SpondyloArthritis international Society; axSpA: Axial spondyloarthritis; BASDAI: Bath Ankylosing Spondylitis Disease Activity Index; BASFI: Bath Ankylosing Spondylitis Functional Index; BASMI: Bath Ankylosing Spondylitis Metrology Index; BME: Bone marrow edema; BMI: Body mass index; CMH: Cochran-Mantel-Haenszel; DVU: Discovertebral unit; HLA: Human leukocyte antigen; IBD: Inflammatory bowel disease; ICC: Intra-class correlation coefficient; MRI: Magnetic resonance imaging; nr-axSpA: Non-radiographic axSpA; ns: Nonsignificant; NSAIDs: Nonsteroidal anti-inflammatory drugs; PsO: Psoriasis; SD: Standard deviation; SIJ: Sacroiliac joint; SPARCC: Spondyloarthritis Research Consortium of Canada; SSS: Sacroiliac joint structural score; STIR: Short tau inversion recovery; T1WSE: T1 weighted spin echo; TNF: Tumor necrosis factor

Acknowledgements

We wish to thank all patients who participated in this study and the investigators and medical staff at all of the participating centers. Editorial/medical writing support was provided by Jennica Lewis, PharmD, CMPP of Engage Scientific Solutions and was funded by Pfizer. The specific ethical bodies that approved the EMBARK study are as follows: Argentina - Comite de Etica en Investigacion Clinica (CEIC), Ciudad Autónoma de Buenos Aires; Belgium - Ethisch Comite Universitair Ziekenhuis Gent; Colombia - Comité de Ética en Investigaciones del Oriente, Bucaramanga, Santander; Comite de ética en Investigación de Servimed E.U, Bucaramanga, Santander; Comite de etica de investigación-Riesgo de Fractura S.A, Bogota, Cundinamarca; Czech Republic - Eticka komise Praha; Finland - Medisiininen Eettinen Toimikunta HUS Konsernihallinto Tutkimuseettiset Toimikunnat, Helsinki; France - CPP Ile-de-France V, Hôpital Saint-Antoine, Paris; Germany - Ethik-Kommission des Landes Sachsen-Anhalt, Dessau-Rosslau; Hungary - Egeszsegugyi Tudomanyos Tanacs Klinikai Farmakologiai Etikai Bizottsaga, Budapest; Republic of Korea - Hanyang University Hospital IRB, Seoul; Chonnam National University Hospital Institutional Review Board, Gwangju; Gachon University Gil Hospital IRB, Incheon; Netherlands - Academisch Medisch Centrum Medisch Ethische Commissie, Amsterdam; Russian Federation - Ethics Committee, Leningrad Regional Clinical Hospital, St. Petersburg; Ethics Council at the Ministry of Healthcare of Russian Federation, Moscow; Ethics Committee at Saint-Petersburg State Budgetary Healthcare Institution, St. Petersburg; Ethics Committee, Rheumatology Research Institute of Russian Academy of Medical Sciences, Moscow; Spain - Comité Coordinador de Ética de la Investigación Biomédica de Andalucía Consejeria de Salud, Sevilla; Taiwan - Kaohsiung Medical University Chung-Ho Memorial Hospital, Institutional Review Board, Kaohsiung; Chung Shan Medical University Hospital Institutional Review Board, Taichung; Taipei Veterans General Hospital Institutional Review Board, Taipei; United Kingdom - National Research Ethics Service, NRES Committee East Midlands, Nottingham.

Funding
This study was funded by Pfizer. Editorial/medical writing support was provided by Jennica Lewis, PharmD, CMPP of Engage Scientific Solutions and was funded by Pfizer.

Availability of data and materials
Pfizer's policies on the provision of clinical trial data are set out on our website: http://www.pfizer.com/research/clinical_trials/trial_data_and_results. In addition to posting clinical trial results on the clinicaltrials.gov registry, Pfizer provides secure access to anonymized patient-level data to qualified researchers in response to scientifically valid research proposals. Further detail can be found at: http://www.pfizer.com/research/clinical_trials/trial_data_and_results/data_requests. Pfizer makes patient-level data available for globally conducted interventional trials in patients that complete after September 27, 2007, or initiated on or before that date and still ongoing as of December 26, 2007, and all such trials initiated after January 2014. Data are made available for trials of authorized medicines/indications, or terminated medicines, two years after clinical trial completion (defined as last subject last visit). Pfizer's practices adhere to the principles for responsible data sharing laid out by the European Federation of Pharmaceutical Industries and Associations (EFPIA) and the Pharmaceutical Research and Manufacturers of America (PhRMA): http://phrma.org/sites/default/files/pdf/PhRMAPrinciplesForResponsibleClinicalTrialDataSharing.pdf.

Authors' contributions
WPM, HJ, AS, JFB, and RGL made substantial contributions to the conception or design of the study. WPM, SW, MD, HJ, AS, JFB, LM, and RGL made substantial contributions to the acquisition, analysis and interpretation of data from the study. AS conducted the statistical analyses. WPM contributed to drafting the manuscript, and WPM, SW, MD, HJ, AS, JFB, LM, and RGL contributed to revising it critically for important intellectual content. All authors read and approved the final manuscript, and all authors agree to be accountable for all aspects of the work.

Authors' information
Not applicable.

Competing interests
WPM has received consulting fees from AbbVie, Amgen, Lilly, Janssen, Pfizer, Sanofi, and UCB, and is the chief medical officer of CaRE Arthritis Ltd. MD is a consultant for and has received research funding/grants from AbbVie, Lilly, Merck, Pfizer, Sanofi, and UCB. HJ, LM, and JFB are employees of, and own stock in Pfizer. AS is an employee of inVentiv Health and was contracted by Pfizer to provide statistical support for the development of this paper. SW and RGL declare that they have no competing interests. No nonfinancial conflict of interest exists for any author.

Author details
[1]Department of Medicine, University of Alberta, 568 Heritage Medical Research Building, Edmonton, AB T6G 2S2, Canada. [2]Paris Descartes University; Department of Rheumatology – Hôpital Cochin, Assistance Publique – Hôpitaux de Paris; INSERM (U1153): Clinical Epidemiology and Biostatistics, PRES Sorbonne Paris-Cité, Paris, France. [3]Pfizer, Collegeville, PA, USA. [4]inVentiv Health, Princeton, NJ, USA. [5]Department of Radiology and Diagnostic Imaging, University of Alberta, Edmonton, AB, Canada.

References
1. Weber U, Lambert RGW, Østergaard M, Hodler J, Pedersen SJ, Maksymowych WP. The diagnostic utility of magnetic resonance imaging in spondylarthritis: an international multicenter evaluation of one hundred eighty-seven subjects. Arthritis Rheum. 2010;62:3048–58.
2. van den Berg R, de Hooge M, van Gaalen F, Reijnierse M, Huizinga T, van der Heijde D. Percentage of patients with spondyloarthritis in patients referred because of chronic back pain and performance of classification criteria: experience from the Spondyloarthritis Caught Early (SPACE) cohort. Rheumatology. 2013;52:1492–9 [Erratum in: Rheumatology. 2015;54:1336].
3. Oostveen J, Prevo R, den Boer J, van de Laar M. Early detection of sacroiliitis on magnetic resonance imaging and subsequent development of sacroiliitis on plain radiography. A prospective, longitudinal study. J Rheumatol. 1999;26:1953–8.
4. Bennett AN, McGonagle D, O'Connor P, Hensor EMA, Sivera F, Coates LC, et al. Severity of baseline magnetic resonance imaging–evident sacroiliitis and HLA–B27 status in early inflammatory back pain predict radiographically evident ankylosing spondylitis at eight years. Arthritis Rheum. 2008;58:3413–8.
5. Heuft-Dorenbosch L, Landewé R, Weijers R, Wanders A, Houben H, van der Linden S, et al. Combining information obtained from magnetic resonance imaging and conventional radiographs to detect sacroiliitis in patients with recent onset inflammatory back pain. Ann Rheum Dis. 2006;65:804–8.
6. Sieper J, Rudwaleit M, Baraliakos X, Brandt J, Braun J, Burgos-Vargas R, et al. The Assessment of SpondyloArthritis international Society (ASAS) handbook: a guide to assess spondyloarthritis. Ann Rheum Dis. 2009;68 Suppl 2:ii1–44.
7. Rudwaleit M, Landewé R, van der Heijde D, Listing J, Brandt J, Braun J, et al. The development of Assessment of SpondyloArthritis international Society classification criteria for axial spondyloarthritis (part I): classification of paper patients by expert opinion including uncertainty appraisal. Ann Rheum Dis. 2009;68:770–6.
8. Rudwaleit M, van der Heijde D, Landewé R, Listing J, Akkoc N, Brandt J, et al. The development of Assessment of SpondyloArthritis international Society classification criteria for axial spondyloarthritis (part II): validation and final selection. Ann Rheum Dis. 2009;68:777–83.
9. Maksymowych WP, Wichuk S, Chiowchanwisawakit P, Lambert RG, Pedersen SJ. Fat metaplasia and backfill are key intermediaries in the development of sacroiliac joint ankylosis in patients with ankylosing spondylitis. Arthritis Rheum. 2014;66:2958–67.
10. Maksymowych WP, Wichuk S, Chiowchanwisawakit P, Lambert RG, Pedersen SJ. Development and preliminary validation of the Spondyloarthritis Research Consortium of Canada Magnetic Resonance Imaging Sacroiliac Joint Structural Score. J Rheumatol. 2015;42:79–86.
11. Rudwaleit M, Jurik AG, Hermann K-GA, Landewé R, van der Heijde D, Baraliakos X, et al. Defining active sacroiliitis on magnetic resonance imaging (MRI) for classification of axial spondyloarthritis: a consensual approach by the ASAS/OMERACT MRI group. Ann Rheum Dis. 2009;68:1520–7.
12. Weber U, Pedersen S, Ostergaard M, Rufibach K, Lambert R, Maksymowych W. Can erosions on MRI of the sacroiliac joints be reliably detected in patients with ankylosing spondylitis? A cross-sectional study. Arthritis Res Ther. 2012;14:R124.
13. Song I-H, Hermann KG, Haibel H, Althoff CE, Poddubnyy D, Listing J, et al. Relationship between active inflammatory lesions in the spine and sacroiliac joints and new development of chronic lesions on whole-body MRI in early axial spondyloarthritis: results of the ESTHER trial at week 48. Ann Rheum Dis. 2011;70:1257–63.
14. Dougados M, van der Heijde D, Sieper J, Braun J, Maksymowych WP, Citera G, et al. Symptomatic efficacy of etanercept and its effects on objective signs of inflammation in early nonradiographic axial spondyloarthritis: a multicenter, randomized, double-blind, placebo-controlled trial. Arthritis Rheum. 2014;66:2091–102.

15. Maksymowych WP, Dougados M, van der Heijde D, Sieper J, Braun J, Citera G, et al. Clinical and MRI responses to etanercept in early non-radiographic axial spondyloarthritis: 48-week results from the EMBARK study. Ann Rheum Dis. 2016;75:1328–35.
16. Maksymowych WP, Inman RD, Salonen D, Dhillon SS, Krishnananthan R, Stone M, et al. Spondyloarthritis Research Consortium of Canada magnetic resonance imaging index for assessment of spinal inflammation in ankylosing spondylitis. Arthritis Rheum. 2005;53:502–9.
17. Maksymowych WP, Inman RD, Salonen D, Dhillon SS, Williams M, Stone M, et al. Spondyloarthritis Research Consortium of Canada magnetic resonance imaging index for assessment of sacroiliac joint inflammation in ankylosing spondylitis. Arthritis Rheum. 2005;53:703–9.
18. Maksymowych WP, Salonen D, Inman RD, Rahman P, Lambert RGW. Low-dose infliximab (3 mg/kg) significantly reduces spinal inflammation on magnetic resonance imaging in patients with ankylosing spondylitis: a randomized placebo-controlled study. J Rheum. 2010;37:1728–34.
19. van der Heijde D, Sieper J, Maksymowych WP, Brown MA, Lambert RGW, Rathmann SS, et al. Spinal inflammation in the absence of sacroiliac joint inflammation on magnetic resonance imaging in patients with active nonradiographic axial spondyloarthritis. Arthritis Rheum. 2014;66:667–73.
20. van den Berg R, de Hooge M, Bakker PAC, van Gaalen F, Navarro-Compán V, Fagerli KM, et al. Metric properties of the SPARCC score of the sacroiliac joints — data from baseline, 3-month, and 12-month follow up in the SPACE cohort. J Rheumatol. 2015;42:1186–93.
21. Pedersen SJ, Wichuk S, Chiowchanwisawakit P, Lambert RG, Maksymowych WP. Tumor necrosis factor inhibitor therapy but not standard therapy is associated with resolution of erosion in the sacroiliac joints of patients with axial spondyloarthritis. Arthritis Res Ther. 2014;16:R100. doi:10.1186/ar4548.
22. Maksymowych WP, Wichuk S, Chiowchanwisawakit P, Lambert RG, Pedersen SJ. Fat metaplasia in the sacroiliac joints on MRI is associated with radiographic status and progression in the spine of patients with axial spondyloarthritis. Ann Rheum Dis. 2014;73 Suppl 2:214. Abstract THU0106.
23. Maksymowych WP, Morency N, Conner-Spady B, Lambert RG. Suppression of inflammation and effects on new bone formation in ankylosing spondylitis: evidence for a window of opportunity in disease modification. Ann Rheum Dis. 2013;72:23–8.

The prevalence and clinical characteristics of nonradiographic axial spondyloarthritis among patients with inflammatory back pain in rheumatology practices

Ruben Burgos-Vargas[1], James Cheng-Chung Wei[2,3,4*], Mahboob U. Rahman[5,6], Nurullah Akkoc[7], Syed Atiqul Haq[8], Mohammed Hammoudeh[9], Ehab Mahgoub[6], Ena Singh[6], Lyndon John Llamado[10], Khalid Shirazy[11], Sameer Kotak[12], Constance Hammond[6], Ron Pedersen[6], Qi Shen[6] and Bonnie Vlahos[6]

Abstract

Background: Patients with ankylosing spondylitis (AS), who by definition have radiographic sacroiliitis, typically experience symptoms for a decade or more before being diagnosed. Yet, even patients without radiographic sacroiliitis (i.e., nonradiographic axial spondyloarthritis [nr-axSpA]) report a significant disease burden. The primary objective of this study was to estimate the prevalence and clinical characteristics of nr-axSpA among patients with inflammatory back pain (IBP) in rheumatology clinics in a number of countries across the world. A secondary objective was to estimate the prevalence of IBP among patients with chronic low back pain (CLBP).

Methods: Data were collected from 51 rheumatology outpatient clinics in 19 countries in Latin America, Africa, Europe, and Asia. As consecutive patients with CLBP ($N = 2517$) were seen by physicians at the sites, their clinical histories were evaluated to determine whether they met the new Assessment of SpondyloArthritis international Society criteria for IBP. For those who did, their available clinical history (e.g., family history, C-reactive protein [CRP] levels) was documented in a case report form to establish whether they met criteria for nr-axSpA, AS, or other IBP. Patients diagnosed with nr-axSpA or AS completed patient-reported outcome measures to assess disease activity and functional limitations.

Results: A total of 2517 patients with CLBP were identified across all sites. Of these, 974 (38.70 %) fulfilled the criteria for IBP. Among IBP patients, 29.10 % met criteria for nr-axSpA, and 53.72 % met criteria for AS. The prevalence of nr-axSpA varied significantly by region ($p < 0.05$), with the highest prevalence reported in Asia (36.46 %) and the lowest reported in Africa (16.02 %). Patients with nr-axSpA reported mean ± SD Ankylosing Spondylitis Disease Activity Scores based on erythrocyte sedimentation rate and CRP of 2.62 ± 1.17 and 2.52 ± 1.21, respectively, indicating high levels of disease activity (patients with AS reported corresponding scores of 2.97 ± 1.13 and 2.93 ± 1.18). Similarly, the overall Bath Ankylosing Spondylitis Disease Activity Index score of 4.03 ± 2.23 for patients with nr-axSpA (4.56 ± 2.17 for patients with AS) suggested suboptimal disease control.
(Continued on next page)

* Correspondence: jccwei@gmail.com
[2]Division of Allergy, Immunology and Rheumatology, Chung Shan Medical University Hospital, No. 110, Sec. 1, Jianguo N. Road, South District, Taichung City 40201, Taiwan
[3]Institute of Medicine, Chung Shan Medical University, Taichung City, Taiwan
Full list of author information is available at the end of the article

(Continued from previous page)

Conclusions: These results suggest that, in the centers that participated in the study, 29 % of patients with IBP met the criteria for nr-axSpA and 39 % of patients with CLBP had IBP. The disease burden in nr-axSpA is substantial and similar to that of AS, with both groups of patients experiencing inadequate disease control. These findings suggest the need for early detection of nr-axSpA and initiation of available treatment options to slow disease progression and improve patient well-being.

Keywords: Nonradiographic axial SpA, Ankylosing spondylitis, Prevalence, Inflammatory low back pain, Chronic low back pain

Background

Spondyloarthritis (SpA) is a constellation of chronic inflammatory conditions that includes ankylosing spondylitis (AS), reactive arthritis, enteropathic arthritis, and psoriatic arthritis, among others [1]. Collectively, the prevalence of SpA varies between 0.5 % and 2 %, making it approximately as common as rheumatoid arthritis [1]. On the basis of their clinical presentation, patients with SpA can be categorized as having axial SpA, in which the spine is predominantly affected, or peripheral SpA, in which the extremities are predominantly affected [2, 3]. According to the 2009 criteria of the Assessment of SpondyloArthritis international Society (ASAS), axial SpA is further categorized into nonradiographic axial SpA (nr-axSpA) and AS, in which the major distinguishing feature is the presence (for AS) or absence (for nr-axSpA) of radiographic sacroiliitis [2, 3].

Approximately 10 % of patients with nr-axSpA develop AS within 2 years and 60 % develop AS within 10 years [4]. Although patients with nr-axSpA may have inflammation detectable by magnetic resonance imaging [5, 6], early detection of axial SpA poses a major challenge to many physicians [2, 3]. Indeed, patients may experience symptoms for a decade or more before receiving a diagnosis [1]. Patients with axial SpA also report a number of impairments in physical functioning and spinal mobility, experience high rates of disability, and contribute to high societal costs [4]. Timely identification of axial SpA may potentially lead to earlier and more effective intervention to delay disease progression [5].

The majority of axial SpA studies have been conducted in Europe, the United States, and Mexico, with information extremely limited in the emerging countries of Latin America, Africa, Central and Eastern Europe, and Asia. The general population prevalence of axial SpA in Europe has been estimated to be between 0.08 % (France) and 0.49 % (Turkey) [6]. The prevalence is slightly higher in the Americas, with researchers in Mexico and the United States reporting rates of 0.60 % and 0.90–1.40 %, respectively [6, 7].

Many of the studies cited above have been focused on AS or axial SpA, leading to a lack of epidemiological and clinical data specific to nr-axSpA. Indeed, even the proportion of axial SpA patients with nr-axSpA is unknown, as estimates vary considerably, ranging from 23 % to 80 % in a recent review of patients with axial SpA [4]. In part, this is due to different methods of assessment and the fact that these studies were not specifically designed to follow patients with undifferentiated SpA and nr-axSpA [4].

The lack of data on nr-axSpA and AS is even more pronounced in emerging countries in Latin America, Europe, Africa, and Asia. The primary objective of this study was to provide prevalence estimates on the presence of nr-axSpA among patients with inflammatory back pain (IBP) in rheumatology clinics across a number of emerging countries. In this study, we also sought to describe the clinical characteristics associated with both nr-axSpA and AS. A secondary objective was to estimate the prevalence of IBP among patients with chronic low back pain (CLBP), given that IBP represents an increasingly important part of identifying patients with axial SpA [2, 3].

Methods

Study design

A noninterventional, cross-sectional study was conducted to estimate the prevalence of nr-axSpA among patients with IBP in 51 rheumatology outpatient clinics from 19 countries in Latin America (Colombia, Costa Rica, Mexico, and Peru), Europe inclusive of western Asia (Hungary, Israel, Kazakhstan, Poland, Romania, Russia, and Turkey), Africa (Algeria, Morocco, and South Africa), and Asia focused on southern and eastern Asia (Bangladesh, China, India, Malaysia, and Taiwan). Patient recruitment took place from January through December 2014. The protocol and study materials received institutional review board approval at each participating site; the specific sites are listed in the Acknowledgements section.

Consecutive patients with CLBP were seen by participating physicians at the study sites and were evaluated clinically to determine whether they met the criteria for IBP. Patients who met 2009 ASAS criteria for IBP had their clinical histories further evaluated to determine their eligibility for the medical record abstraction portion of this study. The inclusion criteria were age ≥18 years, CLBP ≥3 months, and four of five of the following parameters: age of onset <40 years, insidious onset, improvement with exercise, no improvement with rest, and pain at night. The exclusion criteria were noninflammatory back pain, a condition that could mimic IBP (e.g., fibromyalgia), the presence of a neuropathic component, unexplained weight loss of >10 kg within the past 6 months, persistent fever, urinary incontinence or retention, saddle anesthesia, decreased anal sphincter tone or fecal incontinence, bilateral lower extremity weakness or numbness, or progressive neurologic deficit.

For patients who met the appropriate inclusion criteria and provided written informed consent, a medical record abstraction using a case report form (CRF) was performed to determine whether the patients met the criteria for AS, nr-axSpA, or other forms of IBP ("other IBP" hereafter) based on ASAS criteria for axial SpA and the Modified New York (Modified NY) criteria for AS (Fig. 1). More specifically, patients who did not meet ASAS criteria were classified as having other IBP. Patients who met ASAS criteria for axial SpA but did not meet Modified NY criteria were classified as having nr-axSpA. Patients who met both ASAS criteria for axial SpA and Modified NY criteria were classified as having AS.

Patients who were diagnosed with AS or nr-axSpA were provided with a brief survey to evaluate their patient-reported outcomes (PROs). It is important to note that *diagnosed* refers to the physician's classification of that patient as indicated in the medical record. It is not known what information was used to make this assessment. The classification of patients based on ASAS criteria for axial SpA and Modified NY criteria for AS, as described above, was an analytical exercise performed by the authors after data collection; it was not conducted in real time as patients were enrolled into the study. As a result, the study depended upon the physician's classification (referred hereafter as *diagnosis* to distinguish the methods) in order to identify patients eligible to receive the survey, even if this differed from our methods of classification using the ASAS criteria for axial SpA and the Modified NY criteria for AS. This survey was completed entirely by the patient in the waiting room to avoid any influence from the investigator. At the end of subject recruitment, all completed materials were

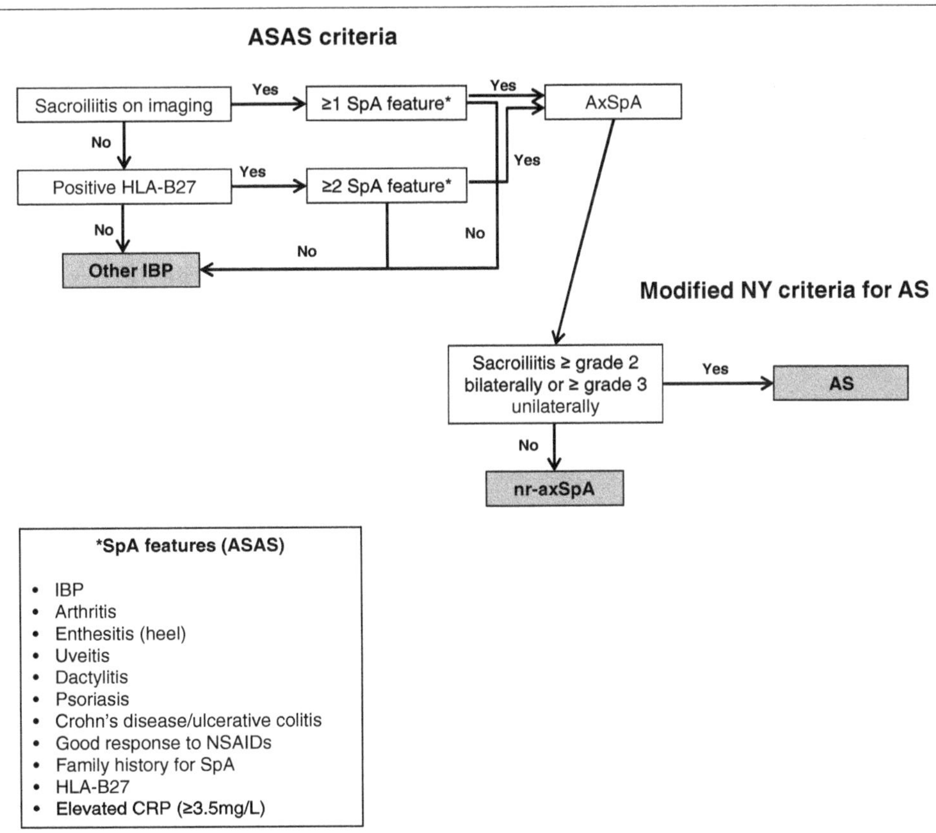

Fig. 1 Summary of inflammatory back pain (IBP) group classifications. *AS* ankylosing spondylitis, *ASAS* Assessment of SpondyloArthritis international Society, *axSpA* axial spondyloarthritis, *CRP* C-reactive protein, *HLA-B27* human leukocyte antigen B27, *Modified NY criteria* Modified New York criteria for ankylosing spondylitis, *nr-axSpA* nonradiographic axial spondyloarthritis, *NSAID* nonsteroidal anti-inflammatory drug, *SpA* spondyloarthritis

collected on-site and checked for completion, with the exception of the patient questionnaire, which remained confidential.

Measures

The CRF assessed information on each patient's demographics (age, sex, race/ethnicity), general health history (body mass index [BMI], years of experienced CLBP), and disease history (human leukocyte antigen B27 [HLA-B27] test results, C-reactive protein [CRP] results, erythrocyte sedimentation rate [ESR] results, family history, nonsteroidal anti-inflammatory drug [NSAID] response). The patient survey included the Ankylosing Spondylitis Disease Activity Score (ASDAS; both ESR and CRP versions), Bath Ankylosing Spondylitis Disease Activity Index (BASDAI), Bath Ankylosing Spondylitis Functional Index (BASFI), and Bath Ankylosing Spondylitis Metrology Index (BASMI).

Statistical analysis

The analysis of the primary objectives (prevalence and clinical characteristics of nr-axSpA) was focused on patients with IBP who met the inclusion or exclusion criteria described above. The analysis of the secondary objective (prevalence of IBP among patients with CLBP) was focused on all patients with CLBP. Frequencies, percentages, and 95 % CIs were reported for binary and/or categorical variables. Counts, means, and SDs were reported for continuous variables. Statistical differences across geographical regions were analyzed using chi-square tests and one-way analysis of variance for categorical and continuous variables, respectively.

Results

Prevalence of nr-axSpA overall, by region, and by sex

A total of 2517 patients with CLBP were identified across all sites (Fig. 2). Of these, 974 (38.70 %) fulfilled the criteria for IBP and were advanced to the CRF portion of the study for assessment of IBP group status (i.e., nr-axSpA, AS, or other IBP). Overall, 29.10 % (95 % CI 26.15–32.05 %) of patients with IBP met the criteria for nr-axSpA (Table 1). The prevalence of AS among patients with IBP was 53.72 % (95 % CI 50.48–56.96 %). The prevalence of nr-axSpA varied significantly by region ($p < 0.05$), with the highest prevalence reported in Asia (36.46 %, 95 % CI 31.64–41.28 %) and the lowest reported in Africa (16.02 %, 95 % CI 11.00–21.04 %). The prevalence of nr-axSpA was similar among males (28.74 %, 95 % CI 25.07–32.41 %) and females (29.75 %, 95 % CI 24.77–34.74 %) with IBP.

Demographic characteristics of patients with nr-axSpA

Patients with nr-axSpA had a mean age of 34.75 years (SD 10.03); 36.47 % were female, and 55.64 % were white (Table 2). These figures contrasted with patients with AS, who had a mean age of 39.03 years (SD 11.38); 28.72 % were female, and 68.23 % were white. Minimal regional differences were observed with respect to the demographic characteristics of patients with nr-axSpA (Table 3). Patients with nr-axSpA were oldest in Africa (36.67 years) and youngest in Asia (33.24 years) ($p < 0.05$); however, no differences in sex, BMI, years since CLBP presentation, or age of IBP onset were observed across regions.

Clinical characteristics of patients with nr-axSpA

Patients with nr-axSpA experienced CLBP for 6.32 ± 7.61 years (compared with 10.91 years for patients with

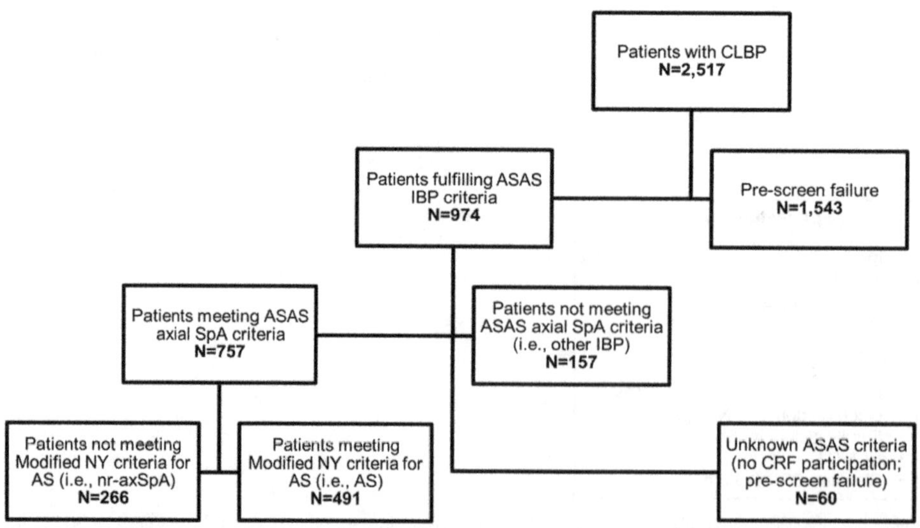

Fig. 2 Study flowchart. *AS* ankylosing spondylitis, *ASAS* Assessment of SpondyloArthritis international Society, *CLBP* chronic low back pain, *CRF* case report form, *IBP* inflammatory back pain, *Modified NY criteria* Modified New York criteria for ankylosing spondylitis, *nr-axSpA* nonradiographic axial spondyloarthritis, SpA spondyloarthritis

Table 1 Prevalence of nonradiographic axial spondyloarthritis among patients with inflammatory back pain across geographic regions

	Total	Latin America	Africa	Europe	Asia	*p* Value
Overall sample						
Number of patients	914	26	206	298	384	
nr-axSpA, *n* (%)	266 (29.10 %)	5 (19.23 %)	33 (16.02 %)	88 (29.53 %)	140 (36.46 %)	<0.001
95 % CI	(26.15–32.05)	(4.05–34.41)	(11.00–21.04)	(24.34–34.72)	(31.64–41.28)	
Among males						
Number of patients	588	12	116	204	256	
nr-axSpA, *n* (%)	169 (28.74 %)	4 (33.33 %)	18 (15.52 %)	57 (27.94 %)	90 (35.16 %)	<0.001
95 % CI	(25.07–32.41)	(6.58–60.08)	(8.91–22.13)	(21.77–34.12)	(29.29–41.02)	
Among females						
Number of patients	326	14	90	94	128	
nr-axSpA, *n* (%)	97 (29.75 %)	1 (7.14 %)	15 (16.67 %)	31 (32.98 %)	50 (39.06 %)	<0.001
95 % CI	(24.77–34.74)	(0.00–20.70)	(8.93–24.41)	(23.42–42.53)	(30.57–47.56)	

nr-axSpA nonradiographic axial spondyloarthritis
The *p* values represent the omnibus statistical comparison of percentages across geographic regions

AS) (Table 2). HLA-B27 test results were available for 71.05 % of those with nr-axSpA, and 82.78 % of them had a positive test result (Table 4). Proportions of 68.14 % and 37.30 % of patients with nr-axSpA had elevated CRP and ESR values, respectively. For context, proportions of 77.20 % and 48.92 % of patients with AS had elevated CRP and ESR values, respectively.

Several clinical characteristics varied across regions among those with nr-axSpA (Table 5). Patients in Europe were the most likely to have a positive HLA-B27 test result (84.85 %), and patients in Asia were the least likely (62.24 %) ($p < 0.05$). Patients in Asia were the most likely to have an elevated ESR value (48.89 %), and patients in Europe were the least likely (20.48 %) ($p < 0.05$). No differences in family history or NSAID response were observed.

Delay from IBP and CLBP to nr-axSpA or AS diagnosis

For patients who received a diagnosis of nr-axSpA, there was a mean delay of 5.21 ± 7.69 years between the presentation of IBP and diagnosis (Table 4). There was a mean delay of 6.48 ± 8.53 years between the presentation of IBP and diagnosis for patients with AS.

Patient-reported outcomes in nr-axSpA and AS

The mean disease activity levels for patients with nr-axSpA were 2.62 ± 1.17 and 2.52 ± 1.21 for the ESR and CRP versions of the ASDAS, respectively, suggesting a high level of disease activity (i.e., ≥2.1) (Table 6). The mean overall BASDAI score was 4.03 ± 2.32 for patients with nr-axSpA, indicating a suboptimal level of disease control. Finally, BASFI score (3.20 ± 2.47) and BASMI scores (11-point version 2.41 ± 1.54, 3-point version 1.62 ± 1.51, linear function version 3.71 ± 2.77) indicated a significant burden for patients with nr-axSpA and were relatively comparable to BASFI score (4.09 ± 2.59) and BASMI scores (11-point version 4.09 ± 2.06, 3-point version 3.40 ± 2.25, linear function version 4.77 ± 2.38) for patients with AS. No differences in PRO measures were observed across regions, with the exception of the 3-point BASMI version (Africa = 2.59 ± 1.52, Europe = 1.46 ± 1.53, Asia = 1.30 ± 1.36; $p < 0.05$).

Discussion

In this study, 39 % of patients referred to rheumatology clinics with CLBP met the ASAS criteria for IBP. Further, 29 % of patients with IBP met the criteria for nr-axSpA. The proportion of axial SpA patients with nr-axSpA was within the range (23–80 %) reported in the literature [4, 8], though on the lower end of prior estimates.

Our data suggest a higher percentage of males among patients with nr-axSpA (64 %) relative to the percentages in other published noninterventional studies (34–50 %) [9, 10] and most clinical trials (48–64 %) [11–16]. There were a number of methodological differences across these studies (e.g., inclusion and exclusion criteria, country), but it is unclear which of these factors would help to explain the differences in results. Further research is necessary.

We found that patients with nr-axSpA were the youngest, and they experienced CLBP for the shortest duration at slightly over 6 years compared with nearly 11 years for patients with AS. Although no age differences were found in past literature reviews between patients with nr-axSpA and those with AS [4, 8], several prior studies have found a longer symptom duration for patients with AS [4–8, 10, 17, 18]. This is to be

Table 2 Demographic characteristics of nonradiographic axial spondyloarthritis, ankylosing spondylitis, and other inflammatory back pain patients

	Total ($N = 914$)	nr-axSpA ($n = 266$)	AS ($n = 491$)	Other IBP ($n = 157$)	p Value
Sex					<0.001
Male, n (%)	588 (64.33 %)	169 (63.53 %)	350 (71.28 %)	69 (43.95 %)	
95 % CI	(61.22–67.44)	(57.74–69.33)	(67.27–75.29)	(36.17–51.73)	
Female, n (%)	326 (35.67 %)	97 (36.47 %)	141 (28.72 %)	88 (56.05 %)	
95 % CI	(32.56–38.78)	(30.67–42.26)	(24.71–32.73)	(48.27–63.83)	
Sex					<0.001
Male, n (row %)	588 (100.00 %)	169 (28.75 %)	350 (59.52 %)	69 (11.73 %)	
95 % CI		(25.08–32.41)	(55.54–63.50)	(9.13–14.34)	
Female, n (row %)	326 (100.00 %)	97 (29.75 %)	141 (43.25 %)	88 (26.99 %)	
95 % CI		(24.78–34.73)	(37.86–48.64)	(22.17–31.82)	
Age, years, mean ± SD	38.68 ± 12.02	34.75 ± 10.03	39.03 ± 11.38	44.26 ± 14.48	<0.001
Race/ethnicity					<0.001
White, n (%)	596 (65.21 %)	148 (55.64 %)	335 (68.23 %)	113 (71.97 %)	
95 % CI	(62.11–68.30)	(49.66–61.62)	(64.10–72.35)	(64.94–79.01)	
Asian, n (%)	116 (12.69 %)	55 (20.68 %)	55 (11.20 %)	6 (3.82 %)	
95 % CI	(10.53–14.85)	(15.80–25.55)	(8.41–14.00)	(0.82–6.83)	
Black, n (%)	12 (1.31 %)	2 (0.75 %)	2 (0.41 %)	8 (5.10 %)	
95 % CI	(0.57–2.05)	(0.00–1.79)	(0.00–0.97)	(1.65–8.54)	
Unknown, n (%)	190 (20.79 %)	61 (22.93 %)	99 (20.16 %)	30 (19.11 %)	
95 % CI	(18.15–23.42)	(17.87–27.99)	(16.61–23.72)	(12.95–25.27)	
BMI category					0.024
Underweight, n (%)	55 (6.02 %)	12 (4.51 %)	38 (7.74 %)	5 (3.18 %)	
95 % CI	(4.47–7.56)	(2.01–7.01)	(5.37–10.11)	(0.43–5.94)	
Normal weight, n (%)	455 (49.78 %)	150 (56.39 %)	236 (48.07 %)	69 (43.95 %)	
95 % CI	(46.53–53.03)	(50.42–62.36)	(43.64–52.49)	(36.17–51.73)	
Overweight, n (%)	279 (30.53 %)	78 (29.32 %)	146 (29.74 %)	55 (35.03 %)	
95 % CI	(27.53–33.52)	(23.84–34.8)	(25.68–33.79)	(27.56–42.51)	
Obese, n (%)	121 (13.24 %)	24 (9.02 %)	70 (14.26 %)	27 (17.20 %)	
95 % CI	(11.04–15.44)	(5.57–12.47)	(11.16–17.36)	(11.28–23.11)	
Unknown, n (%)	4 (0.44 %)	2 (0.75 %)	1 (0.20 %)	1 (0.64 %)	
95 % CI	(0.01–0.87)	(0.00–1.79)	(0.00–0.60)	(0.00–1.88)	
Years since CLBP presentation					<0.001
Number of patients	808	232	435	141	
Mean ± SD, years	9.09 ± 9.07	6.32 ± 7.61	10.91 ± 9.37	8.05 ± 9.10	
Age of IBP onset					<0.001
Number of patients	908	264	488	156	
Mean ± SD, years	28.8 ± 9.7	27.8 ± 7.3	27.0 ± 7.7	36.2 ± 14.2	

Abbreviations: AS ankylosing spondylitis, *BMI* body mass index, *CLBP* chronic low back pain, *CRF* case report form, *IBP* inflammatory back pain, *nr-axSpA* nonradiographic axial spondyloarthritis

Broad race categories (white vs. black vs. Asian vs. unknown) were created on the basis of physician-reported patient ethnicity: white = Indian, Indo-Aryan, Dravidian, Bengali, Arab, Iranian, white, Jewish, Azeri, Mestizo, Amerindian, Berber; black = black, mulatto, mulato, zambo, black African, colored; Asian = Han Chinese, non-Han Chinese, Taiwanese, Chinese, aborigine, Malay, indigenous, mongoloid, Asian; unknown = other or missing

The p values represent the omnibus statistical comparison of percentages (or means) across IBP groups based on the chi-square (or F-test) values

"Other IBP" refers to patients who did not meet the Assessment of SpondyloArthritis international Society classification criteria for axial spondyloarthritis

Table 3 Demographic characteristics of patients with nonradiographic axial spondyloarthritis across geographic regions

	Africa (*n* = 33)	Europe (*n* = 88)	Asia (*n* = 140)	*p* Value
Sex				0.609
Male, *n* (%)	18 (54.55 %)	57 (64.77 %)	90 (64.29 %)	
95 % CI	(37.45–71.64)	(54.73–74.82)	(56.30–72.27)	
Female (%)	15 (45.45 %)	31 (35.23 %)	50 (35.71 %)	
95 % CI	(28.36–62.55)	(25.18–45.27)	(27.73–43.70)	
Age, years mean ± SD	36.67 ± 10.73	36.02 ± 10.56	33.24 ± 9.26	0.035
BMI category				0.21
Underweight, *n* (%)	1 (3.03 %)	4 (4.55 %)	7 (5.00 %)	
95 % CI	(0.00–8.92)	(0.17–8.93)	(1.37–8.63)	
Normal weight, *n* (%)	16 (48.48 %)	51 (57.95 %)	81 (57.86 %)	
95 % CI	(31.32–65.65)	(47.57–68.34)	(49.62–66.09)	
Overweight, *n* (%)	13 (39.39 %)	19 (21.59 %)	44 (31.43 %)	
95 % CI	(22.61–56.17)	(12.94–30.24)	(23.69–39.17)	
Obese, *n* (%)	2 (6.06 %)	14 (15.91 %)	7 (5.00 %)	
95 % CI	(0.00–14.25)	(8.22–23.6)	(1.37–8.63)	
Unknown, *n* (%)	1 (3.03 %)	0 (0.00 %)	1 (0.71 %)	
95 % CI	(0.00–8.92)	–	(0.00–2.12)	
Years since CLBP presentation				0.462
Number of patients	29	74	124	
Mean ± SD, years	8.02 ± 10.01	6.68 ± 9.33	5.67 ± 5.70	
Age of IBP onset				0.115
Number of patients	33	87	139	
Mean ± SD, years	28.4 ± 8.7	28.3 ± 6.5	27.1 ± 7.3	

BMI body mass index, *CLBP* chronic low back pain
The *p* values represent the omnibus statistical comparison of percentages (or means) across regions based on the chi-square (or *F*-test) values

expected, given that nr-axSpA and AS likely represent a progression in the spectrum of the same disease.

Among patients who had been diagnosed with nr-axSpA, there was a delay of approximately 5 years between presentation of IBP and diagnosis. This finding was consistent with the study by Poddubnyy and colleagues, who which also found a gap of slightly more than 5 years between back pain and the assessment of nr-axSpA [17]. However, it should be noted that many patients who met the criteria for nr-axSpA were not diagnosed even after this period of several years, reinforcing the importance of increasing the awareness of, and adherence to, ASAS classification criteria for timely diagnosis and initiation of treatment.

Among those with HLA-B27 test results, 83 % of the patients with nr-axSpA had positive results. This finding is consistent with what was summarized by Boonen et al. [4] and reported directly in two recent noninterventional studies (73 % in a study by Poddubnyy and colleagues [11] and 86 % in a study by Kiltz and colleagues [18]. Over two-thirds (68 %) of patients with nr-axSpA had elevated CRP values (≥3.5 mg/L), which was nearly as high as the percentage of patients with AS who had elevated CRP values (77 %).

Data derived from the patient surveys demonstrated a high level of disease activity and a suboptimal level of disease control, as assessed using the ASDAS and BASDAI, respectively, for patients with nr-axSpA. It is important to note that even patients with nr-axSpA [19], who are in an earlier phase in the course of axial SpA, exhibited a significant burden that was comparable to that of patients with AS. BASDAI scores in our study were lower than those reported in a review of clinical trial results of biologic treatments [8], suggesting a less severe patient-reported burden in this real-world patient population. The levels of functional impairment (BASFI) and limitations (BASMI) were comparable to those reported for clinical trial populations [4]. Given the early age of onset for nr-axSpA, these impairment data suggest that patients can experience a substantial level of burden for many years. This further illustrates the importance of identifying patients early in order to slow disease progression.

Table 4 Clinical characteristics and HLA-B27 test results of patients with nonradiographic axial spondyloarthritis, ankylosing spondylitis, and other inflammatory back pain

	Total ($N = 914$)	nr-axSpA ($n = 266$)	AS ($n = 491$)	Other IBP ($n = 157$)	*p* Value
HLA-B27 test results (when available)					<0.001
Positive, *n* (%)	397 (72.98 %)	135 (71.43 %)	250 (82.78 %)	12 (22.64 %)	
Negative, *n* (%)	147 (27.02 %)	54 (28.57 %)	52 (17.22 %)	41 (77.36 %)	
Years from IBP to SpA diagnosis					0.747
Number of patients	179	98	27	54	
Mean ± SD, years	5.40 ± 7.98	5.21 ± 7.69	6.48 ± 8.53	5.19 ± 8.32	
Family history of SpA					<0.001
Yes, *n* (%)	220 (24.07 %)	70 (26.32 %)	132 (26.88 %)	18 (11.46 %)	
No, *n* (%)	650 (71.12 %)	180 (67.67 %)	343 (69.86 %)	127 (80.89 %)	
Results not available, *n* (%)	44 (4.81 %)	16 (6.02 %)	16 (3.26 %)	12 (7.64 %)	
Family history of SpA (excluding missing)					<0.001
Yes, *n* (%)	220 (25.29 %)	70 (28.00 %)	132 (27.79 %)	18 (12.41 %)	
No, *n* (%)	650 (74.71 %)	180 (72.00 %)	343 (72.21 %)	127 (87.59 %)	
NSAID response					0.125
Positive, *n* (%)	657 (71.88 %)	183 (68.80 %)	358 (72.91 %)	116 (73.89 %)	
Negative, *n* (%)	231 (25.27 %)	72 (27.07 %)	125 (25.46 %)	34 (21.66 %)	
Results not available, *n* (%)	26 (2.84 %)	11 (4.14 %)	8 (1.63 %)	7 (4.46 %)	
Most recent CRP value					0.146
Number of patients	767	226	421	120	
Mean ± SD, mg/L	16.7 ± 26.0	15.8 ± 28.2	18.2 ± 25.3	13.2 ± 23.5	
Most recent CRP level					<0.001
Not elevated (<3.5 mg/L), *n* (%)	219 (23.96 %)	72 (27.07 %)	96 (19.55 %)	51 (32.48 %)	
Elevated (≥3.5 mg/L), *n* (%)	548 (59.96 %)	154 (57.89 %)	325 (66.19 %)	69 (43.95 %)	
Results not available, *n* (%)	147 (16.08 %)	40 (15.04 %)	70 (14.26 %)	37 (23.57 %)	
Most recent CRP level (excluding missing)					<0.001
Not elevated (<3.5 mg/L), *n* (%)	219 (28.55 %)	72 (31.86 %)	96 (22.80 %)	51 (42.50 %)	
Elevated (≥3.5 mg/L), *n* (%)	548 (71.45 %)	154 (68.14 %)	325 (77.20 %)	69 (57.50 %)	
Most recent ESR value					0.009
Number of patients	846	252	464	130	
Mean ± SD, mm/h	29.0 ± 23.6	26.8 ± 23.9	31.2 ± 23.6	25.3 ± 22.8	
Most recent ESR level					<0.001
Not elevated (<28 mm/h), *n* (%)	482 (52.74 %)	158 (59.40 %)	237 (48.27 %)	87 (55.41 %)	
Elevated (≥28 mm/h), *n* (%)	364 (39.82 %)	94 (35.34 %)	227 (46.23 %)	43 (27.39 %)	
Results not available, *n* (%)	68 (7.44 %)	14 (5.26 %)	27 (5.50 %)	27 (17.20 %)	
Most recent ESR level (excluding missing)					<0.001
Not elevated (<28 mm/h), *n* (%)	482 (56.97 %)	158 (62.70 %)	237 (51.08 %)	87 (66.92 %)	
Elevated (≥28 mm/h), *n* (%)	364 (43.03 %)	94 (37.30 %)	227 (48.92 %)	43 (33.08 %)	

Abbreviations: AS ankylosing spondylitis, *CRP* C-reactive protein, *ESR* erythrocyte sedimentation rate, *HLA-B27* human leukocyte antigen B27, *IBP* inflammatory back pain, *nr-axSpA* nonradiographic axial spondyloarthritis, *NSAID* nonsteroidal anti-inflammatory drug, *SpA* spondyloarthritis
The *p* values represent the omnibus statistical comparison of percentages (or means) across IBP groups based on the chi-square values

Limitations

Limitations of this epidemiological study include the use of a single assessment with a questionnaire and CRF that may not adequately capture a comprehensive medical history for a particular patient. It is also important to mention that this was an observational study, so not all patients had complete information available. This could have affected the classification of patients and therefore

Table 5 Clinical characteristics and HLA-B27 test results of patients with nonradiographic axial spondyloarthritis across geographic regions

	Africa ($n = 33$)	Europe ($n = 88$)	Asia ($n = 140$)	p Value
Laboratory-confirmed SpA (HLA-B27)				0.062
Positive, n (%)	15 (45.45 %)	56 (63.64 %)	61 (43.57 %)	
Negative, n (%)	6 (18.18 %)	10 (11.36 %)	37 (26.43 %)	
Results not available, n (%)	12 (36.36 %)	22 (25.00 %)	42 (30.00 %)	
Laboratory-confirmed SpA (excluding missing) (HLA-B27)				0.019
Positive, n (%)	15 (71.43 %)	56 (84.85 %)	61 (62.24 %)	
Negative, n (%)	6 (28.57 %)	10 (15.15 %)	37 (37.76 %)	
Family history of SpA				0.231
Yes, n (%)	9 (27.27 %)	18 (20.45 %)	43 (30.71 %)	
No, n (%)	22 (66.67 %)	67 (76.14 %)	86 (61.43 %)	
Results not available, n (%)	2 (6.06 %)	3 (3.41 %)	11 (7.86 %)	
Family history of SpA (excluding missing)				0.125
Yes, n (%)	9 (29.03 %)	18 (21.18 %)	43 (33.33 %)	
No, n (%)	22 (70.97 %)	67 (78.82 %)	86 (66.67 %)	
NSAID response				0.264
Positive, n (%)	22 (66.67 %)	64 (72.73 %)	93 (66.43 %)	
Negative, n (%)	7 (21.21 %)	22 (25.00 %)	42 (30.00 %)	
Results not available, n (%)	4 (12.12 %)	2 (2.27 %)	5 (3.57 %)	
Most recent CRP level				0.214
Not elevated (<3.5 mg/L), n (%)	10 (30.30 %)	21 (23.86 %)	37 (26.43 %)	
Elevated (≥3.5 mg/L), n (%)	18 (54.55 %)	55 (62.50 %)	80 (57.14 %)	
Results not available, n (%)	5 (15.15 %)	12 (13.64 %)	23 (16.43 %)	
Most recent CRP level (excluding missing)				0.104
Not elevated (<3.5 mg/L), n (%)	10 (35.71 %)	21 (27.63 %)	37 (31.62 %)	
Elevated (≥3.5 mg/L), n (%)	18 (64.29 %)	55 (72.37 %)	80 (68.38 %)	
Most recent ESR level				<0.001
Not elevated (<28 mm/h), n (%)	20 (60.61 %)	66 (75.00 %)	69 (49.29 %)	
Elevated (≥28 mm/h), n (%)	9 (27.27 %)	17 (19.32 %)	66 (47.14 %)	
Results not available, n (%)	4 (12.12 %)	5 (5.68 %)	5 (3.57 %)	
Most recent ESR level (excluding missing)				<0.001
Not elevated (<28 mm/h), n (%)	20 (68.97 %)	66 (79.52 %)	69 (51.11 %)	
Elevated (≥28 mm/h), n (%)	9 (31.03 %)	17 (20.48 %)	66 (48.89 %)	

Abbreviations: CRP C-reactive protein, *ESR* erythrocyte sedimentation rate, *HLA-B27* human leukocyte antigen B27, *NSAID* nonsteroidal anti-inflammatory drug, *SpA* spondyloarthritis

The p values represent the omnibus statistical comparison of percentages (or means) across regions based on the chi-square values

the prevalence estimates. For example, because a positive HLA-B27 test is one way to classify a patient as having nr-axSpA instead of other IBP, missing HLA-B27 data would underestimate the number of nr-axSpA patients relative to other IBP patients. Another limitation was the lack of available information on the other IBP group. Although this group also had poor outcomes based on the PRO data, the explanation for this finding is unclear without knowing more about the composition of the other IBP group. Patient surveys were administered only to patients who were diagnosed with AS and nr-axSpA, so patients who were not diagnosed with either condition, even if they met the appropriate classification criteria, did not provide PRO data. The external validity of the study is dependent on the extent to which patients at the selected rheumatology practices are representative of all IBP patients in these countries. Because these sites were selected for being major centers for the treatment of SpA, it is possible the patients who are managed by these sites are fundamentally different (e.g., more severe disease).

Table 6 Clinical outcomes and patient-reported outcome measures for patients with nonradiographic axial spondyloarthritis, ankylosing spondylitis, and other inflammatory back pain

	Total (*N* = 686)	nr-axSpA (*N* = 188)	AS (*N* = 413)	Other IBP (*N* = 85)	*p* Value
ASDAS score (ESR)					0.003
Number of patients	619	167	378	74	
Mean ± SD	2.87 ± 1.14	2.62 ± 1.17	2.97 ± 1.13	2.92 ± 1.01	
ASDAS score (CRP)					0.002
Number of patients	559	149	346	64	
Mean ± SD	2.81 ± 1.19	2.52 ± 1.21	2.93 ± 1.18	2.81 ± 1.17	
BASDAI					0.010
Number of patients	681	186	412	83	
Mean ± SD	4.44 ± 2.24	4.03 ± 2.32	4.56 ± 2.17	4.77 ± 2.29	
BASFI					<0.001
Number of patients	683	187	411	85	
Mean ± SD	4.09 ± 2.59	3.20 ± 2.47	4.43 ± 2.57	4.38 ± 2.49	
BASMI (11-point)					<0.001
Number of patients	575	154	353	68	
Mean ± SD	3.55 ± 2.03	2.41 ± 1.54	4.09 ± 2.06	3.33 ± 1.75	
BASMI (3-point)					<0.001
Number of patients	564	146	347	71	
Mean ± SD	2.83 ± 2.19	1.62 ± 1.51	3.40 ± 2.25	2.52 ± 2.03	
BASMI (linear function)					<0.001
Number of patients	686	188	413	85	
Mean ± SD	4.44 ± 2.55	3.71 ± 2.77	4.77 ± 2.38	4.47 ± 2.50	

Abbreviation: AS ankylosing spondylitis, *ASDAS* Ankylosing Spondylitis Disease Activity Score, *BASDAI* Bath Ankylosing Spondylitis Disease Activity Index, *BASFI* Bath Ankylosing Spondylitis Functional Index, *BASMI* Bath Ankylosing Spondylitis Metrology Index, *CRP* C-reactive protein, *ESR* erythrocyte sedimentation rate, *IBP* inflammatory back pain, *nr-axSpA* nonradiographic axial spondyloarthritis

The *p* values represent the omnibus statistical comparison of percentages (or means) across IBP groups based on the *F*-test values

Conclusions

The results of the present study suggest that approximately one-third of patients with IBP meet ASAS criteria for nr-axSpA. Patients with nr-axSpA, as compared with patients with AS, tend to be younger and experience symptoms for a shorter time before diagnosis. The PRO data suggest that the overall disease burden in nr-axSpA is substantial and similar to that in AS, with both groups of patients experiencing inadequate disease control. These findings show the continued need for early diagnosis of nr-axSpA across Latin America, Europe, Africa, and Asia. These findings also emphasize the importance of early initiation of available treatment options to slow disease progression and improve patient well-being in these patients' most productive years of life.

Abbreviations

AS, ankylosing spondylitis; ASAS, Assessment of SpondyloArthritis international Society; ASDAS, Ankylosing Spondylitis Disease Activity Score; BASDAI, Bath Ankylosing Spondylitis Disease Activity Index; BASFI, Bath Ankylosing Spondylitis Functional Index; BASMI, Bath Ankylosing Spondylitis Metrology Index; BMI, body mass index; CLBP, chronic low back pain; CRF, case report form; CRP, C-reactive protein; ESR, erythrocyte sedimentation rate; HLA-B27, human leukocyte antigen B27; IBP, inflammatory back pain; Modified NY criteria, Modified New York criteria for ankylosing spondylitis; nr-axSpA, nonradiographic axial spondyloarthritis; NSAID, nonsteroidal anti-inflammatory drug; PRO, patient-reported outcome; SpA, spondyloarthritis95 % CI

Acknowledgements

The authors acknowledge the contributions of the various principal investigators at each site who assisted with the data collection: Drs. Bao, Wang, and Wu (China); Dr. Tsai (Taiwan); Drs. Hussein and Lay (Malaysia); Drs. Islam and Rahman (Bangladesh); Drs. Pulukool, Rajshekhar, Sarkar, and Mouli (India); Drs. Itzhak and Levi (Israel); Drs. Kenar, Ozbek, and Karabulut (Turkey); Drs. Ancuta and Opris (Romania); Drs. Elonakov, Kamalova, Lapshina, Dubinina, and Savinkova (Russia); Drs. Świerkot, Chlebicki, Klama, Krezelok, and Zielinski (Poland); Drs. Széntó, Geher, Keszthelyi, Nagy, and Varga (Hungary); Dr. Tleukulov (Kazakhstan); Drs. Casasola, Flores, Ureña, Fajardo, Martinez (Mexico); Drs. Coto and Mendez (Costa Rica); Dr. Parra (Colombia); Dr. Rojo (Peru); Drs. Djoudi, Ladjouze, Dahou, Benzaoui, and Boudersa (Algeria); Drs. Najia, Toufik, Imane, and Radouane (Morocco); and Drs. Reuter and Plooy (South Africa).

The authors also acknowledge the various institutional review boards and ethics committees of the participating institutions: Shanghai Changhai Hospital Ethics Committee (China), Chung Shan Medical Hospital (Taiwan), Kaohsiung Medical University (Taiwan), Chung-Ho Memorial Hospital (Taiwan), Medical Research & Ethics Committee (Malaysia), Bangabandhu Sheikh Mujib Medical University (Bangladesh), Christian Medical College (India), Nizam's Institute of Medical Sciences (India), Institutional Ethics Committee of Human Research at Medical College (India), KIMS Foundation and Research Center (India), Bnai Zion Medical Center (Israel), Meir Medical Center (Israel), Dokuz Eylul University (Turkey), Warsaw University of Medicine (Poland), University of Szeged Albert Szent-Gyorgyi Clinical Center (Hungary),

Creimed (Colombia), Institutional Ethics Committee of the University of San Martin de Porres (Peru), Ethics Committee for Biomedical Research (Central Ethics Committee of Morocco), National Commission for Personal Data Protection (Central Ethics Committee of Morocco), Medicines Control Council (Central Ethics Committee of South Africa), and Human Research Ethics Committee of Wits Donald Gordon Medical Hospital (South Africa).
The authors also acknowledge Valérie Auclair, PhD, Hélène Kuyas, Xavier Guillaume, MS, MBA, and Geneviève Bonnelye, MS, for their contributions to the study design and data collection, as well as Marco DiBonaventura, PhD, who oversaw the statistical analysis and contributed to the interpretation of the data. Dr. Auclair, Ms. Kuyas, Mr. Guillaume, Ms. Bonnelye, and Dr. DiBonaventura were all full-time employees of Kantar Health at the time of the study, which received funding from Pfizer. Medical writing support was provided by Marco DiBonaventura, PhD, at Kantar Health and was funded by Pfizer.
Finally, the authors acknowledge the participation of all the patients included in the study.

Authors' contributions

RBV, JCCW, MUR, NA, SAH, MH, EM, ES, LJL, KS, SK, CH, RP, QS, and BV participated in the study design. MUR, EM, BV, CH, and QS participated in the study coordination and data collection. BV, CH, RP, and QS led the interpretation of the study results with assistance from the remaining authors. All authors helped to draft the manuscript, and all authors read and approved the final manuscript.

Competing interests

RBV, JCCW, NA, SAH, and MH were paid to participate as site investigators for the study. This study was sponsored by Pfizer. MUR, EM, ES, LJL, SK, CH, RP, QS, and BV were all full-time employees of Pfizer at the time of this study. The authors declare that they have no nonfinancial competing interests.

Author details

[1]Department of Rheumatology, General Hospital of Mexico, Mexico City, Mexico. [2]Division of Allergy, Immunology and Rheumatology, Chung Shan Medical University Hospital, No. 110, Sec. 1, Jianguo N. Road, South District, Taichung City 40201, Taiwan. [3]Institute of Medicine, Chung Shan Medical University, Taichung City, Taiwan. [4]Graduate Institute of Integrated Medicine, China Medical University, Taichung City, Taiwan. [5]University of Pennsylvania, Philadelphia, PA, USA. [6]Pfizer, Collegeville, PA, USA. [7]Dokuz Eylül University, İzmir, Turkey. [8]Bangabandhu Sheikh Mujib Medical University, Dhaka, Bangladesh. [9]Hamad Hospital, Doha, Qatar. [10]Pfizer Asia Pacific Region, Makati, Philippines. [11]Pfizer Africa and Middle East Region, Dubai, UAE. [12]Pfizer, New York, NY, USA.

References

1. Reveille JD. Spondylarthritis (Spondylarthropathy). 2012. http://www.rheumatology.org/I-Am-A/Patient-Caregiver/Diseases-Conditions/Spondyloarthritis. Accessed 2 Jun 2015.
2. Rudwaleit M, Landewé R, van der Heijde D, Listing J, Brandt J, Braun J, et al. The development of Assessment of SpondyloArthritis international Society classification criteria for axial spondyloarthritis (part I): classification of paper patients by expert opinion including uncertainty appraisal. Ann Rheum Dis. 2009;68:770–6.
3. Rudwaleit M, van der Heijde D, Landewé R, Listing J, Akkoc N, Brandt J, et al. The development of Assessment of SpondyloArthritis international Society classification criteria for axial spondyloarthritis (part II): validation and final selection. Ann Rheum Dis. 2009;68:777–83.
4. Boonen A, Sieper J, van der Heijde D, Dougados M, Bukowski JF, Valluri S, et al. The burden of non-radiographic axial spondyloarthritis. Semin Arthritis Rheum. 2015;44:556–62.
5. Huerta-Sil G, Casasola-Vargas JC, Londoño JD, Rivas-Ruíz R, Chávez J, Pacheco-Tena C, et al. Low grade radiographic sacroiliitis as prognostic factor in patients with undifferentiated spondyloarthritis fulfilling diagnostic criteria for ankylosing spondylitis throughout follow up. Ann Rheum Dis. 2006;65:642–6.
6. Stolwijk C, Boonen A, van Tubergen A, Reveille JD. Epidemiology of spondyloarthritis. Rheum Dis Clin North Am. 2012;38:441–76.
7. Peláez-Ballestas I, Navarro-Zarza JE, Julian B, Lopez A, Flores-Camacho R, Casasola-Vargas JC, et al. A community-based study on the prevalence of spondyloarthritis and inflammatory back pain in Mexicans. J Clin Rheumatol. 2013;19:57–61.
8. Sieper J, van der Heijde D. Review: Nonradiographic axial spondyloarthritis: new definition of an old disease? Arthritis Rheum. 2013;65:543–51.
9. Dougados M, d'Agostino MA, Benessiano J, Berenbaum F, Breban M, Claudepierre P, et al. The DESIR cohort: a 10-year follow-up of early inflammatory back pain in France: study design and baseline characteristics of the 708 recruited patients. Joint Bone Spine. 2011;78:598–603.
10. Poddubnyy D, Rudwaleit M, Haibel H, Listing J, Märker-Hermann E, Zeidler H, et al. Rates and predictors of radiographic sacroiliitis progression over 2 years in patients with axial spondyloarthritis. Ann Rheum Dis. 2011;70:1369–74.
11. Althoff CE, Sieper J, Song IH, Haibel H, Weiß A, Diekhoff T, et al. Active inflammation and structural change in early active axial spondyloarthritis as detected by whole-body MRI. Ann Rheum Dis. 2013;72:967–73.
12. Sieper J, van der Heijde D, Dougados M, Mease PJ, Maksymowych WP, Brown MA, et al. Efficacy and safety of adalimumab in patients with non-radiographic axial spondyloarthritis: results of a randomized placebo-controlled trial (ABILITY-1). Ann Rheum Dis. 2013;72:815–22.
13. van der Heijde D, Dijkmans B, Geusens P, Sieper J, DeWoody K, Williamson P, et al. Efficacy and safety of infliximab in patients with ankylosing spondylitis: results of a randomized, placebo-controlled trial (ASSERT). Arthritis Rheum. 2005;52:582–91.
14. Ciurea A, Scherer A, Exer P, Bernhard J, Dudler J, Beyeler B, et al. Tumor necrosis factor α inhibition in radiographic and nonradiographic axial spondyloarthritis: results from a large observational cohort. Arthritis Rheum. 2013;65:3096–106.
15. Dougados M, van der Heijde D, Sieper J, Braun J, Maksymowych WP, Citera G, et al. Symptomatic efficacy of etanercept and its effects on objective signs of inflammation in early nonradiographic axial spondyloarthritis: a multicenter, randomized, double-blind, placebo-controlled trial. Arthritis Rheumatol. 2014;66:2091–102.
16. Landewé R, Braun J, Deodhar A, Dougados M, Maksymowych WP, Mease PJ, et al. Efficacy of certolizumab pegol on signs and symptoms of axial spondyloarthritis including ankylosing spondylitis: 24-week results of a double-blind randomised placebo-controlled phase 3 study. Ann Rheum Dis. 2014;73:39–47.
17. Poddubnyy D, Brandt H, Vahldiek J, Spiller I, Song IH, Rudwaleit M, et al. The frequency of non-radiographic axial spondyloarthritis in relation to symptom duration in patients referred because of chronic back pain: results from the Berlin early spondyloarthritis clinic. Ann Rheum Dis. 2012;71:1998–2001.
18. Kiltz U, Baraliakos X, Karakostas P, Igelmann M, Kalthoff L, Klink C, et al. Do patients with non-radiographic axial spondylarthritis differ from patients with ankylosing spondylitis? Arthritis Care Res. 2012;64:1415–22.
19. Machado P, Landewé R, Lie E, Kvien TK, Braun J, Baker D, et al. Ankylosing Spondylitis Disease Activity Score (ASDAS): defining cut-off levels for disease activity states and improvement scores. Ann Rheum Dis. 2011;70:47–53.

9

Relevance of structural damage in the sacroiliac joints for the functional status and spinal mobility in patients with axial spondyloarthritis: results from the German Spondyloarthritis Inception Cohort

Mikhail Protopopov[1], Joachim Sieper[1], Hildrun Haibel[1], Joachim Listing[2], Martin Rudwaleit[1,3] and Denis Poddubnyy[1,2*]

Abstract

Background: Functional status and spinal mobility in patients with axial spondyloarthritis (axSpA) are known to be determined both by disease activity and by structural damage in the spine. The impact of structural damage in the sacroiliac joints (SIJ) on physical function and spinal mobility in axSpA has not been studied so far. The objective of the study was to analyze the impact of radiographic sacroiliitis on functional status and spinal mobility in patients with axSpA.

Methods: In total, 210 patients with axSpA were included in the analysis. Radiographs of SIJ obtained at baseline and after 2 years of follow up were scored by two trained readers according to the modified New York criteria grading system (grade 0–4). The mean of two readers' scores for each joint and a sum score for both SIJ were calculated for each patient giving a sacroiliitis sum score between 0 and 8. The Bath Ankylosing Spondylitis Functional Index (BASFI) and Bath Ankylosing Spondylitis Metrology Index (BASMI) at baseline and after 2 years were used as outcome measures.

Results: Longitudinal mixed model analysis adjusted for structural damage in the spine (modified Stoke Ankylosing Spondylitis Spine Score - mSASSS), disease activity (Bath Ankylosing Spondylitis Disease Activity Index - BASDAI and C-reactive protein level) and gender, revealed an independent association of the sacroiliitis sum score with the BASFI: $b = 0.10$ (95% CI 0.01–0.19) and the BASMI: $b = 0.12$ (95% CI 0.03–0.21), respectively, indicating that change by one radiographic sacroiliitis grade in one joint is associated with BASFI/BASMI worsening by 0.10/0.12 points, respectively, independently of disease activity and structural damage in the spine.

Conclusion: Structural damage in the SIJ might have an impact on functional status and spinal mobility in axSpA independently of spinal structural damage and disease activity.

Keywords: Axial spondyloarthritis, Ankylosing spondylitis, Structural damage, Sacroiliitis, Physical function, Spinal mobility, BASFI, BASMI

* Correspondence: denis.poddubnyy@charite.de
[1]Department of Gastroenterology, Infectiology and Rheumatology, Charité - Universitätsmedizin Berlin, Hindenburgdamm 30, 12203 Berlin, Germany
[2]German Rheumatism Research Centre, Charitéplatz 1, 10117 Berlin, Germany
Full list of author information is available at the end of the article

Background

Axial spondyloarthritis (axSpA) covers both patients with non-radiographic (nr) axSpA – often the earlier stage of axSpA – and patients with radiographic axSpA, also termed ankylosing spondylitis (AS). The latter is defined by the presence of structural damage in the sacroiliac joints (SIJ) on X-rays according to the modified New York criteria for AS. It was reported previously that functional status and spinal mobility parameters in patients with axSpA are independently determined by irreversible structural damage in the spine, i.e. presence of syndesmophytes and ankylosis, and by potentially reversible disease activity [1–3]. At the same time, structural damage in the SIJ (such as erosions, joint space alteration and especially ankylosis) might also have an impact on mobility and function – a hypothesis that has never been investigated in a wider range of the axSpA spectrum including nr-axSpA and AS.

In the present work, we investigated the association between structural damage in the SIJ and functional status and spinal mobility in patients with axSpA.

Methods

Cohort description and patient selection

The present analysis used the data of the German Spondyloarthritis Inception Cohort (GESPIC). A detailed description of the latter has been reported previously [4, 5]. Briefly, patients included in GESPIC were required to have a definite clinical diagnosis of axSpA according to the treating rheumatologist with symptom duration of up to 5 years for the non-radiographic form and up to 10 years for the radiographic form (AS). Patients with axSpA were classified as having AS if the radiographic criterion of the modified New York Criteria (presence of radiographic changes in the SIJ of at least grade II bilaterally or at least grade III unilaterally) [6] was fulfilled, and as having nr-axSpA otherwise. Overall, 210 patients were included in the present analysis based on the availability of radiographs and clinical data at baseline and after 2 years of follow up.

Clinical assessment

Clinical assessment was performed at baseline and every 6 months thereafter until year 2. Disease activity was assessed by the Bath Ankylosing Spondylitis Disease Activity Index (BASDAI) [7] and level of C-reactive protein (CRP). Functional status was assessed by the Bath Ankylosing Spondylitis Functional Index (BASFI) [8] and spinal mobility by the Bath Ankylosing Spondylitis Metrology Index (BASMI) with an original 2-step method of calculation [9].

Radiographic assessment

Conventional anteroposterior pelvic radiographs and lateral and anteroposterior cervical and lumbar spine radiographs were obtained locally at baseline and after 2 years of follow up. Images were digitized if not available in digitized form, anonymized and subsequently scored by two trained readers (DP and HH) who were blinded to the time point of the investigation and to all clinical data. Grading of radiographic sacroiliitis was performed according to the established scoring system used by the modified New York criteria for AS [6]:

- Grade 0 - normal
- Grade 1 - suspicious changes
- Grade 2 - minimal abnormality, small localized areas with erosion or sclerosis, without alteration in the joint width
- Grade 3 - unequivocal abnormality, moderate or advanced sacroiliitis with one or more of: erosions, evidence of sclerosis, widening, narrowing, or partial ankylosis
- Grade 4 - severe abnormality, total ankylosis

Radiographic changes in hip joints were scored on anteroposterior pelvic radiographs by the same readers using the Bath Ankylosing Spondylitis Radiology Hip Index (BASRI-hip) [10]. Structural damage in the spine was assessed by the same blinded readers according to the modified Stoke Ankylosing Spondylitis Spine Score (mSASSS), as described in detail elsewhere [11].

Statistical analysis

For the current analysis, the mean of the scoring results of the two readers was calculated for each sacroiliac joint. Next, the sum of the two mean sacroiliitis scores (left and right SIJ) was calculated for each patient resulting in a sacroiliitis sum score between 0 (no signs of radiographic sacroiliitis in either SIJ in the opinion of both readers) and 8 (total ankylosis in both SIJ in the opinion of both readers) at baseline and after 2 years. To visualize an association between BASFI/BASMI and the sacroiliitis sum score, combined scatter and cumulative probability plots were created.

The association between the sacroiliitis sum score and BASFI/BASMI was explored first in the linear regression analysis, which was performed with baseline values of the variables of interest. Crude unstandardized parameter estimates (ß coefficients) obtained in the univariable model were then adjusted in the multivariable model for the following factors considered as potential confounders: structural damage in the spine (mSASSS), disease activity (BASDAI and CRP), and sex. In order to address the question of the possible confounding of the association between radiographic sacroiliitis and function/spinal mobility by the damage in the hip joints, models with inclusion of the BASRI-hip as a covariate were built.

Next, linear regression analysis of the association between change in BASFI/BASMI and progression of radiographic sacroiliitis defined as (1) absolute change in the sacroiliitis sum score, (2) worsening of radiographic sacroiliitis by at least one grade in one sacroiliac joint in opinion of both readers and (3) progression from nr-axSpA to AS in the opinion of both readers was performed.

At the final step, both baseline and year-2 parameters were included in a longitudinal linear mixed model analysis that was corrected for the dependencies between the two time-point values of each individual. Crude parameter estimates were adjusted for the same potential confounders as in the linear regression analysis. The latter analysis was performed in the entire group and also separately in the non-radiographic and radiographic subgroups of the patient population in order to address the question of a possibly higher functional relevance of the more advanced structural changes in the SIJ; 95% confidence intervals (CIs) for the parameter estimates were calculated. The inter-reader agreement was assessed by means of the weighted Kappa value. Statistical analysis was performed using SAS v.9.4 (SAS Institute Inc., Cary, NC, USA).

Results

There were no major differences in general baseline characteristics between the included patients (radiographic cohort) and the whole previously described cohort [4], except for a somewhat lower percentage of men in the nr-axSpA subgroup (33.7% in the current study vs 42.9% in the whole cohort). General characteristics of the patients at baseline are presented in Table 1.

Table 1 Baseline disease characteristics of 210 patients with axial spondyloarthritis

Baseline parameters	Nr-axSpA (n = 95)	AS (n = 115)	All patients (n = 210)
Age, years	38.7 ± 9.9	36.8 ± 11.0	37.3 ± 10.6
Male gender, *n* (%)	32 (33.7)	75 (65.2)	107 (51.0)
HLA-B27 positive, *n* (%)	69 (72.6)	97 (84.3)	166 (79.0)
Duration of symptoms, years	3.2 ± 2.2	5.2 ± 2.8	4.2 ± 2.7
BASDAI, points NRS (0–10)	4.2 ± 2.0	3.8 ± 2.2	3.9 ± 2.2
Peripheral arthritis, *n* (%)	16 (16.8)	15 (13.0)	31 (14.8)
BASFI, points NRS (0–10)	2.8 ± 2.2	3.0 ± 2.4	2.9 ± 2.3
BASMI, points (0–10)	1.5 ± 1.5	2.0 ± 1.7	1.8 ± 1.6
CRP, mg/l	6.5 ± 12.8	12.4 ± 16.6	9.7 ± 15.2
mSASSS, points (0–72)	2.3 ± 4.2	5.9 ± 10.3	4.2 ± 8.3
NSAIDs intake, *n* (%)	64 (67.4)	76 (66.1)	140 (66.7)
Systemic steroids intake, *n* (%)	6 (6.3)	6 (5.2)	12 (5.7)
DMARDs intake, *n* (%)	26 (27.4)	35 (30.4)	61 (29.0)
TNFα blocker intake, *n* (%)	1 (1.1)	4 (3.5)	5 (2.4)
Current smoking, *n* (%)	24 (25.3)	39 (33.9)	63 (30.0)

Continuous variables are presented as mean ± standard deviation
AS ankylosing spondylitis, *BASDAI* Bath Ankylosing Spondylitis Disease Activity Index, *BASFI* Bath Ankylosing Spondylitis Functional Index, *BASMI* Bath Ankylosing Spondylitis Metrology Index, *CRP* C-reactive protein, *DMARDs* disease-modifying anti-rheumatic drugs, *mSASSS* modified Stoke Ankylosing Spondylitis Spine Score, *nr-axSpA* non-radiographic axial spondyloarthritis, *NRS* numeric rating scale, *NSAIDs* non-steroidal anti-inflammatory drugs, *TNFα* tumour necrosis factor alpha

Detailed results of the assessment of the SIJ on pelvic radiographs including inter-reader variability and change over time have been reported previously [5, 12]. Briefly, based on the baseline assessment of the SIJ, 115 out of 210 patients were classified as having AS, and 95 as having nr-axSpA. The sacroiliitis sum score distribution at baseline and change in the sacroiliitis sum score after 2 years of follow up are presented in Fig. 1. The mean sacroiliitis sum score at baseline was 4.3 ± 2.0 and the mean change in the sacroiliitis sum score over 2 years was 0.13 ± 0.84. In the entire group of 210 patients, a total of 26 patients (12.4%) had progression of radiographic sacroiliitis by at least one grade after 2 years in the opinion of both readers (16.8% of patients with nr-axSpA and 8.7% of patients with AS). Improvement in radiographic sacroiliitis by at least one grade in the opinion of both readers was observed in 11 patients (5.2%) in the entire group (6.3% and 4.4% of patients with nr-axSpA and AS, respectively). Progression from nr-axSpA to AS after 2 years was observed in the opinion of both readers in 11 out of 95 patients (11.6%), and regression from AS to nr-axSpA was observed in 3 out of 115 patients (2.6%).

There was moderate agreement between the two readers on the fulfilment of the modified New York criteria (weighted Kappa value 0.59 at baseline, and 0.67 and after 2 years of follow up) and on the grade of radiographic sacroiliitis (weighted Kappa values between 0.51 and 0.59 for the left and right SIJ at baseline and year 2) [5]. The combined cumulative probability and scatter plots on Fig. 2 depict the crude relationship between the sacroiliitis sum score and BASFI (Fig. 2a) or BASMI (Fig. 2b).

In the univariable linear regression models, the crude parameter estimates (ß) for the association between sacroiliitis sum score and BASFI/BASMI at baseline were 0.09 (95% CI -0.07 to 0.25) and 0.22 (95% CI 0.12 to 0.33), respectively. After adjustment for the mSASSS, disease activity parameters (BASDAI and CRP), and sex, ß changed to 0.10 (95% CI -0.01 to 0.21) and 0.12 (95% CI 0.01 to 0.22), respectively. These parameter estimates indicate that difference in one sacroiliitis grade is responsible for the difference in 0.10/0.12 points on the BASFI/BASMI, respectively. Adding the BASRI-hip

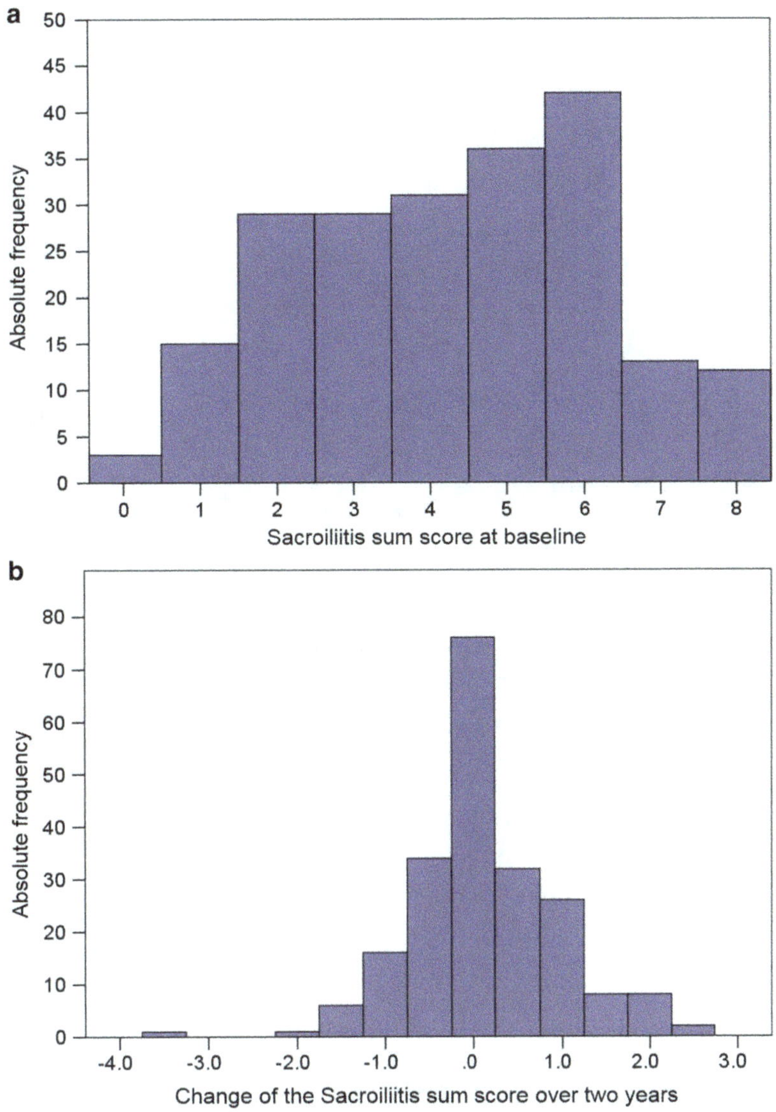

Fig. 1 Distribution of the sacroiliitis sum score at baseline (**a**) and change in the sacroiliitis sum score over 2 years (**b**) in 210 patients with axial spondyloarthritis

score as an additional potential confounder in the models did not substantially affect the parameter estimates for either functional outcome (ß = 0.11, 95% CI -0.01 to 0.23 and 0.13, 95% CI 0.02 to 0.24 for BASFI and BASMI, respectively), therefore, this variable was not included in further analysis.

In the linear regression analysis of the association between BASFI/BASMI change scores over 2 years with the absolute change in the sacroiliitis sum score, ß was 0.03 (95% CI -0.19 to 0.25) and 0.25 (95% CI 0.03 to 0.47), respectively, adjusted for the mSASSS change score, BASDAI change score, time-averaged CRP over two years, and sex.

Worsening of radiographic sacroiliitis by at least one grade in the opinion of both readers was assessed in a similar analysis, with ß of -0.13 (95% CI -0.69 to 0.42) and 0.64 (95% CI 0.09 to 1.19), for BASFI and BASMI, respectively. Progression from nr-axSpA to AS after 2 years was assessed in 95 patients classified as having nr-axSpA at baseline, with ß of 0.79 (95% CI -0.06 to 1.65) and 0.49 (95% CI -0.04 to 1.35), for BASFI and BASMI, respectively.

In the longitudinal mixed model analysis (Table 2) that included values obtained at both time points (baseline and year 2) with correction for dependencies between two values related to the same patient, the sacroiliitis sum score demonstrated stronger association with the BASMI than with the BASFI, with ß = 0.20 (95% CI 0.11 to 0.30) and 0.09 (95% CI -0.05 to 0.22), respectively, in the univariable analysis. However, after adjustment for

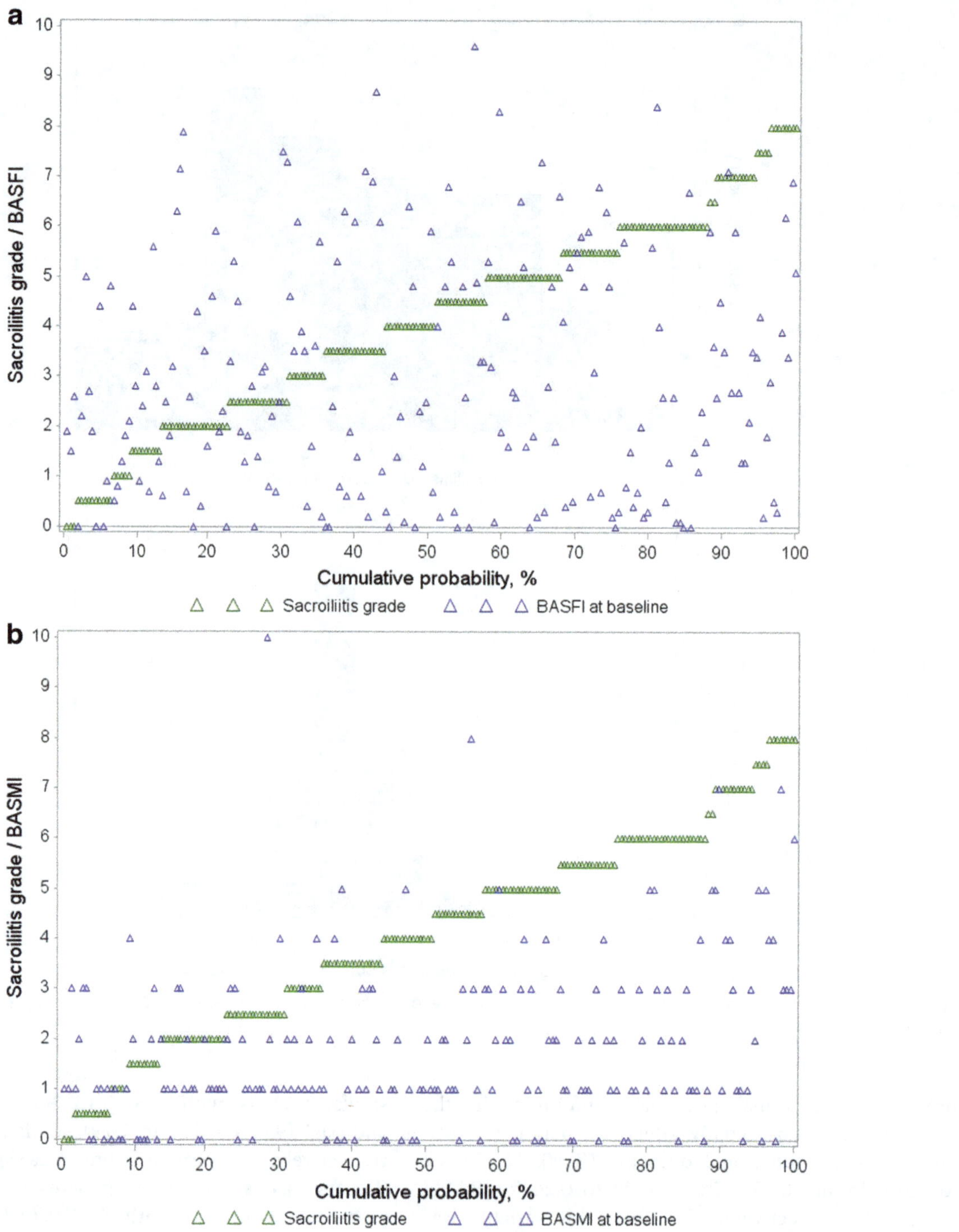

Fig. 2 Combined cumulative probability and scatter plots depicting an association between the sacroiliitis sum score and the Bath Ankylosing Spondylitis Functional Index (BASFI) (**a**) or the Bath Ankylosing Spondylitis Metrology Index (BASMI) (**b**) at baseline in 210 patients with axial spondyloarthritis

the mSASSS, disease activity parameters (BASDAI and CRP) and gender, the strength of association became very similar for both outcomes: ß = 0.10 (95% CI 0.01 to 0.19) for BASFI and ß = 0.12 (95% CI 0.03 to 0.21) for BASMI, indicating that progression by one radiographic sacroiliitis grade would result in a change of 0.10/0.12 points in the BASMI/BASFI. Therefore, progression from grade 0 bilaterally to grade 2 bilaterally or grade 4 bilaterally would result in an increase of 0.40/0.48 or 0.80/0.96 points on the BASFI/BASMI, respectively, independently of structural damage in the spine and disease activity.

Similar analysis performed in the AS and nr-axSpA subgroups resulted in similar results, though the precision of the parameter estimation decreased due to the smaller group size (Table 2).

Discussion

In this work, we showed that structural damage in the SIJ might have an impact, although small, on spinal mobility and physical function in patients with axSpA, independently of other parameters, such as disease activity and structural damage in the spine. To our knowledge, this is the first study that addresses this question in a population of patients with axSpA including non-radiographic and radiographic axSpA (i.e., the full range of radiographic sacroiliitis) and using standardized measures of spinal mobility and functional status assessment – BASMI and BASFI.

Only a few studies have investigated the potential impact of radiographic sacroiliitis on mobility and functional status in patients with axSpA or AS. In a study by Kennedy et al., an association between BASMI score and total radiological score (incorporating the radiographic grade of sacroiliitis) in patients with AS was shown, although the association between radiographic sacroiliitis and spinal mobility measures, regardless of spinal damage, was not investigated [13]. A study by Viitanen et al. showed correlation between radiographic changes in the lumbar spine and in the SIJ and spinal mobility measures, but again the effect of radiographic sacroiliitis alone was not estimated [14]. Taylor et al. also observed correlation between spinal flexion and the SIJ ankylosis score assessed on computed tomography that was, however, not adjusted for any confounders [15]. In a study in reactive arthritis (Reiter's syndrome) radiographic sacroiliitis was found to be mostly asymptomatic and functionally irrelevant, but no standardized methods of spinal mobility and functional status assessment were used [16]. A more recent population-based study revealed no difference in the patient-reported outcome between subjects with and without radiographic sacroiliitis, but again, no standardized methods of spinal mobility and functional status assessment were used, and the number of cases with sacroiliitis was small (n = 14) [17].

Several studies investigated the influence of artificial SIJ ankylosis on spinal mobility. For example, no difference was identified between patients who underwent unilateral and bilateral transsacral-transiliac screw fixation in terms of functional status, indicating that artificial ankylosis of the second SIJ does not reduce the functional parameters (although the outcome was not an objective measurement, but rather a self-reported outcome) [18]. Comparison of quality of life and performance in patients who underwent unilateral SIJ fusion showed results comparable with the average health

Table 2 Association between the sum radiographic sacroiliitis score and functional status/spinal mobility in patients with axial spondyloarthritis

Parameters	Unadjusted mixed model analysis (all patients, n = 210), B (95% CI)	Adjusted mixed model analysis (all patients, n = 210), B (95% CI)	Adjusted mixed model analysis (patients with AS, n = 105), B (95% CI)	Adjusted mixed model analysis (patients with nr-axSpA, n = 95), B (95% CI)
Outcome: BASFI				
Sacroiliitis sum score (0–8)	0.09 (-0.05 to 0.22)	**0.10 (0.01 to 0.19)**	0.16 (-0.03 to 0.36)	0.09 (-0.11 to 0.30)
mSASSS, points (0–72)	-	0.05 (0.03 to 0.07)	0.04 (0.02 to 0.06)	0.08 (0.03 to 0.14)
BASDAI, points NRS (0–10)	-	0.81 (0.74 to 0.88)	0.84 (0.74 to 0.93)	0.75 (0.63 to 0.86)
CRP, mg/l	-	0.00 (-0.01 to 0.01)	0.00 (-0.01 to 0.01)	0.00 (-0.02 to 0.01)
Male sex	-	-0.02 (-0.40 to 0.37)	0.03 (-0.48 to 0.55)	-0.13 (-0.74 to 0.48)
Outcome: BASMI				
Sacroiliitis sum score (0–8)	0.20 (0.11 to 0.30)	**0.12 (0.03 to 0.21)**	0.17 (-0.02 to 0.37)	0.21 (0.01 to 0.40)
mSASSS, points (0–72)	-	0.07 (0.05 to 0.09)	0.07 (0.04 to 0.09)	0.04 (-0.01 to 0.10)
BASDAI, points NRS (0–10)	-	0.22 (0.15 to 0.29)	0.23 (0.14 to 0.32)	0.18 (0.07 to 0.30)
CRP, mg/l	-	0.01 (0.00 to 0.02)	0.01 (0.00 to 0.03)	0.00 (-0.03 to 0.01)
Male sex	-	0.00 (-0.39 to 0.39)	0.32 (-0.21 to 0.85)	-0.35 (-0.92 to 0.22)

mSASSS modified Stoke Ankylosing Spondylitis Spine Score, *AS* Ankylosing Spondylitis, *nr-axSpA* non-radiographic axial spondyloarthritis, *BASFI* Bath Ankylosing Spondylitis Functional Index, *CRP* C-reactive protein, *BASDAI* Bath Ankylosing Spondylitis Disease Activity Index, *NRS* numerical rating scale, *BASMI* Bath Ankylosing Spondylitis Metrology Index

Main results are marked in bold

status of the US population, indicating no significant influence of unilateral SIJ fusion on functional performance [19]. Importantly, SIJ fusion is normally performed in symptomatic patients with mechanical problems in the SIJ and even an improvement in function and spinal mobility could be expected due to pain reduction as an outcome of the intervention.

In our analysis, both cross-sectional and longitudinal models showed a rather small but significant and independent association between radiographic sacroiliitis and spinal mobility/function in patients with axSpA (though the precision of the effect estimation was better in the longitudinal model), indicating that progression from normal (without structural damage visible on radiographs) SIJ to complete bilateral ankylosis would result in a worsening of the BASFI/BASMI by about 1 point (on a 0 – 10 scale), independently of disease activity and structural damage in the spine. For comparison, worsening of the mSASSS score by 1 point (on a scale between 0 and 72) has been reported to result in worsening of the BASFI by 0.06 points, independently of the BASDAI [2].

We hypothesize several explanations for our findings. The first possible explanation would be that the observed independent association between structural damage in the SIJ and spinal mobility/functional status is real. In this case, we have to postulate that the SIJs are indeed relevant for spinal mobility, and structural damage in these joints results in lower function. If so, stopping structural damage in the SIJ might become an additional treatment target in axSpA aiming at preservation of the spinal mobility/functional status in axSpA in a long-term perspective. Nevertheless, a benefit/risk assessment of intensified treatment would be necessary in this case.

An alternative explanation might be related to the fact that the mSASSS score takes into account only structural damage involving the anterior corners of the cervical and lumbar vertebrae. Although mSASSS is considered to be a proxy for the structural damage in the entire spinal column, the fact that assessment of damage to the spinal structures is not included in the mSASSS (i.e. the posterior structures, thoracic spine) might be responsible for the residual confounding causing a significant association between radiographic sacroiliitis and the BASFI/BASMI after adjustment for the mSASSS. We also cannot exclude residual confounding related to other factors, which were not captured and therefore not included in the analysis (e.g. effects of inflammation in the spine as detected by magnetic resonance imaging, which was not performed in GESPIC in the first 2 years).

The clinical significance of our findings is ambiguous. On the one hand, the results expressed in absolute numbers (the change in one sacroiliitis grade in one of the joints is associated with a change of 0.10/0.12 points in the BASFI/BASMI, respectively) seem quite modest, especially considering that the rate of radiographic progression is slow [5, 20–22]. On the other hand, this association is independent from the other factors, somewhat higher than expected and, if true, alongside with other factors it might be a significant contribution to the deterioration of physical function in the long run.

Conclusion

Data from GESPIC indicate that structural damage in the SIJ might have an impact on functional status and spinal mobility independently of structural damage in the spine and disease activity in patients with axSpA – an association that has been mostly neglected previously.

Abbreviations

AS: Ankylosing spondylitis; axSpA: Axial spondyloarthritis; BASDAI: Bath Ankylosing Spondylitis Disease Activity Index; BASFI: Bath Ankylosing Spondylitis Functional Index; BASMI: Bath Ankylosing Spondylitis Metrology Index; BASRI-hip: Bath Ankylosing Spondylitis Radiology Hip Index; CIs: 95% Confidence intervals; CRP: C-reactive protein; GESPIC: German Spondyloarthritis inception cohort; mSASSS: Modified Stoke Ankylosing Spondylitis Spine Score; nr-axSpA: Non-radiographic axial spondyloarthritis; SIJ: sacroiliac joints

Acknowledgements

We thank Prof. M. Leirisalo-Repo, Finland, Prof. D. van der Heijde, The Netherlands, and Prof. M. Dougados, France, for scientific advice on the design of the cohort. We are grateful to Beate Buss and Petra Tietz for monitoring the cohort, Johanna Callhoff, Anja Weiss and Martina Niewerth for the data management support, Joachim Listing for statistical advices, Janis Vahldiek and Georg Heine for the X-ray image handling and for the development of the image-scoring interface, and to all patients who voluntarily participate in this cohort. We further would like to thank the following rheumatologists for inclusion and follow up of their patients: J. Brandt, H. Brandt, J. Braun, G-R. Burmester, H. Deister, E. Edelmann, J. Emmerich, M. Enderlein, E. Feist, A. Gauliard, E. Gromnica-Ihle, F. Heldmann, S. Hermann, U. von Hinüber, Ü. Hübner, K. Karberg, C. Kedor, E. Märker-Hermann, H. Nüßlein, R. Pelle-Lohfink, D. Pick, G. Reichmuth, E. Riehers, M. Rihl, R. Schmidt, S. Schnarr, U. Schneider, I.-H. Song, I. Spiller, U. Syrbe, V. Walz, S. Wassenberg, H. M. Wisseler, H. Zeidler, and S. Zinke.

Funding

GESPIC has been financially supported by the German Federal Ministry of Education and Research (Bundesministerium für Bildung und Forschung – BMBF). As funding by BMBF was reduced according to schedule in 2005 and stopped in 2007, complementary financial support has been obtained also from Abbott/Abbvie, Amgen, Centocor, Schering-Plough, and Wyeth. Since 2010 GESPIC has been supported by Abbvie. Additional support has also been obtained from the ANCYLOSS (grant number FKZ 01EC1002D), ArthroMark (grants numbers FKZ 01EC1009A and FKZ 01EC1401A) and METARTHROS (grant number FKZ 01EC1407A) projects funded by BMBF.

Authors' contributions

DP was responsible for the study design and overseeing the study, participated in patient recruitment, was responsible for scoring of radiographs, performed statistical analysis and data interpretation, and drafted the manuscript. MP performed statistical analysis and data interpretation and drafted the manuscript. JS and MR were responsible for the design of the initial cohort, design of the current study, study recruitment and data collection, contributed to data interpretation, and drafted the manuscript. HH participated in patient recruitment, was responsible for scoring of radiographs, contributed to data interpretation, and drafted the manuscript. JL contributed to statistical analysis and data interpretation and drafted the manuscript. All authors read and approved the final manuscript.

Competing interests
The authors declare that they have no competing interests.

Author details
[1]Department of Gastroenterology, Infectiology and Rheumatology, Charité - Universitätsmedizin Berlin, Hindenburgdamm 30, 12203 Berlin, Germany. [2]German Rheumatism Research Centre, Charitéplatz 1, 10117 Berlin, Germany. [3]Klinikum Bielefeld Rosenhöhe, An der Rosenhöhe 27, 33647 Bielefeld, Germany.

References
1. Machado P, Landewe R, Braun J, Hermann KG, Baker D, van der Heijde D. Both structural damage and inflammation of the spine contribute to impairment of spinal mobility in patients with ankylosing spondylitis. Ann Rheum Dis. 2010;69:1465–70.
2. Landewe R, Dougados M, Mielants H, van der Tempel H, van der Heijde D. Physical function in ankylosing spondylitis is independently determined by both disease activity and radiographic damage of the spine. Ann Rheum Dis. 2009;68:863–7.
3. Wanders A, Landewe R, Dougados M, Mielants H, van der Linden S, van der Heijde D. Association between radiographic damage of the spine and spinal mobility for individual patients with ankylosing spondylitis: can assessment of spinal mobility be a proxy for radiographic evaluation? Ann Rheum Dis. 2005;64:988–94.
4. Rudwaleit M, Haibel H, Baraliakos X, Listing J, Marker-Hermann E, Zeidler H, et al. The early disease stage in axial spondylarthritis: results from the German Spondyloarthritis Inception Cohort. Arthritis Rheum. 2009;60:717–27.
5. Poddubnyy D, Rudwaleit M, Haibel H, Listing J, Marker-Hermann E, Zeidler H, et al. Rates and predictors of radiographic sacroiliitis progression over 2 years in patients with axial spondyloarthritis. Ann Rheum Dis. 2011;70:1369–74.
6. van der Linden S, Valkenburg HA, Cats A. Evaluation of diagnostic criteria for ankylosing spondylitis. A proposal for modification of the New York criteria. Arthritis Rheum. 1984;27:361–8.
7. Garrett S, Jenkinson T, Kennedy LG, Whitelock H, Gaisford P, Calin A. A new approach to defining disease status in ankylosing spondylitis: the Bath Ankylosing Spondylitis Disease Activity Index. J Rheumatol. 1994;21:2286–91.
8. Calin A, Garrett S, Whitelock H, Kennedy LG, O'Hea J, Mallorie P, et al. A new approach to defining functional ability in ankylosing spondylitis: the development of the Bath Ankylosing Spondylitis Functional Index. J Rheumatol. 1994;21:2281–5.
9. Jenkinson TR, Mallorie PA, Whitelock HC, Kennedy LG, Garrett SL, Calin A. Defining spinal mobility in ankylosing spondylitis (AS). The Bath AS Metrology Index. J Rheumatol. 1994;21:1694–8.
10. MacKay K, Brophy S, Mack C, Doran M, Calin A. The development and validation of a radiographic grading system for the hip in ankylosing spondylitis: the Bath Ankylosing Spondylitis Radiology Hip Index. J Rheumatol. 2000;27:2866–72.
11. Creemers MC, Franssen MJ, van't Hof MA, Gribnau FW, van de Putte LB, van Riel PL. Assessment of outcome in ankylosing spondylitis: an extended radiographic scoring system. Ann Rheum Dis. 2005;64:127–9.
12. Poddubnyy D, Haibel H, Listing J, Marker-Hermann E, Zeidler H, Braun J, et al. Baseline radiographic damage, elevated acute-phase reactant levels, and cigarette smoking status predict spinal radiographic progression in early axial spondylarthritis. Arthritis Rheum. 2012;64:1388–98.
13. Kennedy LG, Jenkinson TR, Mallorie PA, Whitelock HC, Garrett SL, Calin A. Ankylosing spondylitis: the correlation between a new metrology score and radiology. Br J Rheumatol. 1995;34:767–70.
14. Viitanen JV, Kokko ML, Lehtinen K, Suni J, Kautiainen H. Correlation between mobility restrictions and radiologic changes in ankylosing spondylitis. Spine (Phila Pa 1976). 1995;20:492–6.
15. Taylor HG, Wardle T, Beswick EJ, Dawes PT. The relationship of clinical and laboratory measurements to radiological change in ankylosing spondylitis. Br J Rheumatol. 1991;30:330–5.
16. McGuigan LE, Hart HH, Gow PJ, Kidd BL, Grigor RR, Moore TE. The functional significance of sacroiliitis and ankylosing spondylitis in Reiter's syndrome. Clin Exp Rheumatol. 1985;3:311–5.
17. Exarchou S, Redlund-Johnell I, Karlsson M, Mellstrom D, Ohlsson C, Turesson C, et al. The prevalence of moderate to severe radiographic sacroiliitis and the correlation with health status in elderly Swedish men–the MrOS study. BMC Musculoskelet Disord. 2013;14:352.
18. Heydemann J, Hartline B, Gibson ME, Ambrose CG, Munz JW, Galpin M, et al. Do transsacral-transiliac screws across uninjured sacroiliac joints affect pain and functional outcomes in trauma patients? Clin Orthop Relat Res. 2016;474:1417–21.
19. Cummings Jr J, Capobianco RA. Minimally invasive sacroiliac joint fusion: one-year outcomes in 18 patients. Ann Surg Innov Res. 2013;7:12.
20. Dougados M, Demattei C, van den Berg R, Vo Hoang V, Thevenin F, Reijnierse M, et al. Rate and predisposing factors for sacroiliac joint radiographic progression after a two-year follow-up period in recent-onset spondyloarthritis. Arthritis Rheumatol. 2016;68:1904–13.
21. Dougados M, Sepriano A, Molto A, van Lunteren M, Ramiro S, de Hooge M, et al. Sacroiliac radiographic progression in recent onset axial spondyloarthritis: the 5-year data of the DESIR cohort. Ann Rheum Dis. 2017; 76:1823-28.
22. Dougados M, Maksymowych WP, Landewe RB, Molto A, Claudepierre P, de Hooge M, et al. Evaluation of the change in structural radiographic sacroiliac joint damage after 2 years of etanercept therapy (EMBARK trial) in comparison to a contemporary control cohort (DESIR cohort) in recent onset axial spondyloarthritis. Ann Rheum Dis. 2017; doi: 10.1136/annrheumdis-2017-212008.

Recurrent anterior uveitis and subsequent incidence of ankylosing spondylitis: a nationwide cohort study from 2002 to 2013

Baek-Lok Oh[1], Jeong Seok Lee[2], Eun Young Lee[2], Hee Young Lee[3] and Hyeong Gon Yu[4*]

Abstract

Background: Anterior uveitis is the most common extra-articular manifestation of ankylosing spondylitis (AS). AS-related anterior uveitis frequently presents as acute, recurrent iridocyclitis; therefore, AS is often initially suspected by an ophthalmologist, not by a rheumatologist. In this study, we aimed to investigate the relationship between the recurrence of anterior uveitis and the subsequent incidence of AS.

Methods: From a national sample cohort, 10,483 patients with new-onset uveitis between 2004 and 2013 and 52415 matched control subjects who had never experienced uveitis were selected. Among the patients with new-onset uveitis, a subpopulation of patients with recurrent uveitis, defined as a minimum 120-day reported interval between consecutive claims of uveitis (based on diagnostic codes) treated with local or systemic steroids or immune-modulating drugs, was identified. The incidence rates of AS were calculated according to the number of episodes of uveitis, and the incidence rate ratios (IRRs) were derived on the basis of the incidence rate in the control group.

Results: The incidence rate per 100,000 person-years of AS after the first uveitis episode was 121.5, whereas the incidence in the control group was 16.9 (IRR, 7.40; 95% CI, 4.99–10.98); after the second uveitis episode, the IRR increased to 17.71 (95% CI, 10.44–30.06). In male and female patients with recurrent uveitis, the incidence rates of AS were 284.1 and 268.7 per 100,000 person-years, respectively. In patients aged under 40 years, the IRR of the recurrent uveitis group was 46.78 (95% CI, 19.61–111.61). In patients aged over 59 years, AS incidence in the recurrent uveitis group did not differ from that in the control group.

Conclusions: The risk of subsequent AS increased with the number of episodes of anterior uveitis. This quantitative evidence could contribute to the establishment of a rationale for ancillary workup for possible systemic associations in patients with recurrent uveitis.

Keywords: Ankylosing spondylitis, Uveitis, Recurrence, Incidence rate

Background

Uveitis is one of the important clinical signs of systemic inflammatory diseases. Identification of systemic associations in patients with uveitis is important not only to determine the etiology of ocular inflammation and improve visual prognosis but also to improve the outcome of the systemic conditions themselves through a targeted therapeutic approach. Bilateral occurrence, granulomatous appearance, or recurrence of anterior uveitis, or posterior extension/involvement of uveitis, might be a clue to a possible systemic association, and ancillary tests should be considered in such cases [1].

Ankylosing spondylitis (AS) is a chronic inflammatory disease with axial spondyloarthritis whose classification criteria include the presence of anterior uveitis [2]. A recent meta-analysis demonstrated that anterior uveitis was the most common extra-articular manifestation of AS, with a prevalence of 25.8% [3]. A rough quantitative estimate of the association between anterior uveitis and the subsequent risk of AS can be obtained from previous

* Correspondence: hgonyu@snu.ac.kr
[4]Department of Ophthalmology, Seoul National University College of Medicine, Seoul National University Hospital, Seoul, South Korea
Full list of author information is available at the end of the article

studies. For example, researchers in a previous study found that the prevalence of AS in the general population varied from < 0.01% to 1.8% globally [4], whereas other studies have shown that AS was prevalent in 4.7–9.3% of patients with anterior uveitis visiting uveitis referral centers [5, 6]. However, these results do not provide quantitative information regarding the risk of subsequent AS in patients with uveitis in the general population.

Therefore, in this study, we investigated the relationship between the recurrence of uveitis and the incidence of subsequent AS in the Korean population by using data from a 12-year national sample cohort. Furthermore, we provide partial quantitative evidence regarding additional workup, including laboratory tests and radiographic imaging, in patients with recurrent anterior uveitis.

Methods

Source population

The present study was exempt from ethical review by the institutional review board because the data originated from de-identified secondary data released by the National Health Insurance Service (NHIS) for research purposes. The NHIS is a compulsory national health insurance that provides universal coverage for almost all residents in Korea. For reimbursement, all healthcare providers submit insurance claims to the NHIS with data including information on demographics, diagnostic codes, prescription records, and healthcare facilities. Therefore, these data have a centralized database structure. The dataset used in this study is an NHIS national sample cohort comprising claims submitted by healthcare providers from 2002 through 2013. The total population of this cohort consisted of 1,025,340 nationally representative random subjects, which represents approximately 2.2% of the total number of patients enrolled in NHIS in 2002. Patients were selected using the stratified random sampling method with 1476 strata according to sex, age, and income level [7].

Study variables

We identified cases of anterior uveitis by identifying specific International Classification of Diseases, Tenth Revision (ICD-10), diagnostic codes (ICD-10 codes H20, H20.0, H20.00, H20.01, H20.04, H20.09, H20.1, H20.8, and H20.9) between January 1, 2002, and December 31, 2013. To specifically include cases of anterior uveitis, we selected patients who were treated using steroids or immunosuppressive agents (Additional file 1: Table S1) on the same day they were diagnosed with a diagnostic code of anterior uveitis. We washed out the first 2 years (2002–2003) for newly detected cases. Among patients diagnosed with AS, those who were diagnosed with anterior uveitis after their AS diagnosis, based on the visitation date, were excluded. Identification of patients with AS using this procedure was based on any claim with a diagnostic code of AS (ICD-10 codes M45.0–45.9). Ultimately, 10,483 patients with incident anterior uveitis in the years 2004–2013 were selected as the study group. The day of the initial diagnosis of uveitis, with treatment, was designated as the index date of the first uveitis episode. We matched up to five control subjects without uveitis from the population cohort to every patient with uveitis according to age, sex, household income level, and the year of uveitis diagnosis. The first day of the year used to match patients with uveitis and control subjects was designated as the index date for the control patients.

According to the Standardization of Uveitis Nomenclature Working Group [8], the term *recurrent uveitis* describes episodes of uveitis separated by at least 3 months of inactivity without treatment. With this claim-based dataset, information about uveitis activity could not be retrieved, and we assumed that uveitis with a prescription of steroid or immunosuppressive agent was active. Details of the prescription provided the duration for which systemic medications, such as oral medication or injection, were supposed to be administered. However, we could not determine the duration for which topical medications, such as steroid ophthalmic solutions, were applied by the patients based on the prescription data. Considering that a bottle of topical steroid is usually used within 1 month, we defined uveitis recurrence as claims of anterior uveitis with treatment separated by at least 120 days. In the uveitis group, patients who experienced recurrence at least once were designated as the recurrent uveitis group and the day of first recurrence was designated as the index date for the second uveitis episode (Fig. 1).

Subsequent AS cases were operationally defined as those involving patients with diagnostic codes of AS (ICD-10 codes M45.0–45.9) claimed at a general hospital or referral center. Any patients who had also been diagnosed with systemic lupus erythematosus (ICD-10 code M32.0) or rheumatoid arthritis (RA; ICD-10 code M05.0 or M06.0) were excluded. Patients diagnosed with AS before 2004 were also excluded to ensure that the AS group included only patients with new episodes. The day of the first visit for AS was designated as the index date. A brief data exploration was conducted to obtain the overall prevalence and sex-specific distribution of AS to confirm the validity of the operational definition. Detailed information of the patients is available in Additional file 2: Table S2.

To aid in the interpretation of the results of this study, we performed an additional analysis with disease controls; patients with RA (ICD-10 codes M05.0–05.9, M06.0–06.9) and herniated intervertebral disc (HIVD;

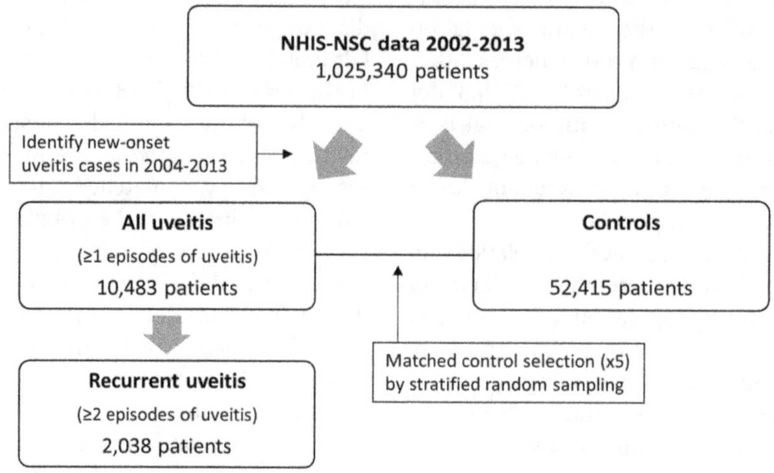

Fig. 1 Flowchart depicting the classification of patients into the "all uveitis," recurrent uveitis, and control groups. *NHIS-NSC* National Health Insurance Service - National Selection Cohort

ICD-10 code M51.2) were included as the disease control subjects. The above-mentioned analysis regarding AS was repeated for RA and HIVD.

Statistical analysis

The primary outcome of this study was the incidence rate ratio (IRR) of AS according to the number of episodes of uveitis: control group (no uveitis), "all uveitis" group (at least one uveitis episode), and recurrent uveitis group (at least two uveitis episodes). The time period was tracked from the index date of each group to (1) the day of AS diagnosis, if any; (2) the day of death, if any; or (3) the last day of the cohort analysis. Incidence rates were calculated as the number of people in whom AS developed after each uveitis episode divided by the total person-time at risk during the study period. The IRR and its 95% CI for AS were calculated using Poisson regression models (i.e., generalized linear models with a Poisson log-linear link function and person-years as the offset variable) based on the incidence rate of AS in the control group. Potential confounding variables such as age, sex, level of income, and year at diagnosis of uveitis episode were included in this model. Separate subgroup analyses with sex and age were performed. Age was stratified into three subgroups: < 40, 40–59, and > 59 years. Statistical analyses were performed using SAS software version 9.3 (SAS Inc., Cary, NC, USA) and R version 3.3.2 (R Foundation for Statistical Computing, Vienna, Austria; http://www.r-project.org). The cutoff for statistical significance was set at $P < 0.05$.

Results

In the present study, 10,483 patients with newly developed anterior uveitis were identified during the period 2004–2013; the average incidence of anterior uveitis was 102.2 per 100,000 person-years. The male/female ratio was 1.14. Table 1 shows the baseline sociodemographic composition of the study population for the three groups: the control group, the "all uveitis" group, and the recurrent uveitis group. We examined 10,483 patients with uveitis and 52,415 sociodemographically matched control subjects. Among the 10,483 patients with uveitis, 2050 (19.6%) experienced at least one or more episodes of uveitis. Excluding the 12 patients who were diagnosed with AS before the second uveitis episode, the recurrent uveitis group comprised 2038 patients. AS developed in 0.08% of the control group subjects, in 0.54% of the patients in the "all uveitis" group, and in 1.03% of those in the recurrent uveitis group ($P < 0.001$). Age, sex, household income, and year of the index date were similar between the control group and uveitis group because these variables were used for matched sampling. The year of the index date in the recurrent uveitis group was later than that in the "all uveitis" group, because the first attacks preceded the second. The median age of the recurrent uveitis group was less than that of the "all uveitis" group (47.5 years vs 52.5 years). For patients with at least one episode of uveitis, the median number of uveitis episodes before AS development was 2 (IQR, 1–3), and the median interval between the first episode of uveitis and AS development was 103.3 weeks (interquartile range, 22.6–214.7 weeks).

Incidence rates per 100,000 person-years of AS in patients in the "all uveitis" group, recurrent uveitis group, and control group are shown in Fig. 2. The IRRs corresponding to each condition are summarized in Table 2. The incidence rate per 100,000 person-years of AS was 16.9 (95% CI, 12.3–22.7) in the control group. Among patients who experienced a uveitis episode at least once, the AS incidence rate increased to 121.5/100,000

Table 1 Baseline demographics of patients with uveitis and matched control subjects

	Control subjects (n = 52,415)	All uveitis (n = 10,483)	Recurrent uveitis (n = 2038)	P value
Ankylosing spondylitis				< 0.001
No	52,371 (99.9%)	10,426 (99.5%)	2017 (99.0%)	
Yes	44 (0.08%)	57 (0.54%)	21 (1.03%)	
Sex				0.983
Male	28,015 (53.4%)	5603 (53.4%)	1085 (53.2%)	
Female	24,400 (46.6%)	4880 (46.6%)	953 (46.8%)	
Age at diagnosis (years)				< 0.001
< 30	9030 (17.2%)	1806 (17.2%)	267 (13.1%)	
30–39	7535 (14.4%)	1507 (14.4%)	360 (17.7%)	
40–49	8980 (17.1%)	1796 (17.1%)	406 (19.9%)	
50–59	8030 (15.3%)	1606 (15.3%)	350 (17.2%)	
60–69	8380 (16.0%)	1676 (16.0%)	322 (15.8%)	
≥ 70	10,460 (20.0%)	2092 (20.0%)	333 (16.3%)	
Household income				> 0.999
First quintile	8760 (16.7%)	1752 (16.7%)	350 (17.2%)	
Second quintile	7510 (14.3%)	1502 (14.3%)	295 (14.5%)	
Third quintile	9650 (18.4%)	1930 (18.4%)	369 (18.1%)	
Fourth quintile	11,200 (21.4%)	2240 (21.4%)	437 (21.4%)	
Fifth quintile (high)	15,295 (29.2%)	3059 (29.2%)	587 (28.8%)	
Year of diagnosis				< 0.001
2004–2005	9020 (17.2%)	1804 (17.2%)	156 (7.67%)	
2006–2007	8980 (17.1%)	1796 (17.1%)	313 (15.4%)	
2008–2009	9920 (18.9%)	1984 (18.9%)	390 (19.2%)	
2010–2011	12,440 (23.7%)	2488 (23.7%)	559 (27.5%)	
2012–2013	12,055 (23.0%)	2411 (23.0%)	617 (30.3%)	

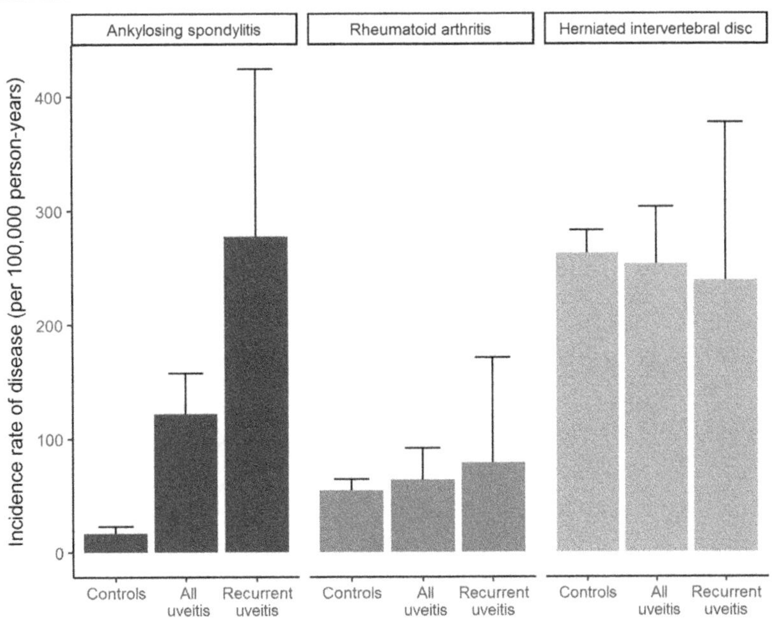

Fig. 2 Incidence of ankylosing spondylitis, rheumatoid arthritis, and herniated intervertebral disc according to uveitis episode numbers

Table 2 Incidence rate ratio of diseases, along with number of episodes of uveitis

Disease	Group	No. of diseases	Person-years	IR	IRR (95% CI)	*P* value
AS	Control subjects	44	52,415	16.9	1 (reference)	
	All uveitis	57	10,483	121.5	7.40 (4.99–10.98)	< 0.001
	Recurrent uveitis	21	2038	277.3	17.71 (10.44–30.06)	< 0.001
RA	Control subjects	141	52,241	54.5	1 (reference)	
	All uveitis	30	10,439	64.0	1.16 (0.78–1.71)	0.473
	Recurrent uveitis	6	2038	78.6	1.45 (0.64–3.28)	0.377
HIVD	Control subjects	671	51,833	262.2	1 (reference)	
	All uveitis	117	10,329	252.9	0.97 (0.80–1.18)	0.757
	Recurrent uveitis	18	2019	238.4	0.93 (0.58–1.48)	0.750

Abbreviations: AS Ankylosing spondylitis, *HIVD* Herniated intervertebral disc, *IR* Incidence rate per 100,000 person-years, *IRR* Incidence rate ratio, *RA* Rheumatoid arthritis

person-years (95% CI, 92.0–157.4). The incidence rates rose to 277.3 (95% CI, 171.6–423.8) in patients who experienced more than two episodes of uveitis. As disease controls, the RA and HIVD incidences did not show a correlation with the occurrence or recurrence of uveitis.

Subgroup analysis for age and sex are provided in Table 3 and Fig. 3. Among the controls, AS occurred predominantly in males (20.4 vs 12.7 per 100,000 person-years). However, among patients with recurrent uveitis, the predilection for male sex was not prominent (284.1 vs 268.7 per 100,000 person-years). In patients aged under 40 years, the IRR for the recurrent uveitis group was 46.78 (95% CI, 19.61–111.61). In contrast, AS incidence in the recurrent uveitis groups aged over 59 years did not differ from that of the controls.

Discussion

In this retrospective, community-based cohort study, we observed that the incidence rate of AS increased with recurrence of episodes of uveitis: 7.4-fold after one uveitis episode and 17.7-fold after two episodes. Furthermore, age and sex had an impact on the association between the number of uveitis episodes and subsequent AS incidence among the groups.

The methodology used for detecting the recurrence of episodes of uveitis is the main highlight of the present study. We had to identify whether a patient with uveitis had a 90-day inactive phase without uveitis treatment during sequential visits with a diagnostic code of uveitis. Considering that claims with a uveitis diagnostic code could not guarantee an active episode, claims with

Table 3 Incidence rate ratio of diseases along with sex and number of episodes of uveitis

Subgroup	Group	No. of AS	Person-years	IR	IRR (95% CI)	*P* value
By age						
< 40 years	Control subjects	11	86,359	12.7	1 (reference)	
	All uveitis	32	15,430	207.4	17.64 (8.87–35.09)	< 0.001
	Recurrent uveitis	12	2461	487.5	46.78 (19.61–111.61)	< 0.001
40–59 years	Control subjects	16	87,723	18.2	1 (reference)	
	All uveitis	19	15,745	120.7	6.70 (3.44–13.06)	< 0.001
	Recurrent uveitis	8	2994	267.2	15.12 (6.41–35.65)	< 0.001
> 59 years	Control subjects	17	85,785	19.8	1 (reference)	
	All uveitis	6	15,739	38.1	1.90 (0.75–4.81)	0.178
	Recurrent uveitis	1	2119	47.2	2.46 (0.33–18.53)	0.382
By sex						
Male	Control subjects	29	142,124	20.4	1 (reference)	
	All uveitis	33	25,678	128.5	6.34 (3.84–10.44)	< 0.001
	Recurrent uveitis	12	4224	284.1	14.38 (7.28–28.41)	< 0.001
Female	Control subjects	15	117,744	12.7	1 (reference)	
	All uveitis	24	21,235	113.0	9.54 (4.99–18.24)	< 0.001
	Recurrent uveitis	9	3350	268.7	23.61 (10.05–55.47)	< 0.001

Abbreviations: AS Ankylosing spondylitis, *IR* Incidence rate per 100,000 person-years, *IRR* Incidence rate ratio

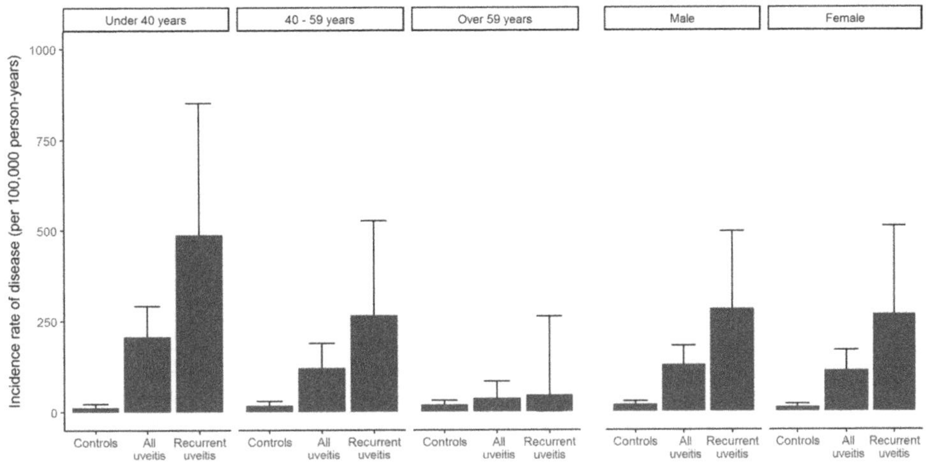

Fig. 3 Incidence of ankylosing spondylitis according to age, sex, and uveitis episode numbers

corresponding diagnostic codes and a prescription code for either steroid or immunosuppressive agents on the same day as the diagnosis were designated active uveitis cases. Thereafter, we defined recurrence of uveitis as cases where the time interval between two episodes of active anterior uveitis was more than 120 days, assuming that a bottle of topical steroid is usually used for 1 month. However, it was possible that the actual duration of application of ophthalmic solutions was less than 1 month, and our criterion of 120 days for defining uveitis recurrence was too long. To confirm whether our study results based on this criterion were stable and robust, we recalculated the primary outcome of the study with different values for time of recurrence interval and found that the results did not vary substantially (Additional file 3: Table S3). Thus, although the criterion for the time interval between claims for identifying recurrence was not indisputably definite, this was estimated to have no significant impact on the results of this study.

We performed additional analyses with disease controls to support the methodology used in this study because the results of a claim-based cohort study could potentially be biased by the increasing annual use of healthcare, especially in chronic diseases, or by the availability of healthcare for only certain diseases. RA is known to be a prevalent inflammatory arthritis that is not associated with uveitis [9]. In our study, RA did not show a correlation with uveitis, either as a single episode or recurrent. HIVD is a representative spondylopathy that is presumably not related to uveitis. If a patient with uveitis had a symptom of spondylopathy and thus the possibility of the patient visiting a spine clinic, the HIVD detection rate hence would have been higher. However, the detected occurrence of HIVD among patients with uveitis was not different from that in the control subjects. On the basis of these results, we assumed that our method of assessing the risk of systemic association in patients with uveitis was not significantly biased.

Male predominance is a well-known characteristic of AS. However, it was not prominent in patients with recurrent uveitis. Therefore, in managing female patients with recurrent uveitis, the possibility of the AS association should not be underestimated. The age-specific subgroup analysis showed that recurrent uveitis was associated with a substantially elevated risk of AS development in younger patients, and additional workup for uveitis should be considered to investigate any systemic association, including AS.

Although a claim data-based epidemiological analysis is advantageous for studying a rare disease and its associations with other diseases, there are certain limitations. First, the diagnoses of uveitis and AS were not clinically confirmed individually according to strict classification criteria, and overestimation or underestimation of the presence of diseases could have occurred. To restrict the overestimation of incident cases, we added the precondition that the identification of a uveitis episode required the simultaneous prescription of a local or systemic steroid or immunosuppressive agent and excluded patients with AS who had diagnostic codes of systemic lupus erythematosus or RA. Underestimation was also possible if a patient with a certain disease did not use the NHIS. In addition, systemic treatment for anterior uveitis might suppress or mask the incidence of subsequent AS. However, because anterior uveitis can usually be managed with topical and oral steroid administration for a limited period, it is unlikely that this treatment can suppress the onset of subsequent AS itself. Second, some potentially useful information was unavailable because medical records and laboratory test results of each patient were not included in the claim data; detailed characteristics of anterior uveitis (e.g., grade of inflammation, granulomatous or nongranulomatous), details of AS manifestation at onset, human leukocyte antigen B27 positivity, and levels of C-reactive protein and acute-phase reactant at the onset of uveitis or AS were not considered. This study would have been more informative if these variables could have been included in the regression model and if the analysis had indicated which variables were valuable in predicting subsequent AS occurrence in patients with uveitis, if any. Inactivity and recurrence of uveitis were also estimated indirectly by the type and schedule of prescribed medication. Although there are some intrinsic limitations of the insurance claim data, the general trend of the association between AS and recurrent uveitis was still obvious.

Conclusions

We evaluated the risk of subsequent AS development after recurrent uveitis among Korean patients during a 10-year follow-up period. The incidence of AS increased proportionally with the number of episodes of uveitis. The estimated incidence of AS increased 7.4- and 17.7-fold after the first and second episodes of uveitis, respectively. This study provides a rationale for ancillary workup for possible systemic associations in patients with recurrent uveitis and emphasizes the importance of multidisciplinary collaboration in the diagnosis and management of AS.

Abbreviations

AS: Ankylosing spondylitis; HIVD: Herniated intervertebral disc; ICD-10: International Classification of Diseases, Tenth Revision; IR: Incidence rate; IRR: Incidence rate ratio; NSC: National Sample Cohort; NHIS: National Health Insurance Service; RA: Rheumatoid arthritis

Acknowledgements

The authors thank the National Health Insurance Service for providing the data regarding the original cohort, which included 1 million Korean individuals.

Funding

This study was supported by a grant from the Korea Health Technology R&D Project through the Korea Health Industry Development Institute (KHIDI), funded by the Ministry of Health & Welfare, Republic of Korea (grant number HI14C1277). The funder had no role in the study design, data collection and analysis, decision to publish, or preparation of the manuscript.

Author's contributions

BLO and HGY participated in the study design, obtained data, conducted statistical analysis, and drafted the manuscript. JSL, EYL, and HYL participated in statistical analysis and revised the manuscript. All authors read and approved the final manuscript.

Consent for publication

All authors gave their consent for publication of the study. No identifiable patient data are contained in this article.

Competing interests

The authors declare that they have no competing interests.

Author details

[1]Department of Ophthalmology, Armed Forces Capital Hospital, Seongnam, Gyeonggi-do, South Korea. [2]Division of Rheumatology, Department of Internal Medicine, Seoul National University College of Medicine, Seoul National University Hospital, Seoul, South Korea. [3]Center for Preventive Medicine and Public Health, Seoul National University Bundang Hospital, Seongnam, Gyeonggi-do, South Korea. [4]Department of Ophthalmology, Seoul National University College of Medicine, Seoul National University Hospital, Seoul, South Korea.

References

1. Wade NK. Diagnostic testing in patients with ocular inflammation. Int Ophthalmol Clin. 2000;40:37–54.
2. Rudwaleit M, van der Heijde D, Landewé R, Listing J, Akkoc N, Brandt J, et al. The development of Assessment of SpondyloArthritis international Society classification criteria for axial spondyloarthritis (part II): validation and final selection. Ann Rheum Dis. 2009;68:777–83.
3. Stolwijk C, van Tubergen A, Castillo-Ortiz JD, Boonen A. Prevalence of extra-articular manifestations in patients with ankylosing spondylitis: a systematic review and meta-analysis. Ann Rheum Dis. 2015;74:65–73.
4. Stolwijk C, Boonen A, van Tubergen A, Reveille JD. Epidemiology of spondyloarthritis. Rheum Dis Clin North Am. 2012;38:441–76.
5. Mathur G, Biswas J. Systemic associations of anterior uveitis in a tertiary care ophthalmic centre in south India. Int Ophthalmol. 2012;32:417–21.
6. Rothova A, Buitenhuis HJ, Meenken C, Brinkman CJ, Linssen A, Alberts C, et al. Uveitis and systemic disease. Br J Ophthalmol. 1992;76:137–41.
7. Lee J, Lee JS, Park SH, Shin SA, Kim K. Cohort Profile: The National Health Insurance Service-National Sample Cohort (NHIS-NSC), South Korea. Int J Epidemiol. 2017;46:e15.
8. Jabs DA, Nussenblatt RB, Rosenbaum JT, Standardization of Uveitis Nomenclature (SUN) Working Group. Standardization of uveitis nomenclature for reporting clinical data: results of the first international workshop. Am J Ophthalmol. 2005;140:509–16.
9. Rosenbaum JT. Round 20: why a rheumatologist needs to understand uveitis. Johns Hopkins Arthritis Center, Physician Corner. Rheumatology Rounds Online. https://www.hopkinsarthritis.org/physician-corner/rheumatology-rounds/round-20-why-a-rheumatologist-needs-to-understand-uveitis/. Accessed 25 Aug 2017.

11

Anti-CD74 antibodies have no diagnostic value in early axial spondyloarthritis: data from the spondyloarthritis caught early (SPACE) cohort

Janneke J. de Winter[1*], Marleen G. van de Sande[1], Niklas Baerlecken[2,6], Inger Berg[3], Roberta Ramonda[4], Désirée van der Heijde[5], Floris A. van Gaalen[5], Torsten Witte[2†] and Dominique L. Baeten[1†]

Abstract

Background: Anti-CD74 IgG antibodies are reported to be elevated in patients with axial spondyloarthritis (axSpA). This study assessed the diagnostic value of anti-CD74 antibodies in patients with early axSpA.

Methods: Anti-CD74 IgG and IgA antibodies were first measured in an exploratory cohort of patients with radiographic axSpA (138 patients with ankylosing spondyloarthritis (AS)) and 57 healthy controls and then were measured in patients with early axSpA (n = 274) and with non-SpA chronic back pain (CBP) (n = 319), participating in the spondyloarthritis caught early (SPACE) prospective cohort study of patients under 45 years old with early back pain (for ≥ 3 months, but ≤ 2 years).

Results: In the exploratory cohort, anti-CD74 IgG antibodies were present in 79.7% of patients with AS vs. 43.9% of healthy controls ($p < 0.001$). Anti-CD74 IgA antibodies were present in 28.5% of patients with AS vs. 5.3% of healthy controls ($p < 0.001$). In the SPACE cohort, anti-CD74 IgG antibody levels were present in 46.4% of the patients with axSpA vs. 47.9% of the patients with CBP ($p = 0.71$). Anti-CD74 IgA antibodies were present in 54.7% of the patients with axSpA and 37.0% of the patients with CBP ($p < 0.001$). This resulted in a positive predictive value of 58.8% (compared to a prior probability of 46.2%) and a negative predictive value of 59.1% (compared to a prior probability of 53.8%). In a regression model, total serum IgA was associated with axSpA odds ratio (OR) 1.19, $p < 0.001$) whereas anti-CD74 IgA was not (OR) 1.01, $p = 0.33$). Furthermore, anti-CD74 IgA was associated with sacroiliitis on magnetic resonance imaging (MRI) (OR) = 2.50, $p = 0.005$) and heel enthesitis (OR) = 2.56, $p = 0.002$).

Conclusions: Albeit anti-CD74 IgA is elevated in patients with early axSpA, this elevation is not sufficiently specific to yield significant diagnostic value in patients under 45 years old presenting with early back pain.

Keywords: Axial spondyloarthritis, Early diagnosis, Biomarker

Background

Axial spondyloarthritis (axSpA) is a prevalent form of chronic inflammatory arthritis, affecting 0.5–1.5% of the Western population [1, 2]. Current biological disease markers in axSpA (human leukocyte antigen (HLA)-B27, C-reactive protein (CRP), sacroiliitis shown on radiography or magnetic resonance imaging (MRI)) have insufficient diagnostic properties to rely on for making a diagnosis, impeding early diagnosis and treatment. Although diagnostic delays have decreased over recent years as a result of modern imaging techniques and more awareness of axSpA, the current diagnostic delay ranging from 5 to 10 years [3–6] prevents treatment in the early disease phase.

Two recent studies provided preliminary evidence that anti-CD74 antibodies are elevated in SpA [7, 8]. CD74, also known as the HLA class II γ-chain or invariant chain,

* Correspondence: j.j.dewinter@amc.uva.nl
†Equal contributors
[1]Department of Clinical Immunology and Rheumatology, Amsterdam Rheumatology and immunology Center, Academic Medical Center/University of Amsterdam, Amsterdam, The Netherlands
Full list of author information is available at the end of the article

is involved in the assembly of major histocompatibility complex II and in preventing premature peptide binding [9]. The extracellular part has two different domains, thyroglobulin type-1 and class II-associated invariant chain peptide (CLIP). Binding of antibodies to CD74 may lead to activation of cells and production of proinflammatory cytokines such as tumor necrosis factor α (TNFα) [10]. The first cross-sectional study showed that anti-CD74 IgG antibodies were present in 67% of the 216 tested patients with axSpA, compared to 6% of 285 non-SpA controls (blood donors or patients with diseases other than axSpA) [8]. The second study showed that IgG anti-CD74 antibodies were detected in 85% of the 145 patients with axSpA and in 8% of the 51 patients without SpA [7].

Although indicating the potential importance of anti-CD74 IgG antibodies in axSpA, the role of anti-CD74 antibodies in a diagnostic setting is still not confirmed. Therefore, the aim of this study was to test the level and diagnostic value of anti-CD74 IgG and IgA antibodies in a "real life" diagnostic setting using patients with axSpA and patients with chronic back pain (CBP) from a cohort of patients with early back pain, the spondyloarthritis caught early (SPACE) cohort.

Methods

Exploratory cohort: patients with radiographic axSpA and healthy controls

Serum from patients with radiographic axSpA (ankylosing spondyloarthritis (AS)) was collected in the Academic Medical Center/University of Amsterdam ($n = 21$) and the Medical University of Hannover ($n = 117$). All patients with AS were diagnosed by a rheumatologist with AS and fulfilled the modified New York (mNY) criteria for AS. Serum from healthy controls was collected in the Academic Medical Center/University of Amsterdam ($n = 19$) and the Medical University of Hannover ($n = 38$). All patients with AS and all healthy controls gave their written informed consent and the studies were approved by the local ethics committees of the Academic Medical Center/University of Amsterdam and the Medical University of Hannover. Serum samples were stored for at least 6 months at − 80 °C.

We included 138 patients with AS and 57 healthy controls. The mean (SD) age was 46.1 (13.1) in patients with AS and 36.7 (13.5) in healthy controls ($p < 0.001$). Of the patients with AS, 92 out of 117 were male vs. 22 out of the 38 healthy controls (78.6% vs. 57.9%, $p = 0.012$). HLA-B27 was determined in 117 out of 138 patients with AS; 108 out of 117 patients were HLA-B27-positive (92.3%). The mean disease duration was 24.3 (13.2) months.

The SPACE cohort

We used baseline serum samples from the SPACE cohort. The SPACE cohort is an ongoing, prospective, multicenter, longitudinal cohort that started in 2009 and has previously been described in detail [11]. In short, the SPACE cohort includes patients aged ≥ 16 years with chronic back pain (for ≥ 3 months, but ≤ 2 years) with onset before the age of 45 years. The local medical ethical committees of the participating sites approved the study and all participants gave their written informed consent. For the present analyses, data and serum from the baseline visit were used. We used the central reading results of radiography and MRI of the sacroiliac joints [11]. The primary outcome was an axSpA diagnosis by a rheumatologist vs. no axSpA diagnosis by a rheumatologist. As secondary outcomes, we used (1) a strict definition of axSpA: patients diagnosed by a rheumatologist as having axSpA plus fulfilling the Assessment of SpondyloArthritis International Society (ASAS) axSpA criteria vs. patients not diagnosed by a rheumatologist as having axSpA and not fulfilling the ASAS axSpA criteria, and (2) patients participating in SPACE diagnosed by a rheumatologist as having axSpA at baseline and after 1 year of follow up vs. patients not diagnosed as axSpA on assessment at these two time points. Serum samples were collected at baseline and stored for at least 6 months at − 80 °C.

We included 593 patients from the SPACE cohort, including 274 patients diagnosed with axSpA at baseline. Table 1 shows baseline characteristics of the study patients. In short, 119 of the patients with axSpA were male vs. 81 of the patients with CBP (43.4% vs. 28.3%, $p < 0.001$). The mean age of the patients with axSpA was 30.7 (7.9) years at inclusion and in the patients with CBP it was 31.4 (8.5) years ($p = 0.83$). Of the axSpA patients, 165 were HLA-B27-positive versus 63 of the patients with CBP (60.7% vs. 22.1%, $p < 0.001$). Of the patients with axSpA, 172 fulfilled the ASAS axSpA criteria and 48 of the patients with CBP fulfilled the ASAS axSpA criteria (62.8% vs. 37.2%, $p < 0.001$).

Missing values were below 5% except for axSpA diagnosis (5.6%), swollen joint count (SJC (5.7%)), C-reactive protein (CRP (7.1%)), sacroiliitis according to the modified New York (mNY) criteria (17.3%), Bath Ankylosing Spondylitis Disease Activity Index (BASDAI) (15.0%)), total serum IgA (9.2%) and the number of patients missing the 1-year evaluation (58.9%). This was mostly due to the study protocol: not all patients were invited for follow up and some patients did not have a 1-year visit due to shorter follow up.

Anti-CD74 antibody detection

Two different enzyme-linked immunosorbent assays (ELISAs) were performed to detect anti-CD74 IgG

Table 1 Demographic and disease characteristics of patients with axial spondyloarthritis (axSpA) and patients with chronic back pain (CBP) participating in the SPACE cohort

	Diagnosed with axSpA		
	Yes (*n* = 274)	No (*n* = 286)	*P* value
Male (*n*, %)	119 (43.4)	181 (28.3)	<0.001
Age (mean, SD)	30.7 (7.9)	31.4 (8.5)	0.83
HLA-B27 positive (*n*, %)	165 (60.7)	63 (22.1)	<0.001
Positive family history (*n*, %)	131 (47.8)	111 (38.8)	0.03
Duration of back pain in months (mean, SD)	13.1 (7.0)	13.5 (7.2)	0.59
Inflammatory back pain (*n*, %)	213 (77.7)	154 (54.0)	<0.001
Peripheral arthritis (*n*, %)	59 (21.6)	23 (8.1)	<0.001
Enthesitis (*n*, %)	91 (33.2)	21 (7.3)	<0.001
Dactylitis (*n*, %)	25 (9.1)	4 (1.4)	<0.001
IBD (*n*, %)	21 (7.7)	16 (5.6)	0.32
Psoriasis (*n*, %)	43 (15.7)	19 (6.6)	0.001
Uveitis (*n*, %)	32 (11.7)	7 (2.4)	<0.001
Tender joint count (mean, SD)	2.2 (5.0)	1.9 (3.7)	0.38
Swollen joint count (mean, SD)	0.6 (2.1)	0.1 (0.6)	0.001
CRP, mg/L (median, IQR)	3.0 (3.0–5.0)	3.7 (3.0–7.0)	0.001
CRP >5 mg/L (*n*, %)	113 (41.7)	70 (26.2)	<0.001
ESR, mm/h (mean, SD)	14.9 (15.8)	9.2 (11.4)	<0.001
ESR >20 mm/h (*n*, %)	63 (23.6)	20 (7.1)	<0.001
ASAS axSpA criteria (*n*, %)	172 (62.8)	48 (16.8)	<0.001
mNY criteria (*n*, %)	33 (14.4)	5 (2.0)	<0.001
Any DMARD use (*n*, %)	38 (14.0)	14 (5.1)	<0.001
NSAID use (*n*, %)	197 (72.4)	172 (60.8)	0.004
BASDAI (mean, SD)	4.2 (2.1)	4.7 (2.0)	0.01
Diagnosed with axSpA at 1-year follow up (*n*, %)	143 (52.2)	16 (5.6)	<0.001

Missing values were below 5% except for axial spondyloarthritis (axSpA) diagnosis (5.6%), SJC (5.7%), C-reactive protein (CRP) (7.1%), modified New York (mNY) criteria (17.3%), Bath Ankylosing Spondylitis Disease Activity Index (BASDAI) (15.0%) and the number of patients still diagnosed as having axSpA after 1 year of follow up (58.9%)

ASAS Assessment of SpondyloArthritis International Society, *DMARD* disease-modifying antirheumatic drug, *ESR* erythrocyte sedimentation rate, *IBD* inflammatory bowel disease, *NSAID* nonsteroidal anti-inflammatory drug

and anti-CD74 IgA antibodies. The Medical University of Hannover developed the ELISAs to detect anti-CD74 IgG and IgA antibodies in cooperation with AESKU Diagnostics (Wendelsheim, Germany), as described earlier by Baerlecken et al. [8]. The originally described ELISAs were improved for the current study as the old (peptide-based) test only worked with serum that had been frozen for a long time. The tests were performed according to the manufacturer's protocol. Anti-CD74 IgG is expressed as optical density (OD), anti-CD74 IgA is expressed as OD (AS vs. healthy controls) or U/mL (in the SPACE cohort, at that time standard serum was available). We also measured the amount of total serum IgA, as earlier studies showed that total serum IgA is elevated in axSpA [12, 13].

Data analysis

The chi-square ($\chi 2$) test and Mann-Whitney U test were used for categorical and continuous data, respectively. Categorical data are presented as number (percent), continuous data are presented as the mean (SD) or as median (interquartile range (IQR)) as appropriate. Statistical tests were two-sided, and p values < 0.05 were considered significant. Only the available data were analyzed. Linear correlation between two continuous variables was calculated by calculating Pearson's correlation coefficient (r). Receiver operating characteristic (ROC) analysis and the maximum value of the Youden index (sensitivity + specificity − 1) [14] was used to evaluate the predictive value of anti-CD74 IgG and IgA antibodies and to calculate the best possible cutoff. These cutoff values were used to calculate the positive predictive value (PPV) and negative predictive value (NPV) and positive and negative likelihood ratios (LR+ and LR-, respectively) of anti-CD74 IgG and IgA antibodies in discriminating between patients with axSpA and patients with CBP.

We explored which characteristics among patients with axSpA were associated with higher anti-CD74 IgA levels by logistic regression. We started with a set of predetermined candidate variables: HLA-B27, disease duration, sacroiliitis on radiography or MRI, peripheral (arthritis, dactylitis and heel enthesitis) and extra-articular (uveitis, psoriasis and inflammatory bowel disease (IBD)) disease manifestations and used backward elimination to create the final model.

We evaluated the association between anti-CD74 IgA and total IgA by univariate and multivariate logistic regression by both forward selection and backward elimination. Besides total IgA and anti-CD74 IgA we added potential confounding variables: HLA-B27, disease duration, sacroiliitis on radiography or MRI, peripheral (arthritis, dactylitis and heel enthesitis) and extra-articular (uveitis, psoriasis and IBD) disease manifestations. Since the interpretation of the regression analysis might be influenced by collinearity between anti-CD74 and total IgA, we first assessed the amount of collinearity by calculating Pearson's correlation coefficient, variance inflating factor (VIF) and tolerance (R^2). Values of Pearson's correlation coefficient >0.7, VIF >5 and tolerance <0.20 were considered problematic for interpreting the regression model [15]. We used IBM SPSS Statistics 24 for all analyses.

Results

Anti-CD74 IgG antibodies

To confirm the earlier results [7, 8], we first measured the level, prevalence and diagnostic value of anti-CD74 IgG antibodies. In the exploratory cohort, median anti-CD74 IgG antibodies (OD) were higher in patients with AS than in healthy controls (0.70 vs. 0.51, $p < 0.001$). The AUC on ROC analysis was 0.70 (95% CI 0.62–0.79) and resulted in a cutoff of 0.52. Using this cutoff, anti-CD74 IgG antibodies were present in 110 out of 138 patients with AS vs. 25 out of 57 healthy controls (79.7% vs. 43.9%, $p < 0.001$).

In the SPACE cohort, median anti-CD74 IgG antibodies (OD) did not differ between patients with axSpA and patients with CBP (0.50 vs. 0.52, $p = 0.15$). The AUC on ROC analysis was 0.47 (95% CI 0.42–0.51). Using a cutoff of 0.52, anti-CD74 IgG antibodies were present in 127 out of 274 patients with axSpA and in 137 out of 286 patients with CBP (46.4% vs. 47.9%, $p = 0.71$) resulting in a PPV of 48.1%, a NPV of 50.3%, a LR+ of 0.97 and a LR- of 1.03.

Anti-CD74 IgA antibodies

Because anti-CD74 IgG antibodies did not have diagnostic value in the SPACE cohort, we explored the level, prevalence and diagnostic value of anti-CD74 IgA antibodies, as earlier research shows that total serum IgA is elevated in axSpA [12, 16] and that IgA is produced at mucosal surfaces, including the gut, which may be inflamed in spondyloarthritis [17].

In the exploratory cohort, median anti-CD74 IgA antibodies (OD) were higher in patients with AS than in healthy controls (0.31 vs. 0.20, $p < 0.001$). The AUC on ROC analysis was 0.78 (95% CI 0.82–0.79) and resulted in a cutoff of 0.22 (Fig. 1). Using this cutoff, anti-CD74 IgA antibodies were present in 39 of 138 patients with AS and in 3 out of 57 healthy controls (28.5% vs. 5.3%, $p < 0.001$.

In the SPACE cohort, median anti-CD74 IgA antibodies (U/mL) were higher in patients with axSpA than in patients with CBP (19.9 vs. 14.0, $p < 0.001$, Fig. 1). The AUC on ROC analysis was 0.60 (95% CI 0.55–0.65). Using a cutoff of 18.0 U/mL, anti-CD74 IgA antibodies were positive in 150 of 274 patients with axSpA vs. 105 of 284 patients with CBP (54.7% vs. 37.0%, $p < 0.001$). Anti-CD74 IgA testing with a pre-test probability of axSpA of 46.2% (and thus 53.8% not having axSpA) resulted in a PPV of 58.8%, a NPV of 59.1%, a LR+ of 1.48 and a LR- of 0.72.

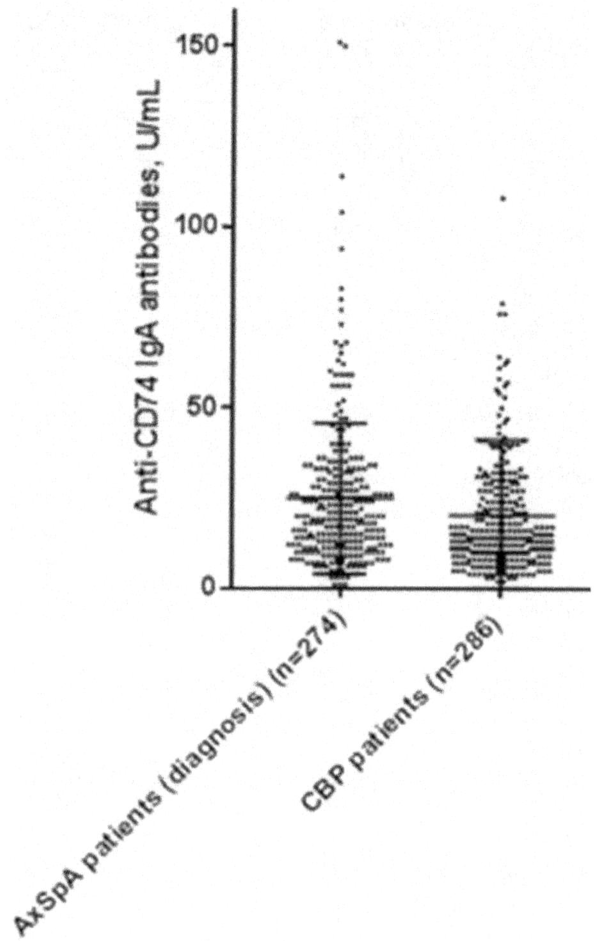

Fig. 1 Anti-CD74 IgA antibody levels measured in serum from participants in the SPACE cohort. Axial spondyloarthritis (axSpA) (diagnosis), participants in SPACE who were diagnosed with axSpA by a rheumatologist at baseline; CBP, patients with chronic back pain. One data point is outside the axis limits

Analyses using different definitions of axSpA

As the results of the diagnostic biomarker analysis may depend on the "gold standard" for diagnosis of axSpA, we also tested the median anti-CD74 IgG and IgA levels looking at (1) patients in the SPACE cohort who were diagnosed using a strict definition of axSpA (diagnosed as by a rheumatologist and also according to the Assessment of SpondyloArthritis International Society (ASAS) criteria) ($n = 172$) versus those not fulfilling either rheumatologist diagnosis or ASAS criteria ($n = 238$) and (2) patients in the SPACE cohort with confirmed diagnosis of axSpA ($n = 143$) or no axSpA ($n = 64$) after 1 of year follow up (1 year follow-up data were available in 244 patients in total). As shown in Table 2, the results of these additional analyses were comparable to the primary analyses.

Anti-CD74 IgA antibodies in axSpA subpopulations

We additionally explored if anti-CD74 IgA antibodies were associated with a specific sub-population of patients with axSpA. In the exploratory cohort, the mean disease duration in patients with AS with or without anti-CD74 IgA antibodies did not differ (24.12 vs. 24.35 months, respectively, p = 0.931).

In the SPACE cohort, on comparison of patients with axSpA with or without HLA-B27, elevated CRP, inflammatory back pain, sacroiliitis shown on MRI and peripheral (enthesitis, arthritis or dactylitis) or extra-articular (psoriasis, uveitis or IBD) manifestations there were no differences (data not shown). Patients with axSpA with radiographic sacroiliitis more often had anti-CD74 IgA antibodies than patients with axSpA without radiographic sacroiliitis (66.7% vs. 46.4%, p = 0.031). In regression analysis within the population of patients with axSpA, sacroiliitis on MRI and heel enthesitis were both significantly associated with elevated anti-CD74 IgA odds ration (OR) = 2.50, p = 0.005 and (OR) = 2.56, p = 0.002, respectively). HLA-B27, CRP, inflammatory back pain, radiographic sacroiliitis and peripheral manifestations other than heel enthesitis or extra-articular manifestations were not associated with anti-CD74 IgA levels.

Total serum IgA

Since earlier studies showed that total serum IgA is elevated in patients with AS [12, 13], we additionally measured total serum IgA in the SPACE cohort. The AUC on ROC curve analysis was 0.59. Total IgA was higher in patients with axSpA than in patients with CBP (4.07 vs. 3.37 g/L, p < 0.001, Table 2). Total serum IgA was higher than the upper reference range (4.0 g/L) in 49.0% of the patients with axSpA and in 35.8% of the patients with CBP (p = 0.008). Anti-CD74 IgA and total IgA were both statistically significant predictors of diagnosis of axSpA, in a univariate logistic regression model (data not shown). We tested for collinearity by first measuring Pearson's correlation coefficient, which was 0.31 for total IgA and anti-CD74 IgA (p < 0.001). Second, we determined the VIF in a linear regression model, showing that the amount of collinearity was low (VIF of 1.11 and R^2 of 0.90). In a multivariate logistic regression model including anti-CD74 IgA and total IgA, total serum IgA was associated with a diagnosis of axSpA (OR) 1.19, p < 0.001), whereas anti-CD74 IgA was not (OR) 1.01, p = 0.33). Adding other potential confounding variables to the model (CRP, inflammatory back pain, HLA-B27, inflammatory bowel disease) did not change the results.

Discussion

The results of our study suggest that (1) serum anti-CD74 IgG and IgA antibodies are elevated in patients with AS compared to healthy controls, (2) serum anti-CD74 IgG antibodies are not elevated in patients with early axSpA compared to patients with CBP, (3) serum anti-CD74 IgA antibody levels are elevated in patients with early axSpA compared to patients with CBP, but (4) serum anti-CD74 IgA antibodies have no diagnostic value in patients with early back pain because of small numerical differences.

Previous studies showed that anti-CD74 IgG antibodies are present in 69% and 85% of patients with (mostly radiographic) axSpA [7, 8] in comparison with 6% and 8% of individuals in control populations without axSpA or back pain. Somewhat lower numbers were obtained in the current study when assessing patients with radiographic axSpA in the SPACE cohort, as 54.5% had anti-CD74 IgG antibodies (data not shown). However, our study revealed two novel pieces of information. First, the percentage of patients with non-radiographic axSpA who were positive for anti-CD74 IgG antibodies was lower (43.9%), suggesting that either the antibodies develop over time or that they are associated with radiographic sacroiliitis rather than with the diagnosis of axSpA per se. Second, the percentage of control patients with elevated

Table 2 Anti-CD74 antibody and IgA levels in serum from patients in the SPACE cohort

	AxSpA (diagnosis)			Diagnosis and ASAS axSpA criteria			AxSpA (diagnosis) confirmed at 1-year follow up		
	Yes (n = 274)	No (n = 286)	*P* value	Yes (n = 172)	No (n = 238)	*P* value	Yes (n = 143)	No (n = 64)	*P* value
Anti-CD74 IgG (OD)	0.50 (0.32–0.65)	0.52 (0.38–0.69)	0.15	0.50 (0.30–0.67)	0.52 (0.39–0.70)	0.075	0.43 (0.30–0.58)	0.48 (0.35–0.61)	0.32
Anti-CD74 IgA (U/mL)	19.9 (11.4–30.6)	14.0 (9.3–26.0)	<0.001	21.8 (11.6–31.9)	13.5 (8.4–22.3)	<0.001	17.6 (9.9–29.0)	13.7 (9.4–23.6)	0.10
Total IgA (g/L)	4.07 (2.90–4.97)	3.37 (2.57–4.66)	<0.001	4.06 (3.01–5.03)	3.29 (2.42–4.62)	0.001	4.02 (2.77–4.78)	3.66 (2.43–4.74)	0.14

Results are shown as median (IQR). Axial spondyloarthritis (axSpA) (diagnosis): SPACE participants diagnosed with axSpA by a rheumatologist at baseline; Assessment of SpondyloArthritis International Society (ASAS) axSpA criteria: SPACE participants fulfilling versus not fulfilling the ASAS axSpA criteria at baseline; Diagnosis and ASAS axSpA: SPACE participants diagnosed as having axSpA and fulfilling the ASAS axSpA criteria versus patients not diagnosed as having axSpA and not fulfilling the ASAS axSpA criteria. Missing values were 5.6% for diagnosis of axSpA, 3% for fulfilling the ASAS axSpA criteria, 30.9% for diagnosis and ASAS axSpA criteria and 58.9% for axSpA diagnosis at 1-year follow up

OD optical density

anti-CD47 IgG antibodies (47.9%) was much higher in our study than in the previous reports. This may be due either to the fact that the antibodies are higher in patients with CBP than in healthy individuals, or may be explained by the fact that the anti-CD74 IgG assay has been modified over time. Indeed, the original assay was sensitive to interference by soluble CD74 in serum, leading to false negative results in samples where sCD74 had not been degraded by freezing-thawing. In contrast, the assay used here is not biased by the presence of sCD74 and should therefore be more reliable.

In contrast with the previous suggestion that the presence of anti-CD74 IgG was especially high in early axSpA and declined with longer disease duration [7, 8], disease duration did not correlate with anti-CD74 IgG but we noted lower presence in non-radiographic axSpA and higher presence in controls with CBP. Collectively, these data indicate that anti-CD74 IgG has no significant diagnostic value in patients under 45 years old presenting with recent-onset back pain.

A second important finding of this study is that anti-CD74 IgA appear better that anti-CD74 IgG antibodies as a biomarker in axSpA. In contrast to IgG, the anti-CD74 IgA antibody levels were indeed higher in patients with axSpA than in patients with CBP. Another study investigating the sensitivity and specificity of anti-CD74 antibodies in a cohort of patients with axSpA (the InterSpA cohort) compared to healthy donors showed that anti-CD74 IgA antibodies were elevated in 65.4% of 104 patients fulfilling the ASAS axSpA criteria [18]. When we used the same cutoff as was used in the InterSpA cohort (15 U/mL), 63.1% of the SPACE patients with axSpA had elevated anti-CD74 IgA antibodies. However, 47.5% of the patients with CBP also had elevated anti-CD74 IgA antibodies when using this cutoff. Despite the numerical differences in the SPACE cohort between patients with axSpA and CBP, testing for anti-CD74 IgA antibodies only modestly increased the pre-test probability of axSpA (46.2%) to 58.8% post-test probability. Similarly, the NPV of anti-CD74 IgA antibodies was low. The LR+ of 1.48 and LR- of 0.72 confirmed that although anti-CD74 is associated with axSpA, their practical significance in diagnostic testing is low. Moreover, the association between axSpA and anti-CD74 IgA antibodies in early back pain may partly be explained by total IgA levels, which have previously been shown to be elevated in patients with axSpA [12, 13]. In the SPACE cohort, total IgA was significantly correlated with CRP and ESR levels (data not shown), showing that IgA levels might be linked to the level of inflammation, which is in line with previous research [19, 20]. In multivariate analysis, the value of anti-CD74 IgA disappeared when adding total IgA levels.

The strengths of our study include the fact that the SPACE cohort is a well-validated "real life", multicenter, multinational cohort with large numbers of patients. The entry criteria for SPACE were designed to reflect at best the clinical practice of patients presenting with chronic back pain to a rheumatologist and in which the rheumatologist considers the possibility of axSpA in his/her differential diagnosis. The work-up of these patients in the SPACE cohort is very similar to what one would do in clinical practice. As such, almost all patients in the SPACE cohort considered as having axSpA (and as indicated (Table 2), to be even more stringent we used not only clinical diagnosis as a reference but also the combination of clinical diagnosis plus diagnosis according to the ASAS axSpA criteria) would also be considered as having SpA in daily practice. Supporting our claim, the percentage of patients with axSpA in SPACE (42% when using both clinical diagnosis and ASAS axSpA criteria) is similar to the percentage of 41.8% in a multicenter study using a referral strategy consisting of the presence of either IBP or HLA-B27 or sacroiliitis on imaging (MRI and/or radiography) [21] and not much higher than the 35.1% in a study using IBP (inflammatory back pain) or a good non-steroidal anti-inflammatory drug (NSAID) response as referral symptom [22]. So percentages around 40% are in line with what one would expect in such "diagnostic" settings.

Furthermore, the meticulous collection of clinical and radiographic data enabled us to define axSpA in several ways and thus correct for potential biases. For example, an accurate clinical diagnosis of axSpA in an early phase remains challenging and the ASAS classification criteria are not appropriate for diagnostic use, questioning the validity of the gold standard for assessment of a potential diagnostic biomarker. The SPACE cohort, however, allowed us to use more strict definitions of diagnosis, either by combining clinical diagnosis and classification criteria or by using clinical diagnosis confirmed at 1 year of follow up. These analyses yielded very similar results to the primary analyses, indicating that it is unlikely that diagnostic biases explain the differences in anti-CD74 IgG between established AS and early axSpA, the relatively high prevalence of anti-CD74 IgG and IgA antibodies in patients with CBP, or the limited PPV and NPV of anti-CD74 IgA in patients with early back pain.

Similarly, the well-documented clinical and imaging data from the SPACE cohort also allowed us to explore if anti-CD74 IgA antibodies were associated with a specific sub-population of patients with axSpA. These analyses showed that anti-CD74 IgA antibodies were not associated with HLA-B27, CRP, disease duration, sacroiliitis on radiography, peripheral manifestations other than heel enthesitis or extra-articular disease manifestations, although they were associated with sacroiliitis on MRI and with heel enthesitis. A longitudinal analysis may be more powerful than our cross-sectional approach to determine whether anti-CD74 antibodies are a useful biomarker for specific features of the disease, for example, to predict radiographic damage.

Although the SPACE cohort is designed to simulate a real-life situation, the generalizability of findings in the SPACE cohort to the intended population could be questioned. First, the SPACE cohort includes patients with chronic back pain for ≥ 3 months but ≤ 2 years, between 16 and 45 years old, in whom the diagnosis of AxSpA was considered. However, patients presenting for diagnostic work-up of potential AxSpA in clinical practice may have significantly longer symptom duration. Although we did not find any correlation between anti-CD74 IgG or IgA antibodies and disease duration in either of our cohorts, we cannot formally exclude a different relationship in patients with longer symptom duration. Second, the SPACE cohort includes patients in secondary and tertiary rheumatology practices, so this is the setting that we tested, and our data are not applicable to a primary care or population-based setting. In the latter settings, however, the pretest probability would be much lower and consequently, the performance of the test would even be worse.

Conclusion

We conclude that anti-CD74 IgG and IgA antibodies are of limited value in diagnosing axSpA in patients with early, chronic back pain. Long-term follow up of patients in the SPACE cohort will show whether anti-CD74 IgA antibodies contribute to predicting certain axSpA characteristics such as radiographic damage, extra-articular manifestations or peripheral joint disease.

Acknowledgements
We acknowledge M.C. Turina for her help in this study.

Funding
DB was supported by a VICI grant from The Netherlands Organization for Scientific Research (NWO), by an ERC grant and by a grant from the Dutch Arthritis Foundation (Reumafonds).

Authors' contributions
JdW: acquisition of data, analysis and interpretation of data, writing and revising the article. MvdS: revising the article, final approval of the version of the article to be published. NB: developing the ELISAs, performing the ELISAs, revising the article, final approval of the version of the article to be published. IB: acquisition of data, revising the article, final approval of the version of the article to be published. RR: acquisition of data, revising the article, final approval of the version of the article to be published. FvG: acquisition of data, revising the article, final approval of the version of the article to be published. DvdH: study conception and design, acquisition of data, revising the article, final approval of the version of the article to be published. TW: developing the ELISAs, revising the article, final approval of the version of the article to be published. DB: study conception and design, writing the article, revising the article, final approval of the version of the article to be published. All authors read and approved the final manuscript.

Competing interests
TW and NB share a patent on the application of CD74 antibodies in diagnosing spondyloarthritis. All other authors declare they have no competing interests.

Author details
[1]Department of Clinical Immunology and Rheumatology, Amsterdam Rheumatology and immunology Center, Academic Medical Center/University of Amsterdam, Amsterdam, The Netherlands. [2]Department of Immunology and Rheumatology, Medical University Hannover, Hannover, Germany. [3]Department of Rheumatology, Diakonhjemmet Hospital, Oslo, Norway. [4]Rheumatology unit, Department of medicine, University of Padua, Padua, Italy. [5]Department of Rheumatology, Leiden University Medical Center, Leiden, The Netherlands. [6]Private Practice, Cologne, Germany.

References

1. Dougados M, Baeten D. Spondyloarthritis. Lancet. 2011;377:2127–37.
2. Reveille JD, Witter JP, Weisman MH. Prevalence of axial spondylarthritis in the United States: estimates from a cross-sectional survey. Arthritis Care Res (Hoboken). 2012;64:905–10.
3. Sykes MP, Doll H, Sengupta R, Gaffney K. Delay to diagnosis in axial spondyloarthritis: are we improving in the UK? Rheumatol (Oxford). 2015;54:2283–4.
4. Feldtkeller E, Rudwaleit M, Zeidler H. Easy probability estimation of the diagnosis of early axial spondyloarthritis by summing up scores. Rheumatology (Oxford). 2013;52:1648–50.
5. Masson Behar V, et al. Diagnostic delay in axial spondyloarthritis: a cross-sectional study of 432 patients. Joint Bone Spine. 2016; https://doi.org/10.1016/j.jbspin.2016.06.005.
6. Rudwaleit M, van der Heijde D, Khan MA, Braun J, Sieper JC. How to diagnose axial spondyloarthritis early. Ann Rheum Dis. 2004;63:535–43.
7. Baraliakos X, Baerlecken N, Witte T, Heldmann F, Braun J. High prevalence of anti-CD74 antibodies specific for the HLA class II-associated invariant chain peptide (CLIP) in patients with axial spondyloarthritis. Ann Rheum Dis. 2014;73:1079–82.
8. Baerlecken NT, et al. Autoantibodies against CD74 in spondyloarthritis. Ann Rheum Dis. 2014;73:1211–4.
9. Neefjes J, Jongsma ML, Paul P, Bakke O. Towards a systems understanding of MHC class I and MHC class II antigen presentation. Nat Rev Immunol. 2011;11:823–36.
10. Starlets D, et al. Cell-surface CD74 initiates a signaling cascade leading to cell proliferation and survival. Blood. 2006;107:4807–16.
11. van den Berg R, et al. Percentage of patients with spondyloarthritis in patients referred because of chronic back pain and performance of classification criteria: experience from the Spondyloarthritis Caught Early (SPACE) cohort. Rheumatology (Oxford). 2013;52:1492–9.
12. Cowling P, Ebringer R, Ebringer A. Association of inflammation with raised serum IgA in ankylosing spondylitis. Ann Rheum Dis. 1980;39:545–9.
13. Wendling D. Spondylarthropathies and the IgA system. Rev Med Interne. 1994;15:55–61.
14. Youden WJ. Index for rating diagnostic tests. Cancer. 1950;3:32–5.
15. O'Brien RM. A caution regarding rules of thumb for variance inflation factors. Qual Quant. 2007;41:673–90.
16. Reynolds TL, Khan MA, van der Linden S, Cleveland RP. Differences in HLA-B27 positive and negative patients with ankylosing spondylitis: study of clinical disease activity and concentrations of serum IgA, C reactive protein, and haptoglobin. Ann Rheum Dis. 1991;50:154–7.
17. Wendling D. The gut in spondyloarthritis. Jt Bone Spine. 2016;83:401–5.
18. Witte T, et al. Sensitivity and specificity of autoantibodies against CD74 in early axial spondyloarthritis [abstract]. Arthritis Rheumatol. 2016;68(suppl 10).

12

The prevalence of depression in axial spondyloarthritis and its association with disease activity

Sizheng Zhao[1,2], Daniel Thong[2], Natasha Miller[1], Stephen J. Duffield[1], David M. Hughes[3], Laura Chadwick[1,2] and Nicola J. Goodson[1,2*]

Abstract

Background: Depression is common among patients with axial spondyloarthritis (axSpA), but reports of its prevalence are highly variable. We performed a systematic review to (i) describe the prevalence of depression in axSpA, (ii) compare its prevalence between axSpA, ankylosing spondylitis (AS) and non-radiographic axSpA (nr-axSpA) cohorts, and (iii) compare disease activity and functional impairment between those with and without depression.

Methods: We searched Medline, PubMed, Web of Science, PsycINFO, CINAHL Plus, the Cochrane library and conference abstracts of the European League Against Rheumatism, British Society for Rheumatology and American College of Rheumatology using a predefined protocol in accordance with Preferred Reporting Items for Systematic reviews and Meta-Analyses (PRISMA) guidelines. Meta-analysis was performed using quality-effects model.

Results: Fifteen original articles and one abstract were included for analysis; 14 studies described AS cohorts and two nr-axSpA. Three screening criteria and one diagnostic criterion were used to define depression. Prevalence ranged from 11 to 64% depending on criteria and thresholds used. Pooled prevalence of at least moderate depression was 15% using the Hospital Anxiety and Depression Scale (HADS) threshold of ≥ 11. The prevalence of depression was similar between axSpA, AS and nr-axSpA cohorts. Patients with depression had significantly worse disease activity, including higher BASDAI by 1.4 units (95% CI 1.0 to 1.9), ASDAS by 0.5 units (95% CI 0.3 to 0.7) and ESR by 3.5 mm/h (95% CI 0.6 to 6.4). They also had greater functional impairment with higher BASFI and BASMI by 1.2 units (95% CI 0.6 to 1.8) and 0.6 units (95% CI 0.3 to 0.8), respectively. Mean age of each study cohort inversely correlated with depression prevalence.

Conclusions: Depression is common among axSpA patients and is associated with more severe disease activity and functional impairment. Identifying and managing depression should form part of their holistic care. Further longitudinal studies are needed to explore the impact of depression on treatment outcomes and axSpA treatment on symptoms of depression.

Keywords: Axial spondyloarthritis, Ankylosing spondylitis, Depression, Prevalence, Mental health, Comorbidity, Meta-analysis, Disease activity, Functional impairment

* Correspondence: ngoodson@liverpool.ac.uk
[1]Musculoskeletal biology I, Institute of Ageing and Chronic Disease, University of Liverpool, Liverpool, UK
[2]Department of Academic Rheumatology, Aintree University Hospital, Liverpool, UK
Full list of author information is available at the end of the article

Background

Axial spondyloarthritis (axSpA) is a chronic inflammatory disease which predominantly affects the axial skeleton. It can be divided into 'radiographic' (ankylosing spondylitis, AS) and 'non-radiographic' (nr-axSpA), depending on whether definitive structural changes are evident on plain radiographs of sacroiliac joints [1, 2]. They are both characterised by inflammatory pain and functional impairment [3].

Like other conditions for which chronic pain is a feature, axSpA is known to be associated with depression [4, 5]. However, quantifying the prevalence of depression is challenging. Formal diagnosis of depression requires expertise and time consuming assessments. Instead, screening questionnaires are often used in both clinical and research settings. There are many different screening tools, each with variable score thresholds to define depression.

Estimating the prevalence of depression in axSpA is further complicated by the distinction of AS and nr-axSpA. Although they can be considered entities along a spectrum, there are key differences: the proportion of male patients is higher in AS than nr-axSpA cohorts, functional impairment is greater in AS cohorts, and AS is more commonly associated with elevated inflammatory markers [6]. Gender, functional impairment and inflammation can all potentially influence the likelihood of developing depression [7–9].

In spite of these challenges, quantifying the prevalence of depression is an important first-step to improve awareness and management of this comorbidity. Depression has direct importance to rheumatologists since current methods of disease severity assessments, on which important treatment decisions are made, rely on subjective patient-reported measures, such as the Bath AS Disease Activity Index (BASDAI) and spinal pain visual analogue scale (spVAS). The presence of depression is known to influence the reporting of pain and impairment [5]. Equally, more severe disease likely increases the risk of developing depression. It has been shown that self-reported anxiety and depression in axSpA have greater associations with disease activity and functional impairment than smoking or deprivation [10].

To date, depression in axSpA has not been systematically reviewed. Our aims were therefore to (i) report pooled prevalence of depression in axSpA, (ii) compare the prevalence of depression between axSpA, AS and nr-axSpA groups, and (iii) compare disease activity and functional impairment between those with and without comorbid depression.

Patients and methods

A systematic review was performed in accordance with the Preferred Reporting Items for Systematic Reviews and Meta-Analyses (PRISMA) guidelines [11]. The protocol for this review was pre-registered in advance (PROSPERO: CRD42017082359). Two reviewers (SZ, DT) searched Medline, PubMed, Web of Science, PsycINFO, CINAHL plus and the Cochrane Library for relevant literature in February 2018. In addition, abstract archives of the European League Against Rheumatism (EULAR), British Society for Rheumatology (BSR) and American College of Rheumatology (ACR) were searched up to, and including, 2017. The following search term was used: depress* AND (ankylosing OR spondyloarthr*). Differential nomenclature for depression (affective disorder, mood disorder, adjustment disorder, dysthymia) did not affect results in preliminary searches.

Studies were included if they: (i) were cross-sectional in design or were longitudinal studies reporting baseline data, (ii) used a validated diagnostic or screening criteria for depression with a defined cut-off threshold, and (iii) recruited adult patients fulfilling the modified New York or ASAS criteria for AS or axSpA, respectively. Studies were excluded if they used non-representative sampling (highly selective recruitment criteria, for example, studies that only recruited women) or had a samples size of less than 30 (to avoid unreliable prevalence estimates). Publications in abstract form only were also considered, as some prevalence studies may not be published as full articles and may have sufficiently described methodology within the restrictions of an abstract. Reviews, comments and editorials were excluded.

Two reviewers (DT, NM) independently assessed study eligibility and extracted data from qualifying studies. Any discrepancies were resolved through discussion moderated by a third reviewer. Information from included studies was extracted into predefined tabulated summaries containing data on: depression criteria and threshold used, study design, sample size, country setting, mean age, percentage of males, and depression prevalence.

Studies were assessed for risk of bias (SZ, NM) using the Health States Quality Index (Additional file 1: Table S1). This is an 11-point scoring system that assesses studies under the following headings: target population and observation period, diagnostic criteria, case ascertainment, measurement administration, catchment area and prevalence measure [12]. For purposes of the below meta-analysis, the score was divided by 10 to derive a quality parameter with an upper limit of 1.

Statistical analysis

Prevalence estimates were reported as percentages (95% confidence interval (CI), I^2 statistic). When performing meta-analysis of proportions (variable bound between 0 and 1), traditional weighting methods based on inverse variance are problematic when the proportions are close to the bound limits, giving more weight to such studies [13]. The double arcsine transformation was therefore used. Results were pooled according to depression criteria and threshold using quality-effects models. This method redistributes weights by accounting for the above quality parameter and can be considered as an extension of the random-effects model. Sub-group meta-analyses by diagnostic category were also performed. All estimates were also presented using random-effects models (DerSimonian-Laird). Heterogeneity of meta-analysis estimates were presented using the I^2 statistic. Funnel plot and the Doi plot/LFK index [13] were used to assess risk of publication bias.

Commonly used thresholds for each screening tool were used to categorise severity of depression. For the Hospital Anxiety and Depression Scale depression subscale (HADS) ≤ 7 was interpreted as no depression, 8 to 10 mild, 11 to 14 moderate and ≥ 15 severe [14]. For the Zung Self-Rating Depression Scale (SDS) ≤ 49 was interpreted as no depression, 50 to 69 depression, ≥ 70 severe depression [15]. The Patient Health Questionnaire (PHQ-9) threshold for depression has been suggested to be between 8 and 11, depending on context [16]. Studies that used similar thresholds were grouped together. If a study reported depression prevalence using two different thresholds, it could contribute to more than one pooled estimate. Sensitivity analyses were performed: studies reporting outlying prevalence estimates were critically reviewed and, if appropriate, excluded to evaluate changes in prevalence and heterogeneity. The association between study characteristics and reported depression prevalence was assessed using Spearman's rank correlation (r_s).

Differences in markers of disease activity and functional impairment were compared between groups with and without depression. Weighted mean difference (WMD) was calculated for each marker of disease activity and functional impairment, with pooled estimates shown in forest plots. Analyses were performed using MetaXL version 5.3 (Sunrise Beach, Australia; http://www.epigear.com/).

Results

A total of 769 full-text publications and 40 conference abstracts were found from the literature search. These titles and abstracts were screened for eligibility. After excluding duplicates and irrelevant studies, 70 studies were assessed for full-text eligibility, from which 15 full-text articles [17–31] and one abstract [32] were included in the analysis. Among the excluded studies, two [33, 34] used the same cohort as the study by Healey et al. [20] and two [35, 36] reported the same cohort as Hakkou et al. [26]. A summary of the selection process is shown in the flowchart (Additional file 1: Figure S1).

Of the 16 included studies, 14 recruited participants with AS (including three axSpA studies which reported on AS participants separately) and two reported on nr-axSpA cohorts (including one axSpA study which reported on nr-axSpA participants separately). Sample size ranged from 60 to 1504. A total of 4753 axSpA patients were included across all studies, including separately described groups of 2857 AS and 334 nr-axSpA patients. Twelve studies were cross-sectional in design, three were longitudinal, and one was a randomised controlled trial (RCT). Four studies were from Turkey, five from China (including one from Hong Kong), three from the UK, and one each from Greece, Morocco and Spain (Canary Islands). The RCT recruited from Europe, Asia and South America.

Three screening criteria and one diagnostic criterion were used for identifying depression. Nine studies used HADS with three different thresholds, five used SDS with three different thresholds, and one used PHQ-9. For the purposes of meta-analyses, HADS ≥ 7/8 were grouped together, and SDS ≥ 50/51/53 were grouped together. Only one study used diagnostic criteria for depression, the Structured Clinical Interview for Diagnostic and Statistical Manual of Mental Disorders (SCID).

Given the strict inclusion criteria employed for this meta-analysis, most studies had high quality scores with one scoring 6, three scoring 8, nine scoring 9 and three scoring ≥ 10 on the Health States Quality Index (Additional file 1: Table S2).

Prevalence of depression

The prevalence of depression ranged from 11 to 64%, depending on criteria and threshold used to identifying disease. Table 1 summarises the study characteristics, depression prevalence and quality score. Funnel/Doi plots and the LFK index suggested no evidence of publication bias (Additional file 1: Figure S2).

Figure 1 shows a forest plot of prevalence estimates using quality-effects models, grouped by criteria and threshold. Pooled prevalence of mild depression (HADS ≥ 7/8) was 38% (95% CI 30 to 45%, I^2 = 85%). Pooled prevalence of at least moderate depression, using HADS ≥ 11, was 15% (95% CI 6 to 25%, I^2 = 89%) and using SDS was 52% (95% CI 29 to 75%, I^2 = 96%). The study by Hyphantis et al. [19] reported 15% depression using PHQ9 ≥ 10. The study by Chan et al. [24] reported a prevalence of 11% for major depressive disorder using the SCID reported. Pooled prevalence using both quality- and random-effects meta-analysis are shown in Table 2.

Two studies reported disproportionately high prevalence of depression. Hakkou et al. [26] attributed this to the cohort's low socioeconomic status. Excluding this study improved the HADS subgroup heterogeneity without altering the pooled estimates significantly (Table 2). The Chinese study by Jiang et al. [31] reported the highest depression prevalence (64%). This cohort had the lowest mean age (27 years) and reported a low participation rate, with only 25% (683/2772) of the total cohort completing

Table 1 Summary of study characteristics, prevalence of depression and quality of studies included in this meta-analysis

Depression criteria (threshold)	Study	Study design	Diagnosis	Sample size	Country	Age, mean (SD)	Males, %	Depression prevalence, %	Quality index
HADS (≥ 7)	Baysal 2011 [27]	Cross-sectional	AS	243	Turkey	34.7 (10.4)	86.4	39.5	0.8
	Kilic 2014 [18]	Cross-sectional	axSpA	316	Turkey	36.3 (9.5)	63.0	44.0	0.9
			AS	174		38.3 (NS)	NS	45.4	
			nr-axSpA	142		33.9 (NS)	NS	42.3	
HADS (≥ 8)	Healey 2011 [20]	Cross-sectional	AS	612	UK	50.8 (12.2)	71.6	32.0	1.0
	Hakkou (a) 2011 [26]	Cross-sectional	AS	110	Morocco	38.5 (12.6)	68.2	55.5	0.9
	Ates 2015 [32]	Cross-sectional	AS	60	Turkey	NS	66.7	43.3	0.7
	Dougados (a) 2017 [25]	RCT	nr-axSpA	192	Europe, Asia, and South America	31.9 (7.8)	60.1	32.3	0.9
HADS (≥ 11)	Martindale 2006 [21]	Longitudinal	AS	89	UK	Median (IQR): 50 (38.5–55.5)	83.1	12.4	0.9
	MacFarlane 2017 [30]	Longitudinal	axSpA	1504	UK	Median (IQR): 51.2 (40.1–63.1)	68	13.8	1.0
	Hakkou (b) 2011 [26]	Cross-sectional	AS	110	Morocco	38.5 (12.6)	68.2	37.3	0.9
	Rodríguez-Lozano 2012 [29]	Cross-sectional	AS	190	Spain	48.4 (11.7)	75.3	10.5	0.9
	Dougados (b) 2017 [25]	Cross-sectional	nr-axSpA	192	Europe, Asia, and South America	31.9 (7.8)	60.1	15.6	0.9
SDS (≥ 50)	Günaydin 2009 [23]	Cross-sectional	AS	62	Turkey	39.6 (10.3)	83.9	27.4	0.9
	Jiang 2018 [31]	Cross-sectional	AS	683	China	27.3 (8.7)	80.4	64.0	1.0
SDS (≥ 51)	Zhang 2016 [17]	Cross-sectional	AS	314	China	27.6 (8.3)	74.5	35.4	0.8
SDS (≥ 53)	Xu 2016 [22]	Cross-sectional	AS	103	China	32.9 (10.7)	75.7	36.9	0.8
	Zou 2016 [28]	Cross-sectional	axSpA	60	China	31.8 (10.1)	73.3	43.3	0.8
			AS	40		31.5 (10.1)	70.0	42.5	
PHQ-9 (≥ 10)	Hyphantis 2013 [19]	Longitudinal	AS	55	Greece	42.9 (10.9)	85.5	14.5	0.9
SCID	Chan 2017 [24]	Cross-sectional	axSpA	160	Hong Kong	46.2 (12.7)	70.6	10.6	0.9
			AS	122		NS	NS	11.5	

HADS Hospital Anxiety and Depression Scale—depression subscale, *SDS* Zung self-rating depression scale, *PHQ9* Patient Health Questionnaire, *SCID* Structured Clinical Interview for Diagnostic and Statistical Manual of Mental Disorders, *AS* ankylosing spondylitis, *axSpA* axial spondyloarthritis, *nr-axSpA* non-radiographic axSpA, *NS* not specified, *IQR* interquartile range

the required assessments. Excluding this study reduced both heterogeneity and prevalence estimate (52 to 36%) for the SDS group.

Prevalence of depression was inversely associated with age ($r_s = -0.71$, $P = 0.003$) but not with study size, BASDAI, year of publication or proportion of males (data not shown).

Comparing axSpA, AS and nr-axSpA cohorts

Fourteen of 16 included studies reported the prevalence of depression for AS cohorts. The pooled prevalences for AS cohorts are shown in Table 2. Again, the studies by Hakkou et al. and Jiang et al. reported high prevalence of depression (Additional file 1: Figure S3) and were excluded in sensitivity analyses.

The studies by Chan et al. [24], Zou et al. [28] and Kilic et al. [18] reported similar prevalence of depression between axSpA and their AS subgroups (Table 1). Kilic et al. also reported similar prevalence between AS and nr-axSpA subgroups (45.4 vs 42.3%, $P = 0.58$).

Two studies reported depression prevalence for nr-axSpA cohorts. Pooled prevalence of mild depression (HADS ≥ 7/8) for nr-axSpA was similar to that of AS cohorts (Table 2).

Comparing markers of disease severity between groups with and without depression

Eight studies compared markers of disease severity between groups with and without depression (Additional file 1:

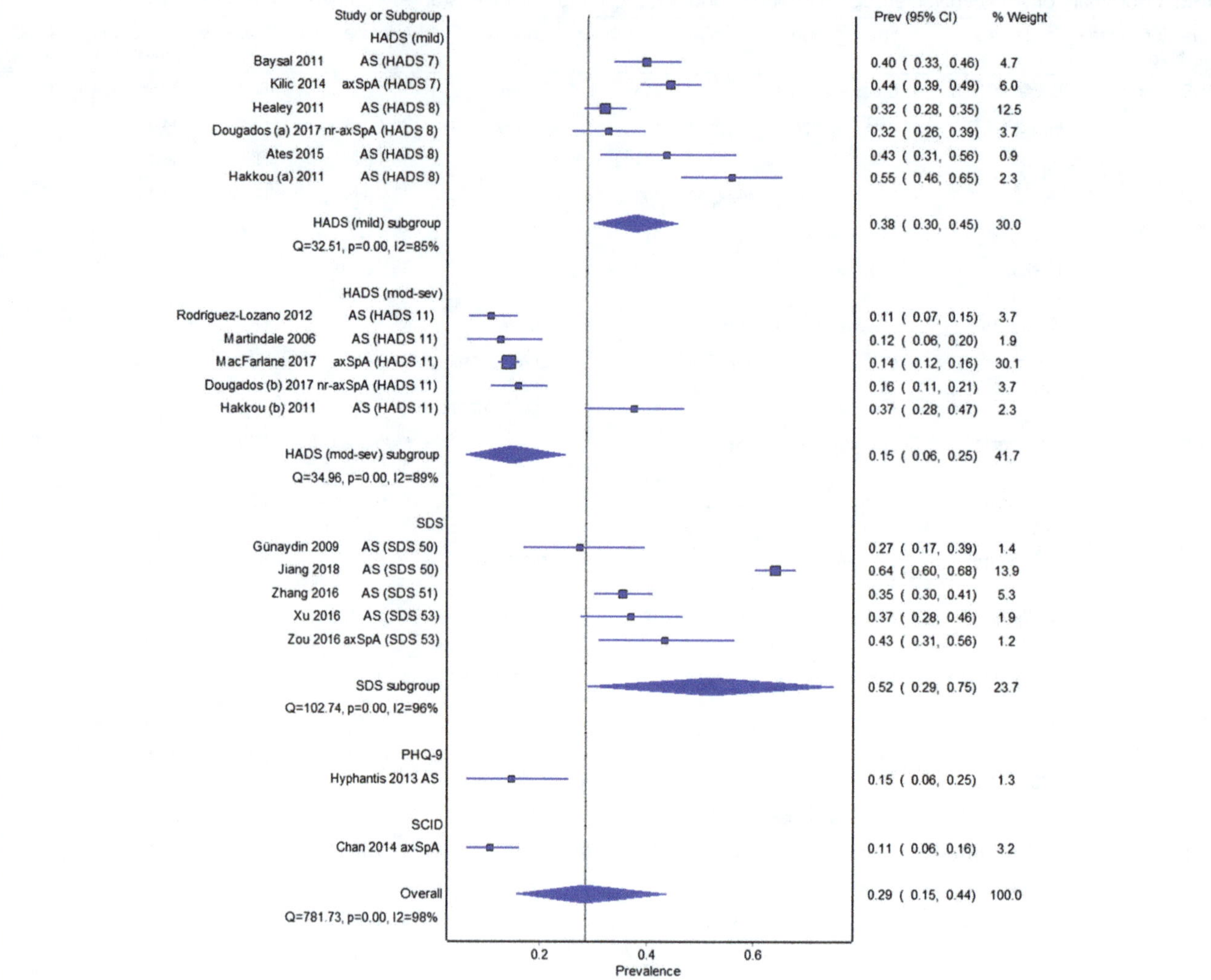

Fig. 1 Pooled prevalence of depression in axSpA cohorts, grouped by criteria and threshold

Table 2 Summaries of pooled depression prevalence grouped by screening criteria and thresholds used

		Quality-effects model		Random-effects model		Sensitivity analysis	
		Pooled prevalence	95% CI, I^2	Pooled prevalence	95% CI, I^2	Pooled prevalence	95% CI, I^2
All studies	HADS (≥ 7/8)	38%	30 to 45%, $I^2 = 85\%$	40%	47 to 33%, $I^2 = 85\%$	36%	30 to 42%, $I^2 = 77\%$
	HADS (≥ 11)	15%	6 to 25%, $I^2 = 89\%$	17%	11 to 24%, $I^2 = 89\%$	14%	12 to 15%, $I^2 = 0\%$
	SDS	52%	29 to 75%, $I^2 = 96\%$	41%	26 to 58%, $I^2 = 96\%$	36%	31 to 40%, $I^2 = 13\%$
AS	HADS (≥ 7/8)	38%	28 to 48%, $I^2 = 86\%$	38%	28 to 48%, $I^2 = 86\%$	36%	28 to 45%, $I^2 = 79\%$
	HADS (≥ 11)	18%	3 to 36%, $I^2 = 94\%$	18%	3 to 36%, $I^2 = 94\%$	11%	8 to 15%, $I^2 = 0\%$
	SDS	52%	28 to 76%, $I^2 = 96\%$	41%	25 to 58%, $I^2 = 96\%$	35%	31 to 39%, $I^2 = 0\%$
nr-axSpA	HADS (≥ 7/8)	36%	27 to 46%, $I^2 = 71\%$	36%	27 to 46%, $I^2 = 71\%$	NA	NA

Estimates were presented by quality-effects model, random-effects model, and sensitivity analysis excluding the studies by Hakkou et al. and Jiang et al.
HADS Hospital Anxiety and Depression Scale—depression subscale, *SDS* Zung self-rating depression scale, *AS* ankylosing spondylitis, *axSpA* axial spondyloarthritis, *nr-axSpA* non-radiographic axSpA, *NA* not applicable

Table S3). For BASDAI, spVAS and BASFI, most studies reported significantly higher scores in the group with depression compared to those without, regardless of criteria or threshold used to define depression (Fig. 2). Across the depressed groups, scores were generally worse for the Bath AS metrology index (BASMI), AS disease activity score (ASDAS), CRP and ESR, but few individual comparisons were statistically significant.

All eight studies reported significantly worse BASDAI in the group with depression. Despite the variety of criteria and thresholds used, the weighted mean differences (WMDs) were similar. Pooling WMDs, BASDAI was 1.4 units (95% CI 1.0 to 1.9) higher in the depressed group. Of the six studies that reported spVAS, the groups with depression scored 1.2 units (95% CI 0.7 to 1.7) higher. Only two studies reported ASDAS, with a pooled WMD of 0.5 units (95% CI 0.3 to 0.7) between the two groups. ESR (3.5 mm/h, 95% CI 0.6 to 6.4 mm/h) was significantly higher in groups with depression, but not CRP (1.3 mg/dl, 95% CI – 0.9 to 3.4).

All studies reported significantly worse BASFI in the group with depression. The pooled difference in BASFI was 1.2 units (95% CI 0.6 to 1.8) but with more variation among the studies. The group with depression in the study by Hakkou et al. had much poorer function (BASFI, BASMI) compared to depressed groups of other studies, despite using a threshold for 'mild' depression. In contrast to other Bath indices, not all studies reported a difference in BASMI when comparing groups with and without depression. Nevertheless, the pooled estimate showed that axSpA patients with comorbid depression had significantly higher BASMI than those without (0.6 units, 95% CI 0.3 to 0.8).

Discussion

This systematic review and meta-analysis of nearly five thousand axSpA patients has shown that depression is highly prevalent and associated with greater disease activity and functional impairment. At least moderate depression was found in 15% of patients, although estimates varied depending on the criteria and thresholds selected; pooled estimates of prevalence of depression in axSpA were 38 to 52% using lower HADS thresholds and the SDS.

The strength of this meta-analysis lies in its strict inclusion criteria, as prevalence estimates can vary

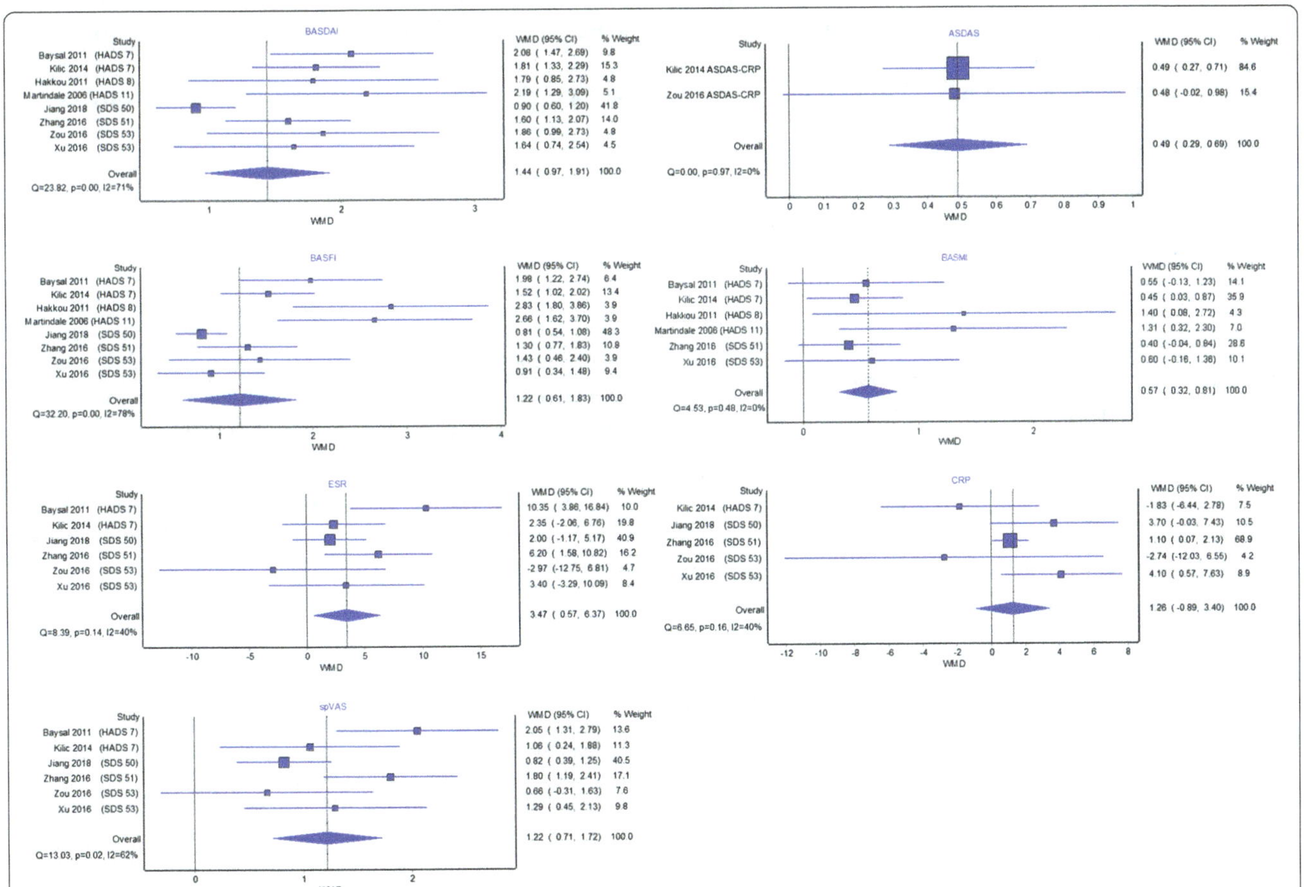

Fig. 2 Measures of disease activity and functional impairment are worse in axial spondyloarthritis patients with comorbid depression. Effect sizes shown as weighted mean difference (*WMD*)

significantly depending on variable sampling methods and definition for depression. The included studies had high quality overall and low risk of publication bias. However, overall heterogeneity of prevalence estimates remained high, largely due to the wide range of screening or diagnostic tools used to define depression. Heterogeneity was improved when estimates were pooled by depression definition, and further reduced in sensitivity analyses excluding the studies by Hakkou et al. and Jiang et al. These two studies highlight the importance of age, which was inversely associated with depression prevalence, and socioeconomic status, which future studies could approximate by grouping by continent or gross domestic product.

The main limitation of the meta-analysis of prevalence was that almost all studies used screening criteria to detect depression. This may lead to over-estimation of the prevalence of true depression. Using diagnostic criteria, Chan et al. found one of the lowest prevalences of depression. However, they reported a sensitivity and specificity of 82 and 79%, respectively, for HADS ≥ 8 in their axSpA cohort, using SCID as the gold standard [24]. Almost all studies described hospital cohorts which are likely to have more severe disease than a random or primary care sample. However, disease activity was not found to be associated with prevalence estimates; although the RCT cohort had much higher disease activity than observational cohorts, it reported similar prevalence of depression. The higher disease activity and functional impairment found in patients with depression were unadjusted for confounders such as smoking and deprivation. It is possible that adjusted effect sizes could be smaller, although data from our own axSpA cohort [10] found that doing so made little difference to the effect size of depression. Lastly, the direction of the causal relationship between depression and axSpA disease severity could only be speculated from these studies of cross-sectional association.

The prevalence of depression in axSpA was higher than that of the general population [37], but very similar to those reported in rheumatoid arthritis (RA) cohorts. A meta-analysis of RA patients reported depression in 15% using HADS ≥ 11 and 34% using HADS ≥ 8 [38]. This similarity was unexpected since the RA cohorts were mostly female. Given that depression is more prevalent in females in the general population [8], it is possible that more male axSpA patients were reporting depression than male RA patients. However, our finding that the prevalence of depression was similar between AS and nr-axSpA groups suggest that gender may not be as significant a risk factor for depression in axSpA.

Patients with depression had significantly worse disease activity and functional impairment across most indices. As an example, the pooled difference in BASDAI was 1.4 units, which is clinically relevant as ≥ 2-unit improvement is considered as response to TNF inhibitors (TNFi) [39]. The direction of this potential causal relationship cannot be inferred from studies included in this meta-analysis. Patients with more severe disease may be at higher risk of developing comorbid depression. Conversely, depression has been shown to exacerbate the perception of pain [40] and may cause axSpA patients with depression to report greater disease severity. This may explain why the differences in subjective indices (BASDAI, spVAS, BASFI) were larger than differences in objective measures (BASMI, ASDAS). It is interesting that the difference in BASDAI between groups with and without depression were similar regardless of severity of depression; the presence of any level of depression may adversely influence response to the BASDAI questionnaire.

In healthcare systems where TNFi can only be continued on the basis of demonstrable response, such as in the UK, efforts should be made to identify and manage comorbid depression to avoid withdrawing efficacious therapy inappropriately. More objective measures of disease activity, such as ASDAS, may be more robust to the influence of depression. Longitudinal axSpA studies are needed to evaluate the impact of depression on treatment outcomes; we have previously demonstrated, in a longitudinal RA cohort, that depression at baseline adversely affects treatment outcomes [41]. Equally, inflammation has been implicated in the pathophysiology of depression and may contribute to non-responsiveness to antidepressant therapies [9]. Longitudinal studies could also shed light on whether TNFi improves severity of depressive symptoms.

Conclusions

Depression is common among axSpA patients and is associated with worse disease activity and functional impairment. Clinicians should be mindful of comorbid depression when managing axSpA patients, especially for younger patients and those with severe disease activity and functional impairment. Patients with depression should be appropriately referred and managed. This is especially pertinent if depressive symptoms are thought to adversely influence assessments of treatment response.

Abbreviations

ACR: American College of Rheumatology; AS: Ankylosing spondylitis; ASAS: Assessment of SpondyloArthritis international Society; ASDAS: Ankylosing Spondylitis Disease Activity Score; axSpA: Axial spondyloarthritis; BASDAI: Bath Ankylosing Spondylitis Disease Activity Index; BASFI: Bath Ankylosing Spondylitis Functional Index; BASMI: Bath Ankylosing Spondylitis Metrology Index; BSR: British Society for Rheumatology; CRP: C-reactive protein; EULAR: European League Against Rheumatism; HADS: Hospital Anxiety and Depression Scale depression subscale; LFK index: Luis Furuya-Kanamori index; PHQ-9: Patient Health Questionnaire; PROSPERO: International prospective register of systematic reviews; SCID: Structured Clinical Interview for Diagnostic and Statistical Manual of Mental Disorders; SDS: Zung Self-Rating Depression Scale; WMD: Weighted mean difference

Authors' contributions
SZ wrote the manuscript with significant contributions from all co-authors. SZ, DT and NM performed the literature search, data extraction and quality assessment. SZ and DMH performed all statistical analysis. SZ and NJG conceived of the project. SJD, LC and NJG participated in its design and coordination. All authors read and approved the final manuscript.

Competing interests
The authors declare that they have no competing interests.

Author details
[1]Musculoskeletal biology I, Institute of Ageing and Chronic Disease, University of Liverpool, Liverpool, UK. [2]Department of Academic Rheumatology, Aintree University Hospital, Liverpool, UK. [3]Department of Biostatistics, Institute of Translational Medicine, University of Liverpool, Liverpool, UK.

References
1. van der Linden S, Valkenburg HA, Cats A. Evaluation of diagnostic criteria for ankylosing spondylitis. A proposal for modification of the New York criteria. Arthritis Rheum. 1984;27(4):361–8.
2. Rudwaleit M, Jurik AG, Hermann KG, Landewe R, van der Heijde D, Baraliakos X, et al. Defining active sacroiliitis on magnetic resonance imaging (MRI) for classification of axial spondyloarthritis: a consensual approach by the ASAS/OMERACT MRI group. Ann Rheum Dis. 2009;68(10):1520–7.
3. van Tubergen A, Weber U. Diagnosis and classification in spondyloarthritis: identifying a chameleon. Nat Rev Rheumatol. 2012;8(5):253–61.
4. Martindale J, Shukla R, Goodacre J. The impact of ankylosing spondylitis/axial spondyloarthritis on work productivity. Best Pract Res Clin Rheumatol. 2015;29(3):512–23.
5. Bair MJ, Robinson RL, Katon W, Kroenke K. Depression and pain comorbidity: a literature review. Arch Intern Med. 2003;163(20):2433–45.
6. Baraliakos X, Braun J. Non-radiographic axial spondyloarthritis and ankylosing spondylitis: what are the similarities and differences? RMD open. 2015;1(Suppl 1):e000053.
7. Prince MJ, Harwood RH, Blizard RA, Thomas A, Mann AH. Impairment, disability and handicap as risk factors for depression in old age. The gospel oak project V. Psychol Med. 1997;27(2):311–21.
8. Piccinelli M, Wilkinson G. Gender differences in depression. Critical review. Br J Psychiatry. 2000;177:486–92.
9. Miller AH, Raison CL. The role of inflammation in depression: from evolutionary imperative to modern treatment target. Nat Rev Immunol. 2016;16(1):22–34.
10. Zhao S, Thong D, Duffield SJ, Hughes D, Goodson NJ. Alcohol and disease activity in axial spondyloarthritis: a cross-sectional study. Rheumatol Int. 2018;38(3):375–81.
11. Moher D, Liberati A, Tetzlaff J, Altman DG, Group P. Preferred reporting items for systematic reviews and meta-analyses: the PRISMA statement. J Clin Epidemiol. 2009;62(10):1006–12.
12. Barendregt JJ, Doi SA. MetaXL user guide (version 5.3). 2016. Available from: http://www.epigear.com/index_files/MetaXL%20User%20Guide.pdf. Accessed Feb 2018.
13. Barendregt JJ, Doi SA, Lee YY, Norman RE, Vos T. Meta-analysis of prevalence. J Epidemiol Community Health. 2013;67(11):974–8.
14. Stern AF. The hospital anxiety and depression scale. Occup Med (Lond). 2014;64(5):393–4.
15. World Health Organization. The Zung Self-Rating Depression Scale. 2018. Available from: http://www.who.int/substance_abuse/research_tools/zungdepressionscale. Accessed Feb 2018.
16. Manea L, Gilbody S, McMillan D. Optimal cut-off score for diagnosing depression with the patient health questionnaire (PHQ-9): a meta-analysis. CMAJ. 2012;184(3):E191–6.
17. Zhang S-L, Gao F, Chen Z-H, Yan Q, Lin H. Influence of psychological status on back pain and clinical assessments in Chinese ankylosing spondylitis patients: a cross-sectional study. Int J Clin Exp Med. 2016;9(12):23624–33.
18. Kilic G, Kilic E, Ozgocmen S. Relationship between psychiatric status, self-reported outcome measures, and clinical parameters in axial spondyloarthritis. Medicine (Baltimore). 2014;93(29):e337.
19. Hyphantis T, Kotsis K, Tsifetaki N, Creed F, Drosos AA, Carvalho AF, et al. The relationship between depressive symptoms, illness perceptions and quality of life in ankylosing spondylitis in comparison to rheumatoid arthritis. Clin Rheumatol. 2013;32(5):635–44.
20. Healey EL, Haywood KL, Jordan KP, Garratt A, Packham JC. Impact of ankylosing spondylitis on work in patients across the UK. Scand J Rheumatol. 2011;40(1):34–40.
21. Martindale J, Smith J, Sutton CJ, Grennan D, Goodacre L, Goodacre JA. Disease and psychological status in ankylosing spondylitis. Rheumatology. 2006;45(10):1288–93.
22. Xu X, Shen B, Zhang A, Liu J, Da Z, Liu H, et al. Anxiety and depression correlate with disease and quality-of-life parameters in Chinese patients with ankylosing spondylitis. Patient Prefer Adherence. 2016;10:879–85.
23. Gunaydin R, Goksel Karatepe A, Cesmeli N, Kaya T. Fatigue in patients with ankylosing spondylitis: relationships with disease-specific variables, depression, and sleep disturbance. Clin Rheumatol. 2009;28(9):1045–51.
24. Chan CYY, Tsang HHL, Lau CS, Chung HY. Prevalence of depressive and anxiety disorders and validation of the hospital anxiety and depression scale as a screening tool in axial spondyloarthritis patients. Int J Rheum Dis. 2017;20(3):317–25.
25. Dougados M, Logeart I, Szumski A, Coindreau J, Jones H. Evaluation of whether extremely high enthesitis or bath ankylosing spondylitis disease activity index (BASDAI) scores suggest fibromyalgia and confound the anti-TNF response in early non-radiographic axial spondyloarthritis. Clin Exp Rheumatol. 2017;35(Suppl 105(3)):50–3.
26. Hakkou J, Rostom S, Aissaoui N, Berrada KR, Abouqal R, Bahiri R, et al. Psychological status in Moroccan patients with ankylosing spondylitis and its relationships with disease parameters and quality of life. J Clin Rheumatol. 2011;17(8):424–8.
27. Baysal O, Durmus B, Ersoy Y, Altay Z, Senel K, Nas K, et al. Relationship between psychological status and disease activity and quality of life in ankylosing spondylitis. Rheumatol Int. 2011;31(6):795–800.
28. Zou Q, Jiang Y, Mu F, Shi Y, Fang Y. Correlation of axial Spondyloarthritis with anxiety and depression. Med Sci Monit. 2016;22:3202–8.
29. Rodriguez-Lozano C, Gantes MA, Gonzalez B, Hernandez-Beriain JA, Naranjo A, Hernandez V, et al. Patient-acceptable symptom state as an outcome measure in the daily care of patients with ankylosing spondylitis. J Rheumatol. 2012;39(7):1424–32.
30. Macfarlane GJ, Barnish MS, Pathan E, Martin KR, Haywood KL, Siebert S, et al. Co-occurrence and characteristics of patients with axial Spondyloarthritis who meet criteria for fibromyalgia: results from a UK National Register. Arthritis Rheum. 2017;69(11):2144–50.
31. Jiang Y, Yang M, Lv Q, Qi J, Lin Z, Liao Z, et al. Prevalence of psychological disorders, sleep disturbance and stressful life events and their relationships with disease parameters in Chinese patients with ankylosing spondylitis. Clin Rheumatol. 2018;37(2):407–14.
32. Ates A, Dortbas F, Karaaslan Y. FRI0202 the relationship between disease activity, functional index, sleep quality, anxiety, depression, fatigue and quality of life in patients with ankylosing spondylitis. Ann Rheum Dis. 2015;74:497–8.
33. Healey EL, Haywood KL, Jordan KP, Garratt AM, Packham JC. Disease severity in ankylosing spondylitis: variation by region and local area deprivation. J Rheumatol. 2010;37(3):633–8.
34. Sandhu J, Packham JC, Healey EL, Jordan KP, Garratt AM, Haywood KL. Evaluation of a modified arthritis self-efficacy scale for an ankylosing spondylitis UK population. Clin Exp Rheumatol. 2011;29(2):223–30.
35. Yacoub YI, Amine B, Abid H, Hajjaj-Hassouni N. Assessment of depression in Moroccan patients with ankylosing spondylitis. Ann Rheum Dis. 2012;71(Supp:3):568.
36. Aissaoui N, Rostom S, Hakkou J, Berrada Ghziouel K, Bahiri R, Abouqal R, et al. Fatigue in patients with ankylosing spondylitis: prevalence and relationships with disease-specific variables, psychological status, and sleep disturbance. Rheumatol Int. 2012;32(7):2117–24.
37. Waraich P, Goldner EM, Somers JM, Hsu L. Prevalence and incidence studies of mood disorders: a systematic review of the literature. Can J Psychiatry. 2004;49(2):124–38.
38. Matcham F, Rayner L, Steer S, Hotopf M. The prevalence of depression in rheumatoid arthritis: a systematic review and meta-analysis. Rheumatology. 2013;52(12):2136–48.
39. Yildiz M, Batmaz I, Sula B, Ucmak D, Sariyildiz MA, Daggulli M, et al. Sexual dysfunction in male patients with Behget's disease. Acta Reumatologica Portuguesa. 2016;41(1):56–61.

Extravascular manifestations of Takayasu arteritis: focusing on the features shared with spondyloarthritis

Oh Chan Kwon[1], Sang-Won Lee[2], Yong-Beom Park[2], Ji Seon Oh[3], Sang Hoon Lee[4], Seokchan Hong[1], Chang-Keun Lee[1], Bin Yoo[1] and Yong-Gil Kim[1*]

Abstract

Background: Takayasu arteritis (TAK) is a systemic disease characterized by large vessel involvement. Although the vascular characteristics of TAK are well characterized, there is no well-organized study demonstrating the extravascular manifestations of TAK. We aimed to evaluate the characteristics of extravascular manifestations of TAK, and to identify the association between vascular and extravascular manifestations of TAK.

Methods: TAK patients from two independent cohorts between January 2012 and October 2017 were included in the study. Patient characteristics were retrospectively collected from the electronic dataset. The computed tomography scans of all subjects were reviewed to evaluate the pattern of vascular involvement and presence of sacroiliitis. Clinical findings including uveitis, skin lesions, oral ulcers, arthritis, and inflammatory bowel disease (IBD) were reviewed. Logistic regression analysis was performed to evaluate the association between vascular and extravascular manifestations.

Results: For the 268 TAK patients, the mean age at diagnosis was 41.2 ± 14.2 years and 88.1% were female. The extravascular manifestation of TAK was observed in 19.0% of patients, the most common being arthritis including sacroiliitis (11.9%) followed by recurrent oral ulcers (8.6%) and IBD (2.6%). A multivariate logistic regression analysis revealed type IIB vascular involvement (adjusted odds ratio (OR) 2.956, 95% confidence interval (CI) 1.337–6.537, $p = 0.007$) and the erythrocyte sedimentation rate (ESR) (adjusted OR 1.014, 95% CI 1.003–1.025, $p = 0.012$) as significantly associated with the presence of axial and peripheral arthritis.

Conclusions: Extravascular manifestations of TAK were observed in up to one-fifth of patients. The most common extravascular manifestation was arthritis, which was associated with a type IIB vascular involvement pattern and a high ESR.

Keywords: Takayasu arteritis, Extravascular manifestation, Arthritis

Background

Takayasu arteritis (TAK) is a systemic vasculitis mainly involving the aorta and its major branches and can cause occlusive or aneurysmal degeneration [1]. The prevalence of TAK in Japan was estimated at 40 per 1 million of population, with a female predominance [2]. The prevalence of TAK in European studies is lower than that in Japan, being 4.7–13.2 per 1 million of population [3–5].

Despite this rarity, based on a number of previous studies [1, 6–11], knowledge regarding TAK has much improved since its first report in Japan in 1908 [12]. In particular, the vascular manifestations of TAK have been well reported in previous studies [1, 6–11]. Although there might be some discrepancies among different ethnic populations, the largest scale observational study conducted in Japan [1] reported that local symptoms and findings attributable to vascular involvement were most commonly observed in the cervicobrachial area.

* Correspondence: bestmd2000@amc.seoul.kr
[1]Division of Rheumatology, Department of Internal Medicine, University of Ulsan, College of Medicine, Asan Medical Center, 88 Olympic-ro 43-gil, Songpa-gu, Seoul 05505, South Korea
Full list of author information is available at the end of the article

Accordingly, the majority of the patients exhibited vascular involvements of the aortic arch or its major branches, which supply the cervicobrachial area. Furthermore, the most common type of angiographic involvement according to Hata's classification [13] was type I (branches of the aortic arch).

Although the vascular manifestations of TAK are well known, the extravascular manifestations of TAK remain unclear. Some recent studies have addressed spondyloarthritis (SpA) [14, 15] and inflammatory bowel disease (IBD) [16, 17] in TAK patients. However, only sporadic case reports regarding other extravascular manifestations such as erythema nodosum [18–20] and uveitis [21, 22] have been reported. Moreover, peripheral arthritis has occasionally been observed in TAK patients, but data concerning these manifestations are not well established. Therefore, we aimed to identify the characteristics of extravascular manifestations of TAK. Furthermore, we evaluated the association between vascular and extravascular manifestations of TAK.

Methods

Study population

Two independent cohorts from two tertiary referral hospitals in South Korea were included. All study subjects were diagnosed with TAK and encoded M314 according to the International Statistical Classification of Diseases and Related Health Problems, Tenth Revision (ICD-10) between January 2012 and October 2017. All patients met the 1990 American College of Rheumatology (ACR) classification criteria for TAK [23]. Computed tomography (CT) scans encompassing the entire aorta and its branches as a diagnostic evaluation were present for all patients. Patients who only underwent localized imaging work-up such as carotid duplex sonography or neck angiography were excluded.

Electronic medical records of the study subjects were reviewed, and information pertaining to age, sex, the presence of hypertension (HTN), clinical symptoms and signs, laboratory data at initial presentation including erythrocyte sedimentation rate (ESR) and C-reactive protein (CRP), and imaging data were collected. Regarding clinical symptoms and signs, those attributable to vascular involvement such as claudication, decreased pulse, and blood pressure difference > 10 mmHg between arms, bruit, and carotidynia were reviewed. The CT scans were utilized to assess the distribution of vascular lesions and categorize them according to Hata's classification [13].

This study was approved by the Institutional Review Board of Asan Medical Center in Seoul, South Korea (IRB No. 2017-0857). The requirement for informed consent was waived due to the retrospective nature of the study.

Extravascular manifestations

The presence of peripheral arthritis, axial arthritis (sacroiliitis), recurrent oral ulcers, erythema nodosum, IBD (Crohn's disease (CD) and ulcerative colitis (UC)), and uveitis were determined from the electronic medical records. A radiologist confirmed the presence of sacroiliitis from the CT scans that were taken for the diagnostic work-up of TAK.

For patients with peripheral arthritis, the number and distribution of joint involvements and positivity of rheumatoid factor (RF), anti-cyclic citrullinated peptide (anti-CCP) antibody, and antinuclear antibody (ANA) (if the laboratory test was performed) were reviewed. The number of joint involvements was classified as monoarthritis (1 joint involved), oligoarthritis (2–3 joints involved), and polyarthritis (≥4 joints involved). The distribution of joint involvement was assessed by the size (small joints, large joints, or both), symmetry, and location (upper extremities, lower extremities, or both) of the joints involved. For patients with sacroiliitis, positivity of HLA-B27 (if the laboratory test was performed) and whether they fulfilled the radiologic 1984 modified New York criteria [24] were reviewed.

Statistical analysis

We described both vascular and extravascular manifestations. Continuous variables were expressed as the mean ± standard deviation (SD) and median (interquartile range (IQR)) for a normal and a non-normal distribution, respectively. Categorical variables were expressed as number (%). To evaluate the association between vascular and extravascular manifestations, we performed logistic regression analysis. Univariate analysis was performed for each variable, and variables determined statistically significant ($p < 0.05$) were included in a multivariate analysis.

Results

Baseline characteristics

During the study period, 268 TAK patients (185 and 83 from each cohort, respectively) with the ICD-10 code M314 who met the 1990 ACR classification criteria for TAK [23] were identified.

The mean age of the study population was 41.2 ± 14.2 years. The patients were predominantly female (88.1%). A blood pressure difference of more than 10 mmHg between both arms, decreased pulse, bruit, HTN, claudication, and carotidynia were observed in 84.1%, 56.7%, 45.8%, 44.8%, 33.9%, and 14.4% patients, respectively. The median ESR result was 24.0 mm/h (IQR 13.0–46.0), and the median CRP serum concentration was 0.17 mg/dl (IQR 0.10–0.70) (Table 1).

Table 1 Baseline characteristics of the 268 Takayasu arteritis patients

Characteristic	N = 268
Age (years), mean (± SD)	41.2 (± 14.2)
Female	236 (88.1%)
Hypertension	120 (44.8%)
Claudication (N^a = 218)	74 (33.9%)
Decreased pulse (N^a = 203)	115 (56.7%)
Blood pressure difference > 10 mmHg (N^a = 239)	201 (84.1%)
Bruit (N^a = 203)	93 (45.8%)
Carotidynia (N^a = 201)	29 (14.4%)
ESR (mm/h), median (IQR)	24.0 (13.0–46.0)
CRP (mg/dl), median (IQR)	0.17 (0.10–0.70)
Vessel involvement	
Common carotid artery	176 (65.7%)
Subclavian artery	170 (63.4%)
Ascending aorta	84 (31.3%)
Aortic arch	100 (37.3%)
Descending aorta	151 (56.3%)
Abdominal aorta	124 (46.3%)
Renal artery	54 (20.1%)
Iliac artery	30 (11.2%)
Pulmonary artery	30 (11.2%)
Hata's classification	
Type I	54 (20.1%)
Type IIA	23 (8.6%)
Type IIB	55 (20.5%)
Type III	10 (3.7%)
Type IV	6 (2.2%)
Type V	120 (44.8%)

Data presented as *n* (%) unless stated otherwise
SD standard deviation, *ESR* erythrocyte sedimentation rate, *IQR* interquartile range, *CRP* C-reactive protein
[a]Patients with missing data excluded

Table 2 Extravascular manifestations of Takayasu arteritis

Manifestation	N = 268
At least one extravascular manifestation present	51 (19.0%)
Arthritis	32 (11.9%)
Axial arthritis (sacroiliitis)	19 (7.1%)
Peripheral arthritis	16 (6.0%)
Recurrent oral ulcers	23 (8.6%)
Inflammatory bowel disease	7 (2.6%)
Crohn's disease	4 (1.5%)
Ulcerative colitis	3 (1.1%)
Erythema nodosum	4 (1.5%)
Uveitis[a]	2 (0.7%)

Data presented as *n* (%)
[a]Both patients had unilateral anterior uveitis

Patterns of vessel involvement

The most frequently involved vessel was the common carotid artery (65.7%), followed by the subclavian artery (63.4%) and the descending aorta (56.3%). The least involved vessels were the iliac and pulmonary arteries (both 11.2%). The most common pattern of vessel involvement according to Hata's classification [13] was type V (44.8%) (Table 1).

Extravascular manifestations

Of the 268 patients, 19.0% displayed at least one extravascular manifestation, the most common being arthritis, followed by recurrent oral ulcers, IBD, and erythema nodosum (11.9%, 8.6%, 2.6%, and 1.5%. respectively). Uveitis (unilateral anterior uveitis) was infrequently detected (0.7%). The 32 arthritic patients comprised 19 with sacroiliitis and 16 with peripheral arthritis (Table 2).

As shown in Table 3, of the 19 patients with sacroiliitis, the majority were female (89.5%) and HLA-B27 negative (85.7%). The 1984 modified New York criteria [24] were met by 68.4% of these patients, and 15.8% exhibited peripheral arthritis. Enthesitis, IBD, and uveitis were present in one patient each. While type V vessel involvement was the most common in the total study population, type IIB was most frequently observed in the patients with sacroiliitis

Table 3 Characteristics of the 19 Takayasu arteritis patients with axial arthritis (sacroiliitis)

Characteristic	N = 19
Age (years), mean (± SD)	38.9 (± 14.9)
Sex	
Male	2 (10.5%)
Female	17 (89.5%)
HLA-B27 (N^a = 7)	1 (14.3%)
Sacroiliitis meeting 1984 modified New York criteria[b] for AS	13 (68.4%)
Peripheral arthritis	3 (15.8%)
Enthesitis	1 (5.3%)
Inflammatory bowel disease	1 (5.3%)
Uveitis	1 (5.3%)
Hata's classification	
Type I	3 (15.8%)
Type IIA	2 (10.5%)
Type IIB	7 (36.8%)
Type III	1 (5.3%)
Type IV	0 (0.0%)
Type V	6 (31.6%)

Data presented as *n* (%) unless stated otherwise
SD standard deviation, *AS* ankylosing spondylitis
[a]Patients with missing data excluded
[b]Radiologic criteria of the 1984 modified New York criteria [24]: sacroiliitis grade ≥ 2 bilaterally or grade 3–4 unilaterally

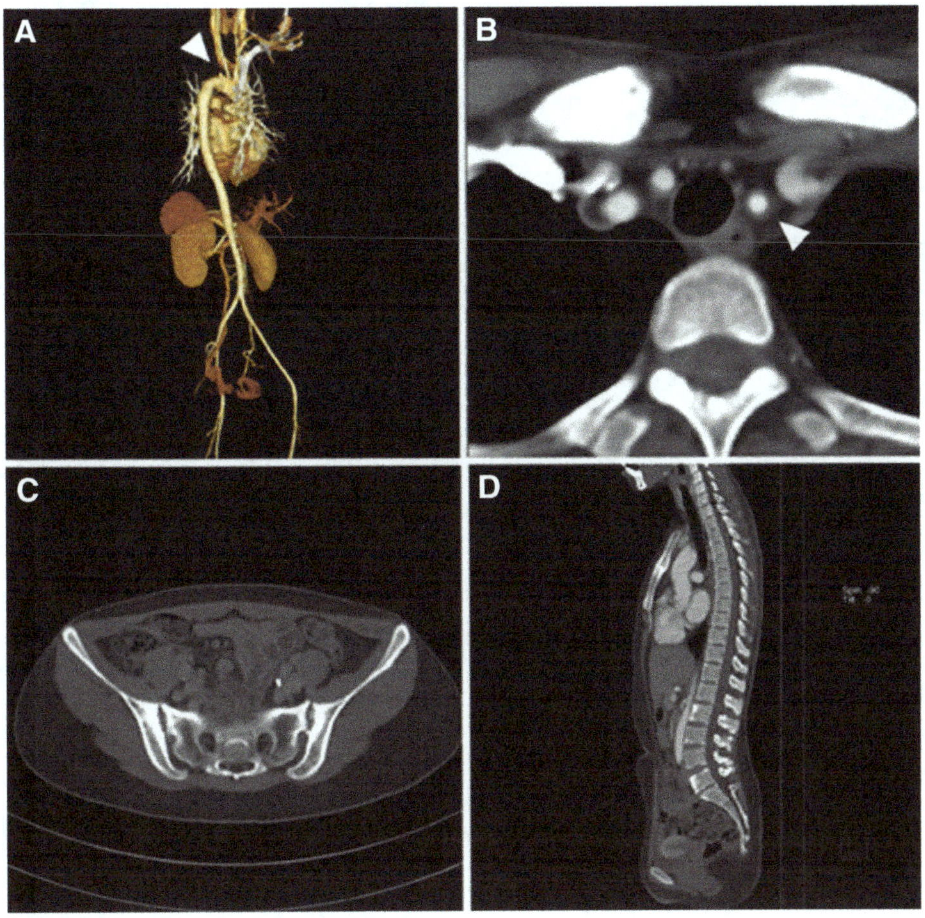

Fig. 1 Computed tomography (CT) images of Takayasu arteritis (TAK) patient who exhibited sacroiliitis as an extravascular manifestation. Female patient, 29 years old, negative for HLA-B27. **a** Complete occlusion in left subclavian artery (arrowhead). **b** Concentric wall thickening in left common carotid artery (arrowhead). **c** Sclerosis in both sacroiliac joints and erosion with joint space widening suggesting grade III sacroiliitis. **d** Vertebral corner inflammations, especially in lumbar spines (L2 and L5)

(36.8%). Representative images of a TAK patient with sacroiliitis are presented in Fig. 1.

The characteristics of the 16 patients with peripheral arthritis are presented in Table 4. Monoarthritis, oligoarthritis, and polyarthritis were observed in 37.5%, 43.8%, and 18.8% of patients, respectively. Regarding joint distribution, large joint involvement was most common (62.5%), and the shoulder joint most frequently affected. The majority of patients exhibited asymmetric joint involvement (87.5%). The locations of involved joints were approximately evenly distributed between the upper extremities, the lower extremities, and both the upper and lower extremities together. RF was positive in 9.1%, and none of the patients were positive for anti-CCP antibody or ANA. The most common vessel involvement was type IIB (50%), which is concordant with that of the study subjects with sacroiliitis.

Vascular manifestations associated with arthritis

Logistic regression analysis was performed to evaluate vascular manifestations associated with arthritis in TAK patients (Table 5). On univariate analysis, ESR, CRP, and type IIB vessel involvement were significantly associated with arthritis ($p = 0.007$, $p = 0.027$, and $p = 0.004$, respectively). Type V vessel involvement was inversely associated with arthritis ($p = 0.048$). On multivariate analysis, ESR ($p = 0.012$) and type IIB ($p = 0.007$) remained significant.

Discussion

In this study, we determined that extravascular manifestations of TAK were not rare, with a prevalence of 19.0%. In particular, arthritis (11.9%) was the most common extravascular manifestation. To the best of our knowledge, this is the first study describing the extravascular manifestations of TAK in detail.

Sacroiliitis was present in 7.1% TAK patients. Considering that the global prevalence of SpA is approximately 1% [25], the proportion of TAK patients with sacroiliitis appears high. Although not clear to date, there might be a shared genetic background between TAK and sacroiliitis,

Table 4 Characteristics of the 16 Takayasu arteritis patients with peripheral arthritis

Characteristic	$N = 16$
Age (years), mean (± SD)	41.6 (± 14.7)
Sex	
Male	2 (12.5%)
Female	14 (87.5%)
Number of joints involved	
Monoarthritis (1 joint)	6 (37.5%)
Oligoarthritis (2–3 joints)	7 (43.8%)
Polyarthritis (≥ 4 joints)	3 (18.8%)
Distribution of joint involvement	
Size	
Small joints	3 (18.8%)
Large joints[a]	10 (62.5%)
Small and large joints	3 (18.8%)
Symmetry	
Symmetric	2 (12.5%)
Asymmetric	14 (87.5%)
Location	
Upper extremities	6 (37.5%)
Lower extremities	5 (31.3%)
Upper and lower extremities	5 (31.3%)
RF ($N^b = 11$)	1 (9.1%)
Anti-CCP antibody ($N^b = 11$)	0 (0.0%)
ANA ($N^b = 11$)	0 (0.0%)
Hata's classification	
Type I	2 (12.5%)
Type IIA	1 (6.3%)
Type IIB	8 (50.0%)
Type III	1 (6.3%)
Type IV	1 (6.3%)
Type V	3 (18.8%)

Data presented as *n* (%) unless stated otherwise
SD standard deviation, *RF* rheumatoid factor, *CCP* cyclic citrullinated peptide, *ANA* antinuclear antibody
[a]Most commonly involved was the shoulder joint
[b]Patients with missing data excluded

Table 5 Vascular manifestations associated with arthritis in Takayasu arteritis

Characteristic	Unadjusted OR	95% CI	*P* value
Univariate analysis			
ESR	1.015	1.004–1.025	0.007*
CRP	1.123	1.013–1.245	0.027*
Claudication	0.687	0.275–1.718	0.422
Decreased pulse	0.816	0.342–1.946	0.646
BP difference > 10 mmHg	1.657	0.474–5.792	0.429
Bruit	1.096	0.459–2.613	0.837
Carotidynia	0.877	0.243–3.163	0.841
Common carotid artery	1.658	0.713–3.853	0.240
Subclavian artery	2.241	0.931–5.394	0.072
Ascending aorta	1.844	0.869–3.913	0.111
Aortic arch	1.567	0.745–3.297	0.236
Descending aorta	2.156	0.957–4.857	0.064
Abdominal aorta	0.486	0.221–1.072	0.074
Renal artery	1.126	0.459–2.761	0.795
Iliac artery	0.230	0.030–1.751	0.156
Pulmonary artery	0.495	0.112–2.186	0.354
Type I	0.707	0.259–1.930	0.498
Type IIA	1.117	0.313–3.994	0.865
Type IIB	3.160	1.448–6.897	0.004*
Type III	0.814	0.100–6.643	0.847
Type IV	1.490	0.169–-13.177	0.720
Type V	0.441	0.196–0.992	0.048*
Multivariate analysis			
ESR	1.014	1.003–1.025	0.012*
CRP	1.052	0.911–1.215	0.489
Type IIB	2.956	1.337–6.537	0.007*
Type V	0.634	0.243–1.652	0.351

OR odds ratio, *CI* confidence interval, *ESR* erythrocyte sedimentation rate, *CRP* C-reactive protein, *BP* blood pressure
*Value considered significant ($p < 0.05$)

which could play a central role in their co-occurrence. Further study regarding this issue could aid in elucidating the pathophysiologic background of these diseases. We discovered that the characteristics of sacroiliitis in TAK differed from SpA patients in general, being predominantly female (89.5%) and exhibiting a low incidence of HLA-B27 positivity (14.3%) [25–27]. This finding is consistent with a previous study [15] that also demonstrated female predominance and low HLA-B27 positivity. Furthermore, the presence of SpA features other than sacroiliitis in these patients was relatively low (peripheral arthritis 15.8%, enthesitis 5.3%, uveitis 5.3%, IBD 5.3%) compared to SpA patients in general (peripheral arthritis 39.8–58.0%, enthesitis 37.8–50.0%, uveitis 8.5–27.0%, IBD 1.8–11.0%) [28]. Considering that aortitis is one of the cardiovascular manifestations observed in ankylosing spondylitis and other forms of SpA [29], it can be challenging to differentiate TAK patients with sacroiliitis from SpA patients with aortitis. The aforementioned differences in the characteristics of sacroiliitis between these two patient types could provide clues in distinguishing one from another.

Peripheral arthritis was observed in 6.0% of TAK patients. This manifestation was characterized by an asymmetric oligoarthritis pattern, mostly involving the large joints. This was similar to the pattern observed in SpA (asymmetric oligoarthritis with lower extremity predominance) [30] except that an even distribution between the upper and lower extremities was observed.

Interestingly, the most common type of vessel involvement in TAK patients with arthritis (axial and/or peripheral arthritis) was type IIB, differing from the total study population where type V was most frequently observed. Furthermore, in the multivariate logistic regression analysis evaluating the association between arthritis and vascular manifestations, type IIB was associated with arthritis approximately three times higher than nontype IIB. Therefore, TAK patients with type IIB should be carefully monitored for arthritis.

In our study, the prevalence of IBD (2.6%) in TAK patients appeared low compared to previous reports (5.8–8.3%) [16, 31]. However, considering that the prevalence of CD and UC are 0.01% and 0.03%, respectively, in the general Korean population [32], a prevalence of 2.6% IBD in our TAK patients is obviously higher than that of the general population. This is consistent with a previous study reporting a higher prevalence of IBD in TAK patients than that in the general population [16, 31].

Recurrent oral ulcers (8.6%) were the second most common extravascular manifestation in our study, whereas erythema nodosum (1.5%) and uveitis (0.7%) were rarely observed. Recurrent oral ulcers, erythema nodosum, and monoarthritis or oligoarthritis are manifestations that are also observed in Behcet's disease, as well as inflammation of large vessels [33]. Thus, it may be confusing to distinguish TAK from Behcet's disease. However, a notable difference between TAK and Behcet's disease is the absence of genital ulcers. In our data, none of the TAK patients exhibited genital ulcers, which have the highest discriminatory value in the International Study Group for Behcet's Disease criteria [34]. Furthermore, occlusion or stenosis due to homogeneous concentric wall thickness favors TAK, whereas thrombotic occlusion or a solitary aneurysm is more likely in Behcet's disease [33].

The present study has some limitations. First, this study was retrospective. Although not many, there were some missing data concerning clinical symptoms and signs. Therefore, there might be other extravascular manifestations that we have not identified. Second, only Korean TAK patients were included, and other ethnic populations could display different results. Thus, further studies with subjects from different ethnic populations are required. Despite these limitations, considering that TAK is such a rare disease, our results are strengthened by the relatively large number of patients.

Conclusions

In summary, we have shown that extravascular manifestations of TAK are observed in up to one-fifth of TAK patients. The most common extravascular manifestation was arthritis (axial arthritis and peripheral arthritis), and Hata's type IIB pattern of vessel involvement and a high ESR were associated with the presence of arthritis. The presented results are meaningful in that they provide clinicians with a better understanding of the accompanying extravascular manifestations of this rare disease.

Funding

This work was supported by grant 2017-655 from the Asan Institute for Life Sciences, Asan Medical Center, South Korea.

Authors' contributions

OCK contributed to the design, acquisition of data, data analyses, data interpretation, and manuscript preparation. S-WL contributed to the acquisition of data, data interpretation, and manuscript preparation. Y-BP contributed to the acquisition of data, data interpretation, and manuscript preparation. JSO contributed to data analyses, data interpretation, and manuscript preparation. SHL contributed to data analyses, data interpretation, and manuscript preparation. SH contributed to the acquisition of data, data analyses, data interpretation, and manuscript preparation. C-KL contributed to the acquisition of data, data analyses, data interpretation, and manuscript preparation. BY contributed to the acquisition of data, data analyses, data interpretation, and manuscript preparation. Y-GK contributed to the study concept and design, acquisition of data, data interpretation, and manuscript preparation. All authors read and approved the final manuscript.

Competing interests

The authors declare that they have no competing interests.

Author details

[1]Division of Rheumatology, Department of Internal Medicine, University of Ulsan, College of Medicine, Asan Medical Center, 88 Olympic-ro 43-gil, Songpa-gu, Seoul 05505, South Korea. [2]Division of Rheumatology, Department of Internal Medicine, Yonsei University College of Medicine, Seoul, South Korea. [3]Clinical Research Center, University of Ulsan College of Medicine, Asan Medical Center, Seoul, South Korea. [4]Department of Radiology and Research Institute of Radiology, University of Ulsan College of Medicine, Asan Medical Center, Seoul, South Korea.

References

1. Watanabe Y, Miyata T, Tanemoto K. Current clinical features of new patients with Takayasu arteritis observed from cross-country research in Japan: age and sex specificity. Circulation. 2015;132:1701–9. https://doi.org/10.1161/circulationaha.114.012547.
2. Terao C, Yoshifuji H, Mimori T. Recent advances in Takayasu arteritis. Int J Rheum Dis. 2014;17:238–47. https://doi.org/10.1111/1756-185x.12309.
3. Mohammad AJ, Mandl T. Takayasu arteritis in southern Sweden. J Rheumatol. 2015;42:853–8. https://doi.org/10.3899/jrheum.140843.
4. Dreyer L, Faurschou M, Baslund B. A population-based study of Takayasu's arteritis in eastern Denmark. Clin Exp Rheumatol. 2011;29:S40–2.
5. Watts R, Al-Taiar A, Mooney J, Scott D, Macgregor A. The epidemiology of Takayasu arteritis in the UK. Rheumatology (Oxford). 2009;48:1008–11. https://doi.org/10.1093/rheumatology/kep153
6. Ueda H, Morooka S, Ito I, Yamaguchi H, Takeda T. Clinical observation of 52 cases of aortitis syndrome. Jpn Heart J. 1969;10:277–88.
7. Jain S, Kumari S, Ganguly NK, Sharma BK. Current status of Takayasu arteritis in India. Int J Cardiol. 1996;54((Suppl)):S111–6.
8. Zheng D, Fan D, Liu L. Takayasu arteritis in China: a report of 530 cases. Heart Vessels Suppl. 1992;7:32–6.
9. Park YB, Hong SK, Choi KJ, Sohn DW, Oh BH, Lee MM, et al. Takayasu arteritis in Korea: clinical and angiographic features. Heart Vessels Suppl. 1992;7:55–9.

10. Kerr GS, Hallahan CW, Giordano J, Leavitt RY, Fauci AS, Rottem M, et al. Takayasu arteritis. Ann Intern Med. 1994;120:919–29.
11. Lupi-Herrera E, Sanchez-Torres G, Marcushamer J, Mispireta J, Horwitz S, Vela JE. Takayasu's arteritis. Clinical study of 107 cases. Am Heart J. 1977;93:94–103.
12. Numano F. The story of Takayasu arteritis. Rheumatology (Oxford). 2002;41:103–6.
13. Moriwaki R, Noda M, Yajima M, Sharma BK, Numano F. Clinical manifestations of Takayasu arteritis in India and Japan—new classification of angiographic findings. Angiology. 1997;48:369–79. https://doi.org/10.1177/000331979704800501.
14. Gan FY, Fei YY, Li MT, Wang Q, Xu D, Hou Y, et al. The characteristics of patients having ankylosing spondylitis associated with Takayasu's arteritis. Clin Rheumatol. 2014;33:355–8. https://doi.org/10.1007/s10067-013-2444-7.
15. Riviere E, Arnaud L, Ebbo M, Allanore Y, Claudepierre P, Dernis E, et al. Takayasu arteritis and spondyloarthritis: coincidence or association? A study of 14 cases. J Rheumatol. 2017;44:1011–7. https://doi.org/10.3899/jrheum.160762.
16. Kilic L, Kalyoncu U, Karadag O, Akdogan A, Dogan I, Bilgen SA, et al. Inflammatory bowel diseases and Takayasu's arteritis: coincidence or association? Int J Rheum Dis. 2016;19:814–8. https://doi.org/10.1111/1756-185x.12837.
17. Terao C, Matsumura T, Yoshifuji H, Kirino Y, Maejima Y, Nakaoka Y, et al. Takayasu arteritis and ulcerative colitis: high rate of co-occurrence and genetic overlap. Arthritis Rheumatol. 2015;67:2226–32. https://doi.org/10.1002/art.39157.
18. Loetscher J, Fistarol S, Walker UA. Pyoderma gangrenosum and erythema nodosum revealing Takayasu's arteritis. Case Rep Dermatol. 2016;8:354–7. https://doi.org/10.1159/000452829.
19. Pascual-Lopez M, Hernandez-Nunez A, Aragues-Montanes M, Dauden E, Fraga J, Garcia-Diez A. Takayasu's disease with cutaneous involvement. Dermatology. 2004;208:10–5. https://doi.org/10.1159/000075039.
20. Gupta M, Singh K, Lehl SS, Bhalla M. Recurrent erythema nodosum: a red flag sign of hidden systemic vasculitis. BMJ Case Rep. 2013;2013 https://doi.org/10.1136/bcr-2013-009507.
21. McDonald MA, Ojaimi E, Favilla I. Anterior uveitis in a child with Takayasu's arteritis. Clin Exp Ophthalmol. 2004;32:336–9. https://doi.org/10.1111/j.1442-9071.2004.00828.x.
22. Becker RW, Sohn RL, Poulik JM, Berguer R. Takayasu's arteritis presenting as uveitis in a 5-year-old girl. Ann Vasc Surg. 2005;19:258–62. https://doi.org/10.1007/s10016-004-0178-3.
23. Arend WP, Michel BA, Bloch DA, Hunder GG, Calabrese LH, Edworthy SM, et al. The American College of Rheumatology 1990 criteria for the classification of Takayasu arteritis. Arthritis Rheum. 1990;33:1129–34.
24. van der Linden S, Valkenburg HA, Cats A. Evaluation of diagnostic criteria for ankylosing spondylitis. A proposal for modification of the New York criteria. Arthritis Rheum. 1984;27:361–8.
25. van Tubergen A. The changing clinical picture and epidemiology of spondyloarthritis. Nat Rev Rheumatol. 2015;11:110–8. https://doi.org/10.1038/nrrheum.2014.181.
26. Rudwaleit M, Haibel H, Baraliakos X, Listing J, Marker-Hermann E, Zeidler H, et al. The early disease stage in axial spondylarthritis: results from the German Spondyloarthritis inception cohort. Arthritis Rheum. 2009;60:717–27. https://doi.org/10.1002/art.24483.
27. Taurog JD, Chhabra A, Colbert RA. Ankylosing spondylitis and axial spondyloarthritis. N Engl J Med. 2016;374:2563–74. https://doi.org/10.1056/NEJMra1406182.
28. Sieper J, Poddubnyy D. Axial spondyloarthritis. Lancet. 2017;390:73–84. https://doi.org/10.1016/s0140-6736(16)31591-4.
29. Palazzi C, DA S, Lubrano E, Olivieri I. Aortic involvement in ankylosing spondylitis. Clin Exp Rheumatol. 2008;26:S131–4.
30. Amor B, Santos RS, Nahal R, Listrat V, Dougados M. Predictive factors for the longterm outcome of spondyloarthropathies. J Rheumatol. 1994;21:1883–7.
31. Gudbrandsson B, Molberg O, Garen T, Palm O. Prevalence, incidence, and disease characteristics of Takayasu arteritis by ethnic background: data from a large, population-based cohort resident in southern Norway. Arthritis Care Res (Hoboken). 2017;69:278–85. https://doi.org/10.1002/acr.22931.
32. Yang SK, Yun S, Kim JH, Park JY, Kim HY, Kim YH, et al. Epidemiology of inflammatory bowel disease in the Songpa-Kangdong district, Seoul, Korea, 1986-2005: a KASID study. Inflamm Bowel Dis. 2008;14:542–9. https://doi.org/10.1002/ibd.20310.

30. Amor B, Santos RS, Nahal R, Listrat V, Dougados M. Predictive factors for the longterm outcome of spondyloarthropathies. J Rheumatol. 1994;21:1883–7.
31. Gudbrandsson B, Molberg O, Garen T, Palm O. Prevalence, incidence, and disease characteristics of Takayasu arteritis by ethnic background: data from a large, population-based cohort resident in southern Norway. Arthritis Care Res (Hoboken). 2017;69:278–85. https://doi.org/10.1002/acr.22931.
32. Yang SK, Yun S, Kim JH, Park JY, Kim HY, Kim YH, et al. Epidemiology of inflammatory bowel disease in the Songpa-Kangdong district, Seoul, Korea, 1986-2005: a KASID study. Inflamm Bowel Dis. 2008;14:542–9. https://doi.org/10.1002/ibd.20310.

14

Detection of high cardiovascular risk patients with ankylosing spondylitis based on the assessment of abdominal aortic calcium as compared to carotid ultrasound

Javier Rueda-Gotor[1*], Fernanda Genre[1†], Alfonso Corrales[1], Ricardo Blanco[1], Patricia Fuentevilla[1], Virginia Portilla[1], Rosa Expósito[2], Cristina Mata[2], Trinitario Pina[1], Carlos González-Juanatey[3], Luis Rodriguez-Rodriguez[4†] and Miguel A. González-Gay[1,5†]

Abstract

Background: This study aimed to determine whether, besides carotid ultrasound (US), a lateral lumbar spine radiography may also help identify ankylosing spondylitis (AS) patients at high risk of cardiovascular (CV) disease.

Methods: A set of 125 AS patients older than 35 years without a history of CV events, diabetes mellitus, or chronic kidney disease was recruited. Carotid US and lateral lumbar spine radiography were performed in all of them. The CV risk was calculated according to the total cholesterol systematic coronary risk evaluation (TC-SCORE) algorithm. Presence of carotid plaques was defined following the Mannheim Carotid Intima-media Thickness and Plaque Consensus. Abdominal aortic calcium (AAC) in a plain radiography was defined as calcific densities visible in an area parallel and anterior to the lumbar spine.

Results: Carotid US showed higher sensitivity than lateral lumbar spine radiography to detect high CV risk in the 54 patients with moderate TC-SCORE (61% versus 38.9%). Using carotid plaques as the gold standard test, a predictive model that included a TC-SCORE ≥ 5% or the presence of AAC in the lateral lumbar spine radiography in patients with both moderate and low CV risk (< 5%) according to the TC-SCORE yielded a sensitivity of 50.9% with a specificity of 95.7% to identify high/very high CV-risk AS patients. A positive correlation between AAC and carotid plaques was observed ($r^2 = 0.49$, $p < 0.001$).

Conclusions: A lateral lumbar spine radiography is a useful tool to identify patients with AS at high risk of CV disease.

Keywords: Ankylosing spondylitis, Cardiovascular disease, Abdominal aortic calcification, Lumbar lateral spine radiography, Carotid ultrasonography

Background

As occurs with other chronic inflammatory conditions, ankylosing spondylitis (AS) is associated with a process of accelerated atherosclerosis [1, 2] which leads to increased rates of subclinical atherosclerosis [3] and cardiovascular (CV) events [4]. A recent meta-analysis of seven longitudinal studies reported an increased frequency of myocardial infarction (odds ratio (OR) 1.60, 95% confidence interval (CI) 1.32–1.93) and stroke (OR 1.50, 95% CI 1.39–1.62) in AS patients when compared to the general population [4]. In a population-based study which included 21,473 AS patients and 86,606 controls matched for age, sex, and location of residence, Haroon et al. [5] found a 36% higher risk of vascular mortality in AS.

Primary prevention strategies designed to avoid atherosclerosis-related CV events in the general population are based on the identification of individuals at high

* Correspondence: ruedagotor@gmail.com
[†]Miguel A. González-Gay, Fernanda Genre and Luis Rodriguez-Rodriguez are contributed equally to this work.
[1]Epidemiology, Genetics and Atherosclerosis Research Group on Systemic Inflammatory Diseases, Division of Rheumatology, Hospital Universitario Marqués de Valdecilla, IDIVAL, University of Cantabria, Avenida de Valdecilla, s/n, 39008 Santander, Spain
Full list of author information is available at the end of the article

CV risk who can benefit from appropriate prevention measures [6]. In this regard, statin use has proved to be very effective, being able to reduce overall mortality by 15% [7]. The benefit may be even greater in AS patients according to a recent study which found a 37% lower risk of all-cause mortality associated with statin initiation [8].

The 2016 "European Guidelines on CV disease prevention in clinical practice" recommended using the total cholesterol systematic coronary risk evaluation (TC-SCORE) to stratify the CV risk and to identify individuals at high CV risk who were candidates for treatment [6]. The TC-SCORE predicts the individual's absolute risk for fatal CV events considering age, sex, total cholesterol levels, smoking, and blood pressure, stratifying the CV risk into low (< 1%), moderate (≥ 1 and < 5%), high (≥ 5 and < 10%), and very high (≥ 10%).

Unfortunately, predictive models designed for the general population do not consider the inflammatory process as a proatherogenic factor, leading to an underestimation of the CV risk when used in inflammatory diseases like AS. In this regard, a recent study disclosed in AS patients a 10-year cumulative incidence of CV events three times higher than that predicted based on the Framingham Risk Score (FRS) [9].

In an attempt to improve the TC-SCORE predictions, the 2016 European Society of Cardiology (ESC) guidelines proposed the use of different imaging techniques to identify high-CV risk individuals with subclinical atherosclerosis [6]. Carotid ultrasonography (US) and multidetector coronary tomography (MDCT) allow one to detect, respectively, carotid plaques and coronary calcifications, which are considered independent predictors of CV events capable of providing additional value to the FRS when estimating CV risk [10, 11]. According to the 2016 ESC guidelines, the presence of both surrogate markers of atherosclerosis automatically implies a very high CV risk [6]. Our group has recently demonstrated that carotid US and MDCT are very useful to redefine the CV risk in AS: up to 63% and 30% of our AS patients with moderate CV risk according to the SCORE risk charts had carotid plaques and coronary calcifications, respectively [12]. However, the restricted availability of MDCT in the daily clinical practice and the considerable amount of radiation associated with the use of this technique may be limitations for to its generalized use.

Abdominal aortic calcium (AAC) constitutes another surrogate marker of atherosclerosis easily detectable in a lateral lumbar spine radiography [13]. Unlike MDTC, it is available in most AS patients. Aortic calcification has been demonstrated to represent true intimal atherosclerosis in postmortem studies [14], correlating with the degree of atherosclerosis in the coronary arterial beds [15]. As occurs with carotid plaques and coronary calcification, AAC deposits constitute an independent predictor of subsequent vascular morbidity and mortality capable of improving the risk prediction based on the FRS [16].

Taking all these considerations into account, the purpose of the present study is to determine whether, besides carotid US, the presence of ACC deposits detected by plain lumbar spine radiographs is able to improve the identification of those AS patients with high/very high CV risk who, therefore, would be candidates to receive intensive preventive therapy.

Methods

Patients

In this cross-sectional study, a set of 125 consecutive AS patients seen over a 5-year period at Hospital Universitario Marqués de Valdecilla and Hospital de Laredo (Cantabria, northern Spain) who fulfilled definitions for AS according to the 1984 modified New York criteria [17] were recruited. Patients with a history of CV events (ischemic heart disease, cerebrovascular accident, peripheral arterial disease, or heart failure) were excluded. This was also the case for those with type 2 diabetes mellitus or with two fasting plasma glucose levels on different days at the time of disease diagnosis or over the extended follow-up > 125 mg/dl as well as those with chronic kidney disease (glomerular filtration rate < 60 ml/min/1.73 m^2) because they are considered as having high or very high CV risk according to current guidelines.

Two clinical indexes of disease activity (Bath Ankylosing Spondylitis Disease Activity Index (BASDAI) and Ankylosing Spondylitis Disease Activity Score (ASDAS)), a functional status index (Bath Ankylosing Spondylitis Functional Index (BASFI)), a metrologic index (Bath Ankylosing Spondylitis Metrology Index (BASMI)), and an enthesitis index (Maastricht Ankylosing Spondylitis Enthesitis Score (MASES)) were evaluated in all patients at the time of the carotid US assessment [18–22].

Information on history of hip involvement, synovitis, enthesitis, extra-articular manifestations (anterior uveitis, psoriasis, and inflammatory bowel disease), syndesmophytes, and HLA-B27 status was also assessed. This was also the case for data on family history of early CV events in first-degree relatives, waist circumference, body mass index, blood pressure at the time of study, and history of traditional CV risk factors (smoking, hypertension, dyslipidemia, and obesity).

Data on C-reactive protein (CRP) and the erythrocyte sedimentation rate (ESR) at the time of recruitment and at disease diagnosis, identification of patients with CRP serum levels higher than 3 mg/L at the time of diagnosis, and total cholesterol, HDL-cholesterol, LDL-cholesterol, and triglycerides at the time of the study were also assessed. Information on therapy including treatment with anti-tumor necrosis factor (anti-TNF) alpha agents from the disease diagnosis was also reviewed.

The TC-SCORE system estimates the 10-year risk of a first fatal atherosclerotic event, whether heart attack, stroke, or other occlusive arterial disease, including sudden cardiac death. Risk estimates have been produced as charts for high and low-risk regions in Europe [6]. Spain was included in the low-risk region of Europe. The risk factors incorporated in the TC-SCORE are those previously described: age, gender, smoking, total cholesterol levels, and systolic blood pressure. Subjects with TC-SCORE < 1% are included in the category of low risk. Those with a TC-SCORE ≥ 1% and < 5% are in the category of moderate risk. When the chart TC-SCORE result is ≥ 5% and < 10% they are classified as having high risk. Finally, those patients with TC-SCORE results ≥ 10% are included in the category of very high CV risk.

The earliest age at which the CV risk scores should be used in the general population has not been rigorously established. Both European [6] and North American [23] guidelines recommend their application in individuals over 40 years old. However, this cutoff point is not uniform and varies across the different CV risk scores: 30 years old for the FRS [24], 40 years old for the TC-SCORE [6], and 45 years old for the Reynolds Risk Score [25], which can only be applied from this age onward. In Spain, the Framingham-based REGICOR adapted function, a CV risk function validated in the Spanish population [26], established its use at an intermediate point of 35 years old. Since patients with AS have early accelerated atherosclerosis, and we observed carotid plaques in patients under 40 years old, we included in the analysis all patients who were age 35 years and older.

Carotid US examination

A set of 125 AS patients underwent carotid US examination to detect focal plaques in the extracranial carotid tree. According to the Mannheim Carotid Intima-media Thickness and Plaque Consensus, a carotid plaque was defined as a focal protrusion in the lumen at least cIMT > 1.5 mm, protrusion at least 50% greater than the surrounding cIMT, or arterial lumen encroaching > 0.5 mm [27]. Carotid US was performed using a commercially available scanner (Mylab 70; Esaote, Genoa, Italy) equipped with a 7–12 MHz linear transducer and the automated software-guided radiofrequency technique Quality Intima Media Thickness in real time (QIMT; Esaote, Maastricht, Holland). Patients with carotid plaques were considered as having very high CV risk.

Evaluation of abdominal aortic calcium deposits

The lateral lumbar spine radiography was performed in the standing position and all X-ray scans were evaluated by an independent reader blinded to the participant's clinical status. We assessed the presence of calcific deposits at each vertebral segment from the first to fourth lumbar vertebrae, both in the posterior and anterior walls of the aorta (Fig. 1). Calcific deposits were regarded as present if densities were visible in an area parallel to the lumbar spine and anterior to the lower part of the spine. Aortic densities at the upper part of the lumbar spine (L1–L2 region) often overlapped the vertebrae as the abdominal aorta in the L1–L2 region is often lateral to the spine. Densities overlapping the vertebrae were deemed present only if they extended from or formed a clear pattern with those of the lower part of the aorta. Since calcific deposits tend to occur first in the lower aorta [28, 29], calcific deposits at the upper levels were almost always accompanied by extensive calcifications in the lower part of the aorta. Other calcific deposits visible in lumbar films, such as intestinal calcifications and calcified costal cartilages, were clearly distinguishable from aortic calcifications (Fig. 1).

The reproducibility of the evaluation of AAC deposits was also evaluated in 20 patients by two investigators (JR-G and AC). The correlation coefficient for AAC was 0.96.

The subject's written consent was obtained for all of the cases. The study was approved by the local ethical committee.

Statistical analysis

Categorical variables were described as percentages and quantitative variables as mean ± standard deviation (SD) or median (interquartile range (IQR)).

Correlation between the presence of carotid plaques and lumbar aortic calcification was analyzed using the Pearson correlation. For each CV risk model, sensitivity, specificity, percentage of correctly classified patients, and area under the receiver operating characteristic (ROC) curve (with 95% CI) were estimated.

Results

Characteristics of AS patients

The main features of the 125 AS patients included in the study are summarized in Table 1.

Men outnumbered women ($n = 78$; 62.4%) and the mean ± SD age at the time of the study was 48.3 ± 9.6 years. HLA-B27 was positive in 92 (74.8%) patients, and syndesmophytes were present in 51 (41.5%) patients. Thirty-eight (30.4%) patients had extra-articular manifestations: uveitis, psoriasis, and inflammatory bowel disease were present in 17.6%, 9.6%, and 8% of patients, respectively. The mean ± SD values of the BASDAI and ASDAS were 3.7 ± 2.0 and 2.4 ± 0.9. Seventy-two (57.6%) patients were found to have CRP > 3 mg/L at the time of disease diagnosis. TNF inhibitors were used in 39.8% of cases. Regarding findings of subclinical atherosclerosis,

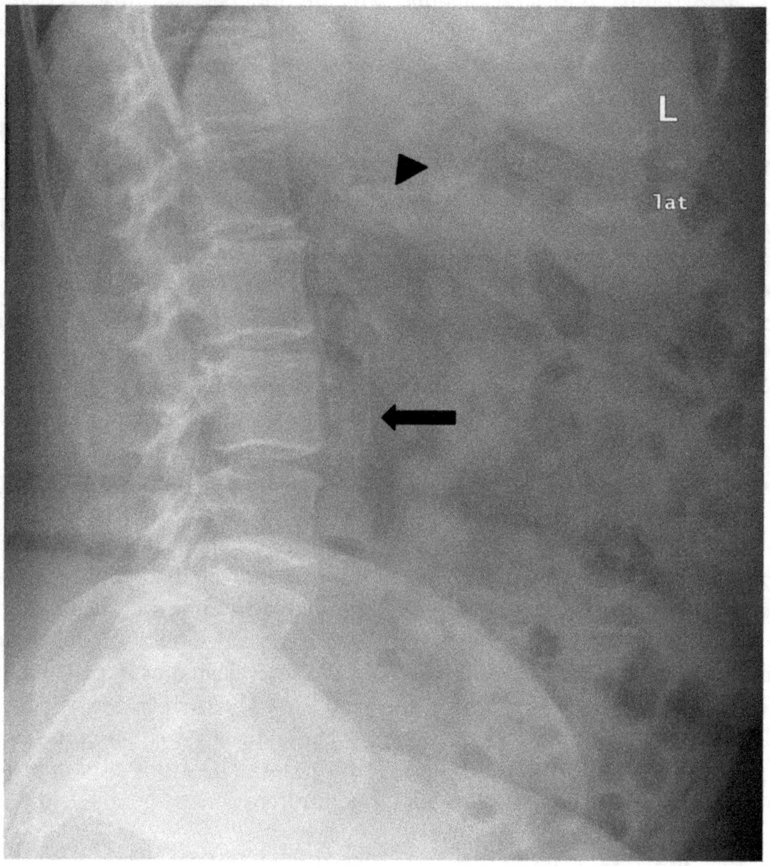

Fig. 1 Abdominal aortic calcifications and calcified costal cartilages. Abdominal aortic calcifications seen as calcium deposits localized in area parallel to lumbar spine and anterior to lower part of spine (long arrow). Calcified costal cartilages have a typical pattern distinguishable from aortic calcifications (arrowhead)

carotid plaques and AAC deposits were found in 55 (44.0%) and 28 (22.4%) patients, respectively. Other characteristics of this series of patients with AS are presented in Table 1.

TC-SCORE risk groups and severe atherosclerotic disease using carotid US and lateral spine radiography

The CV risk was calculated using the TC-SCORE. Based on this algorithm, patients were classified into four different CV risk categories: low, moderate, high, and very high. Then, the frequency of carotid plaques in each category was calculated to assess the ability of the TC-SCORE to correctly classify patients as having high/very high CV risk (Table 2). We also analyzed the prevalence of AAC in the lateral spine radiography in each group of risk (Table 2). Following this approach, 33 of 54 (61.1%) patients classified as having moderate CV according to the TC-SCORE had plaques when the carotid US was performed, whereas 21 of 54 (38.9%) patients with moderate CV risk according to the TC-SCORE also had AAC in the lateral lumbar spine radiography. Moreover, 23.4% and 4.7% of AS patients who fulfilled the category of low CV risk according to the TC-SCORE had carotid plaques and AAC, respectively (Table 2).

Correlation between AAC and carotid US in AS patients

The validity of lateral lumbar spine radiography to identify AS patients at high CV risk was assessed by analyzing the correlation between AAC and carotid plaques (Table 3). We observed that 25 of 28 (89.3%) patients with AAC deposits also had plaques in the carotid US assessment. Regarding patients without AAC deposits in the lateral lumbar spine radiography, 69.1% of them did not have carotid plaques either (Table 3). We observed a positive correlation between AAC and carotid plaques ($r^2 = 0.49$, $p < 0.001$).

Model to establish the presence of high/very high CV risk in patients with AS

Since many patients categorized as having low or moderate CV risk when the TC-SCORE was applied had subclinical atherosclerosis, we set up a predictive model to identify AS patients with high/very high CV risk (Table 4). In this regard, according to the ESC 2016 guidelines, we

Table 1 Features of 125 ankylosing spondylitis (AS) patients

Variable	AS (*n* = 125)
Men/women, *n*	78/47
Age at time of study (years), mean ± SD	48.3 ± 9.6
Age at time of diagnosis (years), mean ± SD	39.5 ± 9.6
HLA-B27 positive, *n* (%)	92 (74.8)
Syndesmophytes, *n* (%)	51 (41.5)
History of synovitis, *n* (%)	35 (28.0)
History of enthesitis, *n* (%)	45 (36.0)
Extra-articular manifestations, *n* (%)	38 (30.4)
Psoriasis	12 (9.6)
Inflammatory bowel disease	10 (8.0)
Uveitis	22 (17.6)
Therapy with TNF inhibitors, *n* (%)	49 (39.8)
ASDAS, mean ± SD	2.4 ± 0.9
BASFI, mean ± SD	3.9 ± 2.5
BASMI, mean ± SD	3.2 ± 1.7
MASES, median (IQR)	1 (0.0–4.0)
BASDAI, mean ± SD	3.7 ± 2.0
CRP (mg/l), median (IQR)	
At time of study	5.2 ± 6.7
At time of disease diagnosis	10.8 ± 19.0
CRP > 3 mg/L at time of disease diagnosis, *n* (%)	72 (57.6)
ESR (mm/1st hour), median (IQR)	
At time of study	12.4 ± 13.4
At time of disease diagnosis	16.1 ± 15.9
History of classic cardiovascular risk factors, *n* (%)	
Current smokers	37 (29.6)
Ex-smokers	31 (24.8)
Obesity	23 (18.4)
Dyslipidemia	40 (32.0)
Hypertension	21 (16.8)
Blood pressure (mmHg), mean ± SD	
Systolic	130.6 ± 15.3
Diastolic	79.5 ± 9.7
Cholesterol and triglycerides (mg/dl), mean ± SD	
Total cholesterol	200.7 ± 34.5
HDL cholesterol	55.6 ± 14.8
LDL cholesterol	124.6 ± 31.7
Triglycerides	97.3 ± 49.4
Carotid plaques, *n* (%)	55 (44.0)
Aortic calcification, *n* (%)	28 (22.4)
TC-SCORE ≥ 5, *n* (%)	7 (5.6)

Main epidemiologic, clinical, radiographic, and ultrasonography features of a series of 125 AS patients older than 35 years of age without history of cardiovascular events, diabetes mellitus, or chronic kidney disease
ASDAS Ankylosing Spondylitis Disease Activity Score, *BASDAI* Bath Ankylosing Spondylitis Disease Activity Index, *BASFI* Bath Ankylosing Spondylitis Functional Index, *BASMI* Bath Ankylosing Spondylitis Metrology Index, *CRP* C-reactive protein, *ESR* erythrocyte sedimentation rate, *HDL* high-density lipoprotein, *IQR* interquartile range, *LDL* low-density lipoprotein, *MASES* Maastricht Ankylosing Spondylitis Enthesitis Score, *SD* standard deviation *TC-SCORE* total cholesterol systematic coronary risk evaluation, *TNF* tumor necrosis factor

Table 2 Prevalence of carotid plaques and abdominal aortic calcium in the different groups of cardiovascular risk

TC-SCORE		Carotid ultrasonography	Lateral lumbar X-ray
		Carotid plaques (*n* = 55, 44%)	AAC deposits (*n* = 28, 22.4%)
Low (< 1%)	*n* = 64	15/64 (23.4%)	3/64 (4.7%)
Moderate (≥ 1% and < 5%)	*n* = 54	33/54 (61.1%)	21/54 (38.9%)
High (≥ 5% and < 10%)	*n* = 7	7/7 (100%)	4/7 (57.1%)
Very high (≥ 10%)	*n* = 0	0 (0%)	0 (0%)

Presence of carotid plaques and AAC deposits in 125 ankylosing spondylitis patients older than 35 years of age without cardiovascular events, diabetes mellitus, or chronic kidney disease, classified according to their cardiovascular risk
AAC abdominal aortic calcium, *TC-SCORE* total cholesterol systematic coronary risk evaluation

classified patients as having high/very high CV risk if they had carotid plaques in the carotid US [6]. Following this approach, 55 of 125 patients fulfilled definitions of high/very high CV risk. However, only 7 (12.7%) of them were detected using the TC-SCORE, without the inclusion in the model of results of imaging techniques (model 1). The detection of aortic atherosclerosis by lateral lumbar spine radiography yielded a high specificity (95.7%) with low sensitivity (45.5%) to identify AS patients with very high CV risk (model 2). A predictive model that included a TC-SCORE ≥ 5% or the presence of AAC in lateral lumbar spine radiography in patients with moderate CV risk according to the SCORE (≥ 1% and < 5%) (model 3) showed the same results as those found in model 2. A higher sensitivity (50.9%) with the same specificity (95.7%) was achieved when the predictive model included TC-SCORE ≥ 5% or the presence of AAC in the lateral lumbar spine radiography in patients with both moderate and low CV risk according to the TC-SCORE (< 5%) (model 4).

Discussion

To the best of our knowledge this is the first study that aimed to assess the ability of the lateral lumbar spine radiography, a diagnostic tool widely available in AS

Table 3 Correlation between abdominal aortic calcium (AAC) deposits and carotid plaques

Lateral lumbar X-ray		Carotid ultrasonography	
		Presence of carotid plaques (*n* = 55/125, 44%)	Absence of carotid plaques (*n* = 70/125, 56%)
Presence of AAC	*n* = 28 (22.4%)	25/28 (89.3%)	3/28 (10.7)
Absence of AAC	*n* = 97 (77.6%)	30/97 (30.9%)	67/97 (69.1%)

Correlation between the presence of AAC deposits and the presence of carotid plaques in 125 patients with ankylosing spondylitis older than 35 years of age without cardiovascular events, chronic kidney disease, or diabetes mellitus

Table 4 Diagnostic models designed to identify ankylosing spondylitis patients with very high cardiovascular risk using presence of carotid plaques as the gold standard test

	Sensitivity (%)	Specificity (%)	Correctly classified (%)	ROC (95% CI)
Model 1. TC-SCORE ≥ 5%	12.7	100	61.6	0.56 (0.52–0.61)
Model 2. Lateral lumbar spine radiography (presence of AAC)	45.5	95.7	73.6	0.71 (0.64–0.78)
Model 3. TC-SCORE ≥ 5% or TC-SCORE ≥ 1% and < 5% plus lateral lumbar spine radiography (presence of AAC)	45.5	95.7	73.6	0.71 (0.64–0.78)
Model 4. TC-SCORE ≥ 5% or TC-SCORE < 5% plus lateral lumbar spine radiography (presence of AAC)	50.9	95.7	76.0	0.73 (0.66–0.80)

AAC abdominal aortic calcium, *CI* confidence interval, *ROC* receiver operating characteristic, *TC-SCORE* total cholesterol systematic coronary risk evaluation

patients, to improve the CV risk stratification in patients with AS. We observed that the presence of AAC deposits detected by a lateral lumbar spine radiography allows one to identify individuals with AS at high risk of CV disease. In this regard, in the present series of 125 AS patients without CV events, chronic kidney disease, or diabetes mellitus, 21 of 54 (38.9%) patients with moderate TC-SCORE and 3 of 64 (4.7%) patients with low TC-SCORE showed AAC in the lateral lumbar spine radiography.

The presence of AAC in a plain radiography has been reported to be associated with an increased risk of CV events, CV mortality [13], and congestive heart failure [30] in the Framingham cohort. Overall, AAC adds to the prediction for intermittent claudication (IC), ischemic stroke (IS), and coronary heart disease over and above traditional CV risk factors in patients with low and intermediate risk [16]. AAC deposits also demonstrated to be a predictor of incident stroke in the Rotterdam study, even stronger than carotid plaques [31]. Both the Rotterdam and the Framingham studies used a quantitative scale to grade the severity of the aortic calcium deposits. It is worth noting that, even though the increase of CV risk was found to be proportional to the extent of the calcifications, AAC demonstrated to be a predictor of CV events and mortality also in cases of reduced calcifications. In keeping with these findings, in a Netherlands population Witteman et al. [32] found a strong independent association between CV deaths and aortic calcifications of any size, regardless of the extent of the calcific deposits. A postmortem study that analyzed the accuracy of the radiologic AAC for the diagnosis of true aortic atherosclerosis confirmed that even the smaller densities indicated the presence of advanced atheromatous plaques, which were almost invariably ulcerated [14]. Witteman et al. [32] also disclosed a high predictive role of AAC for CV death in young individuals, with a six-fold increased risk in men aged 45 years independently of the major CV risk factors, and no excess risk at age 75 years. These findings are particularly relevant in AS patients since the disease typically starts before the age of 45 years and the TC-SCORE tends to underestimate the CV risk, especially in this age group in which practically all patients are classified as having low or moderate CV risk. Indeed, the mean age in our series was 48 years and 118 of the 125 (94%) AS patients were found to have a low or moderate TC-SCORE.

The 2014 ESC guidelines on the diagnosis and treatment of aortic diseases [33] recommended adopting general preventive measures to control risk factors in the presence of aortic atherosclerosis. Treatment with statins led to regression of thoracic aortic and retardation of abdominal aortic atheroma burden assessed by magnetic resonance imaging [34], as well as reduction of the inflammation assessed by PET [35]. In a retrospective study of 519 patients with severe aortic plaque seen on transesophageal echocardiography, only statin treatment was associated with a 70% lower risk of events [36]. A correlation between AAC and atherosclerotic findings in the carotid and coronary arterial beds has previously been reported [15, 37]. This finding constitutes an additional argument to support statin use in AS patients with AAC. The presence of carotid plaques, considered a surrogate marker of subclinical atherosclerosis in the 2016 ESC guidelines, automatically implies a very high CV risk with the consequent indication of statin use. Taking into account these considerations, we can conclude that almost 50% of AS included in the categories of low and moderate CV risk according to the TC-SCORE risk algorithm would benefit from additional primary prevention measures, with special emphasis on the use of statins, if a plain lateral lumbar spine radiography is performed. This is a crucial aspect considering that statins have been shown to decrease mortality by 37% in AS, a figure double that observed in the general population [8].

The major limitation of our study was the absence of prospective follow-up data for the studied patients. Because of this, we dealt with a surrogate outcome based on extrapolation of the data that might not be applicable to AS.

In an attempt to elucidate the best strategy to identify AS patients at high CV risk, we assessed the ability of lateral lumbar spine radiography to detect severe findings of subclinical atherosclerosis. A predictive model that included a TC-SCORE ≥ 5% or the presence of AAC in lateral lumbar spine radiography in patients with a low or moderate TC-SCORE (TC-SCORE < 5%) allowed us to detect half of the AS patients with high/very high CV-risk, also demonstrating a high degree of specificity (95.7%).

Conclusions

When carotid US is not available, plain lateral lumbar spine radiography can be an easy and affordable tool to identify AS patients at high CV risk.

Abbreviations

AAC: Abdominal aortic calcium; AS: Ankylosing spondylitis; ASDAS: Ankylosing Spondylitis Disease Activity Score; BASDAI: Bath Ankylosing Spondylitis Disease Activity Index; BASFI: Bath Ankylosing Spondylitis Functional Index; BASMI: Bath Ankylosing Spondylitis Metrology Index; CRP: C-reactive protein; CV: Cardiovascular; ESR: Erythrocyte sedimentation rate; FRS: Framingham Risk Score; IC: Intermittent claudication; IQR: Interquartile range; IS: Ischemic stroke; MASES: Maastricht Ankylosing Spondylitis Enthesitis Score; MDCT: Multidetector coronary tomography; OR: Odds ratio; ROC: Receiver operating characteristic; SD: Standard deviation; TC-SCORE: Total cholesterol systematic coronary risk evaluation; TNF: Tumor necrosis factor; US: Ultrasonography

Authors' contributions

JR-G made substantial contributions to the conception and design of the manuscript. FG analyzed and interpreted the patient data. AC and RB were involved in acquisition and analysis of data. PF, VP, RE, and CM were involved in acquisition and interpretation of data. TP was involved in acquisition and analysis of data. CG-J revised the manuscript critically for important intellectual content. LR-R analyzed and interpreted the patient data. MAG-G was involved in the conception and drafting and revising the manuscript critically for important intellectual content. All authors read and approved the final manuscript.

Competing interests

The authors declare that they have no competing interests.

Author details

[1]Epidemiology, Genetics and Atherosclerosis Research Group on Systemic Inflammatory Diseases, Division of Rheumatology, Hospital Universitario Marqués de Valdecilla, IDIVAL, University of Cantabria, Avenida de Valdecilla, s/n, 39008 Santander, Spain. [2]Division of Rheumatology, Hospital Comarcal, Laredo, Cantabria, Spain. [3]Division of Cardiology, Hospital Lucus Augusti, Lugo, Spain. [4]Division of Rheumatology, Instituto de Investigación Sanitaria del Hospital Clínico San Carlos (IDISSC), Hospital Clínico San Carlos, Madrid, Spain. [5]Cardiovascular Pathophysiology and Genomics Research Unit, School of Physiology, Faculty of Health Sciences, University of the Witwatersrand, Johannesburg, South Africa.

References

1. Peters MJ, van der Horst-Bruinsma IE, Dijkmans BA, Nurmohamed MT. Cardiovascular risk profile of patients with spondylarthropathies, particularly ankylosing spondylitis and psoriatic arthritis. Semin Arthritis Rheum. 2004;34:585–92.
2. Rueda-Gotor J, Corrales A, Blanco R, Fuentevilla P, Portilla V, Expósito R, et al. Atherosclerotic disease in axial spondyloarthritis: increased frequency of carotid plaques. Clin Exp Rheumatol. 2015;33:315–20.
3. Gonzalez-Juanatey C, Vazquez-Rodriguez TR, Miranda-Filloy JA, Dierssen T, Vaqueiro I, Blanco R, et al. The high prevalence of subclinical atherosclerosis in patients with ankylosing spondylitis without clinically evident cardiovascular disease. Medicine (Baltimore). 2009;88:358–65.
4. Mathieu S, Pereira B, Soubrier M. Cardiovascular events in ankylosing spondylitis: an updated meta-analysis. Semin Arthritis Rheum. 2015;44:551–5.
5. Haroon NN, Paterson JM, Li P, Inman RD, Haroon N. Patients with ankylosing spondylitis have increased cardiovascular and cerebrovascular mortality: a population-based study. Ann Intern Med. 2015;163(6):409–16.
6. Piepoli MF, Hoes AW, Agewall S, Albus C, Brotons C, Catapano AL, et al. 2016 European Guidelines on cardiovascular disease prevention in clinical practice: The Sixth Joint Task Force of the European Society of Cardiology and Other Societies on Cardiovascular Disease Prevention in Clinical Practice (constituted by representatives of 10 societies and by invited experts) Developed with the special contribution of the European Association for Cardiovascular Prevention & Rehabilitation (EACPR). Eur Heart J. 2016;37:2315–81.
7. Taylor F, Huffman MD, Macedo AF, Moore TH, Burke M, Davey Smith G, et al. Statins for the primary prevention of cardiovascular disease. Cochrane Database Syst Rev. 2013;1:CD004816.
8. Oza A, Lu N, Sr S, Fisher MC, Dubreuil M, Rai SK, et al. Survival benefit of statin use in ankylosing spondylitis: a general population-based cohort study. Ann Rheum Dis. 2017;76(10):1737–42.
9. Wright KA, Crowson CS, Michet CJ, Matteson EL. Time trends in incidence, clinical features, and cardiovascular disease in ankylosing spondylitis over three decades: a population-based study. Arthritis Care Res (Hoboken). 2015;67:836–41.
10. Nambi V, Chambless L, Folsom AR, He M, Hu Y, Mosley T, et al. Carotid intima-media thickness and presence or absence of plaque improves prediction of coronary heart disease risk: the ARIC (Atherosclerosis Risk in Communities) study. J Am Coll. 2010;55:1600–7.
11. Detrano R, Guerci AD, Carr JJ, Bild DE, Burke G, Folsom AR, et al. Coronary calcium as a predictor of coronary events in four racial or ethnic groups. N Engl J Med. 2008;358(13):1336–45.
12. Rueda-Gotor J, Llorca J, Corrales A, Parra JA, Portilla V, Genre F, et al. Cardiovascular risk stratification in axial spondyloarthritis: carotid ultrasound is more sensitive than coronary artery calcification score to detect high-cardiovascular risk axial spondyloarthritis patients. Clin Exp Rheumatol. 2018;36(1):73–80.
13. Wilson PW, Kauppila LI, O'Donnell CJ, Kiel DP, Hannan M, Polak JM, et al. Abdominal aortic calcific deposits are an important predictor of vascular morbidity and mortality. Circulation. 2001;103(11):1529–34.
14. Hyman JB, Pstein FN. A study of the correlation between roentgenographic and post-mortem calcification of the aorta. Am Heart J. 1954;48(4):540–3.
15. Eggen DA, Strong JP, Mcgill HC Jr. Calcification in the abdominal aorta; relationship to race, sex, and coronary atherosclerosis. Arch Pathol. 1964;78:575–83.
16. Levitzky YS, Cupples LA, Murabito JM. Prediction of intermittent claudication, ischemic stroke, and other cardiovascular disease by detection of abdominal aortic calcific deposits by plain lumbar radiographs. Am J Cardiol. 2008;101(3):326–31.
17. van der Linden S, Valkenburg HA, Cats A. Evaluation of diagnostic criteria for ankylosing spondylitis. A proposal for modification of the New York criteria. Arthritis. Rheum. 1984;27:361–8.
18. Garrett S, Jenkinson T, Kennedy LG, Whitelock H, Gaisford P, Calin A. A new approach to defining disease status in ankylosing spondylitis: the bath Ankylosing Spondylitis Disease Activity Index. J Rheumatol. 1994;21:2286–91.
19. Lukas C, Landewé R, Sieper J, Dougados M, Davis J, Braun J, et al. Development of an ASAS-endorsed disease activity score (ASDAS) in patients with ankylosing spondylitis. Ann Rheum Dis. 2009;68:18–24.
20. Calin A, Garrett S, Whitelock H, Kennedy LG, O'Hea J, Mallorie P, et al. A new approach to defining functional ability in ankylosing spondylitis: the development of the Bath Ankylosing Spondylitis Functional Index. J Rheumatol. 1994;21:2281–5.
21. Jenkinson TR, Mallorie PA, Whitelock HC, Kennedy LG, Garrett SL, Calin A. Defining spinal mobility in ankylosing spondylitis (AS). The Bath AS Metrology Index. J Rheumatol. 1994;21:1694–8.
22. Heuft-Dorenbosch L, Spoorenberg A, Van Tubergen A, et al. Assessment of enthesitis in ankylosing spondylitis. Ann Rheum Dis. 2003;62:127–32.
23. Goff DC Jr, Lloyd-Jones DM, Bennett G, Coady S, D'Agostino RB Sr, Gibbons R, et al. 2013 ACC/AHA guideline on the assessment of cardiovascular risk: a report of the American College of Cardiology/American Heart Association task force on practice guidelines. J Am Coll Cardiol. 2014;63:2935–59.

24. D'Agostino RB, Vasan RS, Pencina MJ, Wolf PA, Cobain M, Massaro JM, et al. General cardiovascular risk profile for use in primary care: the Framingham Heart Study. Circulation. 2008;117:743–53.
25. Ridker PM, Buring JE, Rifai N, Cook NR. Development and validation of improved algorithms for the assessment of global cardiovascular risk in women: the Reynolds Risk Score. JAMA. 2007;297:611–9.
26. Marrugat J, Subirana I, Comín E, Cabezas C, Vila J, Elosua R, et al. Validity of an adaptation of the Framingham cardiovascular risk function: the VERIFICA study. J Epidemiol Community Health. 2007;61:40–7.
27. Touboul PJ, Hennerici MG, Meairs S, Adams H, Amarenco P, Bornstein N, et al. Mannheim carotid intima-media thickness and plaque consensus (2004-2006-2011). An update on behalf of the advisory board of the 3rd, 4th and 5th watching the risk symposia, at the 13th, 15th and 20th European Stroke Conferences, Mannheim, Germany, 2004, Brussels, Belgium, 2006, and Hamburg, Germany, 2011. Cerebrovasc Dis. 2012;34:290–6.
28. Vihert AM. Atherosclerosis of the aorta in five towns. Bll Wld Hlth Org. 1976; 53:501–8.
29. Mitchell JRA, Adams JH. Aortic size and aortic calcification: a necropsy study. Atherosclerosis. 1977;27:437–46.
30. Walsh CR, Cupples LA, Levy D, Kiel DP, Hannan M, Wilson PW, et al. Abdominal aortic calcific deposits are associated with increased risk for congestive heart failure: the Framingham Heart Study. Am Heart J. 2002; 144(4):733–9.
31. Hollander M, Hak AE, Koudstaal PJ, Bots ML, Grobbee DE, Hofman A, et al. Comparison between measures of atherosclerosis and risk of stroke: the Rotterdam Study. Stroke. 2003;34(10):2367–72.
32. Witteman JC, Kok FJ, van Saase JL, Valkenburg HA. Aortic calcification as a predictor of cardiovascular mortality. Lancet. 1986;2(8516):1120–2.
33. Erbel R, Aboyans V, Boileau C, Bossone E, Bartolomeo RD, Eggebrecht H, et al. 2014 ESC guidelines on the diagnosis and treatment of aortic diseases: document covering acute and chronic aortic diseases of the thoracic and abdominal aorta of the adult. The task force for the diagnosis and treatment of aortic diseases of the European Society of Cardiology (ESC). Eur Heart J. 2014;35(41):2873–926.
34. Yonemura A, Momiyama Y, Fayad ZA, Ayaori M, Ohmori R, Kihara T, et al. Effect of lipid-lowering therapy with atorvastatin on atherosclerotic aortic plaques: a 2-year follow-up by noninvasive MRI. Eur J Cardiovasc Prev Rehabil. 2009;16(2):222–8.
35. Tahara N, Kai H, Ishibashi M, Nakaura H, Kaida H, Baba K, Hayabuchi N, Imaizumi T. Simvastatin attenuates plaque inflammation: evaluation by fluorodeoxyglucose positron emission tomography. J Am Coll Cardiol. 2006; 48:1825–31.
36. Tunick PA, Nayar AC, Goodkin GM, Mirchandani S, Francescone S, Rosenzweig BP, Freedberg RS, Katz ES, Applebaum RM, Kronzon I. Effect of treatment on the incidence of stroke and other emboli in 519 patients with severe thoracic aortic plaque. Am J Cardiol. 2002;90:1320–5.
37. Lewis JR, Schousboe JT, Lim WH, Wong G, Zhu K, Lim EM, et al. Abdominal aortic calcification identified on abdominal aortic calcification identified on lateral spine images from bone densitometers are a marker of generalized atherosclerosis in elderly women. Arterioscler Thromb Vasc Biol. 2016;36(1): 166–73.

15

A single determination of C-reactive protein does not suffice to declare a patient with a diagnosis of axial spondyloarthritis 'CRP-negative'

Robert Landewé[1*], Tommi Nurminen[2], Owen Davies[3] and Dominique Baeten[4]

Abstract

Background: To be eligible to receive treatment with an anti-tumour necrosis factor (TNF), non-radiographic axial spondyloarthritis (nr-axSpA) patients require either elevated levels of C-reactive protein (CRP) (CRP > upper limit of normal (ULN)) or magnetic resonance imaging assessment showing inflammation of the sacroiliac joints, in addition to meeting criteria for high disease activity. Many axSpA patients are classified as 'CRP-negative', or CRP normal, despite having levels close to the ULN, and are therefore formally ineligible for treatment. The aim of this study was to investigate the likelihood of a CRP test indicating elevated levels in axSpA patients that have previously tested CRP normal.

Methods: RAPID-axSpA (NCT01087762) enrolled patients who were either magnetic resonance imaging positive or had elevated CRP (> ULN: 7.9 mg/L). CRP data from the double-blind period for placebo-randomised patients until re-randomisation to certolizumab pegol (week 16 for ASAS20 non-responders/week 24 for ASAS20 responders) were analysed. CRP was assessed at screening, baseline, and nine time points to week 24. Linear mixed models were used to investigate time trends, variability, and correlations of CRP data.

Results: Of 106 placebo-randomised patients with baseline CRP assessments, 26 (25%) tested CRP normal at baseline, of whom 13 (50%) had ≥ 1 test indicating elevated CRP to week 16. Of 80/106 (75%) patients with elevated baseline CRP, 25 (31%) had ≥ 1 normal CRP test to week 16. Linear mixed models did not reveal changes in mean CRP across placebo patients from baseline to week 24.

Conclusions: In axSpA patients with CRP < ULN the CRP test should be repeated after ≥ 4 weeks as there is a substantial chance of finding a positive result for elevated CRP at subsequent testing, thereby allowing the patient access to treatment.

Keywords: C-reactive protein, Non-radiographic axial spondyloarthritis, Inflammation

* Correspondence: landewe@rlandewe.nl
[1]Clinical Immunology and Rheumatology, Amsterdam Rheumatology & Immunology Center and Academic Medical Center, University of Amsterdam, Amsterdam, Netherlands
Full list of author information is available at the end of the article

Background

Axial spondyloarthritis (axSpA) is a chronic inflammatory disease involving the spine and/or sacroiliac joints. Typically, axSpA patients are further classified as having either ankylosing spondylitis (AS) or non-radiographic (nr)-axSpA, depending on the presence or absence of radiographic sacroiliitis, respectively [1]. It is generally accepted that these two subpopulations represent a spectrum of the same disease, and both subgroups have been shown to experience a similar burden of disease and similar clinical response to anti-tumour necrosis factor (TNF) therapy [2, 3]. Nevertheless, concerns have been voiced regarding the possibility of spontaneous remission in nr-axSpA patients, and potential overtreatment with biologics [4]. In the US, anti-TNFs have received Food and Drug Administration (FDA) approval for the treatment of AS [5–8], but are yet to obtain approval for the treatment of nr-axSpA [9]. In contrast, four anti-TNFs have been approved by European regulatory authorities for the treatment of patients with active nr-axSpA on the condition that they must exhibit objective signs of inflammation, demonstrated by magnetic resonance imaging (MRI) and/or elevated levels of C-reactive protein (CRP) [10–12].

The CRP level in axSpA patients is a key indicator of inflammation and is also considered to be a predictor of clinical response to anti-TNF treatment. In a number of studies, patients with elevated CRP at baseline have demonstrated significantly greater responses to anti-TNFs compared with patients with low CRP levels as well as those receiving placebo treatment [13, 14].

To be eligible to receive treatment with an anti-TNF in Europe, Assessment of SpondyloArthritis international Society (ASAS) treatment recommendations state that nr-axSpA patients must have either a positive CRP assessment (elevated CRP greater than the upper limit of normal (ULN)) or a positive MRI showing inflammation of the sacroiliac joints, in addition to meeting criteria for high disease activity [15, 16]. Many axSpA patients with normal CRP levels are classified as CRP 'negative' despite having levels close to the ULN, and are therefore formally ineligible for treatment. The natural degree of CRP fluctuation in patients who have not received anti-TNF therapy is not well understood [17], and should be investigated further.

In this post-hoc analysis of data from a phase 3 randomised controlled trial, we evaluated the consistency of CRP testing in patients with active axSpA.

Methods

Study design

The phase 3 RAPID-axSpA study (NCT01087762) evaluated the efficacy and safety of certolizumab pegol (CZP) in patients with active axSpA. The trial was double-blind and placebo-controlled to week 24, dose-blind to week 48 and open-label to week 204. Data here are taken from the initial 24-week, double-blind, placebo-controlled period.

At week 0, patients were randomised 1:1:1 to placebo, CZP 400 mg every 4 weeks (Q4W), or CZP 200 mg every other week (Q2W). Patients randomised to placebo who did not meet ASAS 20% response criteria (ASAS20) at either weeks 14 or 16 were allocated to escape treatment (re-randomised 1:1 to either CZP 200 mg Q2W or CZP 400 mg Q4W). Placebo-randomised patients who did achieve an ASAS20 response were re-randomised to CZP at week 24 (the end of the double-blind period).

We analysed data only from placebo-randomised patients until their point of re-randomisation to CZP at either week 16 or week 24.

The trial enrolled patients with a clinical diagnosis of axSpA, fulfilling ASAS criteria, with active disease defined by each of the Bath Ankylosing Spondylitis Disease Activity Index (BASDAI) score ≥ 4, spinal pain ≥ 4 on a 0–10 numeric rating scale, CRP > ULN (7.9 mg/L) and/or sacroiliitis on MRI as defined by ASAS classification criteria, within 3 months prior to screening. One re-testing of subjects who failed screening due to the CRP level was permitted. All patients had an inadequate response to, or intolerance of, ≥ 1 non-steroidal anti-inflammatory drug (NSAID). Conventional background medications at stable dose levels were allowed during the screening and double-blind periods of the study. Detailed inclusion and exclusion criteria have been previously presented [18]. Approval from the Independent Ethics Committee or Institutional Review Board was obtained. Informed consent according to the Declaration of Helsinki was collected from all patients.

Study procedures and evaluations

The primary outcome (ASAS20 responder rate at week 12) [18], as well as safety, efficacy, and patient-reported outcomes to week 204, have been reported previously [19]. CRP level was assessed at screening, baseline, and at nine time points (weeks 1, 2, 4, 8, 12, 16, 18, 20, and 24) to week 24. Serum samples were analysed in two central laboratories: the European central laboratory (~ 60% of samples) used a conventional CRP assay with a lower limit of quantification (LLQ) of 3 mg/L, while the samples from North and Latin America (~ 40% of samples) were analysed with a high-sensitivity assay (LLQ 0.1 mg/L). Elevated CRP was defined as CRP > ULN (7.9 mg/L) and values ≤ 7.9 mg/L were considered to have normal CRP levels.

Statistical analysis

Linear mixed models (LMM) were used to investigate time trends, variability, and correlations of CRP data following a Ln(CRP mg/L + 1) transformation [20]. LMM analyses at the group level were used to evaluate possible placebo response, whilst LMM analyses at the patient level allowed auto-correlations (i.e. the similarity of two results depending on the time interval between them) to be quantified. Based upon the results from LMM analyses, simplified descriptive summaries were generated to illustrate reproducibility of CRP tests. Since valid post-week 16 evaluations were available from ASAS20 responders, certain descriptive analyses were restricted up to week 16 a priori to avoid data confoundment. For CRP values below the lower limit of quantification, half the lower limit was used for analysis. Statistical analyses were performed using SAS® version 9.3 (SAS Institute, Cary, NC, USA).

Results

Patient disposition and baseline characteristics

In RAPID-axSpA, a total of 325 patients were randomised to treatment at week 0, 107 to placebo, and 218 to CZP. Of 106 patients receiving placebo with baseline CRP assessments, 26 (25%) had normal CRP tests and 80 (75%) had elevated CRP levels.

Is a patient's CRP status stable?

Of the 26 patients with normal CRP levels at baseline, 13 (50%) subsequently had at least one test indicating elevated CRP levels to week 16, and 1 (4%) patient had elevated CRP for all following assessments to week 16. For the 80/106 patients with elevated CRP at baseline, 25 (31%) subsequently had at least one CRP test with normal CRP levels. No patients exhibited normal CRP levels for all subsequent assessments to week 16 (Table 1).

How does CRP vary over time? Results from LMM analyses

There was no strong evidence of change in mean CRP from baseline to week 24 (note that all patients included were randomised to placebo). However, variation in CRP level was observed over time in individual patients. Analysis of within-subject auto-correlation indicated that short-term assessments (1–2 weeks apart) were strongly correlated, i.e. provided similar results. This correlation decreased in assessments separated by periods of ≥ 4 weeks. Results from LMM analyses are presented in Additional file 1.

Reproducibility of CRP status: what is the likelihood of a change in CRP status at a future assessment?

Given the observed lack of systematic group-level trends in CRP, we calculated how often a value within a given range was followed by an elevated CRP test result at a subsequent assessment (assuming that any available CRP assessments could represent a placebo-randomised patient's first and only available result). Descriptive evaluations demonstrated that 10.8% (n = 7) of ≤ 3 mg/L CRP assessments would result in elevated CRP levels (defined as > 7.9 mg/L) 4 weeks following their initial assessment (Fig. 1). This increased to 53.1% (n = 17) when the original CRP assessment was between ≥ 6 and ≤ 7.9 mg/L. Similarly, 7.0% (n = 15) of CRP assessments ≥ 15 mg/L tested normal after 4 weeks, which increased to 28.3% (n = 13) when the initial CRP test was between > 7.9 and ≤ 10 mg/L. If assessments were repeated 12 weeks later, 62.5% (n = 10) of CRP tests between ≥ 6 and ≤ 7.9 mg/L would be followed by an elevated CRP. For patients with a CRP level between > 7.9 and ≤ 10 mg/L, the likelihood of having normal CRP levels increased to 34.3% (n = 12) after 12 weeks.

Discussion

The results of this study showed that, despite the patient-reported improvements in disease activity in patients treated with placebo [18], CRP levels (as an indicator of inflammation) were not affected. However, fluctuation in CRP levels at the patient level were common: 50% of patients who exhibited normal CRP levels at baseline exhibited at least one elevated CRP result within the following 16 weeks, and 31% changed from elevated to normal CRP levels. In

Table 1 Likelihood of finding elevated C-reactive protein (CRP) tests to week 16 after initial tests at baseline

Proportion of subsequent CRP tests elevated	Baseline CRP test normal (n = 26)	Baseline CRP test elevated (n = 80)
0%	13 (50%)	0 (0%)
> 0–20%	1 (4%)	1 (1%)
> 20–40%	4 (15%)	3 (4%)
> 40–60%	4 (15%)	11 (14%)
> 60–80%	1 (4%)	6 (8%)
> 80–100%	2 (8%)	4 (5%)
100%	1 (4%)	55 (69%)

Data included are from weeks 0, 1, 2, 4, 8, 12, and 16. Elevated CRP was defined as CRP > upper limit of normal (7.9 mg/L) and values ≤ 7.9 mg/L were considered normal

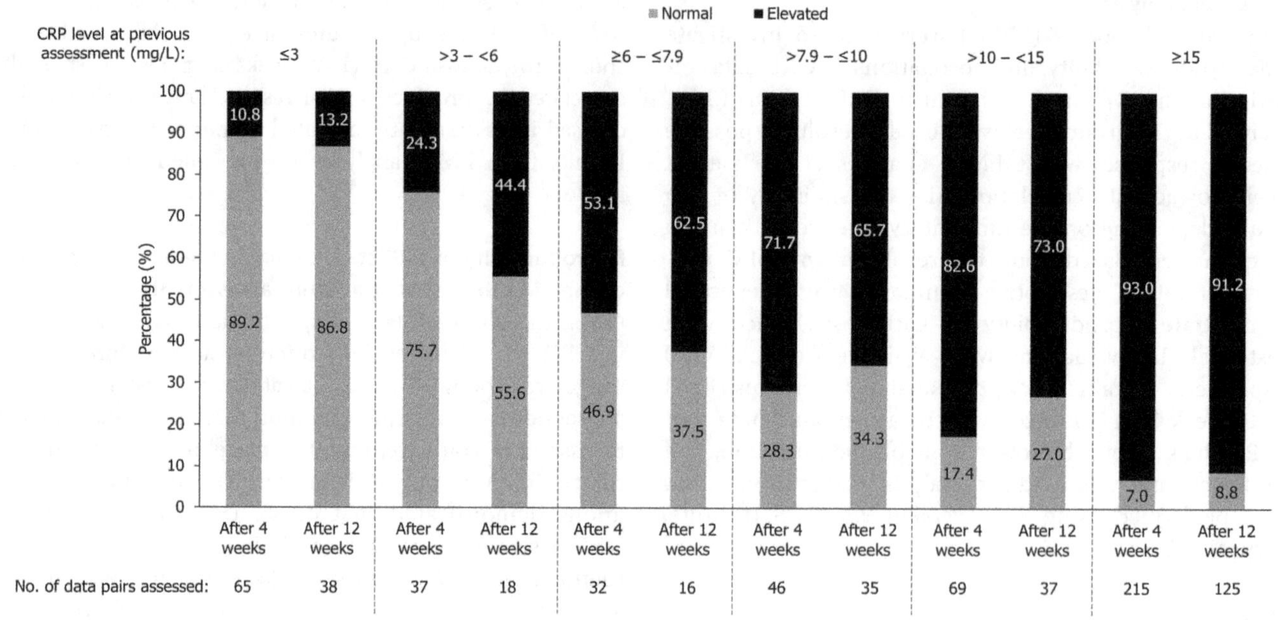

Fig. 1 Percentage of C-reactive protein (CRP) tests subsequently elevated or normal by previous CRP level.
Based on all available within-patient pairs of CRP assessment 4 or 12 weeks apart. Data included are from weeks 0, 4, 8, 12, 16, 20, and 24. Elevated CRP was defined as CRP > ULN (7.9 mg/L) and values ≤ 7.9 mg/L were considered normal

addition, further model-based and descriptive analyses demonstrated that patients with low CRP values at their first evaluation had a realistic chance of exhibiting elevated CRP upon re-evaluation. These results are in agreement with those from the ABILITY-1 study [21], in which 24.6% (14/57) of placebo-treated patients with normal CRP levels at baseline developed elevated CRP levels after 12 weeks, suggesting that a change in a patient's CRP status is more common than previously thought.

Alongside clinical parameters, assessing the likelihood of fluctuation in CRP levels could help inform treatment decisions for nr-axSpA patients. This would be particularly important for those with sacroiliitis on MRI and normal CRP, but high disease activity, suggesting a potential benefit from anti-TNF therapy. Introducing a further CRP test at least 4 weeks after the initial test (due to more short-term test results being highly auto-correlated) could assist with the more accurate categorisation of patient CRP profiles. Furthermore, the likelihood of demonstrating elevated CRP at a later time point is higher in patients with CRP levels just below the ULN.

After 4 weeks, auto-correlation continued to decrease to week 12. Subsequently, an additional assessment after 4 or 12 weeks could theoretically be acceptable, although recommendations should not be made based on these correlation data alone. It may be appropriate to distinguish between these two time points using practical considerations; an assessment at week 4 could be used in cases where rapid initiation of biological therapy is required, whereas week 12 may be more suitable if this time point coincides with a patient's next clinical assessment.

One of the limitations of these post-hoc analyses was that the sample size of the patient population used was relatively small; therefore, the interpretation of these results should be treated with caution. A further limitation was that all patients enrolled in the trial were required to have elevated CRP levels or active inflammation on MRI at screening; patients with elevated CRP at screening would be more likely to have elevated CRP at a later time point. Additionally, a relatively high threshold of ULN (> 7.9 mg/L) was used; different levels of variation may be seen at a lower threshold. Furthermore, the hypothesis that patients with clinically active disease but normal CRP levels at baseline should be re-tested is only relevant for those patients who do not have active inflammation on MRI at baseline. However, all patients in RAPID-axSpA with normal CRP values had demonstrated sacroiliitis on MRI at baseline; therefore, it is unclear whether CRP values in patients with active nr-axSpA who do not show active inflammation on MRI behave in a same manner. To make an evidence-based recommendation regarding the re-testing of CRP levels, it is recommended that additional data are collected to explore whether a patient with clinically active nr-axSpA (without sacroiliitis on MRI) with normal CRP at baseline and elevated CRP levels at a later time point is likely to respond to anti-TNF therapy.

Conclusions

For nr-axSpA patients with no signs of inflammation on MRI and normal CRP levels, in addition to a high disease activity indicative of a potential benefit from anti-TNF treatment, the CRP test should be repeated after at least 4 weeks. There is a substantial chance of finding elevated CRP levels upon subsequent testing, thus making the patient eligible for treatment options such as anti-TNF therapies.

Key messages

- Non-radiographic axSpA patients must exhibit inflammation (via MRI/CRP) to access anti-TNF treatment.
- Non-radiographic axSpA patients with normal CRP levels have a substantial chance of demonstrating elevated CRP at subsequent re-test.
- In non-radiographic axSpA patients, the CRP test should be repeated after at least 4 weeks.

Abbreviations

AS: Ankylosing spondylitis; ASAS: Assessment of SpondyloArthritis international Society; axSpA: Axial spondyloarthritis; BASDAI: Bath Ankylosing Spondylitis Disease Activity Index; CRP: C-reactive protein; CZP: Certolizumab pegol; FDA: Food and Drug Administration; LLQ: Lower limit of quantification; LMM: Linear mixed models; MRI: Magnetic resonance imaging; nr: Non-radiographic; NSAID: Non-steroidal anti-inflammatory drug; Q2W: Every 2 weeks; Q4W: Every 4 weeks; TNF: Tumour necrosis factor; ULN: Upper limit of normal

Acknowledgements

The authors thank the patients, the investigators, and their teams who took part in this study. The authors also acknowledge Alvaro Arjona, PhD, from UCB Pharma, Brussels, Belgium, for publication coordination, and Eleanor Thurtle, MChem, from Costello Medical, Cambridge, UK, for medical writing and editorial assistance in preparing this manuscript for publication, based on the authors' input and direction.

Funding

UCB Pharma sponsored the study and the development of the manuscript/ publication and reviewed the text to ensure that, from a UCB Pharma perspective, the data presented in the publication are scientifically, technically, and medically supportable, that they do not contain any information that has the potential to damage the intellectual property of UCB Pharma, and that the publication complies with applicable laws, regulations, guidelines, and good industry practice.

Authors' contributions

Substantial contributions to study conception/design, or acquisition/analysis/ interpretation of data: RL, TN, OD, and DB; drafting of the publication, or revising it critically for important intellectual content: RL, TN, OD, and DB; final approval of the publication: RL, TN, OD, and DB.

Ethics approval and consent to participate

The study protocol, amendments, and subject informed consent were reviewed by a national, regional, or Independent Ethics Committee (IEC) or Institutional Review Board (IRB). This study was conducted in accordance with the current version of the applicable regulatory and International Conference on Harmonisation (ICH)-Good Clinical Practice (GCP) requirements, the ethical principles that have their origin in the principles of the Declaration of Helsinki, and the local laws of the countries involved. Informed consent was obtained from subjects and documented in accordance with local regulations, ICH-GCP requirements, and the ethical principles that have their origin in the principles of the Declaration of Helsinki.

Competing interests

RL has received consultancy fees and/or research grants and/or speaker's bureau from AbbVie, Ablynx, Amgen, AstraZeneca, Bristol-Myers Squibb, Centocor, GlaxoSmithKline, Novartis, Merck, Pfizer, Roche, Schering-Plough, and UCB Pharma. TN is an employee of UCB Pharma. OD is an employee and stockholder of UCB Pharma. DB has acted as an advisor and/or provided research collaboration for AbbVie, Bristol-Myers Squibb, Boehringer Ingelheim, Eli Lilly, Janssen, MSD, Novartis, Pfizer, Roche, and UCB Pharma, and is an employee of UCB Pharma.

Author details

[1]Clinical Immunology and Rheumatology, Amsterdam Rheumatology & Immunology Center and Academic Medical Center, University of Amsterdam, Amsterdam, Netherlands. [2]UCB Pharma, Monheim, Germany. [3]UCB Pharma, Slough, UK. [4]UCB Pharma, Brussels, Belgium.

References

1. Rudwaleit M, Landewé R, van der Heijde D, et al. The development of assessment of SpondyloArthritis International Society classification criteria for axial spondyloarthritis (part I): classification of paper patients by expert opinion including uncertainty appraisal. Ann Rheum Dis. 2009;68(6):770–6.
2. Sieper J, van der Heijde D, Elewaut D et al. Disease burden is comparable in patients with non-radiographic axial spondyloarthritis and ankylosing spondylitis [abstract]. American College of Rheumatology 2012. November 9–14; Washington, DC. Abstract no. 1361.
3. Baraliakos X, Braun J. Non-radiographic axial spondyloarthritis and ankylosing spondylitis: what are the similarities and differences? RMD Open. 2015;1(Suppl 1):e000053.
4. Sieper J. SP0108 Different approaches to drug approval by EMA and FDA—the example of non-radiographic axial spondyloarthritis. Ann Rheum Dis. 2016;75(Suppl 2):27.
5. U.S. Food and Drug Administration. Center for Drug Evaluation and Research. Cimzia (2008). https://www.accessdata.fda.gov/drugsatfda_docs/label/2017/125160s270lbl.pdf. Accessed 19 June 2017.
6. U.S. Food and Drug Administration. Center for Drug Evaluation and Research. Simponi (2009). https://www.accessdata.fda.gov/drugsatfda_docs/label/2011/125289s0064lbl.pdf. Accessed 19 June 2017.
7. U.S. Food and Drug Administration. Center for Drug Evaluation and Research. Enbrel (2003). https://www.accessdata.fda.gov/drugsatfda_docs/nda/2003/103795_S5097_ENBREL.pdf. Accessed 19 June 2017.
8. U.S. Food and Drug Administration. Center for Drug Evaluation and Research. Remicade (2004). https://www.accessdata.fda.gov/drugsatfda_docs/label/2015/103772s5370lbl.pdf. Accessed 19 June 2017.
9. Corbett M, Jhuti G, Rice S, et al. Tumour necrosis factor-α inhibitors for ankylosing spondylitis and non-radiographic axial spondyloarthritis: a systematic review and economic evaluation. Health Technol Assess. 2016; 20(9):1–334.
10. European Medicine's Agency. Positive recommendations of Committee for Medicinal Products for Human Use (CHMP) on extensions of therapeutic indications for Humira (21 June 2012). http://www.emea.europa.eu/ema/pages/includes/document/open_document.jsp?webContentId=WC500129074. Accessed 13 June 2017.
11. European Medicine's Agency. Positive recommendations of Committee for Medicinal Products for Human Use (CHMP) on extensions of therapeutic

indications for Enbrel (26 June 2014). http://www.ema.europa.eu/docs/en_GB/document_library/EPAR_-_Assessment_Report_-_Variation/human/000262/WC500172150.pdf. Accessed 13 June 2017.
12. European Medicine's Agency. Summary of Product Characteristics for Cimzia (16 May 2014). http://www.ema.europa.eu/docs/en_GB/document_library/EPAR_-_Product_Information/human/001037/WC500069763.pdf. Accessed 13 June 2017.
13. Toussirot E, Vauchy C, Binda D, Michel F. Golimumab in radiographic and nonradiographic axial spondyloarthritis: a review of clinical trials. Drug Des Devel Ther. 2016;10:2087–94.
14. Sieper J, van der Heijde D, Dougados M, et al. Efficacy and safety of adalimumab in patients with non-radiographic axial spondyloarthritis: results of a randomised placebo-controlled trial (ABILITY-1). Ann Rheum Dis. 2013;72(6):815–22.
15. Ward MM, Deodhar A, Akl EA, et al. American College of Rheumatology/Spondylitis Association of America/Spondyloarthritis research and treatment network 2015 recommendations for the treatment of ankylosing spondylitis and nonradiographic axial spondyloarthritis. Arthritis Rheumatol. 2016;68(2):282–98.
16. National Institute for Health and Care Excellence. TNF-alpha inhibitors for ankylosing spondylitis and non-radiographic axial spondyloarthritis (TA383). https://www.nice.org.uk/guidance/ta383. Accessed 6 Mar 2018.
17. Poddubnyy D, Haibel H, Braun J, Rudwaleit M, Sieper J. Brief report: clinical course over two years in patients with early nonradiographic axial spondyloarthritis and patients with ankylosing spondylitis not treated with tumor necrosis factor blockers: results from the German spondyloarthritis inception cohort. Arthritis Rheumatol. 2015;67(9):2369–75.
18. Landewé R, Braun J, Deodhar A, et al. Efficacy of certolizumab pegol on signs and symptoms of axial spondyloarthritis including ankylosing spondylitis: 24-week results of a double-blind randomised placebo-controlled phase 3 study. Ann Rheum Dis. 2014;73(1):39–47.
19. van der Heijde D, Dougados M, Landewé R, et al. Sustained efficacy, safety and patient-reported outcomes of certolizumab pegol in axial spondyloarthritis: 4-year outcomes from RAPID-axSpA. Rheumatology (Oxford). 2017:kex174. https://doi.org/10.1093/rheumatology/kex174.
20. Verbeke G, Molenberghs G. Linear mixed models for longitudinal data. New York: Springer-Verlag; 2000.
21. Baraliakos X, Sieper J, Chen S, Pangan AL, Anderson J. Non-radiographic axial spondyloarthritis patients without initial evidence of inflammation may develop objective inflammation over time. Rheumatology (Oxford). 2017:kex081. https://doi.org/10.1093/rheumatology/kex081.

16

Estrogen attenuates the spondyloarthritis manifestations of the SKG arthritis model

Hyemin Jeong[1], Eun-Kyung Bae[2], Hunnyun Kim[2], Yeong Hee Eun[3], In Young Kim[3], Hyungjin Kim[3], Jaejoon Lee[3], Chan Hong Jeon[1], Eun-Mi Koh[3] and Hoon-Suk Cha[3*]

Abstract

Background: Ankylosing spondylitis (AS) is a male-predominant disease, and radiographic evidence of damage is also more severe in males. Estrogen modulates immune-related processes such as T cell differentiation and cytokine production. This study aimed to evaluate the effect of estrogen on the disease activity of spondyloarthritis (SpA).

Methods: The effects of estrogen on the development of arthritis were evaluated by performing ovariectomy and 17β-estradiol (E2) pellet implantation in zymosan-treated SKG mice. Clinical arthritis scores were measured, and ^{18}F-fluorodeoxyglucose (^{18}F-FDG) small-animal positron emission tomography/computed tomography performed to quantify joint inflammation. The expression of inflammatory cytokines in joint tissue was measured.

Results: E2-treated mice showed remarkable suppression of arthritis clinically and little infiltration of inflammatory cells in the Achilles tendon and intervertebral disc. ^{18}F-FDG uptake was significantly lower in E2-treated mice than in sham-operated (sham) and ovariectomized mice. Expression of TNF, interferon-γ, and IL-17A was significantly reduced in E2-treated mice, whereas expression of sclerostin and Dickkopf-1 was increased in E2-treated mice compared with sham and ovariectomized mice.

Conclusions: Estrogen suppressed arthritis development in SKG mice, a model of SpA. Results of this study suggest that estrogen has an anti-inflammatory effect on the spondyloarthritis manifestations of the SKG arthritis model.

Keywords: Estrogen, Spondyloarthritis, Mice

Background

Ankylosing spondylitis (AS) is a chronic inflammatory disease that primarily affects the sacroiliac joints and spine. Syndesmophytes and ankylosis occur as a consequence of longstanding inflammation, resulting in loss of function and disability. AS is a male-predominant disease and men with this disease also tend to have radiographic evidence of more severe damage [1]. Diagnosing this disease at an early stage is challenging; the classification criteria for axial spondyloarthritis (SpA) were developed by the Assessment of SpondyloArthritis international Society (ASAS) [2] and the ASAS criteria therefore cover both patients with or without established radiographic changes in the sacroiliac joint. The clinical presentation, clinical disease activity, and treatment responses of both groups are similar [3, 4]. However, patients with non-radiographic axial spondyloarthritis (nr-axSpA) have lower C-reactive protein (CRP) [5, 6] and less active inflammation on magnetic resonance imaging (MRI) than patients with AS [6]. Interestingly, the male-to-female ratio of nr-axSpA has been reported to be approximately 1:1, whereas it is 2:1 in patients with AS [5–7]. The proportion of female patients was significantly lower among the group of patients who progressed from nr-axSpA to AS [8]. The female predominance of patients with nr-axSpA can be understood in the same context, as male patients with AS have more severe radiographic damage than female patients with AS [1, 9]. The underlying pathogenesis of the differences between men and women with AS is still unknown.

Jimenez-Balderas et al. reported that 17β-estradiol (E2) levels are lower in patients with active AS than in those with inactive AS. Peripheral arthritis was shown to

* Correspondence: hoonsuk.cha@samsung.com
[3]Division of Rheumatology, Department of Internal Medicine, Samsung Medical Center, Sungkyunkwan University School of Medicine, 81 Irwon-Ro, Gangnam-gu, Seoul 06351, South Korea
Full list of author information is available at the end of the article

subside and the clinical activity of AS was reduced after oral estrogen therapy [10]. Estrogen modulates immune-related processes, such as T cell differentiation and cytokine production [11]. Estrogen is involved in the immune response, characterized by a bias toward type 2 cytokine profiles [12]. Animal model studies have suggested that estrogen can inhibit the differentiation of T helper (Th)17 cells from naïve T cells [13, 14].

Wnt proteins play an important role in the anabolic pattern of joint remodeling in AS. Dickkopf-related protein 1 (Dkk1) is an inhibitor of the Wnt pathway and acts as a master regulator of joint remodeling [15]. Increased Dkk1 is related to bone resorption, whereas decreased Dkk1 is linked to new bone formation [16]. To the best of our knowledge, there are no data about the relationship between estrogen and Wnt inhibitors in patients with AS.

Sakaguchi et al. characterized the SKG mouse strain, which develops spontaneous autoimmune inflammatory arthritis after systemic ß-glucan exposure [17]. Although the SKG mouse model was first used as a rheumatoid arthritis (RA) model, Ruutu et al. reported that SKG mice have clinical characteristics of SpA, including spondylitis, enthesitis, and bowel inflammation [18]. The role of estrogen in the pathogenesis and disease activity of SpA has not been determined. We hypothesized that estrogen has an anti-inflammatory effect on the disease activity of SpA. Therefore, the aim of this study was to investigate the role of estrogen in the disease activity of SpA using the SKG mouse model. We evaluated the effect of estrogen on the development and progression of SpA and investigated the relationship between estrogen and inflammatory cytokines.

Methods

Experimental animals

SKG mice purchased from CLEA Japan were housed in a specific-pathogen-free facility under climate-controlled conditions with a 12-h light/dark cycle and were provided with water and standard diet *ad libitum*. All animal experiments were performed according to the guidelines issued by the Institutional Animal Care and Use Committee in accordance with National Institute of Health (NIH) guidelines. Animals were treated according to the guidelines and regulations of the Laboratory Animal Research Center at Sungkyunkwan University School of Medicine.

Ovariectomy and estrogen pellet insertion

Experiments were performed in three groups: sham-operated (sham (ovary intact)), ovariectomized and ovariectomized + E2. Seven-week-old female SKG mice underwent an ovariectomy (OVx) or a sham operation under anesthesia 2 weeks before arthritis induction. At 8 weeks of age, slow-releasing pellets of E2 (0.72 mg, 60 days release, Innovative Research, Sarasota, FL, USA) were implanted subcutaneously on the neck scruff of mice in the E2-treated group [19]. For these mice, a 0.5-cm incision was made in the loose skin of each mouse's neck, and a small pocket was bluntly dissected caudolaterally. The pellet was installed in the pocket using tweezers. The incision was subsequently closed with a suture.

Induction of arthritis and scoring of clinical signs

Arthritis was induced 2 weeks after ovariectomy or 1 week after E2 pellet implantation. Zymosan A (Sigma, St Louis, MO, USA) was suspended in PBS and incubated for 10 min in boiling water. Then the zymosan A solution was injected intraperitoneally into 9-week-old mice in each of the three groups (3 mg/mouse): sham (ovary intact), ovariectomized and ovariectomized + E2 groups. ^{18}F-fluorodeoxyglucose (^{18}F-FDG) small-animal positron emission tomography (PET)/computed tomography (CT) and cytokine analysis were also compared with the wild-type control group. Clinical scores were monitored following a previously published system [17]: 0, no swelling or redness; 0.1, swelling or redness of the digits; 0.5, mild swelling and/or redness of the wrists or ankle joints; and 1, severe swelling of the larger joints. Scores for the affected joints were totaled for each mouse. The maximum possible score was 6. We defined tail changes as "present" when a mouse developed redness, swelling, hair loss, or bumps along the tail. The presence of periocular changes surrounding the eyeball (blepharitis) was also assessed. Clinical scores were monitored weekly, and mice were sacrificed 8 weeks after zymosan injection.

Measurement of serum estrogen

Serum levels of E2 were measured using a Mouse/Rat Estradiol enzyme-linked immunosorbent assay (ELISA) kit (Calbiotech, CA, USA) according to the manufacturer`s instructions.

^{18}F-FDG PET/CT acquisition and image analysis

Mice were fasted for 5 h before micro-PET/CT studies. A 1.8-MBq injection of ^{18}F-FDG mixed with isotonic saline in a total volume of 150 μL was administered through a tail vein. Imaging was performed 1 h later under isoflurane anesthesia without respiratory gating. Micro-PET images of mice were acquired using an Inveon micro-PET/CT scanner (Siemens Medical Solutions, Malvern, PA, USA) at the Center for Molecular and Cellular Imaging, Samsung Biomedical Research Institute (Seoul, Korea). Acquisition of non-enhanced CT images was followed by PET imaging. Micro-PET images obtained were reconstructed using 3D-ordered subset expectation maximization and then processed using Siemens Inveon Research Workplace 4.1. Three-dimensional regions of interest (ROIs) were drawn over the joints using a threshold range of 70–100% of the maximum intensity, and the average signal level in the ROIs was measured. In the case of the intestine, the ROIs were measured in the abdomen excluding the kidneys and bladder, and percentage injected dose per gram (%ID/g) was measured at a threshold value of 70–100%. Image counts/pixel/s were converted to radioactivity concentrations that were then corrected for injected radioactivity. Researchers were blinded to all clinical data, and ROIs were measured by a technician. Results are expressed as the mean ± SD %ID/g.

Histopathological examination

Mice were anesthetized and euthanized after 8 weeks of zymosan injection. Mouse joint tissues were fixed in 10% formalin, decalcified in ethylenediamine tetraacetic acid (EDTA), and embedded in paraffin. Sections were deparaffinized using xylene, dehydrated in a graded series of alcohol solutions, and stained with hematoxylin and eosin (H&E). Histologic features of the mouse joints were scored as described previously [18]: 1–4, where 1 = few infiltrating immune cells, 2 = 1–2 small patches of inflammation, 3 = inflammation throughout the joint, and 4 = inflammation in soft tissue/entheses/fasciitis. Histologic features of the tail were scored on a scale of 1–4, where 1 = few infiltrating immune cells, 2 = mild inflammation of the discs or along the vertebrae (0–30% of discs), 3 = inflammation of the discs and/or along the vertebrae (30–70% of discs), and 4 = inflammation in > 70% of the discs and along the vertebrae. Microscopic gut inflammation was assessed. Intestines were scored 1 for the presence and 0 for the absence of ileitis or colitis.

RNA isolation and QuantiGene 2.0 Plex assay

Total RNA was extracted from the hind paws and forepaws using a total RNA kit (QuantiGene sample processing kit) according to the manufacturer's protocol. Target hybridization and signal amplification were performed according to the manufacturer's protocol for fresh tissues (QuantiGene 2.0 Plex assay). Signal was detected using a Luminex 100/200 system and reported as median fluorescence intensity (MFI), which is proportional to the number of target RNA molecules present in the sample. Gene expression was first calculated by determining the average signal (MFI) for all genes, and average background signals were subtracted for each gene. Levels of gene expression were then determined by dividing each test gene signal (background subtracted) by the normalization gene signal (background subtracted). Next, fold changes were determined by dividing the normalized value for zymosan-treated samples by the normalized values for the healthy controls. Each sample was assayed using technical duplicates. Target genes were tumor necrosis factor (TNF), IL-6, interferon-γ (IFNγ), IL-4, IL-17A, IL-23, Dkk1, and sclerostin (SOST).

Statistical analyses

One-way analysis of variance (ANOVA) was used to compare normally distributed means. Two-way ANOVA was used to analyze treatment effects on clinical scores over time. Tukey's post hoc test was performed to compare multiple means. Results are presented as mean ± standard error of the mean (SEM). All analyses were performed using SPSS software, version 19.0 (SPSS, Inc., Chicago, IL, USA) and GraphPad Prism (version 5.0, GraphPad Software, San Diego, CA, USA).

Results

Estrogen treatment suppressed arthritis development in SKG mice

The effect of estrogen on arthritis development in female SKG mice was examined. Weekly observations revealed that clinical scores were markedly suppressed in E2-treated mice compared with the sham and ovariectomized groups (Fig. 1a). The onset of arthritis was similar among groups until 24 days after zymosan injection. From 31 days after zymosan injection, arthritis was more aggravated and clinical scores had increased up to 6 points (maximal score) in the sham and ovariectomized groups. However, clinical scores had not increased after 31 days in the E2-treated mice. Clinical scores were significantly lower in E2-treated mice than those in the other two groups from 31 days after zymosan injection until the last observation. The incidence of arthritis was lower in the E2-treated group (Fig. 1b). The incidence of tail changes (Fig. 1c) was higher in the sham and ovariectomized groups than in the E2-treated group. Body weight was significantly higher in the E2-treated group than in the other two groups (Fig. 1d). Mice in the sham and ovariectomized groups achieved a near 100% incidence of blepharitis at an early stage after zymosan injection (Fig. 1e). Mean serum E2 in E2-treated mice was significantly higher than in the other groups (Fig. 1f). There were no significant differences in serum E2 between the sham and ovariectomized groups.

E2 treatment reduced ^{18}F-FDG uptake using micro-PET/CT imaging

Figure 2a shows ^{18}F-FDG uptake in mice spines using micro-PET/CT imaging. The zymosan-treated group had higher ^{18}F-FDG uptake and loss of lordosis than the normal wild-type control group. Quantification of the ROIs of the control, sham, ovariectomy, and

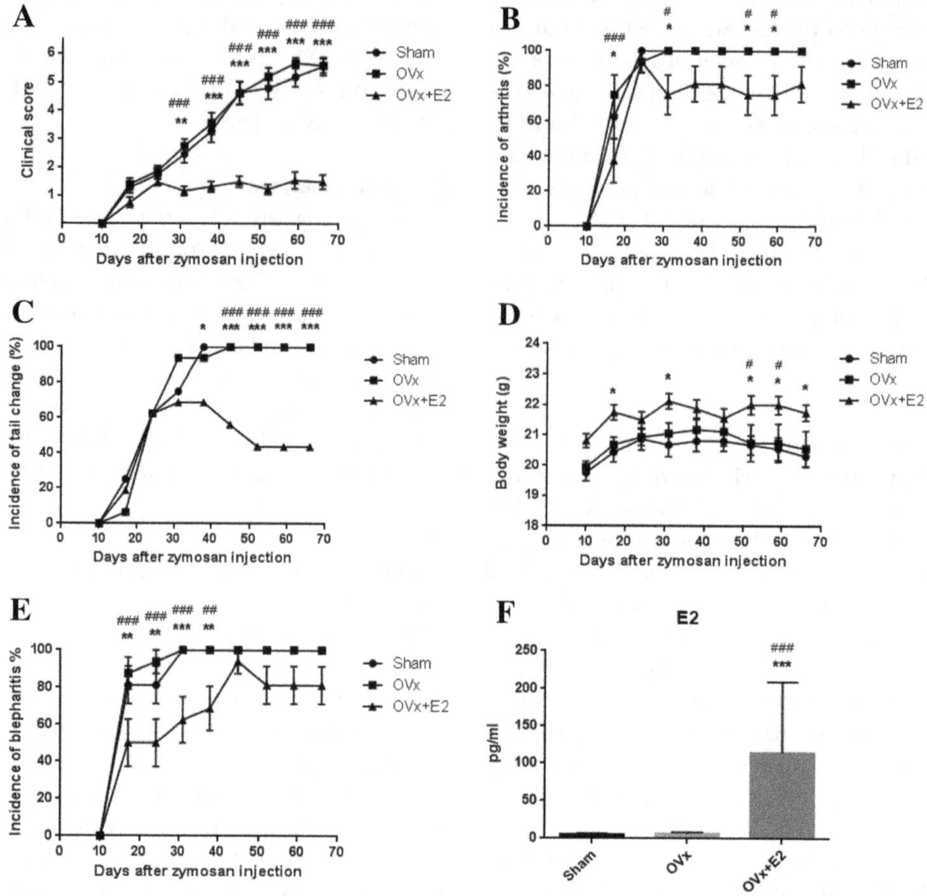

Fig. 1 17β-estradiol (E2) treatment suppressed arthritis development in SKG mice. Clinical scores were markedly suppressed in E2-treated mice compared with mice in the sham-operated (Sham) and ovariectomized (OVx) groups after 31 days of zymosan injection. Clinical scores (**a**), the incidence of arthritis (**b**), the incidence of tail changes (**c**), body weight (**d**), and the incidence of blepharitis (**e**) in the three groups. Serum levels of E2 were measured by ELISA (**f**). Values are mean ± SEM (n = 16 mice per group); $^{*}P < 0.05$, $^{**}P < 0.01$, $^{***}P < 0.001$ (sham vs. OVx + E2); $^{\#}P < 0.05$; $^{\#\#}P < 0.01$; $^{\#\#\#}P < 0.001$ (OVx vs. OVx + E2)

ovariectomy + E2 groups showed that the amount of ^{18}F-FDG uptake was significantly higher in the sham, ovariectomized, and E2-treated groups than in wild-type controls. The E2-treated group had significantly lower ^{18}F-FDG uptake than the sham and ovariectomized groups in both forepaws (Fig. 2b) and hind paws (Fig. 2c). There were no significant differences in the hip joints (Fig. 2d), sacroiliac joints (Fig. 2e), or tail (Fig. 2f) among the sham, ovariectomized, and E2-treated groups. In a total of five joint ROIs, ^{18}F-FDG uptake was significantly lower in the E2-treated group than in the sham and ovariectomized groups (Fig. 2g). ^{18}F-FDG uptake was not significantly different between the sham and ovariectomized groups. In addition, ^{18}F-FDG uptake in the intestine was significantly higher in the ovariectomized and E2-treated groups than the wild-type control group (Fig. 2h). There was no difference between the sham, ovariectomized, and E2-treated groups.

Histologic scores for arthritis and spondylitis were lower in E2-treated mice

Histologic analysis of the mice at 8 weeks after zymosan injection was performed. Inflammation of the ankles, Achilles tendons, plantar fascia, and area around the intervertebral discs was observed. As an extra-articular manifestation, infiltration of inflammatory cells was also seen in the skin of the ears, periorbital soft tissues, and intestines. Figure 3 shows the histologic features of spondylitis and Achilles tendinitis. Inflammation of the intervertebral discs in the tail was prominent in the sham (Fig. 3b) and ovariectomized mice (Fig. 3c). E2-treated mice (Fig. 3d) had a few inflammatory cell infiltrations compared to the wild-type controls (Fig. 3a), but the degree of inflammation was milder than in the sham and ovariectomized mice. The Achilles tendons of both the sham (Fig. 3f) and ovariectomized groups (Fig. 3g) were severely inflamed. E2-treated mice (Fig. 3h) had

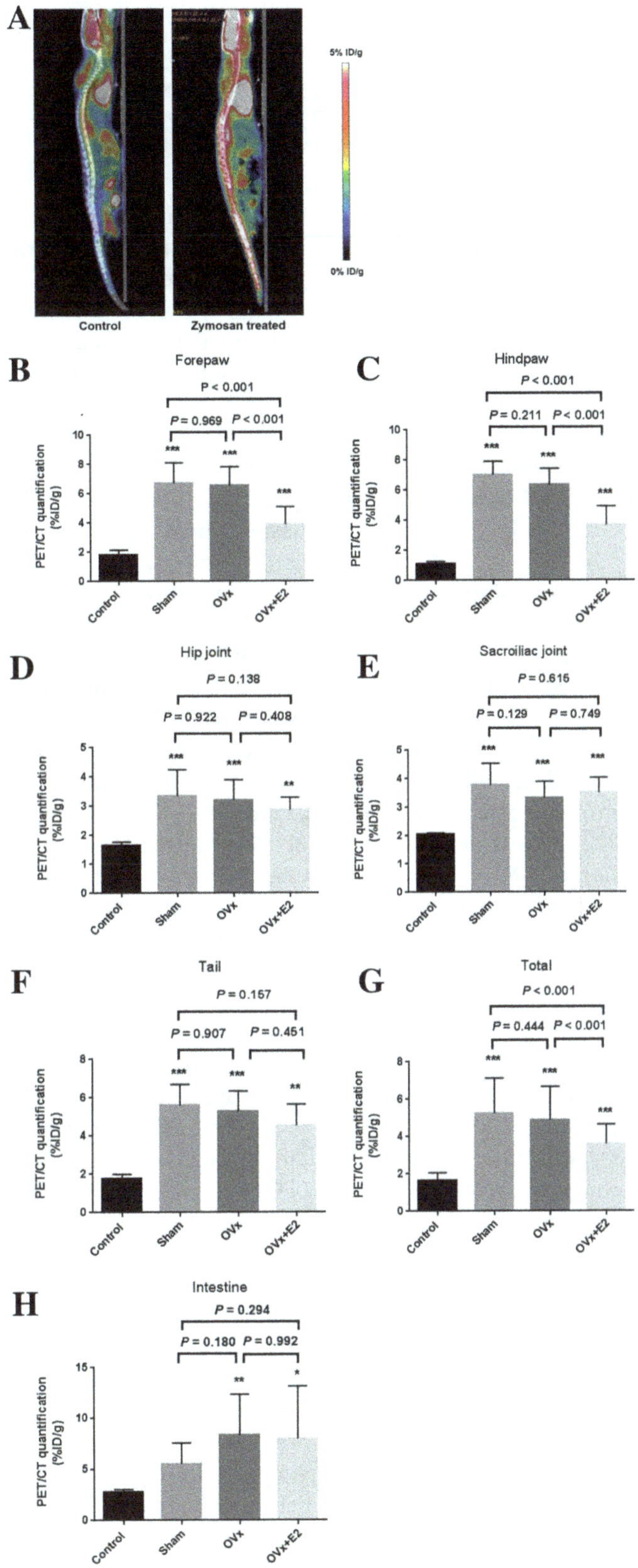

Fig. 2 (See legend on next page.)

(See figure on previous page.)

Fig. 2 Quantitative measurement of ^{18}F-fluorodeoxyglucose (^{18}F-FDG) uptake. Visualization of ^{18}F-FDG uptake in the spine of a wild-type (control) mouse and a mouse 8 weeks after zymosan injection (zymosan-treated) (**a**). Quantification of regions of interest (ROIs) in control, sham-operated (Sham), ovariectomy (OVx), and OVx + 17β-estradiol (OVx + E2) groups. **b-g** Forepaw (**b**), hind paw (**c**), hip joint (**d**), sacroiliac joint (**e**), tail (**f**), total of ROIs of five joints (**g**), and intestine (**h**). Values are mean ± SEM, n = 12 mice per group except for the wild-type control group ($n = 2$); $^{*}P < 0.05$, $^{**}P < 0.01$, $^{***}P < 0.001$ versus controls. PET/CT positron emission tomography/computed tomography

inflammation compared to the wild-type controls (Fig. 3e), but the degree of inflammation was mild compared with the other two groups. Histologic scores for peripheral arthritis (Fig. 3i) and spondylitis (Fig. 3j) were significantly lower in E2-treated mice than in mice in the other groups. Most of the mice in the sham and ovariectomized groups had very severe inflammation. There was no difference between the groups in the presence of enteritis (Fig. 3k). About 70% of mice in the sham, ovariectomized, and E2-treated groups had inflammation of the gut.

Expression of TNFα, IFN-γ, and IL-17A was significantly reduced in E2-treated mice

Local gene expression in the tissues of the hind paws and forepaws, which were harvested at 8 weeks after zymosan injection, was analyzed using the QuantiGene 2.0 Plex assay (Fig. 4). Expression of TNF, IL-6, IL-17A, and IFN-γ was significantly increased in both the sham and ovariectomized groups compared with the wild-type control group. Interestingly, E2 treatment significantly reduced the gene expression of TNF, IL-6, IFN-γ, and IL-17A compared with expression of these genes in the sham and ovariectomized groups (Figs. 4a-c and f). Expression of IL-4 was significantly higher in the E2-treated group than in the ovariectomized group (Fig. 4d). Expression of IL-23 was not significantly different among groups (Fig. 4e). Wnt inhibitors, Dkk1 and SOST, were significantly downregulated in both the sham and ovariectomized groups (Figs. 4g and h). The E2-treated group had significantly increased expression of Dkk1 and SOST compared with the sham and ovariectomized groups.

Discussion

We investigated the role of estrogen in the disease activity of SpA. We found that estrogen suppressed the development of arthritis in SpA, using an animal model. The E2-treated group had significantly suppressed arthritis compared with both the ovariectomized and the sham groups. There was no difference between the ovariectomized and sham groups. We found that arthritis was induced in almost all female mice with normal ovaries, and the clinical score was almost 6 (the maximum score). We could not assess the difference between mice in the ovariectomized group and mice that received a physiologic dose of estrogen (the sham group) because female mice with normal ovaries (the sham group) already had zymosan-induced severe arthritis. A high dose of E2 pellets was used (72 mg, 60 days release), which was higher than the physiologic concentration [19]. The different responses between the E2-treated group and the sham group were likely due to the different estrogen doses received by these two groups.

The current study demonstrated that E2-treated mice had decreased expression of TNF in the joint tissue. These results support the hypothesis that estrogen inhibits the production of TNF [20]. E2 has been shown to downregulate TNF production and reduce the severity of experimental autoimmune encephalomyelitis in cytokine knockout mice [21]. Estrogen-deficient female rats are also reported to have higher bioactive serum TNF than estrogen-supplemented animals [22]. An in vitro study showed that E2 treatment downregulates cytokine-induced TNF gene expression [23]. Considering that TNF is a key cytokine in the pathogenesis of SpA, the results of the current study indicate that transcription of TNF might be regulated by estrogen in patients with SpA.

The current study demonstrated that E2 treatment significantly reduced the gene expression of IFN-γ, whereas the expression of IL-4 increased significantly in the joint tissues in response to E2 treatment. This corresponds well with recent data from a mouse model of autoimmune encephalomyelitis [24]. In that study, high and medium doses of estrogen increased the production of IL-4, IL-10, and transforming growth factor (TGF)-β, whereas estrogen treatment reduced the production of IFN-γ, IL-17, and IL-6. Estrogen triggers a shift in the Th1/Th2 balance toward Th2 production [25]. Thus, in Th1-mediated autoimmune diseases such as RA, symptoms often decrease during pregnancy and flare or initially develop in the postpartum period. In contrast, Th2-mediated diseases such as systemic lupus erythematosus (SLE) often flare during pregnancy [26]. Estrogen also inhibits Th17 cell production. In ovariectomized DBA/1 mice with established collagen-induced arthritis (CIA), E2 treatment reduces the severity of arthritis and results in fewer Th17 cells in the joints compared with controls [27]. Tyagi et al. reported that transcription factors that promote Th17 cell differentiation and IL-17 levels are increased in ovariectomized mice, and that these

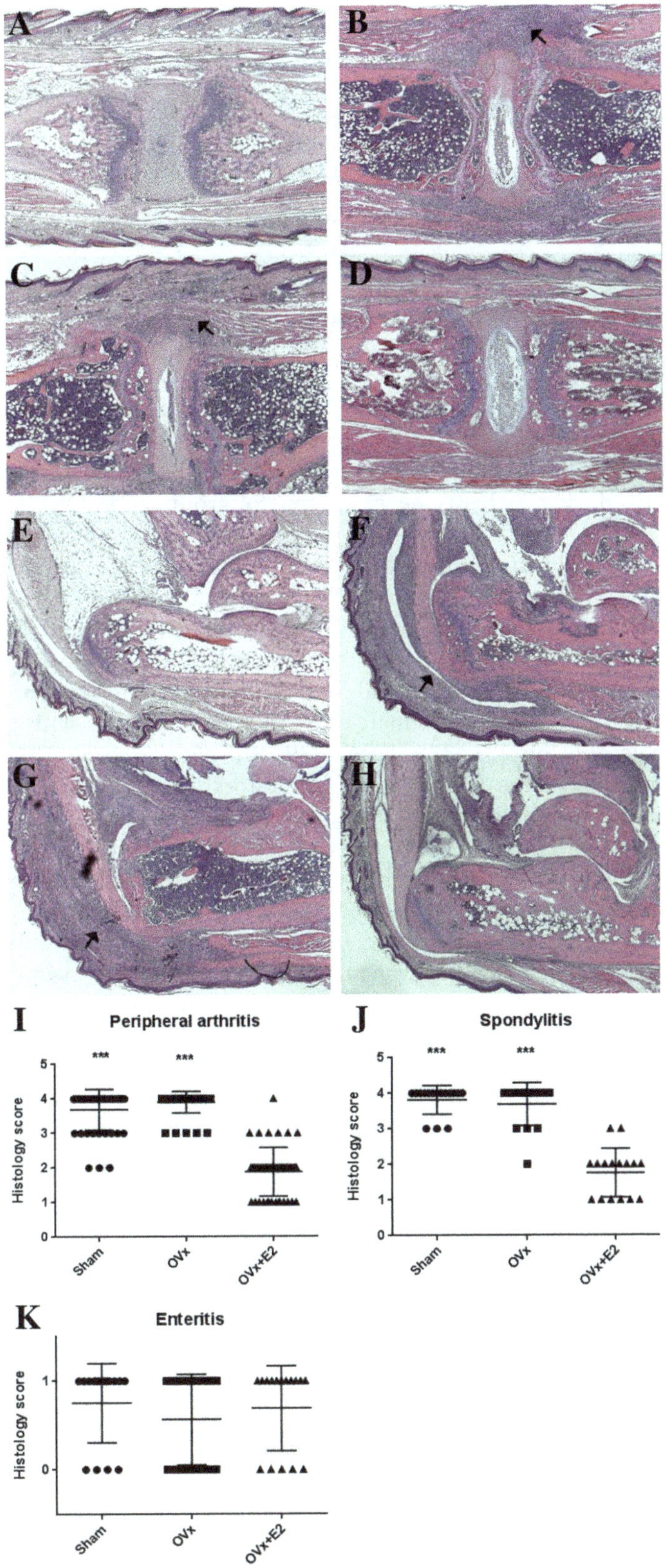

Fig. 3 (See legend on next page.)

(See figure on previous page.)

Fig. 3 The effect of estrogen on microscopic inflammation. **a-d** The intervertebral area of the wild-type control (**a**), sham-operated (Sham) (**b**), ovariectomized (OVx) (**c**), and 17β-estradiol (E2)-treated (OVx + E2) mice (**d**). Arrows in **b** and **c** indicate inflammatory cell infiltration of the intervertebral disc area. **e-f** Achilles tendon of the normal control (**e**), sham (**f**), ovariectomized (**g**), and E2-treated mice (**h**). Arrows in **f** and **g** indicate inflammatory cell infiltration in the Achilles tendon. Inflammatory cell infiltration was not evident in E2-treated mice. Staining with H&E. Original magnification × 40. Histologic severity scores for peripheral joints affected by peripheral arthritis, including the forepaws, hind paws, ankle joints (**i**), tail (**j**), and intestine (**k**). Symbols represent individual mice, horizontal lines represent the mean, and whiskers represent the SEM; $n = 16$ mice per group except for the wild-type control (n = 2); *$P < 0.05$, **$P < 0.01$, ***$P < 0.001$ versus controls

effects are reversed by E2 supplementation [13]. Another study also showed that E2 inhibits arthritis and reduces IL-17-producing γδT cells in the joints of CIA mice [28]. It is well known that the Th17 axis is overactive in patients with AS [29, 30], and the percentage of Th17 cells is significantly lower in nr-axSpA than in AS. Our data suggest that E2 modulates cells with IL-17-producing capacity during arthritis development in SpA.

The mechanism of the relationship between estrogen and T cell differentiation is unknown. In cross-sectional studies, testosterone levels have been found to be similar in patients with AS and controls, but serum dehydroepiandrosterone sulfate (DHEAS) and 17α- hydroxyprogesterone were more elevated in male patients with AS than in male controls [31–33]. The gene for the enzyme, 21-hydroxylase, is located close to the human leukocyte antigen (HLA)-B locus on the short arm of chromosome 6. HLA-B27 might serve as a marker of partial 21-hydroxylase deficiency, resulting in high DHEAS and 17α-hydroxyprogesterone levels. A proinflammatory Th1 phenotype might be enhanced by increased DHEAS, whereas estrogen and progesterone suppress the Th1 phenotype [12]. β-catenin/TCF promotes differentiation of Th2 from naïve CD4 T cells and prevents the differentiation of Th17/Th1. Estrogen might be involved in T cell differentiation via the Wnt/β-catenin pathway [34]. The relationship between estrogen and T cell differentiation in SpA has not been investigated; therefore, further study is needed to determine the role of estrogen in T cell differentiation in SpA.

In the current study, we also evaluated the role of Wnt inhibitors in the disease activity of SpA. The German Spondyloarthritis Inception Cohort (GESPIC) study reported that patients with lower Dkk1 levels were more prone to develop syndesmophytes than those with higher levels [35]. In the present study, expression of Dkk1 was decreased in zymosan-treated mice compared with controls. In addition, expression of Dkk1 was significantly increased in E2-treated mice compared with the ovariectomized and sham groups. This corresponds well with the previous finding that expression of Dkk1 and SOST was reduced in the spine of a proteoglycan-induced spondylitis (PGISp) mouse model of SpA, compared with controls [36]. SOST is another Wnt inhibitor that is a potent suppressor of bone formation, and inhibits bone morphogenic protein. The absence of SOST expression results in increased bone formation and bone mass [37]. In the current study, SOST levels were significantly lower in all of the zymosan-treated groups than in the control group, and SOST levels were higher in the E2-treated group than the other groups. In the cohort study, devenir des spondyloarthrites indifférenciées récentes (DESIR), SOST was significantly lower in patients with SpA than in healthy controls [38]. In addition, SOST was significantly lower in patients with SpA than in control patients, whereas SOST was increased in patients with RA compared with controls [39, 40]. We therefore evaluated the expression of Wnt inhibitors in the SKG mouse model and demonstrated that estrogen inhibited Wnt signaling in SpA. Considering that blockade of Wnt inhibitors induced the fusion of sacroiliac joints and increased bone formation [37, 41], estrogen might be used as a therapeutic target to control the Wnt pathway.

This study had several limitations. First, uterine weights were not measured; rather, we measured the concentration of E2 in mouse serum. The mean concentration of E2 was significantly higher in E2-treated mice than in mice in the other groups, but there was no significant difference between E2 levels in the sham and ovariectomized groups. Inflammation affects ovulation and hormone production. Moreover, 50% of cases of premature ovarian failure have been ascribed to autoimmune disease [42]. Considering that mice in the sham group had severe inflammation in the joints, intestines, and skin at the time of sacrifice, estrogen production might have been decreased due to ovarian failure induced by systemic inflammation. Second, gene expression in the tail was not quantified. However, considering that the incidence of arthritis and the degree of inflammation in the peripheral joints were clinically and histologically closely tied to those of the tail joints, the gene expression patterns found in the joint tissue of the hind paws and forepaws likely reflected those in the tail joints. The strength of this study is that it is one of the few studies to evaluate the role of estrogen in disease activity in SpA. To the best of our knowledge, this is the first

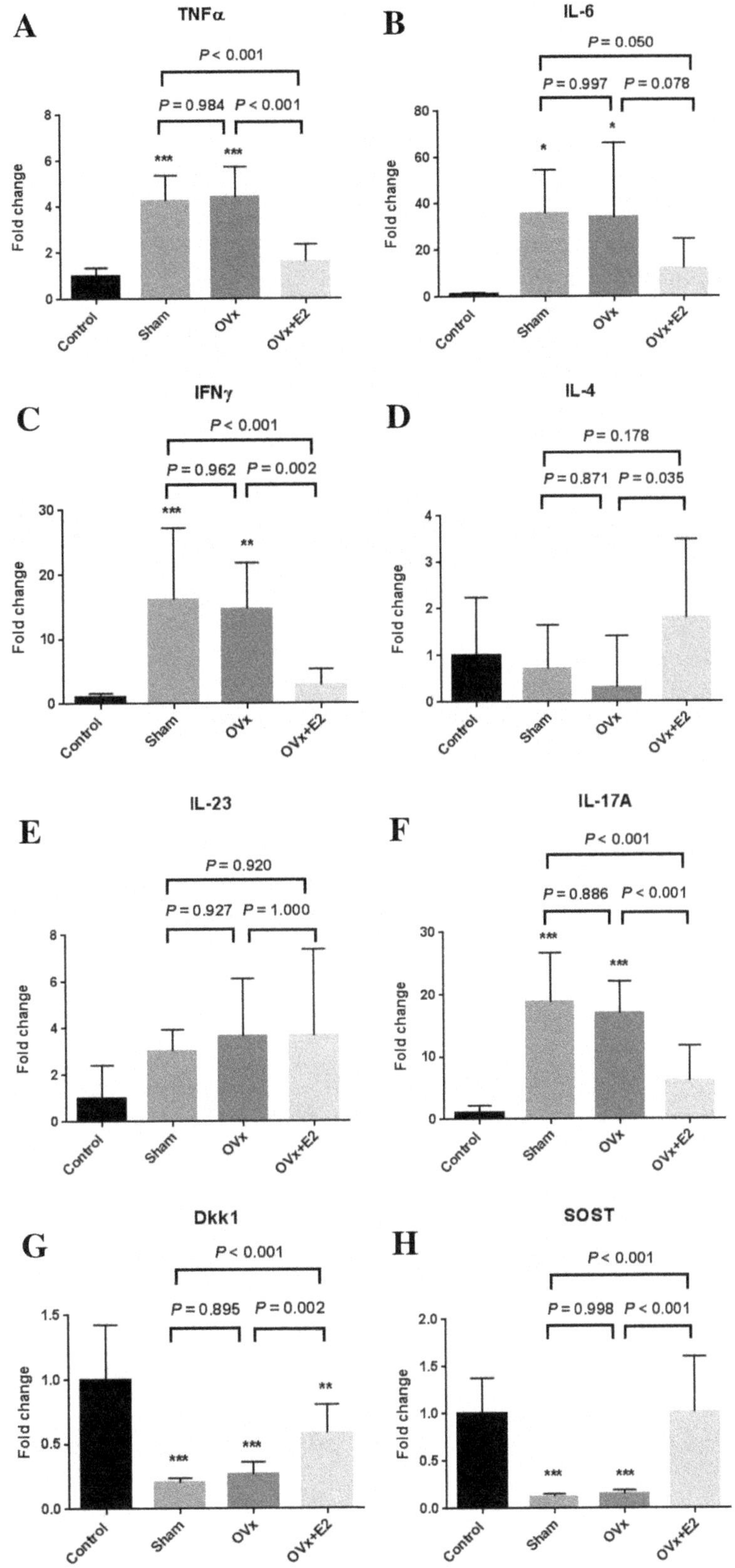

Fig. 4 (See legend on next page.)

(See figure on previous page.)

Fig. 4 Local mRNA expression in the hind paws and forepaws was analyzed using the QuantiGene 2.0 Plex assay. Fold change in gene expression was compared to that in wild-type controls. **a-h** TNFα (**a**), IL-6 (**b**), interferon-γ (IFN-γ) (**c**), IL-4 (**d**), IL-23 (**e**), IL-17A (**f**), dickkopf-related protein 1 (Dkk1) (**g**), and sclerostin (SOST) (**h**). Data are expressed as the average fold change relative to the wild-type control group. Values are mean ± SEM; $n = 12$ mice per group except for the wild-type control ($n = 2$); $^{*}P < 0.05$, $^{**}P < 0.01$, $^{***}P < 0.001$, versus controls. Sham = sham-operated mice, OVx = ovariectomized mice, OVx + E2 = 17β-estradiol-treated ovariectomized mice

study to demonstrate the inhibitory effect of estrogen on SpA, using an animal model of SpA. Furthermore, our results suggest that estrogen might be an effective therapeutic approach to treating SpA. However, hormone treatment has various adverse effects, such as increased risk of breast cancer, endometrial cancer, and thromboembolism. Therefore, selective estrogen receptor modulators (SERMs) were developed to prevent their side effects. Recent studies reported that SERMs inhibit joint inflammation and osteoporosis in female CIA animal models [43, 44]. Further experiments are needed to evaluate the effects of SERMs in the SpA mouse model.

Conclusions

Estrogen suppressed arthritis development in an SpA mouse model. Results of this study suggest that estrogen has an anti-inflammatory effect on the SpA manifestations in the SKG arthritis model. Further study is warranted to determine the molecular mechanisms of estrogen in the pathogenesis of SpA and to evaluate if estrogen is an effective therapeutic treatment option for SpA.

Abbreviations

^{18}F-FDG: ^{18}F-fluorodeoxyglucose; %ID/g: Percentage injected dose per gram; ANOVA: Analysis of variance; AS: Ankylosing spondylitis; ASAS: Assessment of SpondyloArthritis International Society; CIA: Collagen-induced arthritis; CRP: C-reactive protein; CT: Computed tomography; DC: Dendritic cell; DHEAS: Dehydroepiandrosterone sulfate; Dkk1: Dickkopf-related protein 1; E2: 17β-estradiol; EDTA: Ethylenediamine tetraacetic acid; ELISA: Enzyme-linked immunosorbent assay; ER: Estrogen receptor; H&E: Hematoxylin and eosin; HLA: Human leukocyte antigen; IFN: Interferon; IL: Interleukin; MFI: Median fluorescence intensity; MRI: Magnetic resonance imaging; nr-axSpA: Non-radiographic axial spondyloarthritis; OVx: Ovariectomy; PBS: Phosphate-buffered saline; PET: Positron emission tomography; RA: Rheumatoid arthritis; ROI: Region of interest ; SEM: Standard error of the mean ; SERM: Selective estrogen receptor modulator; SOST: Sclerostin; SpA: Spondyloarthritis; Th: T helper; TNF: Tumor necrosis factor

Acknowledgements
Not applicable.

Funding
This study was financially supported by a grant from the Korea Health Industry Development Institute (HI14C2285).

Authors' contributions

HJ designed the study, performed experiments, analyzed the data, and wrote the manuscript; EKB, HK, YHE, and IYK designed the study and performed experiments and interpretation of data; HK, JL, CHJ, and EMK designed the study and revised the article; HSC designed the study, interpreted the data, and wrote the manuscript. All authors read and approved the final manuscript.

Competing interests

The authors declare that they have no competing interests.

Author details
[1]Division of Rheumatology, Department of Internal Medicine, Soonchunhyang University Hospital, Bucheon, South Korea. [2]Samsung Biomedical Research Institute, Seoul, South Korea. [3]Division of Rheumatology, Department of Internal Medicine, Samsung Medical Center, Sungkyunkwan University School of Medicine, 81 Irwon-Ro, Gangnam-gu, Seoul 06351, South Korea.

References

1. Lee W, Reveille JD, Davis Jr JC, Learch TJ, Ward MM, Weisman MH. Are there gender differences in severity of ankylosing spondylitis? Results from the PSOAS cohort. Ann Rheum Dis. 2007;66:633–8.
2. Rudwaleit M, van der Heijde D, Landewe R, Listing J, Akkoc N, Brandt J, et al. The development of Assessment of SpondyloArthritis international Society classification criteria for axial spondyloarthritis (part II): validation and final selection. Ann Rheum Dis. 2009;68:777–83.
3. Sieper J, van der Heijde D. Review: Nonradiographic axial spondyloarthritis: new definition of an old disease? Arthritis Rheum. 2013;65:543–51.
4. Oostveen J, Prevo R, den Boer J, van de Laar M. Early detection of sacroiliitis on magnetic resonance imaging and subsequent development of sacroiliitis on plain radiography. A prospective, longitudinal study. J Rheumatol. 1999; 26:1953–8.
5. Rudwaleit M, Haibel H, Baraliakos X, Listing J, Marker-Hermann E, Zeidler H, et al. The early disease stage in axial spondylarthritis: results from the German Spondyloarthritis Inception Cohort. Arthritis Rheum. 2009;60:717–27.
6. Kiltz U, Baraliakos X, Karakostas P, Igelmann M, Kalthoff L, Klink C, et al. Do patients with non-radiographic axial spondylarthritis differ from patients with ankylosing spondylitis? Arthritis Care Res (Hoboken). 2012;64:1415–22.
7. Dougados M, d'Agostino MA, Benessiano J, Berenbaum F, Breban M, Claudepierre P, et al. The DESIR cohort: a 10-year follow-up of early inflammatory back pain in France: study design and baseline characteristics of the 708 recruited patients. Joint Bone Spine. 2011;78:598–603.
8. Jeong H, Yoon JY, Park EJ, Hwang J, Kim H, Ahn JK, et al. Clinical characteristics of nonradiographic axial spondyloarthritis in Korea: a comparison with ankylosing spondylitis. Int J Rheum Dis. 2015;18:661–8.
9. Ortega Castro R, Font Ugalde P, Castro Villegas MC, Calvo Gutierrez J, Munoz Gomariz E, Zarco Montejo P, et al. Different clinical expression of patients with ankylosing spondylitis according to gender in relation to time since onset of disease. Data from REGISPONSER. Reumatol Clin. 2013;9:221–5.
10. Jimenez-Balderas FJ, Tapia-Serrano R, Madero-Cervera JI, Murrieta S, Mintz G. Ovarian function studies in active ankylosing spondylitis in women. Clinical response to estrogen therapy. J Rheumatol. 1990;17:497–502.
11. Nalbandian G, Kovats S. Estrogen, immunity & autoimmune disease. Curr Med Chem – Immun, Endoc & Metab Agents. 2005;5:85–91.
12. Giltay EJ, van Schaardenburg D, Gooren LJ, Popp-Snijders C, Dijkmans BA. Androgens and ankylosing spondylitis: a role in the pathogenesis? Ann NY Acad Sci. 1999;876:340–64. discussion 65.
13. Tyagi AM, Srivastava K, Mansoori MN, Trivedi R, Chattopadhyay N, Singh D. Estrogen deficiency induces the differentiation of IL-17 secreting Th17 cells: a new candidate in the pathogenesis of osteoporosis. PLoS ONE. 2012;7, e44552.

14. Lelu K, Laffont S, Delpy L, Paulet PE, Perinat T, Tschanz SA, et al. Estrogen receptor alpha signaling in T lymphocytes is required for estradiol-mediated inhibition of Th1 and Th17 cell differentiation and protection against experimental autoimmune encephalomyelitis. J Immunol. 2011;187:2386–93.
15. Diarra D, Stolina M, Polzer K, Zwerina J, Ominsky MS, Dwyer D, et al. Dickkopf-1 is a master regulator of joint remodeling. Nat Med. 2007;13:156–63.
16. MacDonald BT, Joiner DM, Oyserman SM, Sharma P, Goldstein SA, He X, et al. Bone mass is inversely proportional to Dkk1 levels in mice. Bone. 2007;41: 331–9.
17. Sakaguchi N, Takahashi T, Hata H, Nomura T, Tagami T, Yamazaki S, et al. Altered thymic T-cell selection due to a mutation of the ZAP-70 gene causes autoimmune arthritis in mice. Nature. 2003;426:454–60.
18. Ruutu M, Thomas G, Steck R, Degli-Esposti MA, Zinkernagel MS, Alexander K, et al. beta-glucan triggers spondylarthritis and Crohn's disease-like ileitis in SKG mice. Arthritis Rheum. 2012;64:2211–22.
19. Ingberg E, Theodorsson A, Theodorsson E, Strom JO. Methods for long-term 17beta-estradiol administration to mice. Gen Comp Endocrinol. 2012;175:188–93.
20. Roggia C, Gao Y, Cenci S, Weitzmann MN, Toraldo G, Isaia G, et al. Up-regulation of TNF-producing T cells in the bone marrow: a key mechanism by which estrogen deficiency induces bone loss in vivo. Proc Natl Acad Sci USA. 2001;98:13960–5.
21. Ito A, Bebo Jr BF, Matejuk A, Zamora A, Silverman M, Fyfe-Johnson A, et al. Estrogen treatment down-regulates TNF-alpha production and reduces the severity of experimental autoimmune encephalomyelitis in cytokine knockout mice. J Immunol. 2001;167:542–52.
22. Arenas IA, Armstrong SJ, Xu Y, Davidge ST. Chronic tumor necrosis factor-alpha inhibition enhances NO modulation of vascular function in estrogen-deficient rats. Hypertension. 2005;46:76–81.
23. Srivastava S, Weitzmann MN, Cenci S, Ross FP, Adler S, Pacifici R. Estrogen decreases TNF gene expression by blocking JNK activity and the resulting production of c-Jun and JunD. J Clin Invest. 1999;104:503–13.
24. Haghmorad D, Salehipour Z, Nosratabadi R, Rastin M, Kokhaei P, Mahmoudi MB, et al. Medium-dose estrogen ameliorates experimental autoimmune encephalomyelitis in ovariectomized mice. J Immunotoxicol. 2016;13:885–96.
25. Formby B. Immunologic response in pregnancy. Its role in endocrine disorders of pregnancy and influence on the course of maternal autoimmune diseases. Endocrinol Metab Clin North Am. 1995;24:187–205.
26. Wilder RL. Hormones, pregnancy, and autoimmune diseases. Ann NY Acad Sci. 1998;840:45–50.
27. Andersson A, Stubelius A, Karlsson MN, Engdahl C, Erlandsson M, Grahnemo L, et al. Estrogen regulates T helper 17 phenotype and localization in experimental autoimmune arthritis. Arthritis Res Ther. 2015;17:32.
28. Andersson A, Grahnemo L, Engdahl C, Stubelius A, Lagerquist MK, Carlsten H, et al. IL-17-producing gammadeltaT cells are regulated by estrogen during development of experimental arthritis. Clin Immunol. 2015;161:324–32.
29. Shen H, Goodall JC, Hill Gaston JS. Frequency and phenotype of peripheral blood Th17 cells in ankylosing spondylitis and rheumatoid arthritis. Arthritis Rheum. 2009;60:1647–56.
30. Wendling D, Cedoz JP, Racadot E, Dumoulin G. Serum IL-17, BMP-7, and bone turnover markers in patients with ankylosing spondylitis. Joint Bone Spine. 2007;74:304–5.
31. Giltay EJ, Popp-Snijders C, van Schaardenburg D, Dekker-Saeys BJ, Gooren LJ, Dijkmans BA. Serum testosterone levels are not elevated in patients with ankylosing spondylitis. J Rheumatol. 1998;25:2389–94.
32. Tapia-Serrano R, Jimenez-Balderas FJ, Murrieta S, Bravo-Gatica C, Guerra R, Mintz G. Testicular function in active ankylosing spondylitis. Therapeutic response to human chorionic gonadotrophin. J Rheumatol. 1991;18:841–8.
33. Arniaud D, Mattei JP, Boyer J, Roux H. Sex hormones in spondylarthropathies. A study in 57 patients. Rev Rhum Engl Ed. 1998;65:21–6.
34. Bonewald LF, Johnson ML. Osteocytes, mechanosensing and Wnt signaling. Bone. 2008;42:606–15.
35. Heiland GR, Appel H, Poddubnyy D, Zwerina J, Hueber A, Haibel H, et al. High level of functional dickkopf-1 predicts protection from syndesmophyte formation in patients with ankylosing spondylitis. Ann Rheum Dis. 2012;71:572–4.
36. Haynes KR, Pettit AR, Duan R, Tseng HW, Glant TT, Brown MA, et al. Excessive bone formation in a mouse model of ankylosing spondylitis is associated with decreases in Wnt pathway inhibitors. Arthritis Res Ther. 2012;14:R253.
37. Suen PK, Zhu TY, Chow DH, Huang L, Zheng LZ, Qin L. Sclerostin antibody treatment increases bone formation, bone mass, and bone strength of intact bones in adult male rats. Sci Rep. 2015;5:15632.
38. Nocturne G, Pavy S, Boudaoud S, Seror R, Goupille P, Chanson P, et al. Increase in Dickkopf-1 serum level in recent spondyloarthritis. Data from the DESIR cohort. PLoS ONE. 2015;10, e0134974.
39. Appel H, Ruiz-Heiland G, Listing J, Zwerina J, Herrmann M, Mueller R, et al. Altered skeletal expression of sclerostin and its link to radiographic progression in ankylosing spondylitis. Arthritis Rheum. 2009;60:3257–62.
40. Wehmeyer C, Stratis A, Stratis A, Pap T, Dankbar B. The role of the WNT inhibitor sclerostin in rheumatoid arthritis. Ann Rheum Dis. 2010;69:A1–76.
41. Uderhardt S, Diarra D, Katzenbeisser J, David JP, Zwerina J, Richards W, et al. Blockade of Dickkopf (DKK)-1 induces fusion of sacroiliac joints. Ann Rheum Dis. 2010;69:592–7.
42. Weiss G, Goldsmith LT, Taylor RN, Bellet D, Taylor HS. Inflammation in reproductive disorders. Reprod Sci. 2009;16:216–29.
43. Andersson A, Bernardi AI, Nurkkala-Karlsson M, Stubelius A, Grahnemo L, Ohlsson C, et al. Suppression of experimental arthritis and associated bone loss by a tissue-selective estrogen complex. Endocrinology. 2016;157:1013–20.
44. Andersson A, Bernardi AI, Stubelius A, Nurkkala-Karlsson M, Ohlsson C, Carlsten H, et al. Selective oestrogen receptor modulators lasofoxifene and bazedoxifene inhibit joint inflammation and osteoporosis in ovariectomised mice with collagen-induced arthritis. Rheumatology (Oxford). 2016;55:553–63.

17

IL-23/Th17 axis is not influenced by TNF-blocking agents in ankylosing spondylitis patients

Fernanda Manente Milanez[1†], Carla G. S. Saad[1*†], Vilma T. Viana[1], Júlio C. B. Moraes[1], Grégory Vinícius Périco[2], Percival Degrava Sampaio-Barros[1], Célio R. Goncalves[1] and Eloísa Bonfá[1]

Abstract

Background: Advances in pathophysiology and treatment of ankylosing spondylitis (AS) was recently demonstrated. However, the effect of anti-TNF in the newly described inflammatory pathways involved pathogenesis of this disease remains to be determined. The aim of our study was, therefore, to investigate long-term influence of anti-TNF drugs in IL-23/IL-17 axis of AS patients and their possible correlation with treatment, clinical, laboratory and radiographic parameters.

Methods: Eighty-six AS anti-TNF naïve patients, 47 referred for anti-TNF therapy (active-AS; BASDAI ≥ 4) and 39 with BASDAI < 4 (control-AS) were included. The active group was evaluated at baseline, 12-months and 24-months after TNF blockade and compared at baseline to control-AS group and to 47 healthy age- and gender-matched controls. Plasma levels of IL-17A, IL-22, IL-23 and PGE2 were measured. Non-steroidal anti-inflammatory drugs (NSAIDs) intake were recorded every 6 months. Radiographic severity and progression was assessed by mSASSS at baseline and 24 months after therapy.

Results: At baseline, active-AS group presented higher IL-23 and PGE2 levels compared to control-AS group ($p < 0.001$ and $p = 0.008$) and to healthy controls ($p < 0.001$ and $p = 0.02$). After 24-months of TNF blockade, IL-23 and PGE2 remained elevated with higher levels compared with the healthy group ($p < 0.001$ and $p = 0.03$) in spite of significant improvements in all clinical/inflammatory parameters ($p < 0.001$). Further analysis of 27 anti-TNF-treated patients who achieved a good response (ASDAS-CRP < 2.1,with a drop ≥ 1.1) at 24-months revealed that IL-23 plasma levels remained higher than healthy controls ($p < 0.001$) and higher than control-AS group with similar disease activity (ASDAS-CRP < 2.1, $p = 0.01$). In active-AS group ($n = 47$), there was a strong correlation between IL-23 and IL-17A at baseline, 12-months and 24-months after anti-TNF therapy ($p \leq 0.001$).

Conclusion: This study provides novel data demonstrating that the IL-23/IL-17 axis is not influenced by TNF blockade in AS patients despite clinical and inflammation improvements and NSAID intake.

Keywords: Ankylosing spondylitis, Anti-TNF drugs, Inflammation, Interleukin-23, Interleukin-17, Prostaglandin E2

* Correspondence: goncalves-carla@uol.com.br
[†]Equal contributors
[1]Division of Rheumatology, Faculdade de Medicina da Universidade de São Paulo – Reumatologia, Av. Dr. Arnaldo, n° 455, 3° andar, sala 3192, São Paulo, SP 05403-010, Brazil
Full list of author information is available at the end of the article

Background

Spondyloarthritis (SpA) is a group of inflammatory diseases in which ankylosing spondylitis (AS) is the prototype. Despite recent advances in pathophysiology and treatment, this disease group is still a challenge, particularly regarding the understanding of the inflammatory pathways involved, predictors of anti-tumor necrosis factor (anti-TNF) response, and risk factors for radiographic progression.

Recently, the interleukin (IL)-23/IL-17 axis was reported to have a role in SpA pathophysiology because of promising results regarding initial efforts at blocking these pathways in SpA [1–6]. In addition, genetic studies have described interleukin-23 receptor (IL-23R) polymorphisms linked to AS susceptibility [7], and higher IL-23R expression on γ/δ T cells was also associated with increased IL-17 secretion [8]. Evidence from animal studies demonstrated that misfolding of HLA-B27 generates endoplasmic reticulum stress with subsequent unfolded protein response and IL-23 production by activated macrophages and dendritic cells [1, 9]. However, the role of unfolded protein response in modulating the production of IL-23 has not been confirmed in AS patients; instead, recent data suggest that the lipopolysaccharide response and/or autophagy of mononuclear cells may underlie the increased IL production in this disease [10, 11]. Moreover the IL-23/IL-23R complex, in predisposing patients, seems to induce the activation of signal transduction and transcription, with a consequent proliferation and terminal differentiation of Th17 cells, resulting in IL-17 production [1, 12–15]. This overexpression is not only a potent TNFα inducer but also leads to the production of other proinflammatory cytokines and chemokines [14]. Of note, nonsteroidal anti-inflammatory drug (NSAIDs) cyclooxygenase (COX) inhibition may influence prostaglandin E2 (PGE2) levels with a possible impact on the IL-23/IL-17 axis and bone formation in AS. In fact, IL-23 production is affected by various factors, including PGE2 secreted by fibroblasts and/or through its binding to EP-4 receptors [11, 16]. PGE2 seems to have an anabolic effect on bone via EP-2 (Prostaglandin E2 receptor 2) and EP-4 (Prostaglandin E2 receptor 4) receptors and affects human tendon cell differentiation [17, 18].

In this context, clinical practice and registry studies have suggested that the isolated use of anti-TNFα is unable to reduce radiographic progression in AS, suggesting that other pathways may be involved [19–21]. Subsequent studies have inferred a possible benefit of NSAID concomitant use and radiographic progression. In 2005 Wanders et al. [22] demonstrated that the strategy of continuous use of NSAIDs reduces radiographic progression in symptomatic patients with AS, independently of baseline values of radiographic damage or disease activity variables. In addition, a protective effect of a higher NSAID intake over time was associated with retarded radiographic progression in AS patients from a prospective SpA inception cohort in Germany [23].

More recently, Appel et al. [24] described increased IL-23-positive cell expression in subchondral bone marrow and in fibrous tissue in the spine of patients with a longstanding history of AS. In addition, it was demonstrated that the enthesis in a spondyloarthropathy model is a functional IL-23-responsive anatomic site containing primed IL-23 resident cells promoting IL-17 and IL-22 expression [25].

In spite of this compelling evidence regarding the relevance of the IL-23/IL-17 immune axis in AS pathogenesis, there are no data on the long-term influence of TNF blockade in this axis concerning a possible synergistic or independent effect of these cytokines.

This study therefore aims to investigate the influence of anti-TNF therapy in the IL-23/IL-17 axis of AS patients and its possible correlation with clinical, inflammatory markers, treatment, and radiographic parameters.

Methods

Subjects

Eighty-six AS anti-TNF-naïve patients, aged ≥18 to <65 years, who fulfilled the modified AS New York criteria in regular rheumatology outpatient follow-up care were included [26]. At entry, 47 consecutive AS patients (active-AS group) were referred to the Infusion Center to start anti-TNFα therapy, according to the Assessment of SpondyloArthritis International Society (ASAS) consensus statement [27]. They were classified with active disease (Bath Ankylosing Spondylitis Disease Activity Index (BASDAI) ≥4) despite treatment with at least two NSAIDs at a maximal tolerable dose with or without disease-modifying antirheumatic drugs (DMARDs) (methotrexate, sulphasalazine, or leflunomide) at standard doses for at least 6 months [27]. Forty-seven sex-matched and age-matched healthy individuals comprised the healthy control group (healthy controls). Additionally, the AS patient control group of 39 consecutive AS patients with BASDAI <4 under NSAID and/or traditional DMARDS were also evaluated at entry (control-AS group).

Study design

This study comprises: a cross-sectional evaluation comparing 47 active-AS patients (BASDAI ≥4), 39 AS patients with BASDAI <4 (control-AS group), and 47 healthy individuals at baseline (healthy controls); and a longitudinal evaluation of 47 active-AS patients followed with clinical, radiographic, and laboratorial parameters at baseline and 12 and 24 months of anti-TNF therapy.

This study was approved by the Local Ethics Committee on Human Research at the University of São Paulo (CAPPesq). All participants gave written informed consent in accordance with the Declaration of Helsinki.

Clinical outcomes and NSAID use

Clinical outcomes included the C-reactive protein Ankylosing Spondylitis Disease Activity Score (ASDAS-CRP), BASDAI, Bath Ankylosing Spondylitis Functional Index (BASFI), Bath Ankylosing Spondylitis Metrology Index (BASMI), and AS quality-of-life questionnaire (ASQoL) [28]. These clinical parameters were performed at baseline and 12 and 24 months of follow-up. Concomitant medications were recorded every 6 months and NSAID intake (drug, dose, and frequency of use) was standardized to 0–100 as recommended by the ASAS [29].

Definitions of baseline clinical activity and follow-up Anti-TNF response

Active disease was defined as BASDAI ≥4 at entry and, for follow-up, ASDAS-CRP ≥2.1. An anti-TNF response was classified after 24 months of anti-TNF treatment according to ASDAS criteria into responders (ASDAS-CRP <2.1 with a drop ≥1.1 from baseline) and nonresponders (ASDAS-CRP ≥2.1 or a drop <1.1 from baseline) [30].

Laboratory assessment of cytokine levels and inflammation

Plasma samples were obtained from all active-AS patients ($n = 47$) immediately before anti-TNF infusion. The laboratory assessment was performed at baseline and 12 and 24 months after treatment. The control-AS group ($n = 39$) and healthy controls ($n = 47$) underwent a single plasma withdrawal at baseline. All samples were immediately frozen and stored at −80 °C. IL-17, IL-22, and IL-23 were measured by LUMINEX 200™ technology (Luminex B.V., Oosterhout, the Netherlands) using a Millipore kit (EMD Millipore, Darmstadt, Germany) supplied with the following minimal detection concentration (MinDC): IL-17A, MinDC = 2.1 pg/ml; IL-22, MinDC = 0.021 ng/ml; and IL-23, MinDC = 0.098 ng/ml. All samples were tested in duplicate. For PGE2, enzyme-linked immunosorbent assay methodology was employed using a USCN kit (Cloud-Clone Corp, 1304 Langham Creek Dr, Houston, Tx 77084, USA)(sensitivity of 1.52 pg/ml) and a Stat Fax-2.100 (Awareness Technology, Inc. P.O. Drawer 1679 Palm City, FL 34991 USA) reader. Inflammatory response was evaluated by the CRP level (mg/l) and the erythrocyte sedimentation rate (ESR, mm/hour). The frequency of patients' samples ≥ MinDC was 72 % for IL-23, 100 % for PGE2, 36 % for IL-17, and 8 % for IL-22.

Radiological assessment

Structural damage was scored on digital X-ray images of the lumbar and cervical spine according to the modified Stoke Ankylosing Spondylitis Spine Score (mSASSS) at baseline for all AS patients and at 24 months after anti-TNF treatment [31]. Two blinded and independent expert investigators (one musculoskeletal radiologist and one rheumatologist) performed the score evaluation. The baseline and follow-up X-ray images were scored at the same time by two investigators blinded to time point, clinical, and demographic features.

Radiographic spinal progression after 2 years was defined according to an increase by 2 or more units in the mSASSS.

The intraclass correlation coefficients (two-way random and absolute agreement in SPSS 20 (IBM Corporation - 1 New Orchard Road, Armonk, NY, 10504, USA)) between the two readers regarding mSASSS status was 0.997 (95 % confidence interval (CI) 0.995–0.998) at baseline and 0.998 (95 % CI 0.996–0.999) at 24 months. Agreement regarding change in the mSASSS was 0.951 (95 % CI 0.914–0.972).

Statistical analysis

Statistical analysis was performed using SPSS 20. Based on a previous study comparing serum levels of IL-23 and IL-17 in AS patients and healthy controls [32], a minimum sample size of seven individuals per group was calculated. The current study sample size ensured >95 % power to detect similar differences in AS patients and healthy controls. Results are presented as the mean and standard deviation (SD) for continuous variables, the median and 25–75 % interquartile range (IQR) for nonparametric data, and percentages for categorical variables. Data for continuous variables were compared by the t test or Mann–Whitney U test as appropriate. Clinical and laboratorial data at baseline, 12 and 24 months were analyzed by Friedman repeated-measures analysis of variance on ranks followed by a post-hoc analysis by Tukey test to determine which groups in the sample differ. The statistical analysis used the appropriate tests according to data distribution, and for cytokines a nonparametric test was used. Multiple linear regression analysis was performed, including all clinical differences between the active-AS group and the control-AS group, to infer differences in cytokine and PGE2 concentrations. Radiographic progression and anti-TNF response associated factors were analyzed (baseline parameters and their changes after 12 and 24 months of treatment). Spearman's rank was applied for correlation analysis. Statistical significance was established at $p < 0.05$.

Results

Baseline demographic and clinical characteristics of AS patients and healthy controls

Active-AS patients (BASDAI ≥4) and the healthy control group were comparable regarding age (38.02 ± 11.09 years vs. 37.74 ± 10.95 years, $p = 0.90$), male gender (74 % vs. 74 %, $p = 1.00$), and Caucasian predominance (89 % vs. 76 %, $p = 0.17$). The comparison between the control-AS group (BASDAI <4) and the healthy controls showed a similar male gender frequency (74 % vs. 74 %, $p = 1.00$),

Caucasian predominance (74 % vs. 76 %, $p = 1.00$), and a higher mean age (49.51 ± 10.53 years vs. 37.74 ± 10.95 years, $p < 0.001$).

Baseline demographic features for the active-AS and control-AS groups are presented in Table 1. Active-AS patients were younger (p <0.001) and had shorter disease duration ($p = 0.007$), worse clinical outcomes measured by the ASDAS-CRP, BASFI, and ASQoL (p <0.001), higher levels of CRP and ESR (p <0.001), lower mSASSS (p <0.001), and lower BASMI ($p = 0.03$) than control-AS patients. The proportion of patients using methotrexate (mean dose of 20.76 ± 4.67 mg/week) was higher in the active-AS group than the control-AS group (p <0.001).

Baseline cytokine plasma levels in AS patient groups and the healthy control group

The active-AS group presented significantly higher IL-23 and PGE2 plasma levels compared with the control-AS group (p <0.001 and $p = 0.008$) and with healthy controls (p <0.001 and $p = 0.02$). No difference was observed in IL-23 and PGE2 plasma levels comparing the control-AS group with the healthy controls ($p = 0.57$ and $p = 0.99$) (Table 2).

With regard to IL-17 and IL-22, comparable plasma levels were observed evaluating active-AS vs. control-AS groups ($p = 0.45$ and $p = 0.68$), active-AS vs. healthy control groups ($p = 0.48$ and $p = 0.47$), and control-AS vs. healthy control groups ($p = 0.90$ and $p = 0.78$) (Table 2).

Multiple linear regression analysis was performed, including all clinical differences between the active-AS group and the control-AS group (age, disease duration, BASFI, BASMI, ASQoL, mSASSS, and methotrexate use), and no factor was associated with differences in cytokine and PGE2 concentrations.

Longitudinal clinical and laboratorial parameter changes in the active-AS group after 24 months of anti-TNF therapy

At entry, 32 (68 %) patients started with infliximab (the first available TNF blockade at our center during the study period), 13 (28 %) patients with adalimumab, and two (4 %) patients with etanercept at standard doses. Seventeen patients switched to another anti-TNF because of inefficacy or adverse events during the 24 months of follow-up. All patients who started the study were followed until the end (no dropout).

After 2 years of TNF blockade, there was a significant improvement in all clinical parameters evaluated and a concomitant reduction in ESR and CRP was observed (p <0.001) (Table 3). Of note, IL-23 and PGE2 plasma levels remained elevated without significant changes comparing baseline vs. 12 months vs. 24 months ($p = 0.38$ and

Table 1 Clinical and demographic data of ankylosing spondylitis patients at baseline

Variable	Ankylosing spondylitis ($n = 86$)		p value
	Active-AS (BASDAI ≥4; $n = 47$)	Control-AS (BASDAI <4; $n = 39$)	
Gender, male (%)	35 (74 %)	29 (74 %)	1.00
Age (years)	38.0 ± 11.1	49.5 ± 10.5	<0.001
Caucasian (%)	42 (89 %)	29 (74 %)	0.09
Peripheral involvement (%)	31 (66 %)	23 (59 %)	0.65
HLA-B27 positive (%)	82 %	90 %	0.36
Disease duration (years)	10.8 ± 4.5	17.6 ± 8.9	0.007
ASDAS-CRP	3.9 ± 1.0	2.0 ± 0.8	<0.001
BASFI	5.8 ± 2.3	3.8 ± 2.1	<0.001
BASMI	4.5 ± 2.7	5.8 ± 2.7	0.03
ASQoL	12.6 ± 4.8	5.3 ± 4.1	<0.001
CRP (mg/l)	29.7 ± 39.6	4.6 ± 3.5	<0.001
ESR (mm/hour)	29.7 ± 23.3	6.9 ± 6.6	<0.001
mSASSS	15.8 ± 18.9	37.9 ± 25.5	<0.001
NSAID intake score (0–100)	70.3 ± 44.8	68.3 ± 41.4	0.77
Methotrexate (%)	23 (48 %)	2 (0.5 %)	<0.001
Sulphasalazine (%)	27 (57 %)	21 (53 %)	0.83
Leflunomide (%)	2 (4.2 %)	1 (0.02 %)	1.00

All values are expressed as the mean ± standard deviation, except proportions (%)
Nonparametric tests were performed for data that failed the normal distribution
AS ankylosing spondylitis, *ASDAS-CRP* Ankylosing Spondylitis Disease Activity Score-C-reactive protein, *ASQoL* Ankylosing Spondylitis Quality of Life, *BASDAI* Bath Ankylosing Spondylitis Disease Activity Index, *BASFI* Bath AS Functional Index, *BASMI* Bath Ankylosing Spondylitis Metrology Index, *CRP* C-reactive protein, *ESR* erythrocyte sedimentation rate, *mSASSS* modified Stoke Ankylosing Spondylitis Spine Score, *NSAID* nonsteroidal anti-inflammatory drug

Table 2 Baseline cytokine levels in ankylosing spondylitis patients and healthy controls

Cytokine	Ankylosing spondylitis ($n = 86$) Active-AS (BASDAI ≥4; $n = 47$)	Control-AS (BASDAI <4; $n = 39$)	p value[a]	Healthy controls ($n = 47$)	p value[b]	p value[c]
IL-17A (pg/ml)	1.62 (1.06–2.98)	1.57 (1.04–2.17)	0.45	1.57 (1.04–2.17)	0.48	0.90
IL-22 (ng/ml)	0.00 (0.00–0.00)	0.00 (0.00–0.00)	0.68	0.00 (0.00–0.00)	0.47	0.78
IL-23 (ng/ml)	0.08 (0.04–0.17)	0.03 (0.01–0.08)	<0.001	0.02 (0.00–0.05)	<0.001	0.57
PGE2 (pg/ml)	19.46 (5.41–102.58)	7.67 (3.96–24.73)	0.008	7.66 (3.30–30.32)	0.02	0.99

All values are expressed as the median (25–75 % interquartile range)
[a]Active-AS vs. control-AS
[b]Active-AS vs. healthy controls
[c]Control-AS vs. healthy controls
AS ankylosing spondylitis, *BASDAI* Bath Ankylosing Spondylitis Disease Activity Index, *IL* interleukin, *PGE2* prostaglandin E2

$p = 0.98$). Levels of these cytokines at 24 months were higher than those observed for the healthy control group (p <0.001 and $p = 0.03$), whereas no change in IL-17A or IL-22 plasma levels (p >0.05) were detected during TNF blockade, with levels comparable with the healthy control group at 24 months (p >0.05) (Table 3).

The NSAID intake score exhibited a significant decrease after anti-TNF treatment (p <0.01) (Table 3) without a significant correlation between NSAID intake scores and PGE2 plasma levels at baseline ($r = 0.07$), 12 months ($r = -0.20$), and 24 months ($r = -0.28$) of treatment (p >0.05).

After 2 years of treatment with anti-TNF, 27 active-AS patients (57.5 %) achieved a good clinical anti-TNF response (responders). Comparing anti-TNF responders with nonresponders at baseline, there was no significant difference in median (IQR) for IL-17A (2.06 (1.26–3.04) pg/ml vs. 1.53 (0.75–2.17) pg/ml, $p = 0.10$), IL-22 (0.00 (0.00–00) pg/ml vs. 0.00 (0.00–0.00) ng/ml, $p = 0.75$), IL-23 (0.08 (0.04–0.13) pg/ml vs. 0.07 (0.05–0.31) ng/ml, $p = 0.70$), and PGE2 (19.07 (4.25–83.16) pg/ml vs. 36.34 (7.55–127.89) pg/ml, $p = 0.51$).

After 24 months of TNF blockade, active-AS responders (ASDAS-CRP <2.1) had higher plasma levels of IL-17A compared with nonresponders (ASDAS-CRP ≥2.1) ($p = 0.03$). No difference was observed in IL-22, IL-23, and PGE2 plasma levels (p >0.05) (Table 4).

Further analysis of all cytokines levels at 24 months showed that only IL-23 plasma levels were higher in active-AS patients who responded to anti-TNF therapy compared with the control-AS group with similar disease activity

Table 3 Cytokines, inflammatory markers, and clinical parameters in active-AS patients undergoing anti-TNF therapy vs. healthy controls

Variable	Active-AS patients Baseline ($n = 47$)	12 months ($n = 47$)	24 months ($n = 47$)	p value[a]	Healthy controls ($n = 47$)	p value[b]
ESR (mm/hour)	29.70 ± 23.32	9.59 ± 12.10	10.53 ± 13.90	<0.001	NA	
CRP (mg/l)	29.71 ± 39.56	7.57 ± 13.50	5.13 ± 6.23	<0.001	NA	
mSASSS	15.83 ± 18.73	NA	19.49 ± 19.61	<0.001	NA	
ASDAS-CRP	3.93 ± 1.04	2.08 ± 1.12	1.93 ± 1.11	<0.001	NA	
BASFI	5.80 ± 2.33	3.60 ± 2.97	3.18 ± 2.95	<0.001	NA	
BASMI	4.53 ± 2.70	3.70 ± 2.72	3.34 ± 2.56	<0.001	NA	
ASQoL	12.59 ± 4.83	6.57 ± 5.51	5.83 ± 5.81	<0.001	NA	
NSAID intake (0–100)	70.26 ± 44.78	62.43 ± 47.56	45.16 ± 46.37	<0.01	NA	
IL-17A (pg/ml)	1.62 (1.06–2.98)	1.58 (1.14–3.52)	1.69 (0.78–3.46)	0.78	1.57 (1.04–2.17)	0.96
IL-22 (ng/ml)	0.00 (0.00–0.00)	0.00 (0.00–0.00)	0.00 (0.00–0.00)	0.87	0.00 (0.00–0.00)	0.59
IL-23 (ng/ml)	0.08 (0.04–0.17)	0.04 (0.02–0.17)	0.06 (0.03–0.15)	0.38	0.02 (0.00–0.05)	<0.001
PGE2 (pg/ml)	19.46 (5.41–102.58)	23.73 (4.72–102.82)	35.50 (5.88–75.82)	0.98	7.66 (3.30–30.32)	0.03

Values expressed as mean ± standard deviation or median (25–75 % interquartile range)
Nonparametric tests were performed for data that failed the normal distribution
[a]Active-AS at baseline vs. 12 months vs. 24 months by analysis of variance
[b]Active-AS after 24 months TNF blockade vs. healthy controls
AS ankylosing spondylitis, *ASDAS-CRP* Ankylosing Spondylitis Disease Activity Score-C-reactive protein, *ASQoL* Ankylosing Spondylitis Quality of life, *BASFI* Bath Ankylosing Spondylitis Functional Index, *BASMI* Bath Ankylosing Spondylitis Metrology Index, *CRP* C-reactive protein, *ESR* erythrocyte sedimentation rate, *IL* interleukin, *mSASSS* modified Stoke Ankylosing Spondylitis Spine Score, *NA* not analyzed, *NSAID* nonsteroidal anti-inflammatory drug, *PGE2* prostaglandin E2, *TNF* tumor necrosis factor

Table 4 ASDAS-CRP comparison of cytokines in active-AS group responders and nonresponders after 24 months of TNF blockade, control-AS group, and healthy controls

Cytokine	Active-AS patients after anti-TNF			Control-AS group (ASDAS-CRP <2.1; $n = 21$)		Healthy controls ($n = 47$)	
	Responders (ASDAS-CRP <2.1; $n = 27$)	Nonresponders (ASDAS-CRP ≥2.1; $n = 20$)	p value[a]		p value[b]		p value[c]
IL-17A (pg/ml)	2.17 (0.86–3.99)	1.04 (0.66–1.82)	<0.05	1.29 (1.10–2.17)	0.07	1.57 (1.04–2.17)	0.23
IL-22 (ng/ml)	0.00 (0.00–0.00)	0.00 (0.00–0.00)	0.99	0.00 (0.00–0.00)	0.71	0.00 (0.00–0.00)	0.64
IL-23 (ng/ml)	0.09 (0.03–0.21)	0.05 (0.02–0.13)	0.49	0.02 (0.01–0.06)	0.01	0.02 (0.00–0.05)	<0.001
PGE2 (pg/ml)	13.03 (4.30–56.59)	45.17 (10.92–93.76)	0.10	8.13 (4.17–23.07)	0.11	7.66 (3.30–30.32)	0.33

All values are expressed as the median (25–75 % interquartile range)
[a]Active-AS group responders after 24 months of TNF blockade vs. nonresponders
[b]Active-AS group responders after 24 months of TNF blockade vs. control-AS group (ASDAS-CRP <2.1)
[c]Active-AS group responders after 24 months of TNF blockade vs. healthy controls
AS ankylosing spondylitis, *ASDAS-CRP* C-reactive protein Ankylosing Spondylitis Disease Activity Score, *IL* interleukin, *PGE2* prostaglandin E2, *TNF* tumor necrosis factor

(ASDAS-CRP <2.1) ($p = 0.01$) and with the healthy control group ($p < 0.001$) (Table 4).

Correlation analysis of clinical parameters, inflammatory markers, and cytokine plasma levels in active-AS patients

A significant correlation was observed between IL-23 and IL-17 levels at baseline ($r = 0.64$, $p < 0.001$), 12 months ($r = 0.47$, $p = 0.001$), and 24 months ($r = 0.61$, $p < 0.001$). IL-23 was also correlated with PGE2 at 12 months ($r = 0.45$, $p = 0.001$) and 24 months ($r = 0.33$, $p = 0.02$). At 24 months, PGE2 levels were also correlated with the ESR ($r = 0.32$, $p = 0.03$), CRP ($r = 0.32$, $p = 0.03$), and ASDAS-CRP ($r = 0.28$, $p = 0.04$).

Radiographic progression in active-AS patients

There was a significant increase in mSASSS score after 24 months (15.83 ± 18.73 units vs. 19.49 ± 19.61 units, $p < 0.001$) (Table 3). Twenty-seven active-AS patients (57.5 %) increased mSASSS ≥2 units at 24 months (progressors). The progressor group had a mean increase of 6.35 ± 5.88 units in the score, with an initial mSASSS of 18.37 ± 17.93 units and a final score of 24.44 ± 18.61 units ($p < 0.001$). The group of nonprogressors (20 patients) had a mean average increase of 0.67 ± 0.86 units in the score, with an initial mSASSS of 12.40 ± 19.07 units and a final score of 12.80 ± 19.40 units ($p > 0.05$). Initial mSASSS was similar in progressor and nonprogressor patients ($p > 0.05$). Analysis of cytokines, inflammatory markers and clinical parameters (baseline and their changes after 12 and 24 months of treatment) could not identify any risk factors for radiographic progression in this population ($p > 0.05$).

Discussion

This study demonstrated that elevated plasma levels of IL-23 and PGE2 in active-AS patients are independent of TNF blockade and clinical improvement, reinforcing the relevance of these ILs in AS pathogenesis.

The great advantage of this report is the longitudinal follow-up of active-AS patients compared with control-AS (BASDAI <4) and healthy control groups, allowing a more precise definition of the possible association of clinical activity and cytokine levels. We confirmed the previous observation that there are higher levels of IL-23 in AS patients compared with healthy controls supporting a role for these cytokines in AS inflammation [32–34]. Two other investigators reported contrasting data but their analysis did not take into account the distinct levels of disease activity [35, 36]. In fact, we and others have demonstrated that IL-23 levels were higher in active-AS patients compared with the control-AS group (BASDAI <4) and the latter was comparable with the healthy control group [32].

In addition, concomitant evaluation of IL-17A, IL-22, IL-23, and PGE2 in AS patients undergoing anti-TNF therapy performed herein offered a unique opportunity to discriminate how the cytokines interact with the TNF pathway. The lack of information regarding TNF blockade therapy in former studies precludes a definitive conclusion about the relationship with disease progression [32–34]. The only available report of an association between TNF blockade and IL-23/IL-17 is a short-term evaluation with a small sample size of only eight nonpsoriatic SpA patients [35].

A study limitation was the lack of cytokine levels in tissue samples that could have brought additional information about the sites of inflammation. Furthermore, our data may underestimate possible elevations of IL-17 and IL-22 since plasma levels were below the minimal detection concentrations for most patients. In fact, reliable detection of IL-17 and IL-22 plasma levels remains a challenge.

The novel demonstration that PGE2 levels in active-AS patients were higher than those of control-AS patients, in spite of comparable NSAID intake score, supports the notion that PGE2 production does not occur exclusively through COX-1 and COX-2 [16, 17, 37]. Possible significant role of this cytokine in inflammation is evidenced by the fact that active-AS patients had higher levels of PGE2 than healthy controls and that the control-AS group (BASDAI <4) had comparable levels with the healthy group.

Remarkably, levels of IL-23 and PGE2 remained persistently elevated during treatment with anti-TNF drugs, regardless of significant clinical and laboratory parameter improvement. The persistent elevation of these cytokines in the plasma suggests that anti-TNF therapy may not be sufficient for completely blocking the inflammatory process seen in AS. In fact, the relevance of the IL-23/IL-17 pathway in AS pathogenesis is supported by a recent study that demonstrated IL-23-responsive cells (expressing IL-23R) at the tendon/bone interface in a murine model, in which overproduction of IL-23 caused periosteal and entheseal pathology similar to that seen in patients with SpA [25]. Moreover, it was demonstrated that IL-23 is increased locally in involved target organs, such as the gut [38].

Concerning PGE2 levels, there is evidence that prostaglandins, particularly PGE2, have an impact on bone metabolism [17, 39, 40], and two previous genetic studies have demonstrated the association of the *PTGER4* gene with increased predisposition to AS and radiographic progression [41, 42]. The observed PGE2 correlation with disease activity (ASDAS-CRP) and inflammatory markers (ESR and CRP) at 24 months, regardless of a significant reduction in NSAIDs, reinforces the hypothesis of an alternative regulation for this cytokine in the IL-23/IL-17 axis.

Of note, IL-23 can stimulate innate immune cells to produce other proinflammatory cytokines, including TNF, IL-22, and IL-17 family members [15, 43]. Previous studies have also shown an increase of circulating Th17 cells in blood and high levels of IL-17 in AS patients [8, 31–34, 37, 44]. Contrary to expectation, IL-17 and IL-22 were not elevated in the active patients evaluated herein. However, there was a strong correlation of IL-23 with IL-17 plasma levels in active-AS patients undergoing TNF therapy throughout the study. Intriguingly, higher IL-17A levels in active-AS responders compared with nonresponders were observed. However, the interpretation of these data should be made with caution and we should consider that IL-17 is a TNF inducer that could lead to increased TNF production and a possible better response to TNF blockade.

Previous studies showed a high variability in the percentage of progressors and nonprogressors [45, 46]. It was suggested that the presence of prior syndesmophytes, male gender, smoking, HLA-B27 positivity, longer disease duration, and elevated inflammatory markers are possible risk factors for new bone formation in AS [45, 47, 48]. Among the studied variables, we could not identify factors associated with radiographic progression in active-AS under anti-TNF therapy, reinforcing the possibility of multifactorial pathways contributing to this outcome. The sample size of the study did not allow reliable statements about prediction of radiographic progression.

The moderate correlation between IL-23 and PGE2, the persistent high IL-23/PGE2 levels, and the significant radiographic progression in spite of apparent clinical control support the hypothesis that current clinical disease activity and inflammatory markers, such as the ESR and CRP, may not be sufficient to guide treat-to-target therapy in AS [49, 50]. In fact, the lack of magnetic resonance imaging evaluation precluded a more accurate definition about persistent inflammation in these patients.

Of note, even active-AS anti-TNF responders (ASDAS-CRP <2.1) retained high IL-23 levels. This finding strengthens the evidence for a lack of upstream IL-23/IL-17 blockade in AS patients treated with TNF blockade. Moreover, new therapies such as a monoclonal antibody against the common p40 subunit of IL-23 and IL-12 (Ustekinumab) and an anti-IL-17A monoclonal antibody (Secukinumab) show promising results in AS [5, 6].

Conclusions

This study provides novel data demonstrating that the IL-23/IL-17 axis is not influenced by TNF blockade in AS patients despite clinical and inflammation improvements and NSAID intake.

Abbreviations

AS: Ankylosing spondylitis; ASAS: Assessment of SpondyloArthritis International Society; ASDAS-CRP: C-reactive protein Ankylosing Spondylitis Disease Activity Score; ASQoL: Ankylosing Spondylitis quality-of-life questionnaire; BASDAI: Bath Ankylosing Spondylitis Disease Activity Index; BASFI: Bath Ankylosing Spondylitis Functional Index; BASMI: Bath Ankylosing Spondylitis Metrology Index; CI: Confidence interval; COX: Cyclooxygenase; CRP: C-reactive protein; DMARD: Disease-modifying antirheumatic drug; ESR: Erythrocyte sedimentation rate; IL: Interleukin; IL-23R: Interleukin-23 receptor; IQR: 25–75 % interquartile range; MinDC: minimal detection concentration; mSASSS: Modified Stoke Ankylosing Spondylitis Spine Score; NSAID: Nonsteroidal anti-inflammatory drug; PGE2: Prostaglandin E2; SD: Standard deviation; SpA: Spondyloarthritis; TNF: Tumor necrosis factor.

Competing interests

The authors declare that they have no competing interests.

Authors' contributions

FMM was involved in study concept and design, assisting in subject recruitment, acquisition of subjects and data, interpretation of data, and drafting the manuscript. CGSS was involved in study concept and design, assisting in subject recruitment, acquisition of subjects and data, interpretation of data, and drafting the manuscript. VTV was involved in laboratorial data, interpretation of data, and revising the manuscript. JCBM was involved in assisting in subject recruitment, acquisition of data, and revising the manuscript. GVP was involved in radiographic analysis, interpretation of data, and revising the manuscript. PDS-B was involved in assisting in subject recruitment, interpretation of data, and revising the manuscript. CRG was involved in study concept and design, assisting in subject recruitment, and revising the manuscript. EB was involved in study concept and design, acquisition of subject and data, interpretation of data, and drafting the manuscript. All authors read and approved the final manuscript.

Acknowledgements

This study was supported by grants from Fundação de Amparo à Pesquisa do Estado de São Paulo (FAPESP #2009/51897-5 to EB), Conselho Nacional de Desenvolvimento Científico e Tecnológico (#301411/2009-3 to EB), and the Frederico Foundation (to CGSS, PDS-B, and EB).

The authors thank Dr Eduardo Ferreira Borba for helpful discussions, Elaine Leon for laboratory technical support, Claudia Goldenstein-Schainberg and Solange Carrasco for HLA-B27 analysis, and the Centro de Medicação de Alta Complexidade infusion center team.

Author details

[1]Division of Rheumatology, Faculdade de Medicina da Universidade de São Paulo – Reumatologia, Av. Dr. Arnaldo, n° 455, 3° andar, sala 3192, São Paulo, SP 05403-010, Brazil. [2]URC – Unidade Radiológica Criciúma, Rua Antonio de Lucca, 139 - Centro - Criciúma, Santa Catarina, SC 88811-503, Brazil.

References

1. Sherlock JP, Buckley CD, Cua DJ. The critical role of interleukin-23 in spondyloarthropathy. Mol Immunol. 2014;57:38–43.
2. Hreggvidsdottir HS, Noordenbos T, Baeten DL. Inflammatory pathways in spondyloarthritis. Mol Immunol. 2014;57:28–37.
3. Leonardi C, Matheson R, Zachariae C, et al. Anti-interleukin-17 monoclonal antibody ixekizumab in chronic plaque psoriasis. N Engl J Med. 2012;366:1190–9.
4. Papp KA, Leonardi C, Menter A, et al. Brodalumab, an anti-interleukin-17-receptor antibody for psoriasis. N Engl J Med. 2012;366:1181–9.
5. Baeten D, Baraliakos X, Braun J, et al. Anti-interleukin-17A monoclonal antibody secukinumab in treatment of ankylosing spondylitis: a randomised, double-blind, placebo-controlled trial. Lancet. 2013;382:1705–13.
6. Poddubnyy D, Hermann K-GA, Callhoff J, Listing J, Sieper J. Ustekinumab for the treatment of patients with active ankylosing spondylitis: results of a 28-week, prospective, open-label, proof-of-concept study (TOPAS). Ann Rheum Dis. 2014;73:817–23.
7. Wellcome Trust Case Control Consortium (WTCCC), Australo-Anglo-American Spondylitis Consortium (TASC), Burton PR, et al. Association scan of 14,500 nonsynonymous SNPs in four diseases identifies autoimmunity variants. Nat Genet. 2007;39:1329–37.
8. Kenna TJ, Davidson SI, Duan R, et al. Enrichmentof circulating interleukin-17-secreting interleukin-23 receptor-positive γ/δ T cells in patients with active ankylosing spondylitis. Arthritis Rheum. 2012;64:1420–9.
9. Colbert RA, Tran TM, Layh-Schmitt G. HLA-B27 misfolding and ankylosing spondylitis. Mol Immunol. 2014;57:44–51.
10. Ciccia FA, Accardo-Palumbo A, Rizzo A, et al. Evidence that autophagy, but not the unfolded protein response, regulates the expression of IL-23 in the gut of patients with ankylosing spondylitis and subclinical gut inflammation. Ann Rheum Dis. 2014;73:1566–74.
11. Zeng L, Lindstrom MJ, Smith JA. Ankylosing spondylitis macrophage production of higher levels of interleukin-23 in response to lipopolysaccharide without induction of a significant unfolded protein response. Arthritis Rheum. 2011;63:3807–17.
12. Zúñiga LA, Jain R, Haines C, Cua DJ. Th17 cell development: from the cradle to the grave. Immunol Rev. 2013;252:78–88.
13. McGeachy MJ, Chen Y, Tato CM, et al. The interleukin 23 receptor is essential for the terminal differentiation of interleukin17-producing effector T helper cells in vivo. Nat Immunol. 2009;10:314–24.
14. Yeremenko N, Paramarta JE, Baeten D. The interleukin-23/interleukin-17 immune axis as a promising new target in the treatment of spondyloarthritis. Curr Opin Rheumatol. 2014;26:361–70.
15. Smith JA, Colbert RA. Review: The interleukin-23/interleukin-17 axis in spondyloarthritis pathogenesis: Th17 and beyond. Arthritis Rheumatol. 2014;66:231–41.
16. Gagliardi MC, Teloni R, Mariotti S, et al. Endogenous PGE2 promotes the induction of human Th17 responses by fungal β-glucan. J Leukoc Biol. 2010;88:947–54.
17. Blackwell KA, Raisz LG, Pilbeam CC. Prostaglandins in bone: bad cop, good cop? Trends Endocrinol Metab. 2010;2:294–301.
18. Zhang J, Wang JH. Prostaglandin E2 (PGE2) exerts biphasic effects on human tendon stem cells. PLoS One. 2014;9:e87706.
19. van der Heijde D, Landewé R, Baraliakos X, et al. Radiographic findigs following two years of infliximab therapy in patients with ankylosing spondylitis. Arthritis Rheum. 2008;58:3063–70.
20. van der Heijde D, Landewé R, Einstein S, et al. Radiographic progression of ankylosing spondylitis after up to two years of treatment with etanercept. Arthritis Rheum. 2008;58:1324–31.
21. van der Heijde D, Salonen D, Weissman BN, et al. Assessment of radiographic progression in the spines of patients with ankylosing spondylitis treated with adalimumab for up 2 years. Arthrtis Res Ther. 2009;11:R127.
22. Wanders A, Dv H, Landewé R, et al. Nonsteroidal antiinflammatory drugs reduce radiographic progression in patients with ankylosing spondylitis: a randomized clinical trial. Arthritis Rheum. 2005;52:1756–65.
23. Poddubnyy D, Rudwaleit M, Haibel H, et al. Effect of non-steroidal anti-inflammatory drugs on radiographic spinal progression in patients with axial spondyloarthritis: results from the German Spondyloarthritis inception cohort. Ann Rheum Dis. 2012;71:1616–22.
24. Appel H, Maier R, Bleil J, et al. In situ analysis of interleukin-23- and interleukin-12-positive cells in the spine of patients with ankylosing spondylitis. Arthritis Rheum. 2013;65:1522–9.
25. Sherlock JP, Joyce-Shaikh B, Turner SP, et al. IL-23 induces spondyloarthropathy by acting on ROR-γt + CD3+ CD4–CD8– entheseal resident T cells. Nat Med. 2012;18:1069–76.
26. van der Linden S, Valkenburg HA, Cats A. Evaluation of diagnostic criteria for ankylosing spondylitis. A proposal for modification of the New York criteria. Arthritis Rheum. 1984;27:361–8.
27. van der Heijde SJ, Maksymowych WP, Dougados M, et al. Update of the international ASAS recommendations for the use of anti-TNF agents in patients with axial spondyloarthritis. Ann Rheum Dis. 2010;2011:905–8.
28. Sieper J, Rudwaleit M, Baraliakos X, et al. The Assessment of SpondyloArthritis international Society (ASAS) handbook: a guide to assess spondyloarthritis. Ann Rheum Dis. 2009;68 Suppl 2:ii1–44.
29. Dougados M, Simon P, Braun J, et al. ASAS recommendations for collecting, analysing and reporting NSAID intake in clinical trials/epidemiological studies in axial spondyloarthritis. Ann Rheum Dis. 2011;70:249–51.
30. Machado P, Landewé R, Lie E, et al. Ankylosing spondylitis disease activity score (ASDAS): defining cut-off values for disease activity states and improvement scores. Ann Rheum Dis. 2011;70:47–53.
31. Creemers MC, Franssen MJ, van't Hof MA, et al. Assessment of outcome in ankylosing spondylitis: an extended radiographic scoring system. Ann Rheum Dis. 2005;64:127–9.
32. Chen WS, Chang YS, Lin KC, et al. Association of serum interleukin-17 and interleukin-23 levels with disease activity in Chinese patients with ankylosing spondylitis. J Chin Med Assoc. 2012;75:303–8.
33. Wang X, Lin Z, Wei Q, Jiang Y, Gu J. Expression of IL-23 and IL-17 and effect of IL-23 on IL-17 production in ankylosing spondylitis. Rheumatol Int. 2009;29:1343–7.
34. Mei Y, Pan F, Gao J, et al. Increased serum IL-17 and IL-23 in the patient with ankylosing spondylitis. Clin Rheumatol. 2011;30:269–73.
35. Melis L, Vandooren B, Kruithof E, et al. Systemic levels of IL-23 are strongly associated with disease activity in rheumatoid arthritis but not spondyloarthritis. Ann Rheum Dis. 2010;69:618–23.
36. Sveaas SH, Berg IJ, Provan SA, et al. Circulating levels of inflammatory cytokines and cytokine receptors in patients with ankylosing spondylitis: a cross-sectional comparative study. Scand J Rheumatol. 2015;44:118–24.
37. Gaston JS, Goodall JC, Baeten D. Interleukin-23: a central cytokine in the pathogenesis of spondylarthritis. Arthritis Rheum. 2011;63:3668–71.
38. Ciccia F, Bombardieri M, Principato A, et al. Overexpression of interleukin-23, but not interleukin-17, as an immunologic signature of subclinical intestinal inflammation in ankylosing spondylitis. Arthritis Rheum. 2009;60:955–65.
39. Yoshida K, Oida H, Kobayashi T, et al. Stimulation of bone formation and prevention of bone loss by prostaglandin E EP4 receptor activation. Proc Natl Acad Sci U S A. 2002;99:4580–5.
40. Li M, Thompson DD, Paralkar VM. Prostaglandin E(2) receptors in bone formation. Int Orthop. 2007;31:767–72.
41. Chai W, Lian Z, Chen C, et al. JARID1A, JMY, and PTGER4 polymorphisms are related to ankylosing spondylitis in Chinese Han patients: a case-control study. PLoS One. 2013;19:e74794.
42. Cortes A, Maksymowych WP, Wordsworth BP, et al. Association study of genes related to bone formation and resorption and the extent of

radiographic change in ankylosing spondylitis. Ann Rheum Dis. 2015;74(7): 1387-93. doi: 10.1136/annrheumdis-2013-204835. Epub 2014 Mar 20.

43. Miossec P, Kolls JK. Targeting IL-17 and TH17 cells in chronic inflammation. Nat Rev Drug Discov. 2012;11:763–76.
44. Bowness P, Ridley A, Shaw J, et al. Th17 cells expressing KIR3DL2+ and responsive to HLA-B27 homodimers are increased in ankylosing spondylitis. J Immunol. 2011;186:2672–80.
45. Ramiro S, Stolwijk C, van Tubergen A, et al. Evolution of radiographic damage in ankylosing spondylitis: a 12 year prospective follow-up of the OASIS study. Ann Rheum Dis. 2015;74(1):52-9. doi:10.1136/annrheumdis-2013-204055. Epub 2013 Aug 16.
46. Baraliakos X, Listing J, von der Recke A, Braun J. The natural course of radiographic progression in ankylosing spondylitis—evidence for major individual variations in a large proportion of patients. J Rheumatol. 2009;36:997–1002.
47. Poddubnyy D, Haibel H, Listing J, et al. Baseline radiographic damage, elevated acute-phase reactant levels, and cigarette smoking status predict spinal radiographic progression in early axial spondylarthritis. Arthritis Rheum. 2012;64:1388–98.
48. Haroon N, Inman RD, Learch TJ, et al. The impact of tumor necrosis factor α inhibitors on radiographic progression in ankylosing spondylitis. Arthritis Rheum. 2013;65:2645–54.
49. Maksymowych WP. Spondyloarthritis. Treat-to-target in spondyloarthritis—do we have a plan? Nat Rev Rheumatol. 2013;9:507–8.
50. Smolen JS, Braun J, Dougados M, et al. Treating spondyloarthritis, including ankylosing spondylitis and psoriatic arthritis, to target: recommendations of an international task force. Ann Rheum Dis. 2014;73:6–16.

18

Perinatal characteristics, older siblings, and risk of ankylosing spondylitis: a case–control study based on national registers

Ulf Lindström[1*], Helena Forsblad-d'Elia[2], Johan Askling[3], Lars Erik Kristensen[4], Elisabeth Lie[1,5], Sofia Exarchou[6] and Lennart Jacobsson[1]

Abstract

Background: The effect of circumstances and exposures early in life on the risk of developing ankylosing spondylitis (AS) is largely unknown. The purpose of this study was to determine whether perinatal characteristics predict development of AS.

Methods: AS cases (n = 1960; 59 % men) were defined as listed with a diagnosis of AS at least once in the Swedish National Patient Register and registered in the Swedish Medical Birth Register (born ≥1973). Population controls were retrieved from the Swedish Population Register (n = 8378; mean 4.3 controls/case), matched on birth year, sex and county. Odds ratios (OR) for developing AS were determined through conditional logistic regression, with regard to: birth weight, birth order, season of birth, maternal age, gestational length, size for gestational age, type of birth, mode of delivery, congenital malformations, mothers' country of birth, mothers' civil status and size of delivery unit.

Results: In the univariate analyses statistically significant increases in risk for developing AS were observed for having older siblings (OR 1.18; 95 % CI 1.06–1.30). No association was observed for the remainder of analysed exposures, although there was a weak association with birth weight below 3000 g (OR 1.19; 95 % CI 1.04–1.37), though not for "low birth weight" <2500 g (OR 0.90; 95 % CI 0.70–1.16). The increase in risk associated with having older siblings was consistent in a multivariate analysis adjusting for possible confounders (OR 1.23; 95 % CI 1.09–1.39). The direction and magnitude of the point estimates were also consistent in several sensitivity analyses and when stratifying by sex.

Conclusions: Having older siblings was associated with an increased risk for developing AS. These results need to be repeated and confirmed in other cohorts.

Keywords: Ankylosing spondylitis, Epidemiology, Pathogenesis, Spondyloarthritis

Background

Ankylosing spondylitis (AS) is a chronic and progressive inflammatory disease with onset of symptoms before the age of 45 in the majority of cases, and an estimated 1.30–1.56 million prevalent cases in Europe [1, 2]. Other common inflammatory diseases, such as inflammatory bowel disease (IBD), psoriasis, and anterior uveitis are overrepresented in AS, suggesting shared aetiology [3]. The strong correlation between AS and the human leukocyte antigen (HLA) B27 has been extensively investigated [4–8]. Based on twin studies the majority of the susceptibility for AS can be attributed to genetic factors [3], but environmental factors are also likely to contribute to the risk [9, 10], a contribution that may differ depending on phenotype, sex, or age of onset. One proposed hypothesis states that infections may trigger the disease onset in genetically susceptible individuals [10], in similarity to the related disease reactive arthritis [11, 12]. Another hypothesis suggests that mechanical stress

* Correspondence: ulf.lindstrom@gu.se
[1]Department of Rheumatology and Inflammation Research, Institute of Medicine, Sahlgrenska Academy, University of Gothenburg, Guldhedsgatan 10A, 405 30 Gothenburg, Sweden
Full list of author information is available at the end of the article

at the entheses may initiate inflammation and bone remodelling [13]. However, so far the evidence supporting the role of specific environmental risk factors in the development of AS has been limited.

Number of siblings is often applied as a proxy for exposure to childhood infections and has been shown to affect the risk for developing immune-related diseases [14]. Studies have found an inverse relationship between sibship size and risk for allergic diseases, such as childhood asthma and eczema [15–17]. This has been attributed to the "hygiene hypothesis", postulating that an increased exposure to infections during childhood may lead to a lower risk for developing allergy [18]. Two previous studies, investigating the effect of birth order on the risk for developing AS have produced conflicting results [19, 20].

The relationship between exposures even earlier in life, such as factors influencing pregnancy and birth, and later development of disease has been established for diabetes and cardiovascular disease but it has also been implicated in several diseases characterised primarily by inflammation or autoimmunity [21]. Low birth weight has, for example, been associated with a decreased risk for later development of rheumatoid arthritis (RA), and high birth weight with an increased risk [22–24]. High birth weight may also be associated with an increased risk of Sjögren's syndrome [25]. Similarly, season of birth has also been shown to be associated with variations in the risk for subsequent development of certain diseases. For example, children born during autumn and winter months have been shown to have a higher risk for food allergy (suggested to be related to UVB exposure and vitamin D) [26, 27]. Other studies have also indicated a variation in the risk for development of IBD, depending on season or month of birth [28, 29].

No large population-controlled studies have been performed investigating how circumstances and exposures early in life affect the risk of developing AS. The overarching aim of this study was to assess the role of environmental factors, specifically pregnancy and perinatal characteristics, in the pathogenesis of AS, with particular focus on birth order, birth weight and season of birth.

Methods

Setting and data sources

This is a case–control study, based on the Swedish national health care and population registers.

The Swedish National Patient Register (NPR) was initiated in 1964, as an inpatient register collecting administrative and medical data, including diagnoses registered according to the Swedish version of the International Classification of Diseases (ICD) [30] codes at discharge from hospital. Since 1987 the coverage is considered to be close to 100 % [31]. In 2001 an outpatient register was added for outpatient specialized care. The coverage is lower, approximately 80 %, mostly due to missing data from private care [32]. The NPR is considered to have a very high validity in general [33]. Primary care visits are not included in the NPR.

The Swedish population register, managed by Statistics Sweden, contains data on residence, migration and socioeconomic factors for all residents [34].

The Swedish Medical Birth Register (MBR) was initiated in 1973 and includes administrative and medical data related to pregnancy, partum and postpartum neonatal care [35]. It is compulsory for all health care providers involved in prenatal maternity care, delivery or neonatal care to report to the register.

The Prescribed Drug Register contains data on all drugs prescribed in Sweden since July 2005, e.g. date prescribed/dispensed, dose and Anatomical Therapeutic Chemical code (ATC code [36]). The Anti-Rheumatic Therapy in Sweden (ARTIS) Register is a national treatment register, aimed at monitoring disease activity and outcome and safety of pharmacological treatment (including biological drugs) in rheumatic diseases. All public and private rheumatology clinics report to the register, which has an estimated national coverage of 85–95 % for patients treated with tumour necrosis factor inhibitors (TNFi) [37, 38].

All the registers include the individuals personal identification number (PIN), given to all residents in Sweden, enabling cross-linking of different registers [39].

In this study the NPR was used to identify the AS cases and to retrieve data on AS-related inflammatory diseases 1973–2009. Matched controls (see below) were obtained from the population register and data on perinatal characteristics from the MBR. Data on pharmacological treatment were retrieved from the Prescribed Drug Register and the ARTIS register. All ICD and ATC codes used are presented in supplementary Table S1 (Additional file 1).

Study population

AS cases were defined as all individuals registered in the MBR (born in Sweden ≥1973) who at least once up until 2009 had a visit listing an ICD code for AS (ICD-8: 712, 40, ICD-9: 720A, ICD-10: M45) registered in the NPR. We have previously performed a validation study of the AS diagnoses in the NPR and found good validity, with a positive predictive value of at least 80 % for fulfilling the modified New York criteria and 89–97 % fulfilling any of the commonly used classification criteria for spondyloarthritis (SpA) [40].

For each AS case five controls, matched on birth year, sex and county of residence (at the time of their first SpA diagnosis), were retrieved from the population register. Matching at the time of the first SpA diagnosis, rather than the first AS diagnosis, was chosen as the preferred method of matching since a number of cases were expected to first receive another SpA diagnosis before development and subsequent documentation of structural changes of the sacroiliac joints or spine, resulting in a diagnosis of AS. From the population register we also retrieved data on level of formal education and disposable income in 2008, which was used to compare socioeconomic status between cases and controls.

Data on AS-related disease manifestations, conventional synthetic disease-modifying anti-rheumatic drugs (csDMARDs) and TNFi were used for a stratification of disease severity for the AS cases in the sensitivity analyses: from the NPR we collected data on all registered visits to a non-primary care physician with an ICD code attributed to some of the AS-related inflammatory diseases (IBD, psoriasis, and anterior uveitis) for both cases and controls, from birth and up to 2 years after the first AS diagnosis for the index case (at the latest up until 31 December 2011). A 2-year lag period after the first diagnosis of AS was chosen to include patients diagnosed with IBD and psoriasis as a result of medical investigations initiated at the time of the first AS diagnosis.

For the AS cases data on pharmacological treatment, prescribed between 1 January 2011 and 31 December 2011, were obtained from the Prescribed Drug Register for the following csDMARDS: methotrexate and sulphasalazine; and for subcutaneously administered TNFi: etanercept, adalimumab, golimumab and certolizumab pegol. From the ARTIS we obtained data on registered treatment with infliximab for the same time period, since this intravenously administered TNFi is normally not prescribed through a pharmacy and thus not included in the Prescribed Drug Register.

Exposure data

Variables associated with birth characteristics were retrieved from the MBR. The variables assessed were: maternal age, mother's country of birth (Sweden, Nordic or other), mother's civil status (mother married or living with father of the child versus other situation, as recorded in the MBR), number of older siblings, season of birth, mode of delivery (caesarean/vaginal), type of birth (single/multiple), birth weight, birth length, gestational length, birth weight for gestational age [41], congenital malformations, and maternal smoking during pregnancy. In order to adjust for systematic errors arising from possible variations in practice between delivery units, a variable coding for size of delivery unit (based on number of deliveries in the MBR during the study period) was also included. The categories used in the analyses are presented in Table 2. Birth weight was defined as low birth weight <2500 g, normal birth weight 2500–4200 g and high birth weight ≥4300 g. Additional definitions, using alternative cutoffs, were also analysed: <3310 g, 3310–3725 g and ≥3726 g (tertiles) as well as <3000 g, 3000–3999 g and ≥4000 g (to enable comparisons with previous similar studies [24]). Data on a recorded diagnosis of diabetes, among the mothers prior or during the pregnancy, were also obtained from the MBR.

Statistics

Univariate odds ratios (ORs) were computed for the association between exposures (birth characteristics) and the outcome (a diagnosis of AS), by use of conditional logistic regression.

Birth weight and birth order were also assessed in a multivariate conditional logistic regression analysis, which also included possible confounders (gestational length, maternal age and type of birth (single/multiple)). Two measures of socioeconomic status (mother's country of birth and civil status) as well as size of the delivery unit were also included. Season of birth was not entered in the multivariate analysis as the univariate analysis did not reveal any sign of association to development of AS.

The univariate and the main multivariate analyses were also stratified by sex and by birth year above or below the median.

Four sensitivity analyses, essentially subset analyses, were performed, using the same multivariate model as described above. First, excluding all cases and controls with a diagnosis of psoriasis, anterior uveitis, or IBD before or within 2 years after the first AS diagnosis of the index case (excluding 26 % of the entire study population). Second, restricting the analyses to only include cases treated with methotrexate, sulphasalazine, or TNFi during the last year of data collection (2011), limiting the analyses to a presumably more severe subgroup of AS (excluding 64 % of the entire study population). Third, limiting the analysis only to the cases who had received their AS diagnosis at least once from a specialist in rheumatology or internal medicine (excluding 27 % of the entire study population). Fourth, limiting the analysis only to cases who had received an AS diagnosis at least once in outpatient specialized care 2001–2009 (excluding 7 % of the entire study population). An additional analysis, based on only cases and controls still living in their county of birth at the time point of matching, was also performed to minimize the possible influence of migration between regions with different prevalences of ankylosing spondylitis.

Level of formal education and disposable income in 2008 were compared between cases and controls. Level of formal education was categorized as ≤9, 10–12 and >12 years of schooling and compared using a chi-square test. Disposable income in 2008 was only assessed for those ≥30 years old in 2008, an age when most individuals are assumed to have finalized their formal education, and in order to avoid extreme outliers we only included the 0.5^{th} to the 99.5^{th} percentile. Comparison of disposable income was performed using the *t* test. Comparisons of the proportion of mothers with diabetes, between cases and controls, were performed based on Fisher's exact test.

SAS version 9.3 for Windows (SAS Institute, Cary, NC, USA) was used for aggregation of the data, and SPSS version 21 for Windows (IBM Corp., Armonk, NY, USA) was used for the statistical analyses.

Ethical approval

The study was approved by the regional ethics committee in Stockholm, Sweden, 9 September 2011 (number: 2011/29-31/1) and conducted in compliance with the Declaration of Helsinki. Informed consent from individual patients/controls was not required.

Results

Cases and controls

We identified 1960 AS cases (59 % men) and 8377 matched population controls, included in the MBR (born in Sweden after 1972). A total of 95 % of the cases had ≥3 matched controls. Median age at inclusion (matched at first SpA diagnosis) was 25 years (25th-percentile = 20; 75th percentile = 28). Demographics, pharmacological treatment, AS-related inflammatory diseases and level of formal education and disposable income in 2008 are presented in Table 1. No statistically significant difference was observed between cases and controls with respect to level of formal education, disposable income or maternal diabetes prior or during pregnancy.

Table 1 Characteristics of the 1960 cases with ankylosing spondylitis and the 8377 matched population controls

Demographics	Cases n = 1960	Controls n = 8377
Women (%)	801 (41)	346 (41)
Year of birth median (Q1,Q3)	1979 (1975, 1984)	1979 (1975, 1984)
Age at first AS diagnosis median (Q1, Q3)	27 (22, 30)	NA
Living in same county at time of matching and at birth	1299 (66)	5571 (67)
AS-related inflammatory diseases[a]		
Anterior uveitis (%)	337 (17)	22 (0)
Inflammatory bowel disease (%)	108 (6)	58 (1)
Psoriasis (%)	89 (5)	49 (1)
Any of the manifestations above (%)	496 (25)	127 (2)
Rheumatic diagnoses before first AS diagnosis[b]		
Spondyloarthritis diagnosis[c]	627 (32)	NA
Any rheumatic diagnosis[d]	630 (32)	NA
Pharmacological treatment in 2011[e]		
TNF-alpha inhibitor (%)	494 (25)	NA
Methotrexate (%)	161 (8)	NA
Sulphasalazine (%)	217 (11)	NA
Any of the treatments above (%)	700 (36)	NA
Years of formal of education in 2008[f]		
0–9 years	309 (16)	1160 (14)
10–12 years	880 (45)	3705 (44)
>12 years	679 (35)	2993 (36)
Disposable income in 2008 £ mean (SD)[g]	16378 (6797)	16768 (7050)
Maternal diabetes (%)[h]	12 (0.6)	36 (0.4)

AS ankylosing spondylitis. *NA* no data available, *TNF* tumour necrosis factor
[a]AS-related inflammatory diseases are given as cumulative incidence until 2 years after first AS diagnosis for the cases and their matched controls
[b]Rheumatic diagnoses before first AS diagnosis are based on ICD codes in the National Patient Register
[c]Psoriatic arthritis, undifferentiated spondyloarthritis, reactive arthritis and spondyloarthritis associated with inflammatory bowel disease
[d]Any rheumatic disease, see Table S1 in Additional file 1
[e]Pharmacological treatment is based on data in the Prescribed Drug Register for prescriptions during 2011, or in the case of infliximab recoded in the Anti-Rheumatic Therapy in Sweden (ARTIS) register as used during 2011
[f]No statistically significant difference in level of formal education based on chi-square test ($p = 0.115$)
[g]Limited to those ≥30 years old in 2008 and the 0.5^{th} to the 99.5^{th} percentiles (cases = 953; controls = 3977), no statistically significant difference based on *t* test ($p = 0.125$)
[h]Maternal diabetes prior or during pregnancy, as recorded in the Medical Birth Register. No statistically significant difference based on Fisher's exact test ($p = 0.271$)

Univariate analyses

In the univariate analyses a statistically significant association with AS (Table 2) was observed for having older siblings (OR 1.18; 95 % confidence interval (CI) 1.06–1.30). There was no association between season of birth, or birth weight defined as <2500/2500–4200/≥4200 grams, and risk of AS. Categorizing birth weight according to previous similar studies [24] resulted in a weak but significant association for a birth weight <3000 g (OR 1.19; 95 % CI 1.04–1.37; 3000–4000 g: reference; >4000 g: OR 1.04; 95 % CI 0.91–1.19) and categorizing into tertiles resulted in similar, but non-significant point estimates (<3310 g: OR 1.11; 95 % CI 0.99–1.25; 3310–3725 g: reference; >3725 g: OR 1.03 95 % CI 0.91–1.65). For the remainder of the analysed variables there were no statistically significant associations with the outcome of developing AS, although the point estimate for multiple births (OR 1.35; 95 % CI 0.95–1.90) indicated an association, but based on very few events (men = 27 (2.3 %), women = 17 (2.1 %)). Further analysis of multiple births revealed that it was associated with development of AS only for men (OR 1.80; 95 % CI 1.14–2.84) and not for women (OR 0.95; 95 % CI 0.55–1.63). Due to lack of a unique identifier for the mothers, our data did not permit us to identify cases or controls belonging to the same multiple birth (e.g. twins), but eight possible

Table 2 Birth characteristics for ankylosing spondylitis compared to matched population controls, with univariate odds ratios

	Cases (%) (n = 1960)	Controls (%) (n = 8377)	OR (95 % CI)
Maternal age, years			
<25	643 (33)	2676 (32)	1.04 (0.92 to 1.17)
25–29	729 (37)	3156 (38)	1 (reference)
30–34	419 (21)	1815 (22)	1.00 (0.87 to 1.14)
35+	169 (9)	730 (9)	1.01 (0.84 to 1.21)
Missing	0	0	
Mothers' civil status			
Mother married or living with father of the child	1322 (67)	5753 (67)	1 (reference)
Other	463 (24)	1896 (23)	1.06 (0.94 to 1.21)
Missing	175 (9)	728 (9)	
Mothers' country of birth			
Sweden	1762 (90)	7550 (90)	1 (reference)
Nordic	107 (6)	385 (5)	1.17 (0.93 to 1.47)
Other	91 (5)	442 (5)	0.81 (0.64 to 1.03)
Missing	0	0	
Number of older siblings			
0	750 (38)	3550 (42)	1 (reference)
≥1	1210 (62)	4827 (58)	1.18 (1.06 to 1.30)
Missing	0	0	
Type of birth			
Singletons	1916 (98)	8236 (98)	1 (reference)
Multiple birth	44 (2)	141 (2)	1.35 (0.95 to 1.90)
Missing	0	0	
Mode of delivery			
Vaginal	1742 (89)	7544 (90)	1 (reference)
Caesarean	218 (11)	833 (10)	1.14 (0.97 to 1.33)
Missing	0	0	
Season of birth			
March-May	568 (29)	2354 (28)	1 (reference)
June-August	473 (24)	2073 (25)	0.95 (0.83 to 1.09)
September-November	416 (21)	1969 (24)	0.87 (0.76 to 1.00)
December-February	503 (26)	1981 (24)	1.04 (0.91 to 1.19)
Missing	0	0	
Birth weight, g			
<2500	76 (4)	355 (4)	0.90 (0.70 to 1.16)
2500–4200	1764 (90)	7476 (89)	1 (reference)
≥4200	113 (6)	536 (6)	0.90 (0.73 to 1.11)
Missing	7 (0)	10 (0)	
Gestational length, days			
≤258	111 (6)	455 (5)	1.02 (0.82 to 1.27)
259–293	1611 (82)	6846 (82)	1 (reference)
≥294	196 (10)	915 (11)	0.92 (0.78 to 1.08)
Missing	42 (2)	161 (2)	
Birth weight for gestational age[a]			
Small for gestational age	66 (3)	316 (4)	0.89 (0.68 to 1.17)
Appropriate for gestational age	1788 (91)	7652 (91)	1 (reference)
Large for gestational age	49 (3)	227 (3)	0.95 (0.69 to 1.31)
Missing	57 (3)	183 (2)	
Congenital malformation			
No	1829 (93)	7760 (93)	1 (reference)
Yes	75 (4)	354 (4)	0.90 (0.70 to 1.17)
Missing	57 (3)	182 (2)	
Size of delivery unit (no of births ≥1973)			
≥300	484 (25)	2087 (25)	0.91 (0.76 to 1.09)
200–299	581 (30)	2502 (30)	0.92 (0.78 to 1.09)
100–199	598 (31)	2471 (30)	1 (reference)
<100	297 (15)	1317 (16)	0.93 (0.77 to 1.13)
Maternal smoking[b]			
Not smoking during pregnancy	170 (9)	769 (9)	1 (reference)
Smoking during pregnancy	440 (22)	1896 (23)	0.96 (0.78 to 1.17)
Missing	1350 (69)	5713 (68)	

Odds ratios (ORs) determined through conditional logistic regression analyses
[a]Multiple births excluded since reference intervals are not applicable
[b]Only available from 1982, when recording of maternal smoking was initiated

twin pairs (born on the same day, at the same delivery unit) were identified, with no unexpected preponderance for either cases or controls. There was no association between maternal smoking and development of AS (OR 0.96; 95 % CI 0.78–1.17), although this was only available in cases born 1982 and later and in a total for 31 % of the cases. No interactions were observed between maternal smoking and birth weight or having older siblings.

Multivariate analyses

The main multivariate analysis (Fig. 1) confirmed the associations observed in the univariate analyses. The ORs for being diagnosed with AS compared to controls were 1.23 (95 % CI 1.09–1.39) for having older siblings versus not. The ORs for birth weight were also similar in the

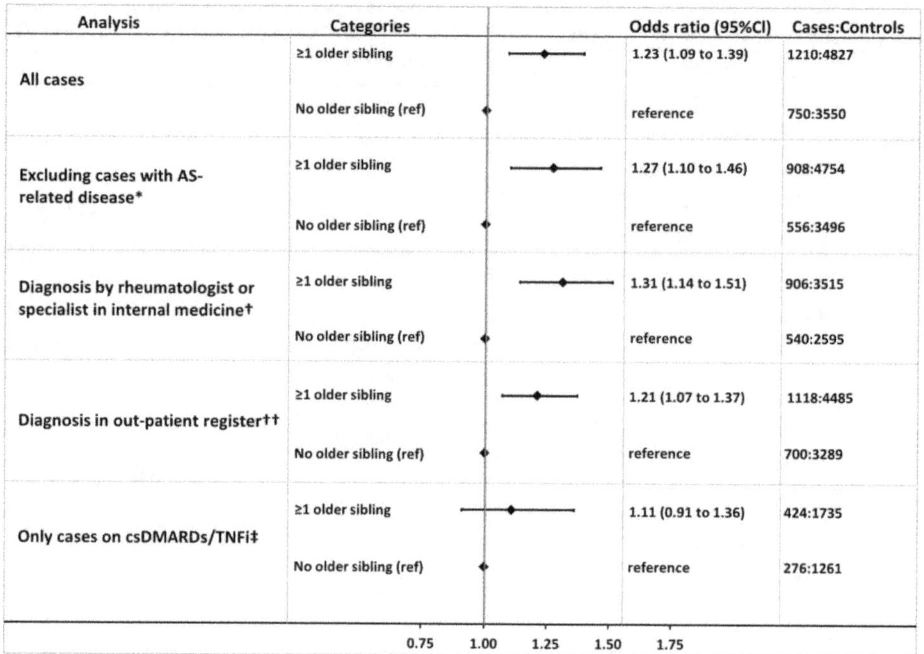

Fig. 1 Odds ratios for developing ankylosing spondylitis with regard to having older siblings. Forest plot presenting odds ratios with 95 % confidence intervals for being diagnosed with ankylosing spondylitis, with regard to having older siblings, in a multivariate conditional logistic regression analysis and four sensitivity analyses. All the analyses were adjusted for birth weight, having older siblings, mother's birth country, mother's civil status, maternal age, gestational length, type of birth (single/multiple) and size of delivery unit. *All cases with an ICD code for psoriasis, anterior uveitis or inflammatory bowel disease before or within 2 years of their AS diagnosis, and their respective controls are excluded. †Including only cases, with their respective controls, who had received ≥1 AS diagnosis at a clinic of rheumatology or internal medicine. ††Including only cases with their respective controls who had received ≥1 AS diagnosis in the outpatient register 2001–2011. ‡Including only cases, with respective controls who were treated with csDMARDs (methotrexate and sulphasalazine) and/or TNFi during any part of 2011. *AS* ankylosing spondylitis, *csDMARDs* conventional synthetic disease-modifying anti-rheumatic drugs, *ICD* International Classification of Diseases, *TNFi* tumour necrosis factor inhibitor

multivariate analysis, compared to the univariate. None of the other exposures in the multivariate analysis were significantly associated with the development of AS and no point estimates except for multiple births (OR 1.25; 95 % CI 0.84–1.84) indicated a possible association.

Sensitivity analyses

Overall, the OR for having older siblings was similar in all sensitivity analyses (Fig. 1), to those in the main analyses. Stratifying the univariate and multivariate analyses by sex and median birth year resulted in overall similar point estimates as in the stratified univariate analyses, supplementary Table S2 (Additional file 2). Multivariate analysis, only including cases and controls still living in their birth county, at the time of matching, revealed no important differences to the main analysis.

Discussion

Principal findings

In this study having older siblings was associated with an increased risk of receiving a diagnosis of AS. There was also a weak increase in risk associated with a birth weight <3000 g, which could not be confirmed in our primary stratifications of birth weight. We found no association between, season of birth, type of birth, mode of delivery, congenital malformations, gestational length or maternal age, and later being diagnosed with AS.

Comparison to previous studies

Birth weight has to our knowledge not been studied as a risk factor for being diagnosed with AS. For IBD, which is associated with AS, one case–control study indicated that cases developing IBD had significantly lower birth weight compared to controls [42], which in that study was probably related to a significantly higher frequency of preterm birth. In our study there was no association between neither birth weight nor gestational length and development of AS in the univariate or any of the multivariate analyses, using the definition for low birth weight set by the World Health Association [43]. However, when using the alternative stratification of birth weight (<3000 g, 3000–4000 g, >4000 g), there was a slight increase in risk for birth weight <3000 g, and similarly so when birth weight was categorized into tertiles. This suggests differences in the distribution of birth weight between those later developing AS compared to controls, although the biological importance of this difference is unclear. Birth weight, in itself, is influenced by a multitude of factors, including gestational length, maternal nutrition [44], maternal diabetes [45], exposure to toxins such as maternal smoking [46], maternal age, sex of the child, socioeconomic status, and birth order [47, 48]. Adjusting for maternal age, gestational length, birth order, civil status of the mothers and type of birth, in the multivariate analyses did not affect the point estimates for birth weight. Maternal diabetes was not linked to the risk of AS in the offspring.

Low birth order was, in a previous study comparing 162 AS cases with their healthy siblings, a risk factor for developing AS [19]. In contrast to this a much larger register-based study of AS cases (4517 patients in the Bath AS register), investigating the position of birth within the family found no statistically significant effect of birth order on the risk of developing AS [20]. Due to their methodology, both of these studies only examined families with more than one child, in order to assess the effect of birth order. In our national case–control study, also including cases without siblings, having older siblings was significantly associated with an increased risk of later receiving a diagnosis of AS. Studies of IBD have indicated that having older siblings may be associated with an increased risk for ulcerative colitis, while having younger siblings may be associated with a decrease in risk for Crohn's disease [49], although results are conflicting [50]. In previous studies, it has been shown that having older siblings constitute a risk for exposure to infections at a very young age [16], and it has been argued that having younger sibling may constitute a risk for exposure to infections during the later years of childhood [14]. In our study the available data did not allow us to assess the effect of having younger siblings. For the related disease – reactive arthritis – the direct pathogenic and temporal association with infectious diseases is well known [11, 12], and for IBD exposure to enteric infections is known to affect the risk of developing both Crohn's disease and ulcerative colitis [50, 51]. Considering the conflicting results concerning the effect of birth order on the risk for developing AS in the current and the two previous studies [19, 20], further studies are needed, preferably also including information regarding type, frequency and severity of infections.

Limitations and strengths of this study

Some limitations should be considered. First, misclassification of cases may be a problem when using health care registers for identification. Previous validation studies performed by our group have, however, demonstrated high validity for ICD codes for AS in the Swedish registers [40]. Furthermore, the proportion of men and women and the frequency of treatment with TNFi were very similar to that found in previous clinical studies on AS in Sweden [52], and the frequencies of IBD, psoriasis and anterior uveitis were also similar to other AS cohorts [53] (although the gender distribution was more equal than in some other cohorts [1, 53], which may to some extent be due to the inclusion of cases with non-radiographic axial SpA in the AS group, as indicated in the validation study [40]), supporting the validity of the case identification. Second, residual or unmeasured confounding could be an issue in all observational studies. We were able to adjust for socioeconomic status to some extent in our main multivariate analysis, and there was no statistically significant difference in level of formal education and disposable income in 2008 between cases and controls. However, other important factors, such as the family income at birth, mother's body mass index (BMI) and the parent's health status (e.g. ankylosing spondylitis), could not be taken into account in the analyses. Third, maternal smoking was only available for 32 % of the cases and during a limited time period. In itself it did not affect the risk of developing AS in the univariate analyses, but due to the limitations in the available data it could not be included in the multivariate analysis. Since smoking is known to be related to both low birth weight [46] and to predict radiographic progression in AS [54] the effect of maternal smoking, or exposure to smoking during childhood, on the risk for developing AS needs to be studied further. Fourth, due to the limited time frame of the study, patients with a long diagnostic delay would not be identified and included as cases [40, 55]. Fifth, using birth order as a possible proxy for childhood infections is inferior to directly recording actual infectious events, which was not possible for the cases/controls in this study.

Our study also has several strengths. First, this is the only study of this research question in AS comparing cases to population controls. Second, it is based on national health care registers, capturing the vast majority of AS cases in Sweden [56], which resulted in relatively large numbers and few missing data for most variables and therefore greater generalizability. This also decreases the risk of selection bias, which may have influenced the results in the previous studies of the effect of birth order on the risk for AS [19, 20]. Third, the consistent magnitudes and directions of the point estimates in the sensitivity analyses suggest that our results were reasonably robust.

Conclusions

Our results point to environmental factors as possible predictors for development of AS. More specifically, we found that having older siblings increased the risk for a

later diagnosis of AS, indicating that factors related to childhood exposure may be of importance in the disease pathogenesis.

Abbreviations

ARTIS: Anti-rheumatic Therapy in Sweden; AS: Ankylosing spondylitis; ATC: Anatomical Therapeutic Chemical; CI: Confidence interval; csDMARDs: Conventional synthetic disease-modifying anti-rheumatic drugs; HLA: Human leukocyte antigen; IBD: Inflammatory bowel disease; ICD: International Classification of Diseases; MBR: Medical Birth Register; NPR: National Patient Register; OR: Odds ratio; PIN: Personal identification number; RA: Rheumatoid arthritis; SpA: Spondyloarthritis; TNFi: Tumour necrosis factor alpha inhibitor.

Competing interests

All authors have completed the Unified Competing Interest form at www.icmje.org/coi_disclosure.pdf (available on request from the corresponding author) and declare that (1) authors have no support from companies for the submitted work; (2) EL has received personal fees from Abbvie, Bristol-Myers Squibb, Hospira and Pfizer (outside the submitted work) and JA and the ARTIS Study Group have or have had agreements with AstraZenica, Pfizer, UCB, Roche, Merck, BMS and Abbvie, outside the submitted work , in the previous 3 years; (3) their spouses, partners, or children have no financial relationships that may be relevant to the submitted work; and (4) authors have no non-financial interests that may be relevant to the submitted work.

EL has received personal fees from AbbVie, personal fees from Bristol-Myers Squibb, personal fees from Hospira, personal fees from Pfizer, personal fees from UCB (outside the submitted work). JA and the ARTIS Study Group have or have had agreements with: AstraZeneca, Pfizer, UCB, Roche, Merck, BMS and Abbvie (outside the submitted work). UL, SE, HF, LEK, and LJ declare that they have no competing interests.

Authors' contributions

All authors have contributed substantially in the process of completing this study and had full access to the data, specified as follows: LJ and JA contributed to the conception and design of the study, as well as interpretation of data and revising the manuscript, LJ also contributed to drafting the manuscript. UL contributed to design, data managing, data analysis/interpretation and writing the manuscript. EL contributed to analysis of data and interpretation of results, as well as revising the manuscript. HF, SE and LEK contributed to design, interpretation of data, drafting and revising the manuscript. All authors have approved the manuscript and agree to be accountable.

Funding

Funding for the study was received from the following sources, which did not influence either the design of the study, the collection and analysis of the data or the preparation of the manuscript: The Swedish Research Council, the Region Västra Götaland (agreement concerning research and education of medical students between the Swedish government and the university hospitals) (HF, LJ, UL, SE, EL), the Stockholm County Council (ALF) (JA), The Swedish National Rheumatism Association (LJ) and the Swedish Foundation for Strategic Research (JA). All researchers assigned as authors state their complete independence from the funders, with regard to this study.

Author details

[1]Department of Rheumatology and Inflammation Research, Institute of Medicine, Sahlgrenska Academy, University of Gothenburg, Guldhedsgatan 10A, 405 30 Gothenburg, Sweden. [2]Institution of Public Health and Clinical Medicine/Rheumatology, Umeå University, Lasarettsgatan 7, 901 87 Umeå, Sweden. [3]Rheumatology Unit and Clinical Epidemiology Unit, Department of Medicine Solna, Karolinska Institutet, Nobels väg 5, Solna 171 76 Stockholm, Sweden. [4]The Parker Institute, Department of Rheumatology, Frederiksberg and Bispebjerg Hospital, Nordre Fasanvej 57, 2000 Frederiksberg, Denmark. [5]Department of Rheumatology, Diakonhjemmet Hospital, Diakonveien 14, Vinderen, 0319 Oslo, Norway. [6]Section of Rheumatology, Department of Clinical Sciences, Lund University, Barngatan 2B, 221 85 Lund, Sweden.

References

1. Braun J, Sieper J. Ankylosing spondylitis. Lancet. 2007;369:1379–90. doi:10.1016/s0140-6736(07)60635-7.
2. Dean LE, Jones GT, MacDonald AG, Downham C, Sturrock RD, Macfarlane GJ. Global prevalence of ankylosing spondylitis. Rheumatology (Oxford). 2014;53:650–7. doi:10.1093/rheumatology/ket387.
3. Reveille JD. The genetic basis of spondyloarthritis. Ann Rheum Dis. 2011;Suppl 1:i44–50. doi:10.1136/ard.2010.140574.
4. Brewerton DA, Hart FD, Nicholls A, Caffrey M, James DC, Sturrock RD. Ankylosing spondylitis and HL-A 27. Lancet. 1973;1:904–7.
5. Calin A, Fries JF. Striking prevalence of ankylosing spondylitis in "healthy" w27 positive males and females. N Engl J Med. 1975;293:835–9. doi:10.1056/NEJM197510232931701.
6. Cohen LM, Mittal KK, Schmid FR, Rogers LF, Cohen KL. Increased risk for spondylitis stigmata in apparently healthy HL-AW27 men. Ann Intern Med. 1976;84:1–7.
7. Christiansen FT, Hawkins BR, Dawkins RL, Owen ET, Potter RM. The prevalence of ankylosing spondylitis among B27 positive normal individuals–a reassessment. J Rheumatol. 1979;6:713–8.
8. van der Linden SM, Valkenburg HA, de Jongh BM, Cats A. The risk of developing ankylosing spondylitis in HLA-B27 positive individuals. A comparison of relatives of spondylitis patients with the general population. Arthritis Rheum. 1984;27:241–9.
9. Brown MA, Kennedy LG, MacGregor AJ, Darke C, Duncan E, Shatford JL, et al. Susceptibility to ankylosing spondylitis in twins: the role of genes, HLA, and the environment. Arthritis Rheum. 1997;40:1823–8. doi:10.1002/1529-0131(199710)40:10<1823::AID-ART15>3.0.CO;2-1.
10. Tam LS, Gu J, Yu D. Pathogenesis of ankylosing spondylitis. Nat Rev Rheumatol. 2010;6:399–405. doi:10.1038/nrrheum.2010.79.
11. Hannu T, Kauppi M, Tuomala M, Laaksonen I, Klemets P, Kuusi M. Reactive arthritis following an outbreak of Campylobacter jejuni infection. J Rheumatol. 2004;31:528–30.
12. Keat AC, Thomas BJ, Taylor-Robinson D, Pegrum GD, Maini RN, Scott JT. Evidence of Chlamydia trachomatis infection in sexually acquired reactive arthritis. Ann Rheum Dis. 1980;39:431–7.
13. Benjamin M, Toumi H, Suzuki D, Redman S, Emery P, McGonagle D. Microdamage and altered vascularity at the enthesis-bone interface provides an anatomic explanation for bone involvement in the HLA-B27-associated spondylarthritides and allied disorders. Arthritis Rheum. 2007;56: 224–33. doi:10.1002/art.22290.
14. Altieri A, Castro F, Bermejo JL, Hemminki K. Association between number of siblings and nervous system tumors suggests an infectious etiology. Neurology. 2006;67:1979–83. doi:10.1212/01.wnl.0000247036.98444.38.
15. Strachan DP. Hay fever, hygiene, and household size. BMJ. 1989;299:1259–60.
16. Strachan DP, Taylor EM, Carpenter RG. Family structure, neonatal infection, and hay fever in adolescence. Arch Dis Child. 1996;74:422–6.
17. Kinra S, Davey Smith G, Jeffreys M, Gunnell D, Galobardes B, McCarron P. Association between sibship size and allergic diseases in the Glasgow Alumni Study. Thorax. 2006;61:48–53. doi:10.1136/thx. 2004.034595.
18. Strachan DP, Ait-Khaled N, Foliaki S, Mallol J, Odhiambo J, Pearce N, et al. Siblings, asthma, rhinoconjunctivitis and eczema: a worldwide perspective from the International Study of Asthma and Allergies in Childhood. Clin Exp Allergy. 2015;45:126–36. doi:10.1111/cea.12349.
19. Baudoin P, van der Horst-Bruinsma IE, Dekker-Saeys AJ, Weinreich S, Bezemer PD, Dijkmans BA. Increased risk of developing ankylosing spondylitis among first-born children. Arthritis Rheum. 2000;43:2818–22. doi:10.1002/1529-0131(200012)43:12<2818::aid-anr23>3.0.co;2-f.
20. Brophy S, Taylor G, Calin A. Birth order and ankylosing spondylitis: no increased risk of developing ankylosing spondylitis among first-born children. J Rheumatol. 2002;29:527–9.

21. Barker DJ, Eriksson JG, Forsen T, Osmond C. Fetal origins of adult disease: strength of effects and biological basis. Int J Epidemiol. 2002;31:1235–9.
22. Mandl LA, Costenbader KH, Simard JF, Karlson EW. Is birthweight associated with risk of rheumatoid arthritis? Data from a large cohort study. Ann Rheum Dis. 2009;68:514–8. doi:10.1136/ard.2007.080937.
23. Jacobsson LT, Jacobsson ME, Askling J, Knowler WC. Perinatal characteristics and risk of rheumatoid arthritis. BMJ. 2003;326:1068–9. doi:10.1136/bmj.326.7398.1068.
24. Carlens C, Jacobsson L, Brandt L, Cnattingius S, Stephansson O, Askling J. Perinatal characteristics, early life infections and later risk of rheumatoid arthritis and juvenile idiopathic arthritis. Ann Rheum Dis. 2009;68:1159–64. doi:10.1136/ard.2008.089342.
25. Mostafavi B, Akyuz S, Jacobsson ME, Nilsen LV, Theander E, Jacobsson LH. Perinatal characteristics and risk of developing primary Sjogren's syndrome: a case–control study. J Rheumatol. 2005;32:665–8.
26. Vassallo MF, Banerji A, Rudders SA, Clark S, Mullins RJ, Camargo Jr CA. Season of birth and food allergy in children. Ann Allergy Asthma Immunol. 2010;104:307–13. doi:10.1016/j.anai.2010.01.019.
27. Mullins RJ, Clark S, Katelaris C, Smith V, Solley G, Camargo Jr CA. Season of birth and childhood food allergy in Australia. Pediatr Allergy Immunol. 2011; 22:583–9. doi:10.1111/j.1399-3038.2011.01151.x.
28. Van Ranst M, Joossens M, Joossens S, Van Steen K, Pierik M, Vermeire S, et al. Crohn's disease and month of birth. Inflamm Bowel Dis. 2005;11:597–9.
29. Shaw SY, Nugent Z, Targownik LE, Singh H, Blanchard JF, Bernstein CN. Association between spring season of birth and Crohn's disease. Clin Gastroenterol Hepatol. 2014;12:277–82. doi:10.1016/j.cgh.2013.07.028.
30. Socialstyrelsen. Internationell statistisk klassifikation av sjukdomar och relaterade hälsoproblem. (Swedish version of International Classification of Diseases and Related Health Problems, Tenth Revision). 2011. http://www.socialstyrelsen.se/klassificeringochkoder/diagnoskodericd-10. Access date Nov 2014.
31. Socialstyrelsen. Inpatient diseases in Sweden 1987–2009. 2009. https://www.socialstyrelsen.se/Lists/Artikelkatalog/Attachments/18152/2010-10-20.pdf. Access date Nov 2014.
32. Socialstyrelsen. Kodningskvalitet i patientregistret. (Quality of coding in the patient register). 2013. http://www.socialstyrelsen.se/publikationer2013/2013-3-10. Access date Nov 2014.
33. Ludvigsson JF, Andersson E, Ekbom A, Feychting M, Kim JL, Reuterwall C, et al. External review and validation of the Swedish national inpatient register. BMC Public Health. 2011;11:450. doi:10.1186/1471-2458-11-450.
34. Statistiska Centralbyrån (Statistics Sweden). http://www.scb.se/en_/. Accessed November 2013.
35. The Swedish Medical Birth Register. Socialstyrelsen. http://www.socialstyrelsen.se/register/halsodataregister/medicinskafodelseregistret/inenglish. Accessed August 2014.
36. World Health Organization: Collaborating Centre for Drug Statistics Methodology. http://www.whocc.no/. Accessed November 2013.
37. Wadstrom H, Eriksson JK, Neovius M, Askling J. How good is the coverage and how accurate are exposure data in the Swedish Biologics Register (ARTIS)? Scand J Rheumatol. 2015;44:22–8. doi:10.3109/03009742.2014.927918.
38. Neovius M, Simard J, Sundstrom A, Jacobsson L, Geborek P, Saxne T, et al. Generalisability of clinical registers used for drug safety and comparative effectiveness research: coverage of the Swedish Biologics Register. Ann Rheum Dis. 2011;70:516–9. doi:10.1136/ard.2010.130914.
39. Ludvigsson JF, Otterblad-Olausson P, Pettersson BU, Ekbom A. The Swedish personal identity number: possibilities and pitfalls in healthcare and medical research. Eur J Epidemiol. 2009;24:659–67. doi:10.1007/s10654-009-9350-y.
40. Lindstrom U, Exarchou S, Sigurdardottir V, Sundstrom B, Askling J, Eriksson JK, et al. Validity of ankylosing spondylitis and undifferentiated spondyloarthritis diagnoses in the Swedish National Patient Register. Scand J Rheumatol. 2015;44:369–76. doi:10.3109/03009742.2015.1010572.
41. Marsal K, Persson PH, Larsen T, Lilja H, Selbing A, Sultan B. Intrauterine growth curves based on ultrasonically estimated foetal weights. Acta Paediatr. 1996;85:843–8.
42. Sonntag B, Stolze B, Heinecke A, Luegering A, Heidemann J, Lebiedz P, et al. Preterm birth but not mode of delivery is associated with an increased risk of developing inflammatory bowel disease later in life. Inflamm Bowel Dis. 2007;13:1385–90. doi:10.1002/ibd.20206.
43. World Health Organization: Low birthweight. Country, regional and global estimates. 2004. http://www.who.int/reproductivehealth/publications/monitoring/9280638327/en/. Accessed November 2015.
44. Wu G, Bazer FW, Cudd TA, Meininger CJ, Spencer TE. Maternal nutrition and fetal development. J Nutr. 2004;134:2169–72.
45. Metzger BE, Lowe LP, Dyer AR, Trimble ER, Chaovarindr U, Coustan DR, et al. Hyperglycemia and adverse pregnancy outcomes. N Engl J Med. 2008;358: 1991–2002. doi:10.1056/NEJMoa0707943.
46. Bernstein IM, Plociennik K, Stahle S, Badger GJ, Secker-Walker R. Impact of maternal cigarette smoking on fetal growth and body composition. Am J Obstet Gynecol. 2000;183:883–6. doi:10.1067/mob.2000.109103.
47. Swamy GK, Edwards S, Gelfand A, James SA, Miranda ML. Maternal age, birth order, and race: differential effects on birthweight. J Epidemiol Community Health. 2012;66:136–42. doi:10.1136/jech.2009.088567.
48. Kramer MS. Determinants of low birth weight: methodological assessment and meta-analysis. Bull World Health Organ. 1987;65:663–737.
49. Montgomery SM, Lambe M, Wakefield AJ, Pounder RE, Ekbom A. Siblings and the risk of inflammatory bowel disease. Scand J Gastroenterol. 2002;37:1301–8.
50. Frolkis A, Dieleman LA, Barkema HW, Panaccione R, Ghosh S, Fedorak RN, et al. Environment and the inflammatory bowel diseases. Can J Gastroenterol. 2013;27:e18–24.
51. Ng SC, Tang W, Leong RW, Chen M, Ko Y, Studd C, et al. Environmental risk factors in inflammatory bowel disease: a population-based case–control study in Asia-Pacific. Gut. 2015;64:1063–71. doi:10.1136/gutjnl-2014-307410.
52. Forsblad-d'Elia H, Wallberg H, Klingberg E, Carlsten H, Bergfeldt L. Cardiac conduction system abnormalities in ankylosing spondylitis: a cross-sectional study. BMC Musculoskelet Disord. 2013;14:237. doi:10.1186/1471-2474-14-237.
53. Rudwaleit M, Haibel H, Baraliakos X, Listing J, Marker-Hermann E, Zeidler H, et al. The early disease stage in axial spondylarthritis: results from the German Spondyloarthritis Inception Cohort. Arthritis Rheum. 2009;60:717–27. doi:10.1002/art.24483.
54. Poddubnyy D, Haibel H, Listing J, Marker-Hermann E, Zeidler H, Braun J, et al. Baseline radiographic damage, elevated acute-phase reactant levels, and cigarette smoking status predict spinal radiographic progression in early axial spondylarthritis. Arthritis Rheum. 2012;64:1388–98. doi:10.1002/art.33465.
55. Feldtkeller E, Erlendsson J. Definition of disease duration in ankylosing spondylitis. Rheumatol Int. 2008;28:693–6. doi:10.1007/s00296-007-0499-y.
56. Jordan KP, Joud A, Bergknut C, Croft P, Edwards JJ, Peat G, et al. International comparisons of the consultation prevalence of musculoskeletal conditions using population-based healthcare data from England and Sweden. Ann Rheum Dis. 2014;73:212–8. doi:10.1136/annrheumdis-2012-202634.

Does the reason for discontinuation of a first TNF inhibitor influence the effectiveness of a second TNF inhibitor in axial spondyloarthritis? Results from the Swiss Clinical Quality Management Cohort

Adrian Ciurea[1*], Pascale Exer[2], Ulrich Weber[3,4], Giorgio Tamborrini[5], Beate Steininger[1], Rudolf O. Kissling[6], Jürg Bernhard[7], Almut Scherer[8] and on behalf of the Rheumatologists of Swiss Clinical Quality Management Program for Axial Spondyloarthritis

Abstract

Background: With regard to switching tumor necrosis factor inhibitors (TNFi) in axial spondyloarthritis (axSpA), conflicting results have been reported as to whether the effectiveness of a second TNFi depends on the reason for discontinuation of the first TNFi.

Methods: Patients with a clinical diagnosis of axSpA starting a second TNFi in the Swiss Clinical Quality Management cohort were included. Effectiveness of treatment at 1 year, as well as drug survival, was compared between subgroups having discontinued the first TNFi because of lack of response, adverse events (AEs), or other reasons. Lack of response was further divided into primary or secondary lack of response (PLR or SLR, respectively), depending on whether the first TNFi was stopped before or after 6 months of treatment.

Results: Among 632 patients with axSpA, median survival of a second TNFi was 1.1 years after PLR and 3.8 years after SLR ($p = 0.003$). At least moderate disease activity as defined by an Ankylosing Spondylitis Disease Activity Score using the erythrocyte sedimentation rate (ASDAS-ESR) <2.1 was achieved after 12 months by 11 %, 39 %, 26 %, and 39 % of patients who discontinued their first TNFi because of PLR, SLR, AEs, and other reasons, respectively ($p = 0.01$). Only 4 % of patients achieved an ASDAS-ESR inactive disease state after PLR, in comparison to 22 % of those after SLR. Similar results were demonstrated in patients fulfilling the Assessment of SpondyloArthritis international Society classification criteria for axSpA ($n = 488$): ASDAS-ESR <2.1 was achieved after 12 months by 9 %, 41 %, 29 %, and 39 % of patients who discontinued their first TNFi because of PLR, SLR, AEs, and other reasons, respectively ($p = 0.01$).

Conclusions: The effectiveness of a second TNFi is significantly impaired in patients with axSpA after PLR to a first TNFi compared with SLR.

Keywords: Axial spondyloarthritis, Tumor necrosis factor inhibitors, Switching, Drug retention

* Correspondence: adrian.ciurea@usz.ch
[1]Department of Rheumatology, University Hospital Zurich, Gloriastrasse 25, CH-8091 Zurich, Switzerland
Full list of author information is available at the end of the article

Background

Although the use of tumor necrosis factor-α inhibitors (TNFi) has revolutionized the treatment of axial spondyloarthritis (axSpA), a significant proportion of patients do not adequately respond [1–5]. Young age, male sex, high baseline Bath Ankylosing Spondylitis Disease Activity Index (BASDAI), low baseline Bath Ankylosing Spondylitis Functional Index (BASFI), high baseline C-reactive protein (CRP), human leukocyte antigen B27 (HLA-B27) positivity, and the absence of enthesitis have been described as predictors of good response to TNFi [6, 7]. We additionally identified smoking to be associated with a worse outcome following TNFi treatment in patients with axSpA [8]. Switching to an alternative TNFi appears to be associated with lower response and/or drug survival rates in patients with ankylosing spondylitis (AS) [9–24]. In patients with rheumatoid arthritis (RA), response to a second TNFi seemed better if the first TNFi was discontinued because of loss of efficacy or adverse events (AEs) in comparison to a primary lack of efficacy [25, 26]. So far, no evidence for a differential response to a second TNFi in dependence on the reason for discontinuation of the first TNFi has been observed in axSpA. As new compounds with different modes of action are currently being tested in axSpA as potential alternatives to TNFi switching [27–29], we explored the effectiveness of switching TNFi in a large real-life observational axSpA cohort.

Methods

Study population

We conducted a longitudinal analysis of data collected annually from patients with a clinical diagnosis of axSpA, including AS, recruited in the ongoing Swiss Clinical Quality Management (SCQM) Cohort from January 2005 to September 2015 [30]. Clinical assessments included a physical examination (spinal and hip mobility according to the Bath Ankylosing Spondylitis Metrology Index, measurement of height and weight, presence of peripheral arthritis, dactylitis as well as enthesitis), laboratory tests (erythrocyte sedimentation rate [ESR] and CRP levels), data on treatment with nonsteroidal anti-inflammatory drugs (NSAIDs) as present or absent, and data on conventional and biologic disease-modifying drugs with dosage and start and stop dates [31]. The following reasons for drug discontinuation were specified in the database by the treating rheumatologist: insufficient effectiveness, AEs, remission, and other reasons. There was no further specification of the "other reasons" category of discontinuation in the SCQM questionnaire, but these reasons may be manifold, such as personal preference by the patient or physician, pregnancy, or elective surgery. As discontinuation due to remission was observed in only 1.9 % of the patients, we pooled this category together with the "other reasons" category for discontinuation. Patient questionnaires included the BASDAI, the BASFI, smoking status (never, previous, or current), and the number of weekly exercise sessions.

Inclusion criteria for the present study

Patients with a clinical diagnosis of axSpA who had initiated a second TNFi after recruitment into the SCQM-axSpA cohort were included. Interruptions of treatment with the same TNFi were not counted as switches. Patients with overlapping TNFi courses or with an unclear start date were excluded. The study was approved by the ethics commission of the Canton of Zurich. Written informed consent was obtained from all patients.

Outcomes

The primary outcome was drug survival of a second TNFi in relation to the reason for discontinuation of the first TNFi. In the case of several reasons for drug discontinuation, the following hierarchy was implemented: lack of effect > AE > other reasons. Only the discontinuation reason highest in hierarchy was used. Lack of efficacy was further divided into primary lack of response (PLR) if the first TNFi was stopped within 6 months after start and in secondary lack of response (SLR) if the first TNFi was discontinued after a 6-month period. The Assessment of SpondyloArthritis international Society (ASAS) recommends assessment of response to treatment after at least 12 weeks [32]. We chose a cutoff of 6 months, however, as clinically relevant improvement may take longer than 3 months [33, 34]. Moreover, the treating rheumatologist has to apply for reimbursement for an alternative TNFi in Switzerland, which may delay the switching process for a couple of weeks. The co-primary outcome of interest was effectiveness of treatment, assessed as the proportion of patients reaching at least an Ankylosing Spondylitis Disease Activity Score (ASDAS) moderate disease activity state (ASDAS <2.1), an ASDAS inactive disease state (ASDAS <1.3), or the ASAS criteria for partial remission (ASAS-PR) at 12 ± 3 months [35, 36]. Achievement of ASDAS cutoffs is primarily presented using the ESR, as CRP levels are registered in SCQM Cohort with the respective reference level and not the detection level, thus impeding the recently proposed ASDAS-CRP imputation [37] in some patients. Results derived using ASDAS-CRP are presented in (see Additional file 2: Table S2) after assuming a constant number of 2 for CRP levels <2. Response was assessed in patients with available outcome values at 12 months. Patients with available outcome measures at this time point who had discontinued the first TNFi but had not started an alternative TNFi were considered nonresponders (response/tolerance analysis). Additionally, response was assessed only among patients still on treatment at 12 ± 3 months (per-protocol response analysis).

Statistical analysis

Baseline characteristics in terms of categorical variables were compared between patients starting a second TNFi after different reasons for discontinuation of the first TNFi using the χ^2 test. For symmetrically distributed discrete or continuous variables, analysis of variance was used for testing whether the means in the different groups were equal. The Kruskal-Wallis test was used for data with skewed distribution. All tests were two-sided, with the significance level set at 0.05.

Drug maintenance was described with Kaplan-Meier plots. The log-rank test was used for testing differences between groups shown in the plots. Multiple adjusted Cox proportional hazards models were set up to estimate a covariate-adjusted effect of the reason for discontinuation of the first TNFi on the drug maintenance of the second TNFi. Ongoing treatments were censored at the last visit in the cohort. The following covariates were used: sex, age, calendar year of switch (to account for the number of various anti-TNF agents available for switch), the individual anti-TNF agents, and the type of TNFi switch (monoclonal antibody [mAb] to mAb versus mAb to soluble receptor anti-TNF agent and vice versa). To assess the significance of differences in response rates after 1 year of treatment with the second TNFi, Fisher's exact test was used. R statistical software was used for all analyses.

Results

Patient disposition and baseline characteristics

A total of 686 patients with axSpA started treatment with a second TNFi after inclusion in the SCQM Cohort. A total of 54 patients lost to follow-up after the start of a second TNFi were excluded from the analyses. The baseline characteristics at the start of the second TNFi in these patients, stratified by the reason of discontinuation of the first TNFi (PLR in 23.1 %, SLR in 42.7 %, AEs in 19.8 %, other in 14.4 %), are shown in Table 1. There was an enrichment of patients with predictors of an impaired response to TNFi in the group having stopped the first TNFi because of PLR: higher proportion of HLA-B27 negativity and presence of enthesitis, higher BASFI, and higher proportions of smokers and of patients classified as having nonresponsive axSpA. Patients in the PLR group also displayed higher baseline BASDAI and ASDAS levels, and a higher percentage were treated with NSAIDs. A similar enrichment of patients with predictors of an unfavorable response, as well as of patients with a higher disease activity, was found in patients who met the ASAS classification criteria for axSpA ($n = 488$) (Table 2). The proportion of patients stopping their first TNFi because of PLR was similar in the groups

Table 1 Characteristics of patients with a clinical diagnosis of axial spondyloarthritis starting a second tumor necrosis factor inhibitor

Parameter	Number of patients	PLR ($n = 146$)	SLR ($n = 270$)	AE ($n = 125$)	Other ($n = 91$)	p Value
Male sex, %	632	47.3	56.3	46.4	52.8	0.20
Age, years	632	43.8 ± 10.5	44.4 ± 11.1	44.1 ± 12.3	45.0 ± 13.1	0.87
Radiographic axSpA, %	454	54.4	69.2	65.8	82.1	0.003
HLA-B27–positive, %	510	43.2	67.1	64.3	71.0	<0.001
Elevated CRP, %	361	30.4	34.2	42.7	29.2	0.33
ASDAS-CRP	316	3.4 ± 0.8	3.1 ± 0.9	3.0 ± 1.1	2.7 ± 1.0	<0.001
ASDAS-ESR	289	3.1 ± 0.8	2.8 ± 0.8	2.8 ± 1.2	2.6 ± 1.2	0.03
BASDAI	348	6.0 ± 1.8	5.2 ± 2.0	4.9 ± 2.3	4.5 ± 2.3	<0.001
BASFI	345	4.6 ± 2.5	4.1 ± 2.5	3.7 ± 2.5	2.8 ± 2.3	0.001
BASMI	288	2.1 ± 1.9	2.3 ± 2.0	2.4 ± 2.1	2.7 ± 1.9	0.36
Peripheral arthritis, %	629	41.4	37.0	31.7	30.8	0.26
Enthesitis heel, %	632	42.5	31.9	26.4	24.2	0.01
Smokers, %	602	67.6	57.2	69.0	50.0	0.01
DMARDs, %	632	21.2	24.1	12.0	24.2	0.03
NSAIDs, %	632	62.3	54.4	48.0	39.6	0.003
BMI, kg/m^2	608	26.3 ± 4.9	25.6 ± 4.9	25.9 ± 4.7	25.7 ± 4.7	0.58
Years of education	596	13.0 ± 3.0	13.5 ± 3.0	13.3 ± 2.9	14.1 ± 3.2	0.07

axSpA axial spondyloarthritis, *ASAS* Assessment of SpondyloArthritis international Society, *ASDAS-CRP* Ankylosing Spondylitis Disease Activity Score using C-reactive protein, *ASDAS-ESR* Ankylosing Spondylitis Disease Activity Score using erythrocyte sedimentation rate, *BASDAI* Bath Ankylosing Spondylitis Disease Activity Index, *BASFI* Bath Ankylosing Spondylitis Functional Index, *BASMI* Bath Ankylosing Spondylitis Metrology Index, *DMARDs* disease-modifying antirheumatic drugs, *NSAIDs* nonsteroidal anti-inflammatory drugs, *BMI* body mass index

Except where indicated otherwise, values for continuous variables are mean (±SD)

Table 2 Characteristics of patients fulfilling the ASAS axial spondyloarthritis classification criteria starting a second tumor necrosis factor inhibitor

Parameter	Number of patients	PLR ($n = 110$)	SLR ($n = 220$)	AE ($n = 88$)	Other ($n = 70$)	p Value
Male sex, %	488	47.3	60.9	53.4	55.7	0.12
Age, years	488	42.8 ± 10.2	43.2 ± 10.9	42.3 ± 11.8	44.2 ± 13.4	0.77
Radiographic axSpA, %	388	66.7	77.4	82.5	87.9	0.02
HLA-B27–positive, %	442	51.6	73.7	75.0	78.3	<0.001
Elevated CRP, %	285	34.8	37.0	52.0	30.8	0.15
ASDAS-CRP	256	3.4 ± 0.9	3.1 ± 0.9	3.0 ± 1.2	2.7 ± 1.1	0.003
ASDAS-ESR	233	3.2 ± 0.8	2.8 ± 0.8	2.8 ± 1.2	2.7 ± 1.2	0.08
BASDAI	275	6.1 ± 1.9	5.1 ± 2.0	4.7 ± 2.4	4.6 ± 2.3	<0.001
BASFI	274	4.7 ± 2.5	4.1 ± 2.5	3.5 ± 2.4	3.0 ± 2.2	0.002
BASMI	228	2.1 ± 1.7	2.3 ± 2.0	2.7 ± 2.3	2.9 ± 2.0	0.27
Peripheral arthritis, %	487	36.7	35.5	26.1	21.4	0.06
Enthesitis heel, %	488	40.0	33.2	26.1	22.9	0.06
Smokers, %	471	73.4	58.4	72.3	55.7	0.01
DMARDs, %	488	20.0	22.7	9.1	17.1	0.03
NSAIDs, %	488	62.7	54.5	50.0	35.7	0.01
BMI, kg/m^2	478	26.1 ± 4.6	25.7 ± 4.8	26.0 ± 4.7	26.2 ± 4.8	0.88
Years of education	463	13.0 ± 3.2	13.5 ± 3.0	13.0 ± 2.9	13.9 ± 3.2	0.23

axSpA axial spondyloarthritis, *ASAS* Assessment of SpondyloArthritis international Society, *ASDAS-CRP* Ankylosing Spondylitis Disease Activity Score using C-reactive protein, *ASDAS-ESR* Ankylosing Spondylitis Disease Activity Score using erythrocyte sedimentation rate, *BASDAI* Bath Ankylosing Spondylitis Disease Activity Index, *BASFI* Bath Ankylosing Spondylitis Functional Index, *BASMI* Bath Ankylosing Spondylitis Metrology Index, *DMARDs* disease-modifying antirheumatic drugs, *NSAIDs* nonsteroidal anti-inflammatory drugs, *BMI* body mass index

Except where indicated otherwise, values for continuous variables are mean (±SD)

with a clinical diagnosis of axSpA, those fulfilling the ASAS criteria, and those who met the modified New York criteria (23.1 %, 22.5 %, and 20.0 %, respectively). A similar proportion of TNFi-treated patients in the PLR and SLR groups was concurrently treated with conventional disease-modifying antirheumatic drugs (Tables 1 and 2).

Drug retention

The median drug retention of the second TNFi was 2.29 years (95 % confidence interval [CI] 1.79–2.97) for all patients with axSpA and 2.61 years (95 % CI 2.05–3.28) in the subgroup fulfilling the ASAS axSpA classification criteria. Drug maintenance depending on the reason for discontinuation of the first TNFi is shown in Fig. 1 for all patients with a clinical diagnosis of axSpA and in Fig. 2 for patients fulfilling the ASAS axSpA classification criteria. Significant differences in retention rates were found between the four groups ($p = 0.001$), with the shortest drug survival observed after previous PLR. The median drug survival of a second TNFi was 1.06 years (95 % CI 0.75–1.96) after PLR and 3.76 years (95 % CI 3.12–4.28) after SLR ($p = 0.003$). This difference remained significant after adjustment for sex, age, the calendar year of switching (reflecting the number of available TNFi at each time point), and the type of TNFi switching (mAb to mAb versus mAb to fusion protein anti-TNF agent and vice versa)

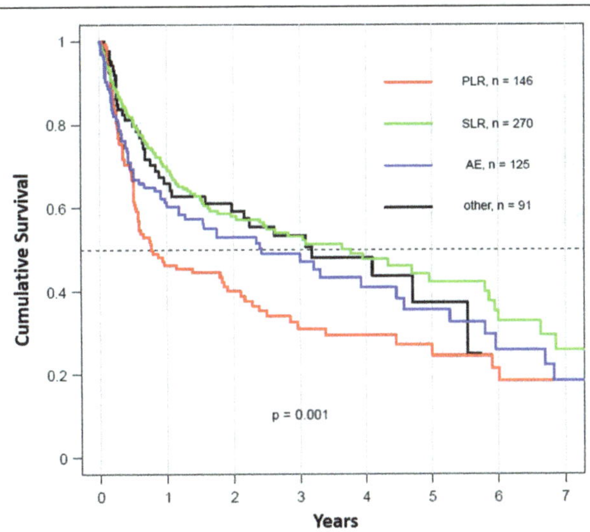

Fig. 1 Drug survival of the second tumor necrosis factor inhibitor (TNFi), stratified by the reason for discontinuation of the first TNFi, in patients with a clinical diagnosis of axial spondyloarthritis. *Other* refers to reason for discontinuation other than lack of effect or intolerance. *AE* adverse events, *PLR* primary lack of response, *SLR* secondary lack of response

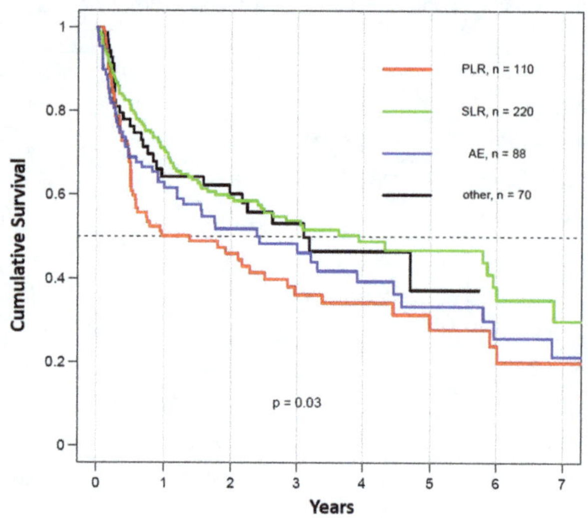

Fig. 2 Drug survival of the second tumor necrosis factor inhibitor (TNFi), stratified by the reason for discontinuation of the first TNFi, in patients fulfilling the Assessment of SpondyloArthritis international Society axial spondyloarthritis classification criteria. *Other* refers to reason for discontinuation other than lack of effect or intolerance. *AE* adverse events, *PLR* primary lack of response, *SLR* secondary lack of response

(Table 3). The hazard ratio for discontinuing the second TNFi after previous SLR in comparison to PLR was 0.56 (95 % CI 0.42–0.75, $p < 0.001$) in all patients diagnosed as having axSpA and 0.58 (95 % CI 0.42–0.81, $p = 0.002$) in those patients fulfilling the ASAS axSpA classification criteria. Similar results were found after replacing the type of TNFi switching by the various anti-TNF agents in the model (adalimumab, certolizumab, etanercept, golimumab, infliximab).

Clinical response

Response to treatment with a second TNFi was assessed in patients with available outcome values at 12 ± 3 months (ASAS-PR [$n = 227$, 36 %] and ASDAS-ESR [$n = 184$, 29 %]). Patients with versus without follow-up at this time point did not differ with regard to important baseline disease characteristics (BASDAI, ASDAS, elevated CRP, HLA-B27, classification as AS, age, peripheral arthritis, enthesitis, smoking, education, reason for discontinuation of first TNFi, physical exercise, body mass index) (see Additional file 1: Table S1).

Response rates to a second TNFi differed significantly between the subgroups, based on the reasons for discontinuation of the first TNFi (Table 4). These were most impaired in the subgroup of patients having discontinued the first TNFi as a consequence of PLR, followed by AEs. At least moderate disease activity (defined by ASDAS-ESR <2.1) was reached by 11 %, 26 %, and 39 % of patients in the PLR, AE, and SLR groups, respectively. Only a negligible proportion of patients achieved ASAS-PR or ASDAS-ESR inactive disease state after PLR (2 % and 4 % of patients, respectively), as opposed to 13 % and 22 %, respectively, after SLR. Similar results were found in patients fulfilling the ASAS axSpA classification criteria (Table 4) and when using the CRP for ASDAS calculation (see Additional file 2: Table S2).

Discussion

Our TNFi switching study in axSpA, which to our knowledge is the largest so far, suggests that the reason for discontinuation of a first TNFi may affect the effectiveness of a second TNFi, as previously reported in RA [25, 26]. Drug retention and treatment responses after switching to a second TNFi in axSpA were impaired in patients having discontinued the first TNFi due to primary lack of effectiveness in comparison to SLR. Earlier investigations had been hampered by the fact that it was often not possible to distinguish between these two reasons for drug discontinuation [18, 22]. As ASAS

Table 3 Cox models for drug retention of a second tumor necrosis factor inhibitor in patients having discontinued the first tumor necrosis factor inhibitor due to primary or secondary lack of response

	Patients with a clinical diagnosis of axSpA[a]			Patients fulfilling the ASAS axSpA classification criteria[b]		
	HR	95 % CI	*p* Value	HR	95 % CI	*p* Value
SLR vs. PLR	0.56	0.42–0.75	<0.001	0.58	0.42–0.81	0.002
Female vs. male	0.94	0.71–1.24	0.65	0.90	0.64–1.25	0.53
Age	1.00	0.99–1.02	0.73	1.00	0.99–1.02	0.93
Cept → mAb[c]	1.11	0.79–1.55	0.56	1.17	0.78–1.73	0.45
mAb → Cept[c]	1.11	0.80–1.56	0.54	1.24	0.84–1.82	0.28
2007–2010 vs. before 2006	1.26	0.50–3.12	0.63	1.18	0.47–2.96	0.73
2010–2015 vs. before 2006	1.58	0.63–3.99	0.33	1.44	0.57–3.67	0.44

ASAS Assessment of SpondyloArthritis international Society, *axSpA* axial spondyloarthritis, *Cept* soluble receptor anti-tumor necrosis factor agent, *mAb* monoclonal antibody anti-tumor necrosis factor agent, *HR* hazard ratio, *CI* confidence Interval, *PLR* primary lack of response, *SLR* secondary lack of response
[a]Total of 416 patients and 207 discontinuation events
[b]Total of 330 patients and 157 discontinuation events
[c]Indicated switch type versus reference category mAb → mAb

Table 4 Response rates after 1 year of treatment with a second tumor necrosis factor inhibitor, stratified by the reason of discontinuation of the first tumor necrosis factor inhibitor

Response criterion	Analysis	Number of patients	All	PLR	SLR	AE	Other	*p* Value[a]	*p* Value[b]
Patients with a clinical diagnosis of axSpA									
ASDAS-ESR <2.1	Response/tolerance	184	28.8	11.1	38.9	26.2	38.9	0.01	0.002
ASDAS-ESR <2.1	Per protocol	124	42.7	21.7	50.8	35.5	63.6	0.04	0.02
ASDAS-ESR <1.3	Response/tolerance	184	14.7	4.4	21.5	9.5	22.2	0.03	0.01
ASDAS-ESR <1.3	Per protocol	124	21.8	8.7	28.8	12.9	36.4	0.07	0.08
ASAS-PR	Response/tolerance	227	11.0	2.0	12.5	13.7	16.7	0.08	0.04
ASAS-PR	Per protocol	146	17.1	4.2	17.4	18.4	33.3	0.12	0.17
Patients fulfilling the ASAS axSpA classification									
ASDAS-ESR <2.1	Response/tolerance	148	31.1	9.1	40.9	29.0	38.9	0.01	0.001
ASDAS-ESR <2.1	Per protocol	100	46.0	18.8	55.1	37.5	63.6	0.04	0.02
ASDAS-ESR <1.3	Response/tolerance	148	16.2	3.0	22.7	12.9	22.2	0.045	0.02
ASDAS-ESR <1.3	Per protocol	100	24.4	6.2	30.6	16.7	36.4	0.13	0.09
ASAS-PR	Response/tolerance	179	11.7	0.0	12.5	16.7	18.5	0.03	0.03
ASAS-PR	Per protocol	106	18.1	0.0	17.5	21.4	35.7	0.05	0.10

axSpA axial spondyloarthritis, *ASDAS-CRP* Ankylosing Spondylitis Disease Activity Score using C-reactive protein, *ASDAS-ESR* Ankylosing Spondylitis Disease Activity Score using erythrocyte sedimentation rate, *AE* adverse events, *PLR* primary lack of response, *SLR* secondary lack of response

Other refers to reason of discontinuation other than lack of effect or intolerance. *Response/tolerance* refers to proportion of patients with a valid follow-up achieving the respective response criterion (with patients having discontinued treatment being defined as nonresponders). *Per protocol* refers to proportion of patients achieving the respective response criterion among those patients still receiving treatment

Except where indicated otherwise, values are percentages

[a] *p* Value overall

[b] *p* Value PLR vs. SLR

recommends assessment of treatment response after at least 12 weeks [32] but time to improvement may be longer than 3 months [33, 34], we have defined a discontinuation due to an insufficient effect after 6 months of treatment as being the consequence of a loss of efficacy. This cutoff allowed us to evaluate drug retention and response rates of the second TNFi. We found a difference of 2.7 years in median retention of the second TNFi between patients in the PLR and SLR groups. Moreover, an ASDAS-ESR inactive disease state was reached by only 4 % of patients after previous PLR in comparison to 22 % after SLR. Thus, PLR may identify a subgroup of patients in whom TNF probably does not play a major role in disease pathogenesis and amplification of inflammation. Whether these patients would experience a superior response to biologics with a different mode of action, as demonstrated for RA [38], remains to be established. An alternative, though mutually not exclusive, reason for impaired effectiveness of the second TNFi in the PLR group is a higher proportion of patients with predictors of an impaired response to anti-TNF agents [7] in our study (normal CRP, HLA-B27 negativity, high BASFI levels, and frequent enthesitis). Furthermore, misdiagnosis in some patients in the PLR group cannot be ruled out in the PLR group, given the low percentage of HLA-B27–positive patients (43 %). We expected a lower proportion of PLR patients in the groups fulfilling the ASAS classification criteria or the modified New York classification criteria, which was not the case, however. Finally, even with a correct diagnosis of axSpA, patients may have additional reasons for back pain (e.g., degenerative spinal disease or fibromyalgia [39–41]), which may be misinterpreted as axSpA activity, prompting the initiation of anti-TNF treatment. Reassessment of a diagnosis of axSpA and of musculoskeletal comorbidities in patients having experienced PLR to a first TNFi seems advisable before initiating a next biologic.

The results were very similar in patients with a clinical diagnosis of axSpA made by their treating rheumatologist and those fulfilling the ASAS classification criteria for axSpA. The presentation of patients with axSpA diagnosed on clinical grounds also allows comparison with TNFi switching in other observational cohorts [18, 22], where the proportion of patients fulfilling the modified New York criteria or the ASAS axSpA classification criteria was not reported. The median drug survival of a second TNFi was 2.3 years in SCQM and 1.6 years in the Danish DANBIO registry [22]. In DANBIO, the proportion of patients with a clinical diagnosis of AS treated for at least 2 years with a second TNFi who reached an ASDAS-CRP <2.1 was 37 %. We found a similar proportion of patients with axSpA (43 %) with an ASDAS-ESR <2.1 at 1 year of treatment with a second TNFi. Our result differed significantly in dependence on the reason for discontinuation of the first TNFi: only 22 % after previous PLR, 36 % after AEs and 51 % after SLR.

Over 75 % of the patients in the SCQM Cohort met the ASAS classification criteria for axSpA. Patients fulfilling the ASAS criteria showed comparable response rates (with 19 %, 38 %, and 55 % reaching an ASDAS-ESR <2.1 in the PLR, AE, and SLR groups, respectively) to those of the patients in the entire cohort defined by the treating rheumatologists.

A limitation of our response analyses is that follow-up data of ASDAS at 12 months was available for only approximately one-third of patients. However, patients with versus without follow-up at this time point did not differ with regard to clinically relevant baseline disease characteristics. The limitation of incomplete follow-up is inherent to observational registries. In the NOR-DMARD registry [18], ASDAS responses were available in 25 % of patients at 3 months and 29 % at the last observation and in DANBIO in 45 % of patients at 2 years [22]. There was no difference in response rates among the various anti-TNF agents used as second-line treatment in DANBIO, while drug survival of second treatment courses was longer in adalimumab-treated patients previously treated with infliximab [22]. In RA, drug survival of infliximab was shown to be inferior to adalimumab or etanercept [26], although other comparisons yielded a similar maintenance of various TNFi [42]. Moreover, the type of TNFi switch was shown to affect the effectiveness of a second TNFi in RA: Switching from an anti-TNF mAb to a soluble TNF receptor yielded better results than vice versa [26]. We were unable to confirm differences between individual anti-TNF agents or between various types of switching with regard to drug maintenance.

Conclusions

Our findings suggest that the effectiveness of a second TNFi is impaired in patients with axSpA who have experienced a PLR to a first TNFi during the first 6 months of treatment.

Abbreviations

AE: adverse event; AS: ankylosing spondylitis; ASAS: Assessment of SpondyloArthritis international Society; ASDAS: Ankylosing Spondylitis Disease Activity Score; axSpA: axial spondyloarthritis; BASDAI: Bath Ankylosing Spondylitis Disease Activity Index; BASFI: Bath Ankylosing Spondylitis Functional Index; BASMI: Bath Ankylosing Spondylitis Mobility Index; BMI: body mass index; CI: confidence interval; CRP: C-reactive protein; DMARD: disease-modifying antirheumatic drug; ESR: erythrocyte sedimentation rate; HLA-B27: human leukocyte antigen B27; HR: hazard ratio; mAb: monoclonal antibody; NSAID: nonsteroidal anti-inflammatory drug; PLR: primary lack of response; PR: partial remission; RA: rheumatoid arthritis; SCQM: Swiss Clinical Quality Management; SLR: secondary lack of response; TNFi: tumor necrosis factor inhibitor.

Competing interests

JB has received consulting fees from Merck Sharp & Dohme, Pfizer, and Roche. AC has received consulting and/or speaking fees from AbbVie, Celgene, Eli Lilly, Janssen-Cilag, Merck Sharp & Dohme, Novartis, Pfizer, and UCB. PE has received speaking fees from AbbVie and Merck Sharp & Dome. UW has received speaking fees from AbbVie. The other authors declare that they have no competing interests.

Authors' contributions

AC made substantial contributions to study conception and design and to data acquisition, analysis, and interpretation, and drafted the manuscript. PE, GT, and JB made substantial contributions to data acquisition, analysis, and interpretation and revised the manuscript critically for important intellectual content. UW made substantial contributions to study design and to acquisition and interpretation of data, and helped to draft the manuscript. BS made substantial contributions to data acquisition, analysis, and interpretation and revised the manuscript. ROK made substantial contributions to study conception as well as to analysis and interpretation of data, and revised the manuscript. AS made substantial contributions to study design, performed the statistical analyses, and helped with data interpretation and drafting of the manuscript. All authors read and approved the final manuscript.

Acknowledgments

We thank all the rheumatologists and patients involved in the study for their participation, the members of the SCQM axSpA scientific board for contribution to pelvic x-ray scoring and helpful discussions, and the entire SCQM staff for data management and support. A list of rheumatology offices and hospitals that are contributing to the SCQM registries can be found at http://www.scqm.ch/institutions. The SCQM Foundation is supported by the Swiss Society of Rheumatology and by AbbVie, Bristol-Myers Squibb, Merck Sharp & Dohme, Pfizer, Roche, UCB, and Janssen and has received project-based financial support from the Arco Foundation, Switzerland, as well as from the Swiss Balgrist Society, Switzerland. This study was supported by an investigator-initiated study grant from AbbVie and by a grant from the "Stiftung für Rheumaforschung." The study sponsors had no role in the study design or in the collection, analysis, or interpretation of the data; the writing of the manuscript; or the decision to submit the manuscript for publication. Publication of this article was not contingent upon approval by the study sponsors.

Author details

[1]Department of Rheumatology, University Hospital Zurich, Gloriastrasse 25, CH-8091 Zurich, Switzerland. [2]Private Rheumatology Practice, Basel, Switzerland. [3]King Christian 10th Hospital for Rheumatic Diseases, Gråsten, Denmark. [4]South Jutland Hospital, Denmark Institute of Regional Health Research, University of Southern Denmark, Odense, Denmark. [5]Department of Rheumatology, Bethesda Hospital, Basel, Switzerland. [6]Department of Rheumatology, Balgrist University Hospital, Zurich, Switzerland. [7]Department of Rheumatology and Rehabilitation, Bürgerspital, Solothurn, Switzerland. [8]Swiss Clinical Quality Management Foundation, Zurich, Switzerland.

References

1. van der Heijde D, Dijkmans B, Geusens P, Sieper J, DeWoody K, Williamson P, et al. Efficacy and safety of infliximab in patients with ankylosing spondylitis: results of a randomized, placebo-controlled trial (ASSERT). Arthritis Rheum. 2005;52:582–91.
2. Davis JC, van der Heijde D, Braun J, Dougados M, Cush J, Clegg D, et al. Sustained durability and tolerability of etanercept in ankylosing spondylitis for 96 weeks. Ann Rheum Dis. 2005;64:1557–62.
3. van der Heijde D, Kivitz A, Schiff MH, Sieper J, Dijkmans BA, Braun J, et al. Efficacy and safety of adalimumab in patients with ankylosing spondylitis: results of a multicenter, randomized, double-blind, placebo-controlled trial. Arthritis Rheum. 2006;54:2136–46.

4. Inman RD, Davis Jr JC, van der Heijde D, Diekman L, Sieper J, Kim SI, et al. Efficacy and safety of golimumab in patients with ankylosing spondylitis: results of a randomized, double-blind, placebo-controlled, phase III trial. Arthritis Rheum. 2008;58:3402–12.
5. Landewé R, Braun J, Deodhar A, Dougados M, Maksymowych WP, Mease PJ, et al. Efficacy of certolizumab pegol on signs and symptoms of axial spondyloarthritis including ankylosing spondylitis: 24-week results of a double-blind randomised placebo-controlled phase 3 study. Ann Rheum Dis. 2014;73:39–47.
6. Maneiro JR, Souto A, Salgado E, Mera A, Gomez-Reino JJ. Predictors of response to TNF antagonists in patients with ankylosing spondylitis and psoriatic arthritis: systematic review and meta-analysis. RMD Open. 2015;1:e000017.
7. Vastesaeger N, van der Heijde D, Inman RD, Wang Y, Deodhar A, Hsu B, et al. Predicting the outcome of ankylosing spondylitis therapy. Ann Rheum Dis. 2011;70:973–81.
8. Ciurea A, Scherer A, Weber U, Exer P, Bernhard J, Tamborrini G, et al. Impaired response to treatment with tumour necrosis factor α inhibitors in smokers with axial spondyloarthritis. Ann Rheum Dis. 2015. doi:10.1136/annrheumdis-2013-205133.
9. Gomez-Reino JJ, Carmona L, BIOBADASER Group. Switching TNF antagonists in patients with chronic arthritis: an observational study of 488 patients over a four-year period. Arthritis Res Ther. 2006;8:R29.
10. Delaunay C, Farrenq V, Marini-Portugal A, Cohen JD, Chevalier X, Claudepierre P. Infliximab to etanercept switch in patients with spondyloarthropathies and psoriatic arthritis: preliminary data. J Rheumatol. 2005;32:2183–5.
11. Cantini F, Niccoli L, Benucci M, Chindamo D, Nannini C, Olivieri I, et al. Switching from infliximab to once-weekly administration of 50 mg etanercept in resistant or intolerant patients with ankylosing spondylitis: results of a fifty-four-week study. Arthritis Rheum. 2006;55:812–6.
12. Conti F, Ceccarelli F, Marocchi E, Magrini L, Spinelli FR, Spadaro A, et al. Switching tumour necrosis factor α antagonists in patients with ankylosing spondylitis and psoriatic arthritis: an observational study over a 5-year period. Ann Rheum Dis. 2007;66:1393–7.
13. Pradeep DJ, Keat AC, Gaffney K, Brooksby A, Leeder J, Harris C. Switching anti-TNF therapy in ankylosing spondylitis. Rheumatology (Oxford). 2008;47:1726–7.
14. Coates LC, Cawkwell LS, Ng NW, Bennett AN, Bryer DJ, Fraser AD, et al. Real life experience confirms sustained response to long-term biologics and switching in ankylosing spondylitis. Rheumatology (Oxford). 2008;47:897–900.
15. Rudwaleit M, Van den Bosch F, Kron M, Kary S, Kupper H. Effectiveness and safety of adalimumab in patients with ankylosing spondylitis or psoriatic arthritis and history of anti-tumor necrosis factor therapy. Arthritis Res Ther. 2010;12:R117.
16. Spadaro A, Punzi L, Marchesoni A, Lubrano E, Mathieu A, Cantini F, et al. Switching from infliximab or etanercept to adalimumab in resistant or intolerant patients with spondyloarthritis: a 4-year study. Rheumatology (Oxford). 2010;49:1107–11.
17. Haberhauer G, Strehblow C, Fasching P. Observational study of switching anti-TNF agents in ankylosing spondylitis and psoriatic arthritis versus rheumatoid arthritis. Wien Med Wochenschr. 2010;160:220–4.
18. Lie E, van der Heijde D, Uhlig T, Mikkelsen K, Rodevand E, Koldingsnes W, et al. Effectiveness of switching between TNF inhibitors in ankylosing spondylitis: data from the NOR-DMARD register. Ann Rheum Dis. 2011;70:157–63.
19. Paccou J, Solau-Gervais E, Houvenagel E, Salleron J, Luraschi H, Philippe P, et al. Efficacy in current practice of switching between anti-tumour necrosis factor-α agents in spondyloarthropathies. Rheumatology (Oxford). 2011;50:714–20.
20. Plasencia C, Pascual-Salcedo D, Garcia-Carazo S, Lojo L, Nuno L, Villalba A, et al. The immunogenicity to the first anti-TNF therapy determines the outcome of switching to a second anti-TNF therapy in spondyloarthritis patients. Arthritis Res Ther. 2013;15:R79.
21. Spadaro A, Lubrano E, Marchesoni A, D'Angelo S, Ramonda R, Addimanda O, et al. Remission in ankylosing spondylitis treated with anti-TNF-α drugs: a national multicentre study. Rheumatology (Oxford). 2013;52:1914–9.
22. Glintborg B, Ostergaard M, Krogh NS, Tarp U, Manilo N, Loft AG, et al. Clinical response, drug survival and predictors thereof in 432 ankylosing spondylitis patients after switching tumour necrosis factor α inhibitor therapy: results from the Danish nationwide DANBIO registry. Ann Rheum Dis. 2013;72:1149–55.
23. Gulyas K, Bodnar N, Nagy Z, Szamosi S, Horvath A, Vancsa A, et al. Real-life experience with switching TNF-α inhibitors in ankylosing spondylitis. Eur J Health Econ. 2014;15 Suppl 1:S93–100.
24. Fabbroni M, Cantarini L, Caso F, Costa L, Pagano VA, Frediani B, et al. Drug retention rates and treatment discontinuation among anti-TNF-α agents in psoriatic arthritis and ankylosing spondylitis in clinical practice. Mediators Inflamm. 2014;2014:862969.
25. Remy A, Avouac J, Gossec L, Combe B. Clinical relevance of switching to a second tumour necrosis factor-α inhibitor after discontinuation of a first tumour necrosis factor-α inhibitor in rheumatoid arthritis: a systematic literature review and meta-analysis. Clin Exp Rheumatol. 2011;29:96–103.
26. Chatzidionysiou K, Askling J, Eriksson J, Kristensen LE, van Vollenhoven R, ARTIS group. Effectiveness of TNF inhibitor switch in RA: results from the national Swedish register. Ann Rheum Dis. 2015;74:890–6.
27. Baeten D, Baraliakos X, Braun J, Sieper J, Emery P, van der Heijde D, et al. Anti-interleukin-17A monoclonal antibody secukinumab in treatment of ankylosing spondylitis: a randomised, double-blind, placebo-controlled trial. Lancet. 2013;382:1705–13.
28. Poddubnyy D, Hermann KG, Callhoff J, Listing J, Sieper J. Ustekinumab for the treatment of patients with active ankylosing spondylitis: results of a 28-week, prospective, open-label, proof-of-concept study (TOPAS). Ann Rheum Dis. 2014;73:817–23.
29. Pathan E, Abraham S, Van Rossen E, Withrington R, Keat A, Charles PJ, et al. Efficacy and safety of apremilast, an oral phosphodiesterase 4 inhibitor, in ankylosing spondylitis. Ann Rheum Dis. 2013;72:1475–80.
30. Ciurea A, Scherer A, Exer P, Bernhard J, Dudler J, Beyeler B, et al. Tumor necrosis factor-α inhibition in radiographic and non-radiographic axial spondyloarthritis: results from a large observational cohort. Arthritis Rheum. 2013;65:3096–106.
31. Sieper J, Rudwaleit M, Baraliakos X, Brandt J, Braun J, Burgos-Vargas R, et al. The Assessment of SpondyloArthritis international Society (ASAS) handbook: a guide to assess spondyloarthritis. Ann Rheum Dis. 2009;68 Suppl 2:ii1–44.
32. van der Heijde D, Sieper J, Maksymowych WP, Dougados M, Burgos-Vargas R, Landewé R, et al. Update of the international ASAS recommendations for the use of anti-TNF agents in patients with axial spondyloarthritis. Ann Rheum Dis. 2011;70:905–8.
33. Braun J, van der Horst-Bruinsma IE, Huang F, Burgos-Vargas R, Vlahos B, Koenig AS, et al. Clinical efficacy and safety of etanercept versus sulfasalazine in patients with ankylosing spondylitis: a randomized, double-blind trial. Arthritis Rheum. 2011;63:1543–51.
34. Breban M, Vignon E, Claudepierre P, Devauchelle V, Wendling D, Lespessailles E, et al. Efficacy of infliximab in refractory ankylosing spondylitis: results of a six-month open-label study. Rheumatology (Oxford). 2002;41:1280–5.
35. Machado P, Landewé R, Lie E, Kvien TK, Braun J, Baker D, et al. Ankylosing Spondylitis Disease Activity Score (ASDAS): defining cut-off values for disease activity states and improvement scores. Ann Rheum Dis. 2011;70:47–53.
36. Anderson JJ, Baron G, van der Heijde D, Felson DT, Dougados M. Ankylosing spondylitis assessment group preliminary definition of short-term improvement in ankylosing spondylitis. Arthritis Rheum. 2001;44:1876–86.
37. Machado P, Navarro-Compan V, Landewé R, van Gaalen FA, Roux C, van der Heijde D. Calculating the Ankylosing Spondylitis Disease Activity Score if the conventional C-reactive protein level is below the limit of detection or if high-sensitivity c-reactive protein is used: an analysis in the DESIR cohort. Arthritis Rheumatol. 2015;67:408–13.
38. Finckh A, Ciurea A, Brulhart L, Moller B, Walker UA, Courvoisier D, et al. Which subgroup of patients with rheumatoid arthritis benefits from switching to rituximab versus alternative anti-tumour necrosis factor (TNF) agents after previous failure of an anti-TNF agent? Ann Rheum Dis. 2010;69:387–93.
39. Roussou E, Ciurtin C. Clinical overlap between fibromyalgia tender points and enthesitis sites in patients with spondyloarthritis who present with inflammatory back pain. Clin Exp Rheumatol. 2012;30(6 Suppl 74):24–30.
40. Almodovar R, Carmona L, Zarco P, Collantes E, Gonzalez C, Mulero J, et al. Fibromyalgia in patients with ankylosing spondylitis: prevalence and utility of the measures of activity, function and radiological damage. Clin Exp Rheumatol. 2010;28(6 Suppl 63):S33–9.
41. Salaffi F, De Angelis R, Carotti M, Gutierrez M, Sarzi-Puttini P, Atzeni F. Fibromyalgia in patients with axial spondyloarthritis: epidemiological profile and effect on measures of disease activity. Rheumatol Int. 2014;34:1103–10.
42. Fisher A, Bassett K, Wright JM, Brookhart MA, Freeman H, Dormuth CR. Comparative persistence of the TNF antagonists in rheumatoid arthritis – a population-based cohort study. PLoS One. 2014;9(8):e105193.

20

Patient-reported impact of spondyloarthritis on work disability and working life: the ATLANTIS survey

Roberta Ramonda[1*], Antonio Marchesoni[2], Antonio Carletto[3], Gerolamo Bianchi[4], Maurizio Cutolo[5], Gianfranco Ferraccioli[6], Enrico Fusaro[7], Salvatore De Vita[8], Mauro Galeazzi[9], Roberto Gerli[10], Marco Matucci-Cerinic[11], Giovanni Minisola[12], Carlomaurizio Montecucco[13], Raffaele Pellerito[14], Fausto Salaffi[15], Giuseppe Paolazzi[16], Piercarlo Sarzi-Puttini[17], Raffaele Scarpa[18], Gianfilippo Bagnato[19], Giovanni Triolo[20], Guido Valesini[21], Leonardo Punzi[1], Ignazio Olivieri[22] and ATLANTIS study group

Abstract

Background: The aim was to establish how patients experience the impact of spondyloarthritis (SpA) on work disability and working life.

Methods: The survey was performed in 17/20 regions in Italy (1 January to 31 March 2013). A multiple-choice questionnaire was published on the official website of the sponsor - the National Association of Rheumatic Patients (ANMAR) - and hard-copies were distributed at outpatient clinics for rheumatic patients.

Results: Respondents (n = 770) were of both sexes (56 % men), educated (62 % at high school or more), of working age (75 % aged ≤60 years), and affected by SpA. The most common types diagnosed were ankylosing spondylitis (AS) (39 %) and psoriatic arthritis (PsA) (36 %). Respondents were working full-time (45 %), part-time (8 %) or had retired (22 %); 15 % were unemployed (for reasons linked to the disease or for other reasons, students or housewives). Patients reported disability (39 %), were receiving disability benefits (34 %), were experiencing important limitations that were hindering their professional development/career (36 %) and some had to change/leave their job or lost it because of SpA (21 %). Employed respondents (n = 383) had worked on average 32.2 h in the last 7 days. More hours of work were lost over the last 7 days due to SpA (2.39 h vs 1.67 h). The indirect costs of the disease amounted to €106/week for patients reporting well-being/good physical conditions/improvement and €216/week for those reporting permanent impairment.

Conclusions: Most patients were in the midst of their productive years and were experiencing considerable difficulties in carrying out their job because of the disease: half of them reported disability and one third were experiencing important limitations in their career perspective.

Keywords: Spondyloarthritis, Survey, Absenteeism, Presenteeism, WPI

Background

Major advances have occurred in the diagnosis and classification of spondyloarthritis (SpA) over the last 10 years, especially since spinal inflammation was demonstrated on magnetic resonance imaging (MRI) in the absence of radiographic evidence of change [1]. The changes were formalized in the revised versions of the Assessment of SpondyloArthritis International Society (ASAS) classification criteria for axial (ax) [2] and peripheral SpA [3]. Thanks to these criteria, patients with axial SpA without radiographic evidence of sacroiliitis can now be classified as having non-radiographic axSpA, a form which does not appear to differ significantly from radiographic axSpA in terms of the main clinical manifestations, disease activity, pain, quality of life and response to anti-tumor necrosis factor (anti-TNF) therapy [4–6]. Differences between patients with non-radiographic and radiographic axSpA have been found in age, symptom duration, human leukocyte

* Correspondence: roberta.ramonda@unipd.it
[1]Rheumatology Unit, Department of Medicine DIMED, University of Padova, Via Giustiniani, 2, Padova 35128, Italy
Full list of author information is available at the end of the article

antigen (HLA)-B27 positivity [7] and gender distribution. Although less inflammation (i.e., lower C-reactive protein and less evidence of spinal inflammation on MRI) and less impairment in spinal mobility have been observed in non-radiographic axSpA than in the axSpA, the two conditions are associated with a similar burden in terms of disease activity, physical function and health ratio quality of life (HR-QoL) impairment [8]. ASAS classification criteria are also important because they enable detection of early SpA, so that treatment can be introduced earlier than in the past when the average delay in diagnosis was about 10 years [9]. Of course, former classification criteria for specific subtypes of SpA, such as the modified New York Criteria for ankylosing spondylitis (AS) [10] or Classification Criteria for Psoriatic Arthritis (CASPAR) for psoriatic arthritis (PsA) [11] remain valid to classify particular forms of the disease.

Before the introduction of the ASAS criteria, the global prevalence of SpA was calculated to be approximately 1 %, with notable variability, ranging from 0.01 % in Japan to 2.5 % in Northern Arctic populations. The recognition of non-radiographic axSpA will have a considerable impact on the prevalence of SpA, because many patients who had an unclassifiable axSpA can now be classified according to the ASAS criteria [1, 8].

The increase in the prevalence of SpA has notable socioeconomic implications. By definition, SpA is a disease that occurs in young adults at the peak of their productive lifespan [2]. Moreover, it is associated with a considerable burden in terms of restrictions in activities of daily living [12, 13], reduction in health-related quality of life (HR-QoL) [13, 14] and in work productivity, and in terms of unemployment [15–17].

The reduction in work productivity is an important component of the indirect costs of SpA, which are typically calculated in terms of absenteeism and presenteeism using tools such as the Work Productivity and Activity Impairment Questionnaire in AS (WPAI) [18]. Absenteeism is defined as the quantity of sick leave either specifically due to the disease itself or, in the event that it is difficult to distinguish between sick leave due to the disease itself and sick leave due to concomitant or incident diseases, the total amount of sick leave expressed as days in a year or hours per week. Presenteeism is defined as patient-reported reduced productivity at work [18]. Caution is required in the extrapolation of data from one country to another, because findings on work productivity and unemployment are affected by a number of local factors, primarily the local unemployment/disability benefit system [19].

We carried out a survey in Italy called Atlantis (an underwater world that we would like to bring to light), which was designed to establish how the diagnostic work-up and management of SpA in Italy is experienced by the patients, and assess the impact of SpA on daily living, personal relationships, work disability and working life. This paper reports findings on work disability and working life.

Methods

Study characteristics

This was a cross-sectional survey sponsored by the Italian National Association of Rheumatic Patients (ANMAR). It was carried out in 17 out of the 20 regions in Italy from 1 January to 31 March 2013 by Doxa-Pharma, a company experienced in carrying out surveys in the healthcare field,

Table 1 Main features of survey respondents

Sociodemographic characteristics	Respondents, %
Gender	
Male	56 %
Female	44 %
Age, years	
≤30	8 %
31–40	17 %
41–50	26 %
51–60	27 %
61–70	17 %
>70	4 %
Not specified	1 %
Education	
Degree/Master's degree	17 %
High school	45 %
Junior high school	28 %
Primary school	8 %
Not specified	2 %
Marital status	
Married/living with partner	64 %
Single	20 %
Divorced/separated/widow(er)	12 %
Not specified	4 %
Residence	
North-West	24 %
North-East	26 %
Central regions	26 %
South and Islands	24 %
Diagnosis	
Ankylosing spondylitis	41 %
Psoriatic arthritis	39 %
Spondyloartritis with inflammatory bowel disease	10 %
Undifferentiated spondyloarthritis	6 %
Reactive arthritis	4 %

under the guidance of an experienced rheumatologist (RR, author), who was the scientific coordinator of the project. According to Italian regulations, the study did not require written informed consent because the questionnaire was completed anonymously. Additional sensitive data were not collected.

Patients and methods

The survey was conducted on patients with a defined diagnosis of SpA made by a rheumatologist and the questionnaire was drafted with five sections: (1) personal details and diagnosis of the patient, including information on work status and any welfare benefits granted; (2) the diagnostic work-up; (3) follow up; (4) impact of the disease on quality of life; and (5) impact on working life, including absenteeism and presenteeism. We considered the indirect costs of the disease in terms of sick leave, which was defined as the weekly cost due to the hours of absence from the job because of the disease, and in terms of presenteeism, which was defined as the quantification of the weekly cost due to the lower job performance of the patients because of the disease. The sum of these two indices, termed the time loss, was defined as the weekly income that was not produced (indirect cost), considering the Italian weekly per capita income in euros in 2012 divided by the standard 44 weeks of work. The multiple-choice questions focused on work status and working life (see Additional file 1 for all questions in detail). Data were collected through two parallel channels: (1) the survey questionnaire was published on the web, with a link placed at the official ANMAR website (www.anmar-italia.it), to be completed by patients who were willing to do so, and (2) hard copies of the survey questionnaire were distributed throughout the Italian regions of interest by ANMAR volunteers, with the support of specialists at the hospitals with clinics dedicated to the management of rheumatic patients.

Data analysis

The data were analyzed descriptively. For the open questions we read all the answers and encoded various items. Data were expressed in terms of frequency and averages. Electronic software (SAS and DIANA) was used to perform an interpretative reading of these data. Collected data were analyzed in relation to sociodemographic variables (sex, age, area of residence) and the type of specific SpA disease.

Results

A total of 770 subjects took part in the survey. Their main features are summarized in Table 1.

More respondents were men (56 %). Most of them were married or living with a partner (64 %), were of working age (78 % aged ≤60 years; mean age = 50 years) and educated (62 % had completed high school or had a university degree). Their distribution throughout Italy was homogeneous, ranging from 24–26 % in the four main Italian geographical areas. The subjects were suffering from AS (41 %), PsA (39 %) SpA with inflammatory bowel diseases (IBD) (10 %), undifferentiated SpA (6 %) and reactive arthritis (4 %) (Fig. 1). Many patients reported that they had contacted other specialists after the diagnosis: ophthalmologists 50 %, cardiologists 45 %, dermatologists 43 %, gastroenterologists 37 %, psychologists

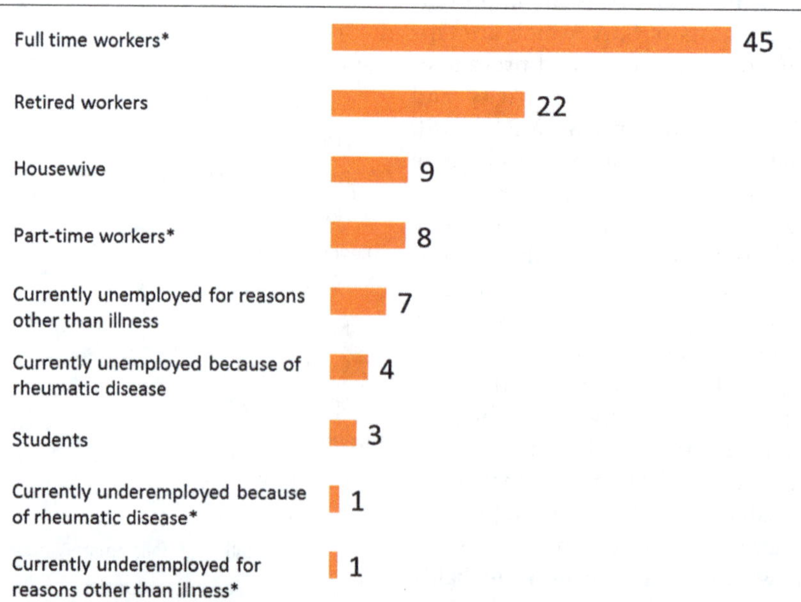

Fig. 1 Main work status in patients with spondyloarthritis

10 %, specialists in infectious diseases 8 %, pulmonologists 2 %, neurologists 2 %, gynecologists 1 %, endocrinologists 1 %, and neurosurgeons 1 % [20].

Slightly below half of the respondents were working either full-time (45 %) or part-time (8 %). Nearly one fourth had retired (22 %) and 15 % were unemployed (for reasons linked to SpA in 4 % of the cases; the remaining were students, housewives or individuals who were unemployed due to reasons other than SpA) (Fig. 1). Half of the respondents (49 %) reported that they were disabled (Table 2) and had to cancel or postpone commitments because of their disease (50 %) and 13 % declared that they had to do this at least half of the time. This depended on symptom control.

One third of patients (36 %) experienced important limitations that hindered their professional development/career. Of these, 19 % had controlled symptoms, 32 % were improving and 50 % had uncontrolled symptoms. One in five patients actually had to change or leave their job or had actually lost it because of SpA (21 %). Discrimination may have played a role in some cases, because 14 % of subjects reported this, and another 14 % believed that SpA had had an impact on their salary (Table 2). The impact on salary also depended on symptom control: 12 % of the patients with controlled symptoms believed that their disease had had a negative effect on their salary compared to 20 % with uncontrolled symptoms. The 383 respondents (49.7 % of the total sample) who were employed had worked on average 32.2 h in the last 7 days. Approximately 60 % had actually worked full-time (31 h or more) (Fig. 2).

Questions about absenteeism revealed that more hours had been lost over the previous 7 days due to SpA (on average 2.39 h vs 1.67 h), than for other reasons such as vacation or family commitments. The hours of absence because of SpA amounted to 59 % of the hours of absence from the work place and to 7 % of weekly working hours. The time loss cost was €216 per week for the patients reporting permanent impairment and €106 euros for the patients who reported well-being or an improvement in their physical condition.

Table 2 Impact on working life

Reported consequences of SpA	Respondents, %
Disability	49 %
Receives disability benefits	34 %
Has applied for disability benefits	8 %
Cannot work full-time, but does not meet criteria for disability benefit	7 %
Has to cancel or postpone work commitments because of SpA	50 %
Does not apply	27 %
Never	23 %
Sometimes	37 %
About half the time	7 %
Most of the time	4 %
All the time	2 %
Limitations to work projects or career in general because of SpA	48 %
Does not apply	20 %
None	12 %
Negligible	20 %
Minor limitations	12 %
Tangible limitations	15 %
Major limitations	21 %
Had to change/leave a job or lost a job because of SpA	21 %
Yes	21 %
Does not apply	24 %
No	55 %
Has felt discriminated at work because of SpA	14 %
Yes	14 %
Does not apply	31 %
No	55 %
Fewer raises in salary because of SpA	14 %
Does not apply	44 %
Not at all	36 %
Negligible	6 %
A little	4 %
Quite a bit	7 %
A lot	3 %

SpA spondyloarthritis

Discussion

This survey spearheaded by ANMAR has shown that patients with SpA experience major disadvantages in their working life: one half of the respondents claimed that they were disabled, and one half reported that SpA interfered significantly with their work commitments; SpA was the main source of absenteeism and presenteeism. What is more, the survey identified a number of issues that, to our knowledge, have not been investigated to date: one half experienced restrictions in their work prospects and career, 21 % had had to change/leave a job or had lost a job because of SpA, and 14 % had experienced discrimination at the workplace.

The sample was representative of the SpA population in terms of gender, age and diagnosis, [1, 21, 22]. Participation from all four main geographical areas of Italy was almost the same for each (24–26 %). The collection of data both via the website and distribution at hospital outpatient clinics ensured that there was no

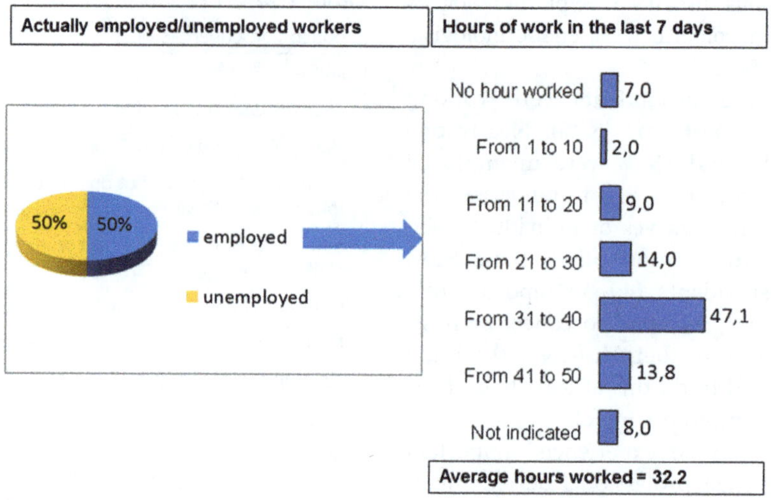

Fig. 2 Results (employed/unemployed workers) by the survey

pre-selection of computer-literate patients [23]. Even so, the survey did include patients who were more educated than average, as only 28 % of respondents had not continued after junior high school, whereas the national average in 2013 was 44 % [23]; this is probably due to the fact that the elderly (a less educated generation) were under-represented in the sample (patients over 60 years of age represented 21 % vs the 27.2 % in the general population [24].

The employment rate was slightly lower than in the general population, being 53 % instead of the expected rate of 58 %, according to the official employment statistics in the general population in Italy in 2013 [25], after correction for the higher percentage of male individuals in the survey than in the general population. Discrimination may have played a role in some cases; in fact, 14 % of the patients reported having the impression of being treated differently from other colleagues due to their rheumatic disease. The proportion of SpA patients receiving disability benefits was nearly five times higher than the proportion in the general population (34 % vs 7.3 %) [24, 26].

One of our study limitations was the use of a non-validated questionnaire. However, our findings on work disability and reduction in productivity, both in terms of absenteeism and presenteeism, are consistent with similar published studies, which all report that SpA is associated with disability and reduction in productivity. Nevertheless, comparisons between different studies is difficult because of the differences in patient populations (e.g., the proportions with manual vs non-manual occupations, proportions with non-SpA-related comorbidities), and in the definition of endpoints (e.g., sick leave may be total or restricted to leave due to SpA), and, above all, differences in local employment and benefit systems [25]. The mean total sick leave was 4 hours per week, which amounts to 26 days of sick leave a year, which is well within the range reported in the literature mentioned above.

In our results we also included an assessment of indirect costs, in terms of time loss, which is the sum of sick leave and presenteeism costs. In this study time loss cost was €216 per week for the patients with permanent impairment and €106 euros for the patients who were well or claimed that their physical conditions had improved.

Another limitation of this survey is the lack of information on disease duration. However, it has been shown that productivity is substantially reduced, even in patients with early SpA (mean disease duration 4.8 years) [27]. This evidence is cause for major concern, because the onset of the disease is in young adulthood and it therefore results in limitations during patients' most productive years. Indeed, this prospect was emphasized by the fact that nearly half of the respondents had the perception of a loss in their work prospects.

To our knowledge, this is the first survey that documents the perception of limitations in work prospects and career, and discrimination at the workplace. A number of factors have been found to be associated with work disability and loss of productivity at work. Unemployment is associated with older age, social deprivation, longer disease duration, functional impairment, and depression, whereas absenteeism is associated only with disease activity and depression, and presenteeism with older age, disease activity, anxiety, and depression [28]. In particular, in a cross-sectional self-reported postal survey examining 1447 Swedish respondents with SpA, presenteeism was associated with a series of disease activity and quality of life measures, including the Bath Ankylosing Spondylitis Activity Index (BASDAI), the Bath Ankylosing Spondylitis

Functional Index (BASFI), the EuroQoL (EQ)-5D pain and symptom, and the ASAS scores [17]. Findings were similar within the more rigorous context of a randomized, controlled clinical trial (ATLAS) in which there was significant correlation between the Short Form (SF)-36/Ankylosing Spondylitis Quality of Life (ASQoL), BASDAI/BASFI,/ Health Utility Index (HUI)-3 scores and WPAI-Specific Health Problem (SHP) scores, and between the patient's and the physician's global assessment of disease activity and WPAI-SHP scores [29]. The correlation between the level of disease activity and work productivity suggests that treatments able to control disease activity would also reduce disability and loss of productivity [30–34].

Conclusions

As SpA impacts productivity mainly in the prime of patients' working lives, it is important to increase public awareness, so that patients will be in a position to seek timely, appropriate care, which will undoubtedly optimize their diagnostic and therapeutic outcome.

Abbreviations

ANMAR: Italian National Association of Rheumatic Patients; AS: ankylosing spondylitis; ASAS: Assessment of SpondyloArthritis International Society; ASQoL: Ankylosing Spondylitis Quality of Life; Ax: axial; BASDAI: Bath Ankylosing Spondylitis Activity Index; BASFI: Bath Ankylosing Spondylitis Functional Index; EQ-5D: EuroQoL-5D; HR-QoL: health-related quality of life; HUI-3: Health Utility Index scores; IBD: inflammatory bowel disease; MRI: magnetic resonance imaging; PsA: psoriatic arthritis; SF-36: Short Form-36; SpA: spondyloarthritis; TNF: tumor necrosis factor; WPAI: Work Productivity and Activity Impairment Questionnaire.

Competing interests

The authors declare that they have no competing interests.

Authors' contributions

RR designed the study, participated in the acquisition of data, performed the statistical analysis, made a substantial contribution to the interpretation of data, and drafted and revised the manuscript. AM participated in the acquisition of data, performed the statistical analysis, made a substantial contribution to the interpretation of data, and revised the manuscript. AC, GB, MC, GF, EF, MG, SDV, RG, MMC, GM, CMM, RP, FS, GP, PSP, RS, GFB, GT, and GV participated in the acquisition of data and helped revise the manuscript. LP participated in the acquisition of data, made a substantial contribution to the interpretation of data and helped revise the manuscript. IO participated in the design of the study, acquisition of data, made a substantial contribution to the interpretation of data, and revised the manuscript. All authors read and approved the final manuscript and they agreed to be accountable for all aspects of the work.

Acknowledgements

Collaborators: the ATLANTIS study Group - Augusta Ortolan[1], Mariagrazia Lorenzin[1], Paola Frallonardo[1], Alessandro Giollo[3], Antonella Locaputo[4], Sabrina Paolino[5], Davide Simone[6], Luca Quartuccio[8], Elena Bartoloni[10], Rossella De Luca[11], Francesca Bartoli[11], Felice Sensi[12], Roberto Caporali[13], Marco Di Carlo[15], Bortolotti Roberto[16], Fabiola Atzeni[17], Luisa Costa[18], Francesco Ciccia[20], Fabio Perrotta[21], Michele Gilio[22]. Coordinator - Italian National Association of Rheumatic Patients (ANMAR) on the Doxa-Pharma organization.

Author details

[1]Rheumatology Unit, Department of Medicine DIMED, University of Padova, Via Giustiniani, 2, Padova 35128, Italy. [2]Division of Rheumatology, Day Hospital Unit, Istituto Ortopedico G. Pini, Milano, Italy. [3]Rheumatology Unit, University of Verona, Verona, Italy. [4]Department of Locomotor System, Division of Rheumatology, ASL3-Azienda Sanitaria Genovese, Arenzano, Genova, Italy. [5]Research Laboratory and Academic Division of Clinical Rheumatology, Department of Internal Medicine, IRCCS A.O.U. San Martino-IST, University of Genova, Genova, Italy. [6]Division of Rheumatology, Institute of Rheumatology & Affine Sciences, Catholic University School of Medicine, Roma, Italy. [7]Rheumatology Unit, Città della Salute e della Scienza, University Hospital of Torino, Torino, Italy. [8]Rheumatology Clinic, Department of Medical and Biological Sciences, Azienda Ospedaliero-Universitaria S. Maria della Misericordia, Udine, Italy. [9]Research Center of Systemic Autoimmune and Autoinflammatory Diseases, University of Siena, Siena, Italy. [10]Rheumatology Unit, Department of Medicine, University of Perugia, Perugia, Italy. [11]Department of Experimental and Clinical Medicine, Division of Rheumatology, Azienda Ospedaliero-Universitaria Careggi (AOUC), University of Firenze, Firenze, Italy. [12]Division of Rheumatology, San Camillo Hospital, Roma, Italy. [13]Department of Rheumatology, University of Pavia, IRCCS San Matteo Foundation, Pavia, Italy. [14]Rheumatology Unit, Ospedale Mauriziano, Torino, Italy. [15]Rheumatology Department, Polytechnic University of the Marche Region, Jesi, Italy. [16]Department of Rheumatology, Santa Chiara Hospital, Trento, Italy. [17]Rheumatology Unit, L. Sacco University Hospital, Milano, Italy. [18]Rheumatology Research Unit, Department of Clinical and Experimental Medicine, University Federico II, Napoli, Italy. [19]Department of Clinical and Experimental Medicine, University of Messina, Messina, Italy. [20]Department of Internal Medicine, Rheumatology Unit, University of Palermo, Palermo, Italy. [21]Rheumatology Unit, La Sapienza University of Roma, Roma, Italy. [22]Rheumatology Department, San Carlo Hospital, Potenza, Italy.

References

1. Van Tubergen A. The changing clinical picture and epidemiology of spondyloarthritis. Nature Rev Rheumatol. 2015;11:110–8.
2. Rudwaleit M, van der Heijde D, Landewè E, Listing J, Akkoc N, Brandt J, et al. The development of Assessment of SpondyloArthritis International Society classification criteria for axial spondyloarthritis (part II): validation and final selection. Ann Rheum Dis. 2009;68:777–83.
3. Rudwaleit M, van der Heijde D, Landewè E, Akkoc N, Brandt J, Chou CT, et al. The Assessment of SpondyloArthritis International Society classification criteria for peripheral spondyloarthritis and for spondyloarthritis in general. Ann Rheum Dis. 2011;70:777–83.
4. Kiltz U, Baraliakos X, Karakostas P, Igelmann M, Kalthoff L, Klink C, et al. Do patients with non-radiographic axial spondylarthritis differ from patients with ankylosing spondylitis? Arthritis Care Res. 2012;64:1415–22.
5. Rudwaleit M, Haibel H, Baraliakos X, Listing J, Märker-Hermann E, Zeidler H, et al. The early disease stage in axial spondylarthritis. Results from the German Spondyloarthritis Inception Cohort. Arthrits Rheum. 2009;60:717–27.
6. Wallis D, Haroon N, Ayearst R, Listing J, Märker-Hermann E, Zeidler H, et al. Ankylosing Spondylitis and nonradiographic axial spondyloarthritis: part of a common spectrum or distinct disease? J Rheumatol. 2013;40: 2038–4.
7. Robinson PC, Wordsworth BP, Reveille JD, Brown MA. Axial spondyloarthritis: a new disease entity, not necessarily early ankylosing spondylitis. Ann Rheum Dis. 2013;72(2):162–4.
8. Boonen A, Sieper J, van der Heijde D, Dougados M, Bukowski JF, Valluri S, et al. The burden of non-radiographic axial spondyloarthritis. Semin Arthritis Rheum. 2014;44(5):556–62.
9. Song IH, Sieper J, Rudwaleit M. Diagnosing early ankylosing spondylitis. Curr Rheumatol Rep. 2007;9:367–74.
10. van der Linden S, Valkenburg HA, Cats A. Evaluation of diagnostic criteria for ankylosing spondylitis. A proposal for modification of the New York criteria. Arthritis Rheum. 1984;27:361–8.
11. Taylor W, Gladman D, Helliwell P, Marchesoni A, Mease P, Mielants H, et al. Classification criteria for psoriatic arthritis: development of new criteria from a large international study. Arthritis Rheum. 2006;54:2665–73.

12. Dagfinrud H, Kjeken I, Mowinckel P, Hagen KB, Kvien TK. Impact of functional impairment in ankylosing, spondylitis: impairment, activity limitation and participation restriction. J Rheumatol. 2005;32:516–23.
13. Singh JA, Strand V. Spondyloarthritis is associated with poor function and physical health-related quality of life. J Rheumatol. 2009;36:1012–20.
14. Lee S, Mendelsohn A, Sarnes E. The burden of psoriatic arthritis. A literature review from a global health systems perspective. P T. 2010;53(12):680–9.
15. Boonen A. A review of work-participation, cost-of-illness and cost-effectiveness studies in ankylosing spondylitis. Nat Clin Pract Rheum. 2006;2:546–53.
16. Tillett W, de-Vries C, McHugh NJ. Work disability in psoriatic arthritis: a systematic review. Rheumatology. 2012;51:275–83.
17. Haglund E, Bremander A, Bergman S, Jacobsson LT, Petersson IF. Work productivity in a population-based cohort of patients with spondyloarthritis. Rheumatology. 2013;52:1708–14.
18. Reilly MC, Gooch KL, Wong RL, Kupper H, van der Heijde D. Validity, reliability and responsiveness of the Work Productivity and Activity Impairment Questionnaire in ankylosing spondylitis. Rheumatology. 2010;49:812–9.
19. Boonen A, van der Heijde D, Landewè R, Spoorenberg A, Schouten H, Rutten-van Mölken M, et al. Work status and productivity costs due to ankylosing spondylitis: comparison of three European countries. Ann Rheum Dis. 2002;61:429–37.
20. Moltó A, Etcheto A, van der Heijde D, Landewé R, van den Bosch F, Bautista Molano W, et al. Prevalence of comorbidities and evaluation of their screening in spondyloarthritis: results of the international cross-sectional ASAS-COMOSPA study. Ann Rheum Dis 2015 pii: annrheumdis-2015-208174. doi: 10.1136/annrheumdis-2015-208174. [Epub ahead of print].
21. Sieper J, Rudwaleit M, Khan M, Braun J. Concepts and epidemiology of spondyloarthritis. Best Pract Res Clin Rheumatol. 2006;20:401–17.
22. Liu JT, Yeh HM, Liu SY, Chen KT. Psoriatic arthritis: epidemiology, diagnosis and treatment. World J Orthop. 2014;5:637–543.
23. ISTAT Noi Italia 100 statistics to understand the country we live in. http://noi-italia2013en.istat.it/. Accessed 27 Mar 2015.
24. Statistiche demografiche ISTAT. http://demo.istat.it/pop2013/index.html. Accessed 27 Mar 2015.
25. Tasso di occupazione. http://dati.istat.it/Index.aspx?DataSetCode=DCCV_TAXOCCU&Lang=. Accessed 27 Mar 2015.
26. Trattamenti pensionistici e beneficiari 2013. https://www.inps.it/docallegati/Mig/Doc/sas_stat/BeneficiariPensioni/Trattamenti_pensionistici_beneficiari-2013.pdf. Accessed 27 Mar 2015.
27. Boonen A, de Vet H, van der Heijde D, van der Linden S. Work status and its determinants among patients with ankylosing spondylitis. A systematic literature review. J Rheumatol. 2001;28:1056–62.
28. Healey EL, Haywood KL, Jordan KP, Garratt A, Packham JC. Impact of ankylosing spondylitis on work in patients across the UK. Scand J Rheumatol. 2011;40:34–40.
29. van der Heijde DM, Revicki DA, Gooch KL, Wong RL, Kupper H, Harnam N, ATLAS Study Group. Physical function, disease activity, and health-related quality-of-life outcomes after 3 years of adalimumab treatment in patients with ankylosing spondylitis. Arthritis Res Ther. 2009;11:R124.
30. Maksymowych WP, Gooch KL, Wong RL, Kupper H, van der Heijde D. Impact of age, sex, physical function, health-related quality of life, and treatment with adalimumab on work status and work productivity of patients with ankylosing spondylitis. J Rheumatol. 2010;37:385–92.
31. Keat AC, Gaffney K, Gilbert AK, Harris C, Leeder J. Influence of biologic therapy on return to work in people with work disability due to ankylosing spondylitis. Rheumatology. 2008;47:481–3.
32. Van der Heijde D, Han C, DeVlam K, Burmester G, van den Bosch F, Williamson P, et al. Infliximab improves productivity and reduces workday loss in patients with ankylosing spondylitis: results from a randomized, placebo-controlled trial. Arthritis Rheum. 2006;55:569–74.
33. Kristensen LE, Englund M, Neovius M, Askling J, Jacobsson LT, Petersson IF. Long-term work disability in patients with psoriatic arthritis treated with anti-tumour necrosis factor: a population-based regional Swedish cohort study. Ann Rheum Dis. 2013;72:1675–9.
34. Prince DS, McGuigan LE, McGirr EE. Working life and physical activity in ankylosing spondylitis pre and post anti-tumor necrosis factor-alpha therapy. Int J Rheum Dis. 2014;17:165–72.

21

Evaluation of treatments for sacroiliitis in spondyloarthropathy using the Spondyloarthritis Research Consortium Canada scoring system

Yang Cui[1†], Jinping Zheng[1†], Xiao Zhang[1*], Hui Zeng[2] and Riqiang Luo[1]

Abstract

Background: In this study, the Spondyloarthritis Research Consortium Canada (SPARCC) scoring method was used to compare treatment methods in patients with axial spondyloarthritis (SpA), a form of sacroiliitis. MRI abnormalities in bone marrow edema (BME) were compared before and after treatment in order to compare the efficacy of anti-TNF-α and DMARD, alone or in combination, as treatments for sacroiliitis.

Methods: Fifty-six Chinese patients with axial SpA (mean age 22.6 years) were recruited. Patients were divided into three groups according to different treatments (anti-TNF-α alone vs. DMARDs alone vs. combined anti-TNF-α and DMARDs). MRI examinations were performed before and after treatment. The SPARCC score, clinically relevant AS Disease Activity (ASDAS) indices, erythrocyte sedimentation rate (ESR), and C-reactive protein (CRP) were analyzed.

Results: After treatment, ASDAS and SPARCC scores, ESR, and CRP were significantly improved ($P < 0.05$) in the anti-TNF-α monotherapy and combination groups; however, there were no statistically significant differences ($P > 0.05$) in clinical disease activity and radiological inflammation of sacroiliac joint (SIJ) in patients in the DMARDs alone group. SPARCC showed a correlation with ASDAS score pre-treatment, but not post-treatment. Furthermore, there were significant changes ($P < 0.05$) in these patients with axial SpA after only 3 months of treatment. Follow-up studies of patients who continued therapy for 4-6 months and 9-12 months revealed statistically significant differences from baseline ($P < 0.05$).

Conclusions: SPARCC can be used to assess severity of disease pre-treatment. Anti-TNF-α treatment resulted in effective reduction of disease activity and BME of SIJ after 3 months of therapy.

Keywords: spondyloarthritis, sacroiliitis, imaging studies, scoring, biologics, disease-modifying anti-rheumatic drugs

Background

Spondyloarthritis (SpA) is a chronic, debilitating inflammatory rheumatic disease that affects axial and peripheral joints, organs, and other tissues. Epidemiology surveys of patients with SpA in China have reported a prevalence of SpA in the military of 0.45 %; however, the pooled incidence and prevalence of SpA from studies performed in civilian populations is 0.93 %. These numbers are similar to the prevalence found in Caucasian populations in Europe or the United States [1–11]. Sacroiliitis is the pathological sign and one of the early manifestations of SpA [12]. The management of SpA is extremely difficult. The traditional anti-rheumatic drugs (disease-modifying anti-rheumatic drugs (DMARDs)) are not clearly effective towards improving arthropathy of the central axis. In addition, numerous adverse reactions limit their clinical application. Biological agents such as tumor necrosis factor alpha (TNFα) inhibitor have been used in clinical research to treat ankylosing spondylitis (AS), showing efficacy against disease reactiveness and positive effects on joint function.

* Correspondence: xiaozhang640@sohu.com
[†]Equal contributors
[1]Department of Rheumatism, Guangdong General Hospital, Guangdong Academy of Medical Sciences, No. 106, Zhongshaner Road, Guangzhou, China
Full list of author information is available at the end of the article

During the 2013 European League against Rheumatism (EULAR) meeting on spondyloarthropathy, it was determined that inflammation demonstrated by magnetic resonance imaging (MRI) and radiographic progression should be considered when determining therapeutic goals. Therefore, a standard assessment system is necessary for evaluating imaging changes in the sacroiliac joint (SIJ) in patients with SpA. In a study by Landewe et al. [13], the Spondyloarthritis Research Consortium Canada (SPARCC) system had a high level of inter-reader variability and sensitivity to change. The AS working group of the International Association for the Evaluation of Spinal Arthritis/Outcome Measures in Rheumatology (ASAS/OMERACT) proposed that MRI should be used as the first choice for evaluation of spinal arthritis [14].

More and more studies have used the SPARCC scoring system [15] to evaluate the efficacy of treatments in reducing joint inflammation of patients with SpA. Previous studies have shown a correlation between SPARCC scores and clinical disease activity. Zhang et al. [16] determined a correlation between the apparent diffusion coefficient (ADC) and SPARCC scores. However, little attention has been focused on the period in which bone marrow edema (BME) of the SIJ should be evaluated and the differences in joint inflammation changes between different therapies. Therefore, this study aimed to investigate the value of the SPARCC scoring system in evaluating the treatment of patients with axial SpA. Specifically, the efficacy of anti-TNFα and DMARDs as treatments for sacroiliitis was assessed with both drugs alone or in combination.

Methods

Patient eligibility

Fifty-six patients with SpA treated at the Guangdong General Hospital between September 2012 and March 2014 were recruited. Inclusion criteria included meeting the ASAS classification criteria for axial SpA [17]. The Bath Ankylosing Spondylitis Disease Activity Index (BASDAI) score had to be ≥4 [18]. No patient had been treated with systemic glucocorticoids for a period of 3 months prior to the trial. Participation required that patients had no active infectious diseases or severe organ function failure.

The 56 patients were divided into three groups according to therapy type. There were 18 patients with SpA treated using anti-TNFα alone, 21 patients treated using anti-TNFα combined with DMARDs, and 17 patients treated with DMARDs alone. All patients were allowed to use nonsteroidal anti-inflammatory drugs (NSAIDs) during the study as needed. The dose of anti-TNFα was gradually reduced as the disease became under better control (Ankylosing Spondylitis Disease Activity (ASDAS) indices <1.3) [19]. The reduction in dosage was as follows: if the patient's ASDAS was <1.3 after 3 months of adequate therapeutic dosage of anti-TNFα, the interval between injections was extended (from 50 mg every week down to 50 mg every 10 days); and when ASDAS remained <1.3 after another 3 months of treatment, the interval was extended to 50 mg every 15 days. No patient discontinued treatment before the end of the study, and the dose for those who had undergone DMARD treatment remained the same as at the beginning of the study. Patients underwent MRI before and within 12 months after treatment.

Patients ever treated with anti-TNFα (total 39 patients, including anti-TNFα monotherapy and anti-TNFα combined with DMARDs) were divided into three subgroups according to the period of MRI examination: Group A, patients underwent MRI in their 3rd month of treatment ($n = 10$); group B, patients underwent MRI during their 4th–6th month of treatment ($n = 17$); and group C, patients underwent MRI during their 9th–12th month of treatment ($n = 12$).

The study was approved by the ethical committee of Guangdong General Hospital, China (approval No. 2013005H(RE)). Written informed consents were obtained from the participants.

MRI scan

All patients' SIJs were examined using T1-weighted images (T1WI), T2 fast-suppressed (T2-fs), and short-tau inversion recovery (STIR). The BME of the SIJ was scored by two experienced radiologists (10 and 2 years of experience, respectively) according to the SPARCC sacroiliitis scoring system. Readers were blinded to treatment and time sequence of the images. Final scores were taken as the average of the two readers.

SPARCC scoring system

The radiologists observed an increased signal in the iliac bone and sacrum in six consecutive slices through the SIJ on T2-fs images or STIR sequences on oblique coronal slices. These slices comprise most of the synovial compartment. Each SIJ is divided into four quadrants, and each quadrant has 1 point for the presence of an increased STIR signal. Next, a total score of 48 is obtained from the six slices of the two SIJs. Then, 1 point is added for each SIJ exhibiting an intense signal (compared with the signal from adjacent blood vessels) or depth of BME ≥1 cm for the six slices, bringing the total score to 72.

Clinical evaluation

The ASDAS [19] included back pain, general condition, and stiffness using a visual analog score, which was determined by doctor inquiry and patient self-reporting. C-reactive protein (CRP) and the erythrocyte sedimentation rate (ESR) were determined for all patients. For assessment of the ESR, 5 ml blood were obtained from the

Table 1 Patient characteristics and disease parameters

	All	Anti-TNF alone	Anti-TNF + DMARDs	DMARDs alone
Age (years)	21 (15–36)	23 (15–29)	27 (18–32)	28 (22–36)
Gender (male/female)	12/44	3/15	6/15	3/14
Disease duration	2 (0.17–10)	0.67 (0.17–3)	2 (0.75–6)	7.5 (3.5–10)
HLA-B27-positive	91.1 % (51/56)	88.9 % (16/18)	90.5 % (19/21)	94.1 % (16/17)
Baseline				
SPARCC	32.45 ± 18.71	27.76 ± 18.38	39.53 ± 19.21	28.67 ± 15.51
ASDAS	2.84 ± 1.26	2.56 ± 1.24	3.58 ± 1.05	2.21 ± 1.03
ESR[a]	27.10 ± 32.39	27.94 ± 33.24	38.49 ± 38.50	12.14 ± 8.43
CRP[a]	17.50 ± 23.07	16.29 ± 23.05	26.29 ± 28.02	7.919 ± 5.60

[a]Not normally distributed, compared by paired rank test
ASDAS Ankylosing Spondylitis Disease Activity Indices, *CRP* C-reactive protein, *DMARD* disease-modifying anti-rheumatic drug, *ESR* erythrocyte sedimentation rate, *SPARCC* Spondyloarthritis Research Consortium Canada, *TNF* tumor necrosis factor

median antebrachial vein of each patient after a 12-hour fast and kept at 4 °C. Then, a 1.6 ml blood sample was combined with 0.4 ml sodium citrate (10^9 mmol/l) and the mixture was placed into an ESR tube taking care not to create bubbles. The tube was placed vertically on the ESR stand and the ESR was read after an hour. For CRP, the blood sample underwent coagulation and was centrifuged. The serum was taken and kept at 4 °C. CRP levels were measured using a Roche Cobas 6000 c501 automatic analyzer (Roche Diagnostics, Laval, Canada) based on an immunoturbidimetry method, using the reagents and instructions provided by the manufacturer.

Treatment adverse effects were recorded based on the reports from the patients, clinical examination, and relevant biochemistry indexes.

Statistical analysis

Factorial analysis was used for inter-group comparisons using SPSS 16.0 (IBM, Armonk, NY, USA). Intragroup comparisons were performed with a paired *t* test or rank

Table 2 Differences of indexes in patients with different treatment method

Index	Baseline (mean ± SD)	Post-treatment (mean ± SD)	*t/Z*	*P*
Patients treated by anti-TNF alone (*n* = 18)[a]				
SPARCC	27.76 ± 18.38	14.38 ± 14.91	2.681	**0.011**
ASDAS	2.56 ± 1.24	1.83 ± 0.71	4.231	**0.006**
ESR[b]	27.94 ± 33.24	5.72 ± 7.06	−2.763	**0.009**
CRP[b]	16.29 ± 23.05	2.70 ± 2.55	−2.470	**0.022**
Patients treated by anti-TNF combined with DMARDs (*n* = 21)[c]				
SPARCC	39.53 ± 19.21	20.71 ± 15.98	5.110	**0.000**
ASDAS	3.58 ± 1.05	1.88 ± 0.74	4.278	**0.003**
ESR[b]	38.49 ± 38.50	9.02 ± 13.29	−2.703	**0.010**
CRP[b]	26.29 ± 28.02	8.43 ± 15.79	−2.329	0.053
Patients treated by DMARDs alone (*n* = 17)[d]				
SPARCC	28.67 ± 15.51	21.66 ± 11.23	0.820	0.419
ASDAS	2.21 ± 1.03	1.99 ± 0.47	1.301	0.261
ESR[b]	12.14 ± 8.43	4.65 ± 4.27	−2.396	**0.013**
CRP[b]	7.919 ± 5.60	5.55 ± 4.46	−1.911	0.056

[a]Baseline of clinical practices from patients in anti-TNF group: 85.7 % male; age, 23.3 ± 6.43; symptom duration, 3.15 ± 2.98; HLA-B27-positive, 100 %
[b]Not normally distributed, compared by paired rank test
[c]Baseline of clinical practices from patients in combination group: 82.35 % male; age, 21.6 ± 3.36; symptom duration, 2.97 ± 2.69; HLA-B27-positive, 88.2 %
[d]Baseline of clinical practices from patients in DMARD group: 80 % male; age, 20.5 ± 2.75; symptom duration, 3.0 ± 2.66; HLA-B27-positive, 90 %
ASDAS Ankylosing Spondylitis Disease Activity Indices, *CRP* C-reactive protein, *DMARD* disease-modifying anti-rheumatic drug, *ESR* erythrocyte sedimentation rate, *SD* standard deviation, *SPARCC* Spondyloarthritis Research Consortium Canada, *TNF* tumor necrosis factor

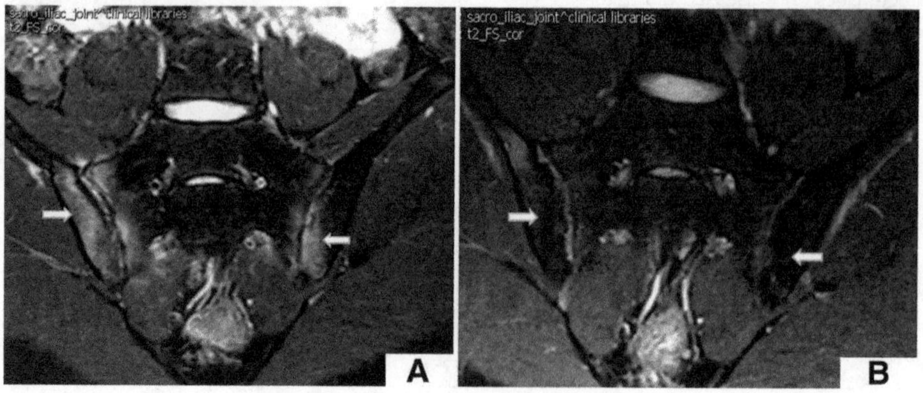

Fig. 1 BME changes **a** before (SPARCC score 65) and **b** after 6 months of anti-TNFα monotherapy (SPARCC score 22)

sum test and nonparametric test. Two-sided P <0.05 was considered statistically significant.

Results

Patient age ranged from 15 to 45 years; average patient disease duration was from 2 months to 10 years. Characteristics of the patients are presented in Table 1.

MRI scans

For the seven (17.9 %) patients treated with anti-TNFα, BME completely disappeared within 12 months. Similar outcomes were observed in patients treated with anti-TNFα alone or in combination with DMARDs; for these patients, there was a significant decrease in their SPARCC scores within 12 months of treatment (P < 0.05) (Table 2 and Figs. 1 and 2). Nevertheless, for patients treated by DMARDs, SPARCC scores did not change after treatment (P = 0.419) (Table 2 and Fig. 3).

Patients treated with anti-TNFα alone showed decreased SPARCC scores, ASDAS indices, ESR, and CRP within 12 months of starting treatment. SPARCC scores, ASDAS indices, and ESR were significantly decreased within 12 months after treatment with anti-TNFα combined with DMARD therapy. However, there were no significant differences in SPARCC scores, ASDAS indices, ESR, or CRP for patients treated with DMARDs alone within the 12-month study period (Table 3).

In detail, SPARCC scores in Group A were significantly decreased after 3 months of full-dose anti-TNFα (P = 0.012). In Group B (4–6 months of full-dose anti-TNFα), SPARCC values were reduced (P = 0.001). In Group C, patients were treated 9–12 months of anti-TNFα, and the values were also reduced (P = 0.038). The correlation between ASDAS values and MRI values was assessed, showing good correlation pre treatment but not after treatment (Fig. 4).

Adverse effects

Two patients experienced adverse reactions in the form of a temporary rash at the area of injection. One subject experienced a mild rash after oral sulfasalazine (SASP) intake. The diameters of the rashes were less than 5 mm, mild, without skin ulceration, and lasted for only 2 days without any treatment. One patient experienced a urinary tract infection during the second month of anti-TNFα treatment, caused by *Escherichia coli*. The patient

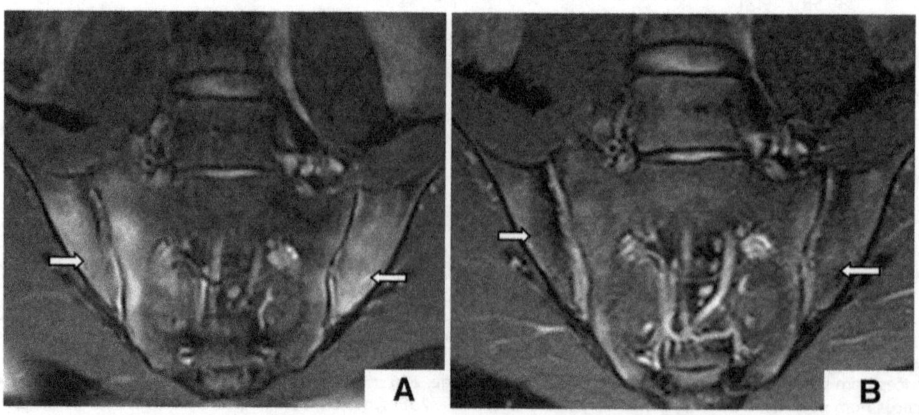

Fig. 2 BME changes **a** before (SPARCC score 72) and **b** after 6 months of treatment with anti-TNFα combined with DMARDs (SPARCC score 13)

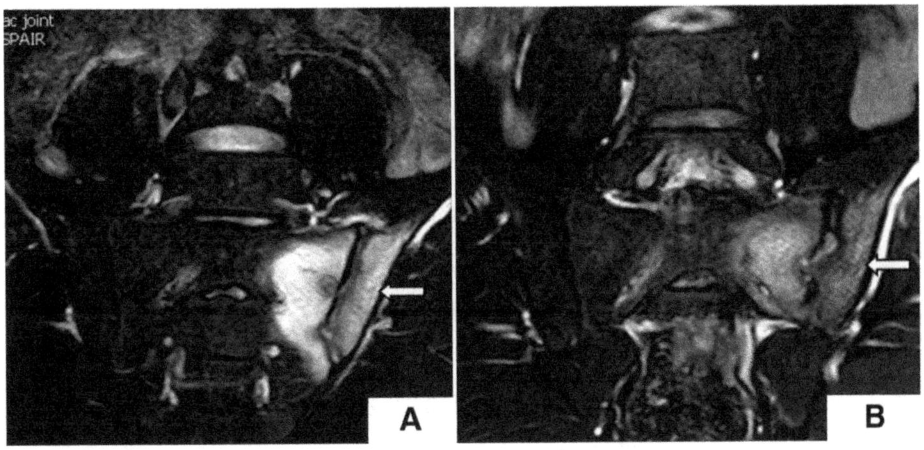

Fig. 3 BME changes **a** before (SPARCC score 36) and **b** after 8 months of DMARDs monotherapy (SPARCC score 33)

was treated with levofloxacin for 2 weeks based on results from a bacterial culture. Two patients experienced mild liver function abnormalities (patient 1, ALT = 42 U/l; patient 2, AST = 57 U/l). Liver function returned to normal after 2 weeks of liver treatment.

Discussion

NSAIDs and anti-rheumatic drugs are the primary treatment for SpA. SASP is believed to reduce the ESR and morning stiffness [20]. The pathogenesis of SpA is complex. Recent studies have revealed that TNFα plays a key role in the development of the disease. Studies have shown that TNF antagonists can significantly improve both disease activity and joint function [20–25].

In this study, patients with high SpA activity treated by targeted therapy (including etanercept, infliximab, and adalimumab) for 3 months showed significantly decreased ASDAS indices, SPARCC scores, and ESR ($P < 0.05$), indicating that 3 months of full-dose anti-TNFα therapy have significant efficacy as treatment against SpA. Furthermore, there was obvious resorption of SIJ acute inflammatory lesions observed from MRI examination. In 2013, an expert advisory committee advised the use of etanercept for the treatment of rheumatoid

Table 3 Differences of indexes in patients at different treatment periods

Index	Baseline (mean ± SD)	Post-treatment (mean ± SD)	*t/Z*	*P*
Group A: 3 months of full-dose anti-TNFα ($n = 10$; $n = 6$ for anti-TNFα alone, $n = 4$ for combination)[a]				
ASDAS	3.43 ± 1.55	1.66 ± 0.40	2.675	**0.043**
SPARCC	31.67 ± 18.64	14.50 ± 18.41	3.768	**0.012**
ESR[b]	52.00 ± 43.83	5.00 ± 5.55	−2.023	**0.046**
CRP[b]	36.58 ± 40.37	1.92 ± 1.09	−1.782	0.083
Group B: 4–6 months of anti-TNFα ($n = 17$; $n = 4$ for anti-TNFα alone, $n = 13$ for combination)[c]				
ASDAS	2.46 ± 0.58	1.58 ± 0.69	4.920	**<0.001**
SPARCC	34.98 ± 18.93	18.54 ± 15.72	4.285	**0.001**
ESR[b]	27.77 ± 34.95	7.22 ± 12.31	−2.749	**0.007**
CRP[b]	16.34 ± 23.11	4.37 ± 17.87	−2.283	**0.025**
Group C: 9–12 months of anti-TNFα ($n = 12$; $n = 6$ for anti-TNFα alone, $n = 6$ for combination)[d]				
ASDAS	2.91 ± 0.89	2.05 ± 1.21	2.517	**0.042**
SPARCC	38.24 ± 15.39	23.09 ± 15.65	2.527	**0.038**
ESR[b]	28.29 ± 27.77	12.43 ± 13.57	−1.498	0.128
CRP[b]	14.43 ± 11.65	10.81 ± 16.54	−1.529	0.134

[a]Baseline of clinical practices from patients in Group A: 85.7 % male; age, 23 ± 5.62; symptom duration, 2.6 ± 3.25; HLA-B27-positive, 85.7 %
[b]Not normally distributed, compared by paired rank test
[c]Baseline of clinical practices from patients in Group B: 85.7 % male; age, 23.3 ± 6.43; symptom duration, 3.15 ± 2.98; HLA-B27-positive, 100 %
[d]Baseline of clinical practices from patients in Group C: 80 % male; age, 21.3 ± 2.53; symptom duration, 3.97 ± 3.52; HLA-B27-positive, 90 %
ASDAS Ankylosing Spondylitis Disease Activity Indices, *CRP* C-reactive protein, *DMARD* disease-modifying anti-rheumatic drug, *ESR* erythrocyte sedimentation rate, *SD* standard deviation, *SPARCC* Spondyloarthritis Research Consortium Canada, *TNFα* tumor necrosis factor alpha

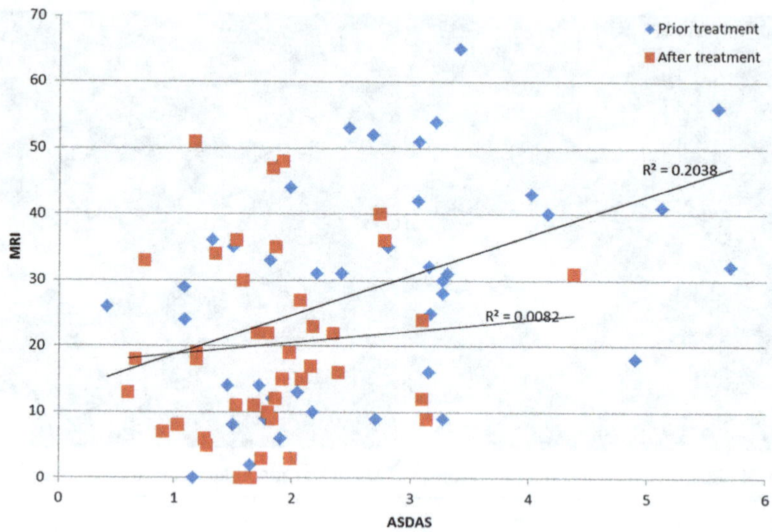

Fig. 4 Correlations between ASDAS values and MRI values in all patients before treatment. *ASDAS* Ankylosing Spondylitis Disease Activity, *MRI* magnetic resonance imaging

arthritis and AS [26], and suggested that assessment of treatment efficacy in patients with AS should be performed at least 3 months after starting the treatment. Based on the present study, anti-TNFα could be of great help in improving the symptoms of SpA. After 3 months of anti-TNFα, the clinical activity and BME of the SIJ in patients with SpA showed significant improvement, and patients might maintain remission with continued use, even with a reduction in treatment dose. As shown in this study, both anti-TNFα alone and in combination with DMARDs showed significant changes in SPARCC scores, ASDAS indices, and ESR. Previous studies [26–28] showed that there were differences of SPARCC score in disease-dormant patients and in disease-active patients. Furthermore, the SPARCC score has been proven to be positively correlated with the BASDAI, suggesting that the SPARCC scoring system can be used to assess inflammation activity in SpA. The SPARCC scoring system therefore plays an important role in evaluating treatment efficacy. The SPARCC scoring system provides a reference for imaging and evaluating the efficacy of different therapies. SIJ MRI examination has high sensitivity for the early stages of sacroiliitis [29], and it is safer and easier to repeat than X-ray or computed tomography scan.

There were some limitations to this study. The sample size was small and the timing of MRI examinations was not similar for all patients. Furthermore, the treatment dose levels varied between participants. In this study, DMARDs seem to have a modest effect at best on SpA, but this study was not designed to examine the efficacy of DMARDs. The results suggest that only a 3-month follow-up might be necessary to assess the response to treatment, and that subsequent follow-ups are relatively optional. However, this study was not designed to address this issue, and we cannot draw any conclusion on this point. Additional multicenter trials are necessary to determine adequately the usefulness of anti-TNFα and the SPARCC scoring system in patients with SpA.

Conclusions

The SPARCC scoring system is a good index for showing the severity of sacroiliitis pre treatment. In addition, this study showed that anti-TNFα was effective in reducing BME of the SIJ examined by MRI.

Abbreviations

ADC: Apparent diffusion coefficient; AS: Ankylosing spondylitis; ASAS/OMERACT: International Association for the Evaluation of Spinal Arthritis/Outcome Measures in Rheumatology; ASDAS: Ankylosing Spondylitis Disease Activity; BASDAI: Bath Ankylosing Spondylitis Disease Activity Index; BME: Bone marrow edema; CRP: C-reactive protein; DMARD: Disease-modifying anti-rheumatic drug; ESR: Erythrocyte sedimentation rate; EULAR: European League against Rheumatism; MRI: Magnetic resonance imaging; NSAID: Nonsteroidal anti-inflammatory drug; SIJ: Sacroiliac joint; SASP: Sulfasalazine; SpA: Spondyloarthritis; SPARCC: Spondyloarthritis Research Consortium Canada; STIR: Short-tau inversion recovery; T1WI: T1-weighted images; T2-fs: T2 fast-suppressed; TNFα: Tumor necrosis factor alpha.

Competing interests

The authors declare that they have no competing interests.

Authors' contributions

YC, JPZ, and XZ contributed to study conception and design. YC, JPZ, XZ, HZ, and RQL contributed to data acquisition, or data analysis and interpretation. YC, JPZ, XZ, HZ, and RQL were involved in drafting the manuscript or revising it critically for important intellectual content. All authors have given final approval of the version to be published.

Author details

[1]Department of Rheumatism, Guangdong General Hospital, Guangdong Academy of Medical Sciences, No. 106, Zhongshaner Road, Guangzhou, China. [2]Medical Imaging Centre, Guangdong General Hospital, Guangdong Academy of Medical Sciences, Guangzhou 510010, China.

References

1. Ng SC, Liao Z, Yu DT, Chan ES, Zhao L, Gu J. Epidemiology of spondyloarthritis in the People's Republic of China: review of the literature and commentary. Semin Arthritis Rheum. 2007;37:39–47.
2. Wigley RD, Zhang NZ, Zeng QY, Shi CS, Hu DW, Couchman K, et al. Rheumatic diseases in China: ILAR-China study comparing the prevalence of rheumatic symptoms in northern and southern rural populations. J Rheumatol. 1994;21:1484–90.
3. Zhang NZ, Zeng QY, Zhang FS, Chen JB, Shi QS, Yao QP. An epidemiology study of rheumatic diseases in China. Chin J Rheumatol. 1997;1:31–5.
4. Chen R, Wang QW, Lin QQ, Wu XR, Xu JC, Xie SH. Epidemiological study of spondyloarthropathies. Chin J Rheumatol. 2000;4:240–1.
5. Chao TM, Han QW, Duan YC, Ji YB, Chen LZ, Dong DX. Epidemiological study of ankylosing spondylitis among some of the male soldiers stationed in the northeast military zone. Chin J Rheumatol. 2000;4:307–8.
6. Liu ZF, Liu JM, Liu JZ, Zhao RM, Zhang HK. Epidemiological study of spondyloarthropathies in the rural areas of Shandong province. Chin J Rheumatol. 2001;5:181–2.
7. Chen R, Du LC, Lin QQ, Chen SB, Lin L, Xu JC. Epidemiological study of seronegative spondyloarthropathies in a particular Beijing factory. Chin J Prim Med Pharm. 2002;9:593–4.
8. Shi F, Gu K, Lu W, Weng WF, Zhu MY, Peng YY, et al. Study on the prevalence of arthritis and relevant factors in Shanghai. Zhonghua Liu Xing Bing Xue Za Zhi. 2003;24:1136–40.
9. Dai SM, Han XH, Zhao DB, Shi YQ, Liu Y, Meng JM. Prevalence of rheumatic symptoms, rheumatoid arthritis, ankylosing spondylitis, and gout in Shanghai, China: a COPCORD study. J Rheumatol. 2003;30:2245–51.
10. Wu ZB, Zhu P, Wang HK, Zheng ZH, Jia Y, Ding J. Prevalence of seronegative spondyloarthritis in the army force of China. Chin J Epidemiol. 2004;25:753–5.
11. Dong HY, Zang CH, Zhang AL, Zheng JZ. Epidemiological study of seronegative spondyloarthropathies in Taiyuan. Chin Remedies Clin. 2006;6:262–5.
12. Gladman DD. Clinical aspects of the spondyloarthropathies. Am J Med Sci. 1998;316:234–8.
13. Landewe RB, Hermann KG, van der Heijde DM, Baraliakos X, Jurik AG, Lambert RG, et al. Scoring sacroiliac joints by magnetic resonance imaging. A multiple-reader reliability experiment. J Rheumatol. 2005;32:2050–5.
14. van der Heijde D, Landewe R. Selection of a method for scoring radiographs for ankylosing spondylitis clinical trials, by the Assessment in Ankylosing Spondylitis Working Group and OMERACT. J Rheumatol. 2005;32:2048–9.
15. Maksymowych WP, Inman RD, Salonen D, Dhillon SS, Williams M, Stone M, et al. Spondyloarthritis research Consortium of Canada magnetic resonance imaging index for assessment of sacroiliac joint inflammation in ankylosing spondylitis. Arthritis Rheum. 2005;53:703–9.
16. Zhang P, Yu K, Guo R, Shah S, Morelli JN, Runge VA, et al. Ankylosing spondylitis: correlations between clinical and MRI indices of sacroiliitis activity. Clin Radiol. 2015;70:62–6.
17. Rudwaleit M, van der Heijde D, Landewe R, Akkoc N, Brandt J, Chou CT, et al. The Assessment of SpondyloArthritis International Society classification criteria for peripheral spondyloarthritis and for spondyloarthritis in general. Ann Rheum Dis. 2011;70:25–31.
18. Calin A, Garrett S, Whitelock H, Kennedy LG, O'Hea J, Mallorie P, et al. A new approach to defining functional ability in ankylosing spondylitis: the development of the Bath Ankylosing Spondylitis Functional Index. J Rheumatol. 1994;21:2281–5.
19. Lukas C, Landewe R, Sieper J, Dougados M, Davis J, Braun J, et al. Development of an ASAS-endorsed disease activity score (ASDAS) in patients with ankylosing spondylitis. Ann Rheum Dis. 2009;68:18–24.
20. Chen J, Lin S, Liu C. Sulfasalazine for ankylosing spondylitis. Cochrane Database Syst Rev. 2014;11:CD004800.
21. Lee J, Noh JW, Hwang JW, Oh JM, Kim H, Ahn JK, et al. Extended dosing of etanercept 25 mg can be effective in patients with ankylosing spondylitis: a retrospective analysis. Clin Rheumatol. 2010;29:1149–54.
22. Lee SH, Lee YA, Hong SJ, Yang HI. Etanercept 25 mg/week is effective enough to maintain remission for ankylosing spondylitis among Korean patients. Clin Rheumatol. 2008;27:179–81.
23. Cantini F, Niccoli L, Cassara E, Kaloudi O, Nannini C. Duration of remission after halving of the etanercept dose in patients with ankylosing spondylitis: a randomized, prospective, long-term, follow-up study. Biologics. 2013;7:1–6.
24. Navarro-Compan V, Moreira V, Ariza-Ariza R, Hernandez-Cruz B, Vargas-Lebron C, Navarro-Sarabia F. Low doses of etanercept can be effective in ankylosing spondylitis patients who achieve remission of the disease. Clin Rheumatol. 2011;30:993–6.
25. Song IH, Althoff CE, Haibel H, Hermann KG, Poddubnyy D, Listing J, et al. Frequency and duration of drug-free remission after 1 year of treatment with etanercept versus sulfasalazine in early axial spondyloarthritis: 2 year data of the ESTHER trial. Ann Rheum Dis. 2012;71:1212–5.
26. Experts on etanercept treating rheumatoid arthritis and ankylosing spondylitis. Advices on etanercept treating rheumatoid arthritis and ankylosing spondylitis (2013). Chin J Intern Med. 2013;93:1363–9.
27. Weber U, Maksymowych WP, Jurik AG, Pfirrmann CW, Rufibach K, Kissling RO, et al. Validation of whole-body against conventional magnetic resonance imaging for scoring acute inflammatory lesions in the sacroiliac joints of patients with spondylarthritis. Arthritis Rheum. 2009;61:893–9.
28. Francois RJ, Gardner DL, Degrave EJ, Bywaters EG. Histopathologic evidence that sacroiliitis in ankylosing spondylitis is not merely enthesitis. Arthritis Rheum. 2000;43:2011–24.
29. Puhakka KB, Jurik AG, Schiottz-Christensen B, Hansen GV, Egund N, Christiansen JV, et al. Magnetic resonance imaging of sacroiliitis in early seronegative spondylarthropathy. Abnormalities correlated to clinical and laboratory findings. Rheumatology (Oxford). 2004;43:234–7.

Sponyloarthritis features forecasting the presence of HLA-B27 or sacroiliitis on magnetic resonance imaging in patients with suspected axial spondyloarthritis: results from a cross-sectional study in the ESPeranza Cohort

Victoria Navarro-Compán[1,2*], Eugenio de Miguel[1], Désirée van der Heijde[2], Robert Landewé[3,4], Raquel Almodóvar[5], Carlos Montilla[6], Emma Beltrán[7] and Pedro Zarco[5]

Abstract

Introduction: Chronic back pain (CBP) is frequently the presenting symptom in patients with suspected axial spondyloarthritis (axSpA). Presence of sacroiliitis on magnetic-resonance-imaging (MRI) or HLA-B27 adds to diagnostic certainty. However, these costly tests cannot be applied in all patients with CBP. This study aims to investigate which SpA features increase the likelihood of a positive HLA-B27 or positive MRI of the sacroiliac-joints (MRI-SI) in patients with suspected axSpA.

Methods: Data from 665 patients with CBP within the ESPeranza Programme were analysed. Diagnostic utility measures (LR+, LR−) for a positive MRI-SI or HLA-B27 were calculated for various definitions of inflammatory back pain (IBP), their separate items and for other SpA features.

Results: Pretest probabilityies of a positive result was 41 % for MRI-SI and 40 % for HLA-B27. For a positive MRI-SI result the most useful IBP characteristic was alternating buttock pain (LR + =2.6). Among the IBP-criteria, fulfillment of the 'ASAS criteria' (LR + =2.1) was most contributory. Interestingly, the addition of alternating buttock pain to the Calin/ASAS-IBP criteria (LR + =6.0 and 5.5, respectively) or the addition of awakening at second half of night to the Calin-IBP criteria (LR + =5.5) increased the pre-test probability of MRI-sacroiliitis from 41 % to 79–80 %. Dactylitis (LR + =4.1) and inflammatory bowel disease (IBD) (LR + =6.4) increased this probability to 73 % and 81 %, respectively. To forecast HLA-B27 positivity, awakening at the second half of the night, fulfillment of the ASAS-IBP definition and uveitis were the most useful, but only marginally predictive (LR + = 1.3, 1,6 and 2.6, respectively).

Conclusions: If patients with suspected axial SpA have either 1) IBP according to Calin/ASAS definition plus alternating buttock pain, or 2) IBP according to Calin definition plus awakening at night, or 3) dactylitis or 4) IBD, the probability of finding a positive MRI-SI increases significantly.

* Correspondence: mvictoria.navarroc@gmail.com
[1]Department of Rheumatology, IdiPaz, University Hospital La Paz, Madrid, Spain
[2]Department of Rheumatology, Leiden University Medical Center, Leiden, The Netherlands
Full list of author information is available at the end of the article

Introduction

Axial spondyloarthritis (axSpA) has a major impact on physical function and quality of life [1]. Nevertheless, despite these important consequences patients with axSpA have been traditionally diagnosed after several years of symptoms [2]. In this sense, magnetic resonance imaging of sacroiliac joints (MRI-SI) has become important in the last decade, especially in the early stages of the disease. Nowadays, performing imaging, and testing human leucocyte antigen B27 (HLA-B27) are among the most important diagnostic procedures in patients with (suspicion of) axSpA. Accordingly, imaging and HLA-B27 results are also the entry criterion for classifying patients with chronic back pain (CBP) as having axSpA based on the classification criteria of the Assessment of SpondyloArthritis International Society (ASAS) [3].

Furthermore, in patients with suspected axSpA the starting point of the disease is usually the presence of CBP. However, CBP is one of the most prevalent symptoms in the general population and therefore it is essential to be able to select which patients with CBP have the highest chance of being diagnosed with axSpA. For this purpose, several referral strategies including different manifestations at the beginning of the disease have been developed for primary physicians, but [4–6] in clinical practice most patients are referred from primary care to rheumatologists because of inflammatory back pain (IBP) [4]. However, despite the publication of several IBP definitions [7–9], there is only poor agreement between primary physicians and rheumatologists about the presence of IBP. In addition to this, the original algorithm for diagnosing axSpA has been recently modified, excluding IBP as an obligatory entry criterion. This modification has been applied based on the finding that up to 30 % of patients with axSpA do not have IBP, and therefore its inclusion as an obligatory entry criterion results in too many misdiagnoses [10]. According to the modified algorithm, complementary examinations (HLA-B27 and MRI) need to be considered in those patients without sacroiliitis on conventional x-rays or with fewer than four featuresof SpA, which usually comprises most of the referred patients. But in clinical practice, due to efficiency reasons these tests must usually be restricted to patients with higher probability of a positive result. Based on clinical features, it would be very helpful for rheumatologists to identify which referred patients have the highest likelihood of ultimately being diagnosed as having axSpA. Such features of SpA that can be obtained by taking history or by simple physical examination, could potentially contribute to an efficient test-sequence to be applied in patients presenting with CBP and to optimise the use of supplementary tests in these patients. Based on this, this study aims to investigate which features of SpA may increase the pre-test probability of a positive test result of HLA-B27 or MRI-SI in patients with suspected axSpA, which is a step forward in making a diagnosis of axSpA.

Methods

Study design and population

This study was performed within the context of the ESPeranza Programme. The details from this initiative have been previously reported [11–13]. In summary, the ESPeranza Programme is a Spanish prospective multicentre national health programme aiming to facilitate early diagnosis of patients with spondyloarthritis. The programme was designed in compliance with the Helsinki Declaration and approved by the Ethical Committee of Research Unit of Hospital Reina Sofía in Córdoba. Over 3 years from April 2008, primary physicians and other specialists were asked by rheumatologists to refer patients meeting the following criteria: 1) age from 18 to 45 years; 2) symptom duration between 3 and 24 months; and 3) fulfilling one of the following three symptoms: IBP, asymmetrical arthritis or spinal/joint pain plus the presence of at least one of the following features: psoriasis, inflammatory bowel disease (IBD), anterior uveitis, radiographic sacroiliitis, HLA-B27 positivity, or a family history of spondylitis. All patients provided signed informed consent. In total, 25 centres across the country participated in the programme and 775 patients met the inclusion criteria. For the current study, only those patients referred with axial symptoms (n = 665) were selected.

Data collection and clinical measures

In the ESPeranza programme, sociodemographic and disease data were collected including age, sex, symptom duration, family history of SpA or related diseases, peripheral manifestations (enthesitis, dactylitis and/or arthritis) and extra-articular manifestations (psoriasis, uveitis, IBD). In addition, all typical characteristics of IBP were separately collected including: morning stiffness, improvement of back pain with exercise and not with rest, alternating buttock pain, insidious onset and awakening during the second half of the night. Moreover, the SpA feature related with CBP and CBP, "Good response to nonsteroidal anti-inflammatory drugs (NSAIDs)" were collected too. Based on this information, the fulfilment of the different existing IBP criteria was established as follows: Calin (at least four out of the following five criteria: age <40 years, insidious onset, duration >3 months, morning stiffness, improvement with exercise); Berlin (at least two out of the following four: morning stiffness, improvement with exercise and not with rest, awakening during the second half of the night, alternating buttock pain) and ASAS (at least four out of the following five: age <40 years, insidious onset, improvement with exercise, no improvement with rest, night pain).

Clinical assessments were also performed, including disease activity (Bath ankylosing spondylitis disease activity index, BASDAI), function (Bath ankylosing spondylitis functional index, BASFI), and laboratory tests (C-reactive protein (CRP)). The presence of HLA-B27 was tested in the local laboratory of each centre according to the standard procedure. The evaluation of conventional radiographs of the cervical and lumbar spine and of the pelvis was part of the protocol. MRI-SI was not included in the protocol as mandatory. Nevertheless, all rheumatologists were asked to perform MRI-SI if possible. However, due to existing differences between centres in accessibility to MRI, including budget limitations and waiting lists for MRI, MRI-SI was not performed all patients. MRI-SI was evaluated locally by one reader at each hospital, who evaluated the presence or absence of sacroiliitis according to the ASAS definition [14].

Statistical analysis

For descriptive purpose, results for continuous variables are presented as mean and standard deviation (SD) and for categorical variables are shown as percentage and relative frequencies. The diagnostic utility of each IBP characteristic, good response to NSAIDs, IBP definitions (Calin, Berlin, ASAS) and other features of SpA for a positive MRI-SI or HLA-B27 was calculated. Diagnostic utility was assessed based on sensitivity, specificity, positive and negative predictive values (PPV and NPV) and especially, positive and negative likelihood (LR+ and LR−). Importantly, a cutoff value of 4.0 was used for LR+ to define a feature of SpA as useful. The reason for the selection of this cutoff is that it has been associated with a moderate increase (approximately 25 %) in the likelihood of disease [15]. Finally, post-test probability was calculated based on the positive and negative likelihood ratios using the following conversion formula:

$$\text{Odds} = \text{Probability}/(1 - \text{Probability}).$$

According to Bayes' law (post-test odds = pre-test odds* LR, in which LR− is used if a feature is absent and the LR+ if a feature is present) the likelihood of finding a positive MRI/HLAB27 was estimated in patients with this particular feature present or absent.

Results

Baseline characteristics

A total of 665 patients with axial symptoms were referred and included in ESPeranza. Fifty five percent were male, mean (SD) age was 33.2 (7.1) years and mean (SD) symptom duration was 12.6 (6.6) months. For most of them (n = 653; 98.2 %) data was also available on HLA-B27 testing, and these were included in the analysis to evaluate the association between IBP characteristics and the presence of HLA-B27. Approximately half of the patients (n = 326; 49 %) had MRI-SI performed and were included in the analysis to investigate the association between IBP characteristics and positive MRI-SI. Demographic and disease characteristics were similar for patients in the whole cohort compared with patients in whom MRI-SI had been performed (Table 1). In total, 270 (41 %) patients were HLA-B27 positive and 130 (40 %) patients had a positive MRI-SI result (pre-test probabilities).

Table 1 Baseline characteristics for all patients with axial symptoms included in Esperanza (left column) and for the subgroup of patients who underwent MRI-SI (right column)

Characteristic	Patients with axial symptoms referred to Esperanza (n = 665)	Patients with axial symptoms and SIJ MRI available (n = 326)
Age, years	33.2 ± 7.1	32.8 ± 7.0
Male	363 (54.6)	175 (53.7)
Symptoms duration, months	11.9 ± 6.6	12.6 ± 6.4
Morning stiffness	393 (59.1)	195 (59.8)
Improve with exercise, not with rest	208 (31.3)	97 (29.8)
Alternating buttock pain	197 (29.6)	98 (30.1)
Insidious onset	430 (64.7)	256 (78.5)
Awakening at second half of night	315 (47.4)	169 (51.8)
Response to NSAIDs	407 (61.2)	200 (61.3)
Enthesitis	107 (16.1)	45 (13.8)
Psoriasis	82 (12.3)	35 (10.7)
Dactylitis	26 (3.9)	14 (4.3)
IBD	26 (3.9)	10 (3.1)
Uveitis	34 (5.1)	16 (4.9)
Arthritis	95 (14.3)	37 (11.3)
Family history	170 (25.6)	89 (27.3)
HLA-B27	270 (40.6)	144 (44.2)
Elevated CRP, mg/L	177 (26.6)	89 (27.3)
BASDAI	4.0 ± 2.3	3.9 ± 2.3
BASFI	2.5 ± 2.4	2.3 ± 2.4
ASAS criteria for axial SpA	291 (43.8)	167 (51.2)
Imaging arm	194 (29.2)	132 (40.5)
MRI-SI positive	85 (12.8)	85 (26.1)
mNY-positive[a]	109 (16.4)	47 (14.4)
Clinical arm only	97 (14.6)	35 (10.7)

Results are presented as mean ± SD or number (%). [a]Patients who were both magnetic resonance imaging of sacroiliac joints (MRI-SI)-positive and modified New York criteria for ankylosing spondylitis (mNY)-positive) are included. *NSAIDs* nonsteroidal anti-inflammatory drugs, *IBD* inflammatory bowel disease, *HLA-B27* human leucocyte antigen B27, *CRP* C-reactive protein, *BASDAI* Bath ankylosing spondylitis disease activity index, *BASFI* Bath ankylosing spondylitis functional index, *ASAS* Assessment of SpondyloArthritis International Society, *SpA* spondyloarthritis

IBP characteristics forecasting the presence of sacroiliitis on MRI or HLA-B27

Table 2 shows the results for the diagnostic utility of these characteristics. While alternating buttock pain was most contributory in predicting a positive MRI-SI result (LR + = 2.6; LR – = 0.6), awakening during the second half of the night was the most contributory in predicting a positive HLA-B27 result (LR+ =1.3; LR – = 0.8). However, individually none of the characteristics made a very strong contribution.

IBP definitions forecasting the presence of sacroiliitis on MRI or HLA-B27

The three multi-item IBP definitions performed more or less similarly in terms of a LR+. To forecast a positive MRI-SI, the ASAS criteria performed slightly better but still produced very low LRs (LR + = 2.1; LR – = 0.7) (Table 3). Based on these results, it was decided to assess whether or not the addition of other IBP characteristics (or good response to NSAID) which were not included in the definitions of IBP increased their diagnostic utility. This means that patients had to fulfil the specific IBP definition plus the additional characteristic. The results for this analysis are depicted in Table 3. Of all possible combinations, the ones that performed better were the combination of the Calin/ASAS definition and alternating buttock pain (LR + = 6.0 and 5.5, respectively; LR – = 0.7 for both combinations) and the combination of the Calin definition and awakening in the second half of the night (LR + = 5.5; LR – = 0.8). These combinations had a post-test probability of sacroiliitis on MRI of 79–80 % if the combined criterion was present, and 32–35 %, if the combined criterion was absent.

Similar to sacroiliitis, the three IBP definitions performed similarly well to predict a positive HLA-B27 result (Table 3). The ASAS criteria performed best but the LR+ (1.6) and LR– (0.9) was poor. On the other hand, and in contrast to the results for sacroiliitis, the addition of other IBP characteristics (or good response to NSAIDs) to the existing IBP definitions only slightly increased their diagnostic utility.

Other features of SpA forecasting the presence of sacroiliitis on MRI or HLA-B27

The utility of features of SpA other than IBP in helping to anticipate a positive (or a negative) MRI-SI or a positive (or negative) HLA-B27 test result was also evaluated. These SpA features included peripheral and extra-articular manifestations, family history of SpA or related diseases, elevated CRP and HLA-B27 (only for MRI-SI). While dactylitis and IBD appeared to be the most useful features of SpA for forecasting positive MRI-SI (LR + = 4.1 and 6.4, respectively), uveitis was the best for a positive HLA-B27 test, but had a LR+ of only 2.6 (Table 3). The presence or history of dactylitis or IBD resulted in a post-test probability for positive MRI of 73 % and 81 %, respectively, compared with the pre-test probability of 40 %. The post-test probability decreased from 40 % to 35 % if both dactylitis and IBD were confirmed absent.

Discussion

This study evaluates the utility of IBP characteristics, separately and combined, as well as other features of SpA to anticipate the presence of sacroiliitis on MRI or a positive result in HLA-B27 testing in patients with suspected axSpA.

In contrast to most prediction analyses, we have adopted a Bayesian approach based on likelihood ratios, rather than a 'frequentist approach' with odds ratios focusing on positive test results. The Bayesian approach is far closer to clinical reality because it directly visualizes the consequences of a positive test result (here, IBP criteria present) and a negative test result (here, IBP criteria absent) on the likelihood of the outcome (here, positive MRI-SI result) in a cohort with a given prevalence of the outcome. In contrast, the effects of odds ratios obtained with regular regression analysis (either significant or not) on the outcome of interest are entirely dependent

Table 2 Values for diagnostic utility measures for each of the inflammatory back pain characteristics in relation to the presence of sacroiliitis on MRI, and positive HLA-B27 testing

	Sacroiliitis on MRI						HLA-B27					
	Sen	Spe	LR+	LR–	PPV	NPV	Sen	Spe	LR+	LR–	PPV	NPV
Morning stiffness for >30 minutes	68.5	45.9	1.3	0.7	45.6	68.7	63.3	43.6	1.1	0.8	44.2	62.8
Improvement with exercise, not with rest	31.5	71.4	1.1	0.1	42.3	61.1	33.7	70.2	1.1	0.9	44.4	60.0
Alternating buttock pain	47.7	81.6	2.6	0.6	63.3	70.2	31.9	71.3	1.1	0.9	43.9	59.7
Insidious onset	87.7	27.6	1.2	0.4	44.5	77.1	68.1	37.1	1.1	0.9	43.3	62.3
Awakening in second half of the night	64.6	56.6	1.5	0.6	49.7	70.7	55.2	57.4	1.3	0.8	47.8	64.5
Response to NSAIDs	69.2	43.9	1.2	0.7	45.0	68.3	67.4	43.3	1.2	0.8	45.6	65.4

MRI magnetic resonance imaging, *HLA-B27* human leucocyte antigen B27, *Sen* sensitivity, *Spe* specificity, *LR+* positive likelihood ratio, *LR–* negative likelihood ratio, *PPV* positive predictive value, *NPV* negative predictive value, *NSAIDs* nonsteroidal anti-inflammatory drugs

Table 3 Values for diagnostic utility measures for each of the inflammatory back pain definitions and other features of SpA in relation to the presence of sacroiliitis on MRI and positive HLA-B27 testing

	Sacroiliitis on MRI						HLA-B27					
	Sen	Spe	LR+	LR−	PPV	NPV	Sen	Spe	LR+	LR−	PPV	NPV
IBP definition												
Calin criteria	51.5	70.9	1.8	0.7	54.0	68.8	36.3	74.2	1.4	0.9	49.7	62.3
Berlin criteria	72.3	50.5	1.5	0.6	49.2	73.3	64.1	49.3	1.3	0.7	47.1	66.1
ASAS criteria	47.7	77.0	2.1	0.7	57.9	68.9	31.5	80.7	1.6	0.9	53.5	62.3
IBP definition plus other IBP characteristics												
Calin + alt. buttock	30.8	94.9	6.0	0.7	80.0	67.4	17.4	86.4	1.3	1.0	51.0	56.3
Calin + NSAIDs	36.2	80.1	1.8	0.8	54.7	65.4	28.5	75.7	1.2	0.9	48.8	56.5
Calin + night	28.0	94.9	5.5	0.8	77.8	67.4	16.2	87.9	1.3	1.0	52.3	56.3
Calin + alt. buttock + night	26.9	94.9	5.3	0.8	77.8	66.2	16.0	88.1	1.3	1.0	52.3	56.3
Calin + alt. buttock + NSAIDs	20.0	96.9	6.5	0.8	81.3	64.6	10.4	91.0	1.2	1.0	48.4	55.5
Calin + Night + NSAIDs	29.2	87.2	2.3	0.8	60.3	65.0	21.5	88.3	1.8	0.9	56.3	61.5
Berlin + Insidious	64.6	62.2	1.7	0.6	53.1	72.6	50.7	53.1	1.1	0.9	46.8	57.0
Berlin + NSAIDs	53.8	68.4	1.7	0.7	53.0	69.1	48.9	66.1	1.4	0.8	50.4	64.7
Berlin + insidious + NSAIDs	47.7	76.0	2.0	0.7	56.9	68.7	34.0	67.2	1.0	1.0	45.8	55.6
ASAS + alt. Buttock	30.8	94.4	5.5	0.7	78.4	94.4	18.1	86.4	1.3	0.9	52.0	56.5
ASAS + NSAIDs	36.9	86.2	2.7	0.7	64.0	67.3	24.4	82.0	1.4	0.9	56.4	61.9
ASAS + stiffness	39.2	81.1	2.1	0.7	58.0	66.8	31.3	76.3	1.3	0.9	51.7	57.7
ASAS + alt. Buttock + NSAIDs	21.5	96.4	6.0	0.8	80.0	64.9	10.7	94.3	1.9	0.9	56.9	94.3
ASAS + stiffness + NSAIDs	28.5	88.8	2.5	0.8	62.7	65.2	19.4	83.1	1.1	1.0	48.3	55.9
ASAS + stiffness + alt. buttock	26.9	94.9	5.3	0.8	77.8	66.2	16.0	88.1	1.3	1.0	52.3	56.3
Other SpA features												
Enthesitis	11.5	84.7	0.8	1.0	33.3	59.1	17.8	85.1	1.2	0.9	85.1	45.7
Peripheral arthritis	13.8	90.3	1.4	0.9	48.6	61.2	16.7	87.7	1.4	0.9	87.7	48.9
Dactylitis	23.1	94.4	4.1	0.8	21.4	59.3	4.8	96.9	1.6	09	96.9	52.0
Uveitis	6.2	95.9	1.5	0.9	50.0	60.6	8.1	96.9	2.6	0.9	96.9	64.7
Psoriasis	10.0	88.8	0.9	1.0	37.1	59.8	7.0	83.8	0.4	1.1	83.8	23.5
Inflammatory bowel disease	23.1	96.4	6.4	0.8	30.0	59.8	1.5	94.5	0.3	1.0	94.5	16.0
Family history of SpA	27.7	73.0	1.0	0.9	40.4	60.3	33.7	80.2	1.7	0.8	80.2	54.5
Elevated CRP	40.8	77.5	1.8	0.8	55.1	66.0	38.5	77.1	1.7	0.8	77.1	54.6
HLA-B27	59.7	65.1	1.7	0.6	53.5	70.6	–	–	–	–	–	–

MRI magnetic resonance imaging, *HLA-B27* human leucocyte antigen B27, *Sen* sensitivity, *Spe* specificity, *LR+* positive likelihood ratio, *LR–* negative likelihood ratio, *PPV* positive predictive value, *NPV* negative predictive value, *ASAS* Assessment of SpondyloArthritis International Society, *Alt.* alternating, *NSAIDs* nonsteroidal anti-inflammatory drugs, *SpA* spondyloarthritis, *CRP* C-reactive protein

on the prevalence of the outcome, and the clinical value is difficult to disentangle (and often disappointingly low).

To predict the presence of sacroiliitis on MRI, we have found that alternating buttock pain and the ASAS-definition for IBP are the most useful characteristic and criterion, respectively, but neither of them performed sufficiently well when tested alone. Interestingly, the addition of the criterion of alternating buttock pain to the Calin or ASAS definition increased the positive likelihood ratio for MRI-SI notably compared to the Calin or ASAS definition alone (LR+ 6.0 vs 1.8 respectively for the Calin definition and 5.5 vs 2.1, respectively, for the ASAS definition). When the Berlin algorithm had been designed, the criterion of alternating buttock pain also increased the specificity for axSpA but at the cost of a very low sensitivity (because alternating buttock pain was a rare finding) [16]. When the ASAS definition for IBP was later developed, it therefore did not contribute independently to the presence of IBP according to expert opinion and therefore was not included in the proposed definition [7]. In the current study, we decided to re-examine the performance of the criterion of alternating buttock pain, because of the high cost associated with MRI-SI: we were searching for a criterion that could help us in deciding which patients should undergo MRI-SI. Moreover, the addition of the IBP characteristic of awakening in the second half of the night to the Calin criteria also increased significantly the likelihood ratio of having a positive MRI-SI compared to the performance of the Calin criteria alone (LR+ 5.5 vs 1.8, respectively). Furthermore, in addition to IBP, other features of SpA have been identified for predicting the presence of sacroiliitis on MRI in patients with suspected axSpA. The most useful features we observed were dactylitis and IBD.

In addition, in order to recommend a tool as diagnostically relevant in the context of a Bayesian approach, both positive and negative LR should be explored [15]. It is obvious that single features fall short in this regard. But if a patient with CBP has any of the four following characteristics: 1) IBP according to the Calin or ASAS definition plus alternating buttock pain; 2) IBP according to the Calin definition plus awakening in the second half of the night; 3) dactylitis; or 4) IBD, the probability of having a positive MRI-SI is very high (73–81 %). So in the case of limited resources, the presence of any of these three characteristics may help to increase the diagnostic efficiency of the MRI-SI.

Forecasting a positive HLA-B27 test result is more difficult: neither the individual IBP characteristics, nor the existing or other possible combinations were found useful to predict a positive HLA-B27 test. Among other SpA features, uveitis appeared to be the most closely related to a positive HLA-B27, but it is not sufficiently useful.

To our knowledge, this is the first study investigating this topic. This study has a few strengths: first, many patients with suspected axSpA were included from all over Spain. Second, the mean symptom duration in these patients was very short compared to most diagnostic utility studies and this is an advantage in the referral of patients to early axSpA clinics. Most importantly, patients included in this analysis came from a national health programme representing a typical scenario of common clinical practice that involved primary physicians, rheumatologists and other specialists who usually take care of patients with suspected axSpA. Relying on the conclusions of a local reader (radiologist or rheumatologist) rather than on a report of a central reading committee (as in clinical trials) should also be interpreted in this context, but this is exactly the clinical situation that we wanted to address.

Limitations should be considered too: the most important limitation is the possibility of confounding by indication. For the analysis of the association between IBP characteristics, or other features of SpA, and the presence of sacroiliitis on MRI, data were only included for those patients in whom MRI-SI was ordered by the rheumatologist. As there is always a reason to do so, patient selection is very likely, which may have implications for the external validity of this study. On the other hand, patients included in this analysis (because they had MRI ordered) had similar characteristics to the overall group of patients. Second, inter-reader variation by 25 different local readers who assessed the MRI may have influenced this study too. In this sense, it can be argued that the results of this study are applicable to clinical practice where many different readers are usually involved. Third, all patients included in this study came from the same country and the same cohort, which may limit the extrapolation of the results to other countries. However, in a sub-analysis of Spanish patients participating in the international study evaluating several referral strategies for diagnosis of axSpA, the national results were very similar to those observed in the global population [17]. Fourth, It should be pointed out that the diagnostic performance is dependent on the prior probability of the outcome of interest: While the diagnostic performance in terms of likelihood ratios is considered to be rather stable across cohorts, the application of these likelihood ratios in cohorts with other prior probabilities are very different. A final limitation is obviously that we failed to frame a group of patients in whom the likelihood of a positive MRI and/or positive HLAB27 was very low, as the negative likelihood ratios of all features tested fell short as the lowest LR– was 0.6.

Conclusions

In summary, if a patient has IBP according to the Calin or ASAS definition plus alternating buttock pain or IBP according to the Calin criteria plus awakening in the second half of the night, or dactylitis or IBD, the probability of positive MRI-SI increases from 40 to approximately 75 %. So in the case of limited resources, the presence of any of these four characteristics may improve the efficiency of ordering MRI in patients with suspected axSpA. None of the IBP definitions or any of the other SpA features appear to be useful to forecasting a positive HLA-B27 test.

Abbreviations

ASAS: Assessment of SpondyloArthritis International Society; AxSpA: axial spondyloarthritis; BASDAI: Bath ankylosing spondylitis disease activity index; BASFI: Bath ankylosing spondylitis functional index; CBP: chronic back pain; CRP: C-reactive protein; HLA-B27: Human leucocyte antigen B27; IBD: inflammatory bowel disease; IBP: inflammatory back pain; LR–: negative likelihood ratio; LR+: positive likelihood ratio; MRI-SI: magnetic resonance imaging of sacroiliac joints; NPV: negative predictive value; NSAID: nonsteroidal anti-inflammatory drug; PPV: positive predictive value.

Competing interests

The authors declare that they have no competing interests.

Authors' contributions

VNC performed the statistical analysis, critically interpreted the results and wrote the first draft of the manuscript. EdM, RL, DvdH and PZ participated in the design of the study, critically interpreted the results and revised the manuscript. RA, CM and EB substantially contributed to the acquisition of data and critically revised the draft of the manuscript. All authors read and approved the final version of the manuscript.

Acknowledgements

The authors would like to thank all patients participating in the Esperanza Programme as well as all members of the Esperanza Study Group. Members of the Esperanza Study Group are as follows. Coordinators: E Collantes, H Reina Sofía, Córdoba; L Carmona and M Gobbo, Research Unit, Sociedad Española de Reumatología (SER), Madrid. Scientific commitee: J Mulero, H. Puerta de Hierro, Madrid; E de Miguel, H. U. La Paz, Madrid; S Muñoz-Fernández, H. Infanta Sofía, Madrid; P Zarco, F. H. Alcorcón, Madrid; Collaborators: J Rivera, H. Gregorio Marañón, Madrid; JC López Robledillo, H. Niño Jesús, Madrid; C Castillo Gallego, H.U. La Paz, Madrid; J Rosas, G Santos, H. Marina Baixa, Villajoyosa; JL Fernández Sueiro, J Pinto Tasende, E González Díaz de Rabago, H. U. Juan Canalejo, La Coruña; C Montilla, S Gómez Castro, López R, J del Pino Montes, H. U. de Salamanca, Salamanca; IP Granados Bautista, A Hernández Sanz, H. Virgen de la Salud, Toledo; J Sanz Sanz, H. Puerta de Hierro, Majadahonda, Madrid; M Fernández Prada, J Tornero, H.U. de Guadalajara, Guadalajara; C Campos, J Calvo, H.G.U. de Valencia, Valencia; X Juanola, V Ríos, H.U. de Bellvitge, Barcelona; E Moreno, MI Rotés, H. de San Rafael, Barcelona; I Ibero, C Fernández Carballido, V Jovaní, N Martínez Alberola, H.G.U. de Elda, Alicante; LF Linares, MJ Moreno Ramos, A Uceda, MJ Moreno Martínez, MD Beteta, H.U. Virgen de la Arrixaca, Murcia; JC Quevedo, C Rodríguez Lozano, H.U. Dr Negrín, Las Palmas de Gran Canaria; E Trujillo, S Bustabad, H.U. de Canarias, Santa Cruz de Tenerife; JA Román Ivorra, S Muñoz Gil, H. U. Dr Peset, Valencia; A Juan Mas, I Ros Vilamajó, M Ibáñez Barceló, H. Son Llatzer, Mallorca; MC Castro Villegas, H.U. Reina Sofía, Córdoba; J Gratacós Matmija, M Moreno Martínez-Loza, H. Sabadell Corp. Parc Taulí, Barcelona; R Almodóvar, H. Fundación Alcorcón, Madrid; E Rejón, S Rodríguez Montero, H.U. Virgen de Valme, Sevilla; T Ruiz Jimeno, H. Sierrallana, Torrelavega; JJ Aznar, E Chamizo Carmona, N Garrido Puñal, H. de Mérida, Mérida; P Fernández Dapica, H. 12 de Octubre, Madrid; E Brito Brito, H. Ramón y Cajal, Madrid; E Pérez Pampín, H. Clínico Universitario de Santiago, Santiago de Compostela. VNC received one of the ASAS research grants on call 2013 to perform this study. The Spanish Foundation of Rheumatology received funding from Pfizer to develop the Esperanza Programme. Nowadays, the programme is supported by a restricted grant of the Institute Carlos III (FIS PI13/02034). The sponsor had no role in the study design, the collection, analysis or interpretation of the data, in the writing of the report, or in the decision to submit the article for publication.

Author details

[1]Department of Rheumatology, IdiPaz, University Hospital La Paz, Madrid, Spain. [2]Department of Rheumatology, Leiden University Medical Center, Leiden, The Netherlands. [3]Department of Clinical Immunology & Rheumatology, Academic Medical Center, University of Amsterdam, Amsterdam, The Netherlands. [4]Department of Rheumatology, Atrium Medical Center Heerlen, Heerlen, The Netherlands. [5]Department of Rheumatology, University Hospital Foundation Alcorcón, Madrid, Spain. [6]Department of Rheumatology, Hospital Clínico Universitario de Salamanca, Salamanca, Spain. [7]Department of Rheumatology, Hospital Universitario General de Valencia, Valencia, Spain.

References

1. Landewe R, Dougados M, Mielants H, van der Tempel H, van der Heijde D. Physical function in ankylosing spondylitis is independently determined by both disease activity and radiographic damage of the spine. Ann Rheum Dis. 2009;68:863–7.
2. Feldtkeller E, Bruckel J, Khan MA. Scientific contributions of ankylosing spondylitis patient advocacy groups. Curr Opin Rheumatol. 2000;12:239–47.
3. Rudwaleit M, van der Heijde D, Landewe R, Listing J, Akkoc N, Brandt J, et al. The development of Assessment of SpondyloArthritis international Society classification criteria for axial spondyloarthritis (part II): validation and final selection. Ann Rheum Dis. 2009;68:777–83.
4. Sieper J, Srinivasan S, Zamani O, Mielants H, Choquette D, Pavelka K, et al. Comparison of two referral strategies for diagnosis of axial spondyloarthritis: the Recognising and Diagnosing Ankylosing Spondylitis Reliably (RADAR) study. Ann Rheum Dis. 2013;72:1621–7.
5. Braun A, Saracbasi E, Grifka J, Schnitker J, Braun J. Identifying patients with axial spondyloarthritis in primary care: how useful are items indicative of inflammatory back pain? Ann Rheum Dis. 2011;70:1782–7.
6. Poddubnyy D, Vahldiek J, Spiller I, Listing J, Rudwaleit M, Sieper J. Evaluation of 2 screening strategies for early identification of patients with axial spondyloarthritis in primary care. J Rheumatol. 2011;38:2452–60.
7. Sieper J, van der Heijde D, Landewe R, Brandt J, Burgos-Vagas R, Collantes-Estevez E, et al. New criteria for inflammatory back pain in patients with chronic back pain: a real patient exercise by experts from the Assessment of SpondyloArthritis international Society (ASAS). Ann Rheum Dis. 2009;68:784–8.
8. Calin A, Porta J, Fries JF, Schurman DJ. Clinical history as a screening test for ankylosing spondylitis. JAMA. 1977;237:2613–4.
9. Rudwaleit M, Metter A, Listing J, Sieper J, Braun J. Inflammatory back pain in ankylosing spondylitis: a reassessment of the clinical history for application as classification and diagnostic criteria. Arthritis Rheum. 2006;54:569–78.
10. van den Berg R, de Hooge M, Rudwaleit M, Sieper J, van Gaalen F, Reijnierse M, et al. ASAS modification of the Berlin algorithm for diagnosing axial spondyloarthritis: results from the SPondyloArthritis Caught Early (SPACE)-cohort and from the Assessment of SpondyloArthritis international Society (ASAS)-cohort. Ann Rheum Dis. 2013;72:1646–53.
11. Fernandez Carballido C, en nombre del Grupo E. Diagnosing early spondyloarthritis in Spain: the ESPeranza program. Reumatol Clin. 2010;6:6–10.
12. Munoz-Fernandez S, Carmona L, Collantes E, Mulero J, García-Yébenes MJ, de Miguel E, et al. A model for the development and implementation of a national plan for the optimal management of early spondyloarthritis: the Esperanza Program. Ann Rheum Dis. 2011;70:827–30.
13. Villaverde V, Carmona L, Lopez Robledillo JC, Serrano S, Gobbo M, Grupo de Estudio E. Motivations and objections to implement a spondyloarthritis integrated care pathway. A qualitative study with primary care physicians. Reumatol Clin. 2013;9:85–9.
14. Rudwaleit M, Jurik AG, Hermann KG, Landewé R, van der Heijde D, Baraliakos X, et al. Defining active sacroiliitis on magnetic resonance imaging (MRI) for classification of axial spondyloarthritis: a consensual approach by the ASAS/OMERACT MRI group. Ann Rheum Dis. 2009;68:1520–7.
15. McGee S. Simplifying likelihood ratios. J Gen Intern Med. 2002;17:646–9.
16. Rudwaleit M, van der Heijde D, Khan MA, Braun J, Sieper J. How to diagnose axial spondyloarthritis early. Ann Rheum Dis. 2004;63:535–43.
17. Juanola X, Fernandez-Sueiro JL, Torre-Alonso JC, Miguelez R, Munoz-Fernandez S, Ballina J, et al. Comparison of 2 referral strategies for the diagnosis of axial spondyloarthritis in Spain. The RADAR study. Reumatol Clin. 2013;9:348–52.

23

Inflammation-driven bone formation in a mouse model of ankylosing spondylitis: sequential not parallel processes

Hsu-Wen Tseng[1], Miranda E. Pitt[1], Tibor T. Glant[2], Allan F. McRae[1,3], Tony J. Kenna[1], Matthew A. Brown[1], Allison R. Pettit[4*] and Gethin P. Thomas[1*]

Abstract

Background: Ankylosing spondylitis (AS) is an immune-mediated arthritis particularly targeting the spine and pelvis and is characterised by inflammation, osteoproliferation and frequently ankylosis. Current treatments that predominately target inflammatory pathways have disappointing efficacy in slowing disease progression. Thus, a better understanding of the causal association and pathological progression from inflammation to bone formation, particularly whether inflammation directly initiates osteoproliferation, is required.

Methods: The proteoglycan-induced spondylitis (PGISp) mouse model of AS was used to histopathologically map the progressive axial disease events, assess molecular changes during disease progression and define disease progression using unbiased clustering of semi-quantitative histology. PGISp mice were followed over a 24-week time course. Spinal disease was assessed using a novel semi-quantitative histological scoring system that independently evaluated the breadth of pathological features associated with PGISp axial disease, including inflammation, joint destruction and excessive tissue formation (osteoproliferation). Matrix components were identified using immunohistochemistry.

Results: Disease initiated with inflammation at the periphery of the intervertebral disc (IVD) adjacent to the longitudinal ligament, reminiscent of enthesitis, and was associated with upregulated tumor necrosis factor and metalloproteinases. After a lag phase, established inflammation was temporospatially associated with destruction of IVDs, cartilage and bone. At later time points, advanced disease was characterised by substantially reduced inflammation, excessive tissue formation and ectopic chondrocyte expansion. These distinct features differentiated affected mice into early, intermediate and advanced disease stages. Excessive tissue formation was observed in vertebral joints only if the IVD was destroyed as a consequence of the early inflammation. Ectopic excessive tissue was predominantly chondroidal with chondrocyte-like cells embedded within collagen type II- and X-rich matrix. This corresponded with upregulation of mRNA for cartilage markers *Col2a1*, *sox9* and *Comp*. Osteophytes, though infrequent, were more prevalent in later disease.

Conclusions: The inflammation-driven IVD destruction was shown to be a prerequisite for axial disease progression to osteoproliferation in the PGISp mouse. Osteoproliferation led to vertebral body deformity and fusion but was never seen concurrent with persistent inflammation, suggesting a sequential process. The findings support that early intervention with anti-inflammatory therapies will be needed to limit destructive processes and consequently prevent progression of AS.

Keywords: Ankylosing spondylitis, Proteoglycan-induced spondylitis mouse model, Enthesis, Intervertebral disc destruction, Chondroidal bone formation, Spondyloarthropathy, Arthritis, Osteoproliferation

* Correspondence: allison.pettit@mater.uq.edu.au; gethin.thomas@uq.edu.au
[4]The University of Queensland-Mater Research Institute, Translational Research Institute, 37 Kent Street, Woolloongabba, QLD 4102, Australia
[1]The University of Queensland Diamantina Institute, Translational Research Institute, 37 Kent Street, Woolloongabba, QLD 4102, Australia
Full list of author information is available at the end of the article

Background

Ankylosing spondylitis (AS) is a chronic inflammatory arthritis predominantly affecting the axial skeleton, particularly the spine and pelvis. The disease is characterised by inflammation at the entheses, which is followed by uncontrolled osteoproliferation that often leads to fusion (ankylosis) of affected joints. There is ongoing debate regarding whether inflammation is the direct trigger of the osteoproliferation seen in AS. Whilst there is evidence that the anti-inflammatory treatments of non-steroidal anti-inflammatory drugs (NSAIDs) and tumour necrosis factor (TNF)-inhibitor biologic therapies can slow osteoproliferative disease, the outcome is variable and the effect is at best partial with ankylosis still progressing. Ankylosis in patients with AS results from the development and fusion of syndesmophytes, defined as bony bridges growing at the vertebral corners. Multiple mechanisms of bone formation have been proposed to underlie the osteoproliferation in AS, including intramembranous, endochondral and chondroidal ossification [1, 2]. The causative pathological mechanism that initiate and perpetuate the excessive bone formation and subsequently ankylosis remain unknown.

In patients with AS, longitudinal magnetic resonance imaging (MRI) and radiographic imaging can be used to follow disease progression, but the resolution and sensitivity of these imaging modalities are insufficient to show correlations of specific pathological processes at a detailed anatomical level. Collection of serial biopsies from spinal lesions of patients with AS would substantially aid elucidation of mechanistic changes underlying the inflammatory response and the mechanism(s) of bone formation. However, this approach is constrained because of ethical limitations and biopsy collection challenges. A few studies have been performed on sacroiliac joint biopsies from patients undergoing hip replacement and in zygapophyseal joints from spinal surgeries [2–6]. Such studies, though informative, are limited by sample size and anatomical location, coupled with being predominantly obtained from late-stage disease patients in whom the inflammation-osteoproliferative transition has already occurred. Disease-relevant animal models thus present the only viable approach to elucidate mechanisms underlying disease progression in the axial skeleton. Time course studies in spinal samples from animal models present a powerful approach to biologically map the full progression of AS, particularly to investigate the mechanistic link between inflammation and osteoproliferation.

We aimed to delineate the disease progression and causal association between inflammation, destruction and osteoproliferation in AS by undertaking a comprehensive time course study in the proteoglycan (PG)-induced spondylitis (PGISp) mouse model. The PGISp mouse model was chosen for its recapitulation of AS clinical features, including development of both inflammation and osteoproliferation in the spine in response to an immune stimulus [7, 8]. These previous studies in the PGISp model demonstrated intervertebral disc (IVD) destabilization, cartilage damage, chondrophyte/osteophyte formation and their subsequent fusion. However, these studies were qualitative and the inter-dependence between these features was not assessed.

We performed a 6-month time course in PGISp mice spanning from the onset to advanced disease with regular sampling occurring throughout disease progression. We developed a novel histological scoring system that measured the full breadth of disease features. Unbiased computational modelling of these scores allowed us to determine the key features differentiating different disease stages and predict associations. We used histology, immunohistochemistry, and gene expression data to precisely characterise the timing and morphology of pathological events within affected joints.

Methods

Mouse model, immunization and collection

The PGISp model was established by treating 3-month-old female IL-$4^{-/-}$ BALB/c mice with 2 mg of human cartilage extract (PG) together with 2 mg of dimethyl dioctadecyl ammoniumbromide (DDA) (Sigma-Aldrich, St. Louis, MO, USA) as described previously [8]. IL-$4^{-/-}$mice were used because of the higher disease incidence and severity over wild-type BALB/c mice [9]. PG was administered via intraperitoneal injections at week 0, 3 and 6 of the study. Age-matched naïve female IL-$4^{-/-}$ BALB/c mice were used as controls.

Spine samples, including thoracic and lumbar spine, from 12 to 17 mice were collected 6, 8, 10, 12, 16 and 24 weeks after the first PG injection. All experiments were approved by the University of Queensland animal ethics committee.

Histology

Spine samples from 5 to 10 mice per group were fixed in 4 % paraformaldehyde (Sigma-Aldrich) for 48–72 hours followed by decalcification in 14 % ethylenediaminetetraacetic acid disodium salt dihydrate (EDTA) (Sigma-Aldrich) for 3–4 weeks. Embedded spine samples were cut into 5-μm serial sections along the sagittal plane using a standard rotary microtome. Sections were deparaffinised with xylene and graded ethanol, rehydrated in tris-buffered saline (TBS) (50 mM Tris, 150 mM NaCl, pH = 7.4), stained with Mayer's haematoxylin and eosin (H&E) or toluidine blue (0.01 % toluidine blue O (Sigma-Aldrich) in 0.1 % sodium chloride solution, pH = 2.0) and mounted.

Semi-quantitative histological scoring

Histological scoring criteria outlined in Table 1 were developed to capture the broad range of inflammatory, catabolic and anabolic changes that occur within the vertebral joints of the spine in this AS model. Scoring was performed on one H&E and one toluidine blue stained section from each sample. Only samples with correct sagittal orientation and at least six IVDs in the section plane were included in the analysis. On average, nine vertebral joints were scored in each mouse. Anterior and posterior sides of each joint were scored separately and then averaged to generate the final score for any given joint. Joints with a score above zero within any of the criteria categories were defined as affected joints, and mice that had at least one affected IVD were defined as affected mice. PGISp mice with normal spine morphology and no evidence of disease were excluded from further spinal disease incidence and progression analysis. The disease progression was measured by averaging scores of all vertebral joints.

Immunohistochemistry

Sagittal sections (4-μm) were rehydrated and subjected to different antigen retrieval processes depending on the primary antibody. For type I and II collagen, spine sections were digested in pre-warmed 25 % trypsin (Biocare Medical, Concord, NSW, Australia) for 10 min at room temperature (RT). For type X collagen, sections were incubated in 0.1 U/ml chondroitinase ABC (Sigma-Aldrich) in tris-acetate buffer (0.1 M Tris, 30 mM Acetate buffer, 10 mM EDTA, pH 6.5) for 2 hours at 37 °C. No antigen retrieval was performed for osterix antibody. All sections were incubated in 3 % H_2O_2 for 30 min at RT and blocked in Sniper Blocking Reagent (Biocare Medical) for 10 min followed by 10 % foetal bovine serum for 1 hour at RT. For type I or II collagen and osterix staining, sections were incubated with rabbit anti-type I or II collagen or osterix antibodies or equivalent concentration of normal rabbit IgG for 1 hour at RT. For type X collagen staining, sections were incubated with rabbit anti-type X collagen antiserum or equivalent concentration of rabbit serum overnight at 4 °C. After washing in TBS, sections were incubated in MACH1 HRP polymer reagent (Biocare Medical) for 30 min and detected by using diaminobenzidine (DAB) chromogen (Biocare Medical). Sections were counterstained in acidified haematoxylin

Table 1 Histological score criteria

Category	Score	Criteria
Inflammation	0	Normal
	1	Minor infiltration of inflammatory cells at periphery of the joint
	2	Moderate infiltration – inflammatory pannus < 50 % joint area
	3	Marked infiltration – inflammatory pannus > 50 % joint area
Intervertebral disc destruction	0	Normal
	1	Less than 50 % disc destruction
	2	More than 50 % disc destruction
	3	Total disc destruction/only necrotic disc left
Cartilage damage	0	Normal
	1	Some loss of articular cartilage or growth plate cartilage or both
	2	Severe loss of articular cartilage and some growth plate cartilage damage
	3	Severe loss of articular cartilage and severe growth plate cartilage damage
Bone erosion	0	Normal
	1	One or a few small areas of resorption in original vertebral bone.
	2	Numerous areas of obvious focal resorption in original vertebral bone or several areas of severe destruction.
Excess tissue formation (excluding inflammatory infiltrate)	0	Normal
	1	Mesenchymal cell invasion or expansion or both
	2	Moderate fibrocartilage formation (<50 % of the original disc area)
	3	Extensive fibrocartilage formation (>50 % of the original disc area)
Ectopic chondrocytes/chondrophyte	0	Normal
	1	Single small area
	2	Single large area
	3	Multiple areas

(Sigma-Aldrich). Reagent details are listed in Additional file 1: Table S1.

RNA extraction and quantitative real-time polymerase chain reaction

Spine samples from five to eight PGISp or from five to seven age-matched naïve female mice at each time point were flash-frozen in liquid nitrogen and stored at −80 °C. Spine samples were homogenized separately in Trizol (Life Technologies, Mulgrave, Victoria, Australia), and RNA extracted as described previously [8]. Synthesis of cDNA was conducted by using a Tetro cDNA synthesis kit (Bioline, Alexandria, NSW, Australia) in accordance with the instructions of the manufacturer. Gene expression was measured by SYBR Green-based quantitative real-time reverse transcription polymerase chain reaction (qPCR) using the Sensimix SYBR kit and run on a ViiA7 Real-Time PCR System (Life Technologies). Primer sequences are listed in Additional file 1: Table S2. PCR conditions were 10 min at 95 °C followed by 50 cycles of 15 sec at 95 °C and 45 sec at 60 °C. The expression of individual genes was normalized to β-actin and gene expression quantified by using the ΔCT equation.

Statistics

Data was analysed by Mann-Whitney or Kruskal-Wallis tests analysis by using PRISM 6 (GraphPad Software, La Jolla, CA, USA). *P* values of less than 0.05 were considered significant. Unsupervised analysis was conducted by using the hclust function in R. Histological scores of affected IVD of affected mice were averaged and computed by using hierarchical cluster analysis with Ward's method.

Results

PGISp axial joint histopathology progresses from inflammation to osteoproliferation

To characterise axial disease progression in PGISp mice, H&E stained sections from spines collected across a 24-week disease time course were semi-quantitatively scored in accordance with the criteria outlined in Table 1. These criteria scored inflammation, vertebral disc destruction, bone erosion, excess tissue formation (mesenchymal tissue expansion or fibrocartilage formation) and ectopic chondrocyte/chondrophyte formation in the vertebral joints. Histological scoring of these major disease features was used to model axial disease progression in the PGISp mice. All the vertebral joints and IVD in naïve mice appeared normal throughout the time course and were treated as a single mouse group for statistical analysis.

The PGISp mice exhibited early disease by 6 weeks post-PG priming, and 60 % of mice had either one or two mildly affected vertebral joints. By 8 weeks after the first PG injection, every PGISp mouse had at least one affected vertebra, and 50 % of all vertebral joints were affected (Fig. 1a). The majority of joints were only mildly affected at 8 weeks, but severe inflammation was observed in a small percentage (Fig. 1a). Averaging the inflammatory scores of all the vertebral joints in individual affected PGISp mice and comparing this average inflammation score across the time course showed that inflammation peaked at 12 weeks (Fig. 1b), and 18–19 % of affected joints were severely inflamed (Fig. 1a). At both 10 and 12 weeks after PG priming, the inflammation score was significantly elevated (Fig. 1b). There was heterogeneity in inflammation severity at any time point both between and within individual animals, and some vertebral joints showed no inflammation whereas others had significant inflammatory infiltrates (Fig. 1b). Average inflammation severity decreased from 16 weeks after PG priming, and by 24 weeks the majority of joints had no or only very minor associated inflammation (Fig. 1a). When compared with all other histopathological features scored (Fig. 1c–g), inflammation was the earliest detectable axial histopathological feature in the PGISp model but was a transient disease process (Fig. 1b).

Histopathological features of the disease reflecting destruction (Fig. 1c–e) or tissue formation (Fig. 1f and g) demonstrated a sustained or progressive disease pattern. Most reached maximal score at 24 weeks after priming (Fig. 1c–e), much later than was observed for inflammation scores (Fig. 1b). Initiation of disc destruction (Fig. 1c), bone erosion (Fig. 1d), cartilage damage (Fig. 1e) and excessive tissue formation (Fig. 1f) were evident from 8 weeks after priming. Disc destruction and bone erosion were significantly increased from week 10 onwards in PGISp compared with naïve mice (Fig. 1c and d, respectively). Disc destruction (Fig. 1c) and bone erosion (Fig. 1d) peaked at the same time as inflammation (Fig. 1b) but subsequently plateaued, consistent with their being irreparable tissue changes driven by the inflammatory processes. Excessive tissue (Fig. 1e) and ectopic chondrocyte formation (Fig. 1f) increased steadily from week 10 through to week 24.

A notable feature was that, in all the mice analysed, severe inflammation and significant excessive tissue formation did not occur simultaneously within the same joint, consistent with these features representing distinct early and late stages of PGISp progression, respectively. Another feature of late-stage disease was cartilage damage, which was not significantly elevated compared with naïve or 6-week mice until 16 weeks after PG priming. This suggests that this destructive event is more likely a secondary consequence of other joint changes initiated by the inflammatory process, rather than a direct consequence of the inflammation.

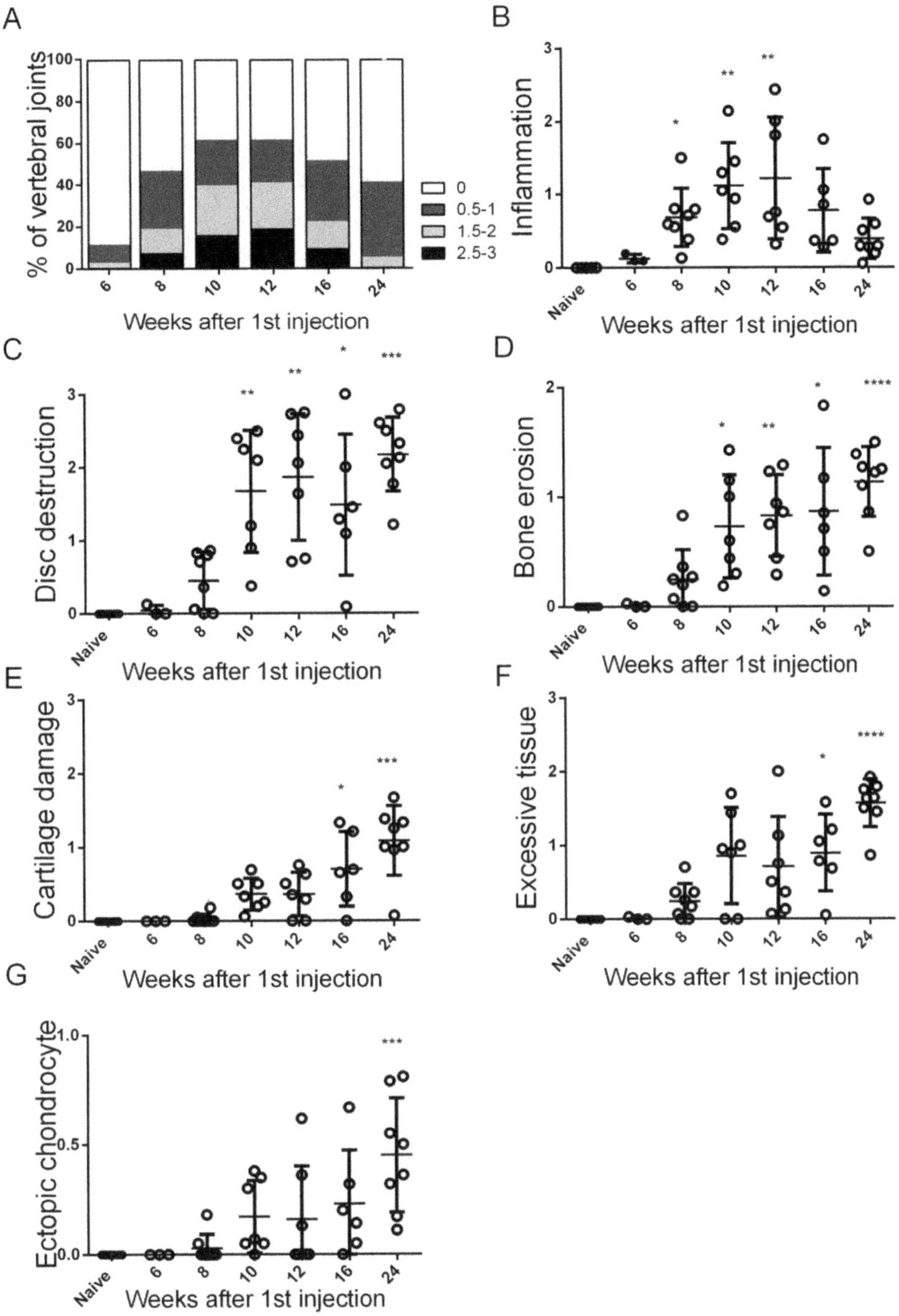

Fig. 1 PGISp mouse model disease progression. **a** The severity of inflammatory infiltrate is represented by the percentages of different scores at each time point. Axial disease progression is described by the features of (**b**) inflammation, (**c**) disc destruction, (**d**) bone erosion, (**e**) cartilage damage, (**f**) excessive tissue formation and (**g**) ectopic chondrocyte formation. Each point represents the average scores of all vertebral joints within each affected mouse at the particular time points (3–10 mice per time point). The results are shown as mean ± standard deviation and analysed by Kruskal-Wallis test followed by Dunn's multiple comparison test. ****$P < 0.0001$, ***$P < 0.001$, **$P < 0.01$, *$P < 0.05$ compared with naïve

Inflammation drives tissue damage and disc destruction in PGISp mice

Detailed histological assessment across the time course exemplified the heterogeneity of disease progression between different animals and even between individual vertebral joints, similar to that reported previously in this model [7, 8] and in AS [10]. At the 6-week time point, the earliest detected feature of inflammation was accumulation of inflammatory cells at the periphery of the IVD adjacent to the annulus fibrosus (AF) (Fig. 2a). At 8 weeks

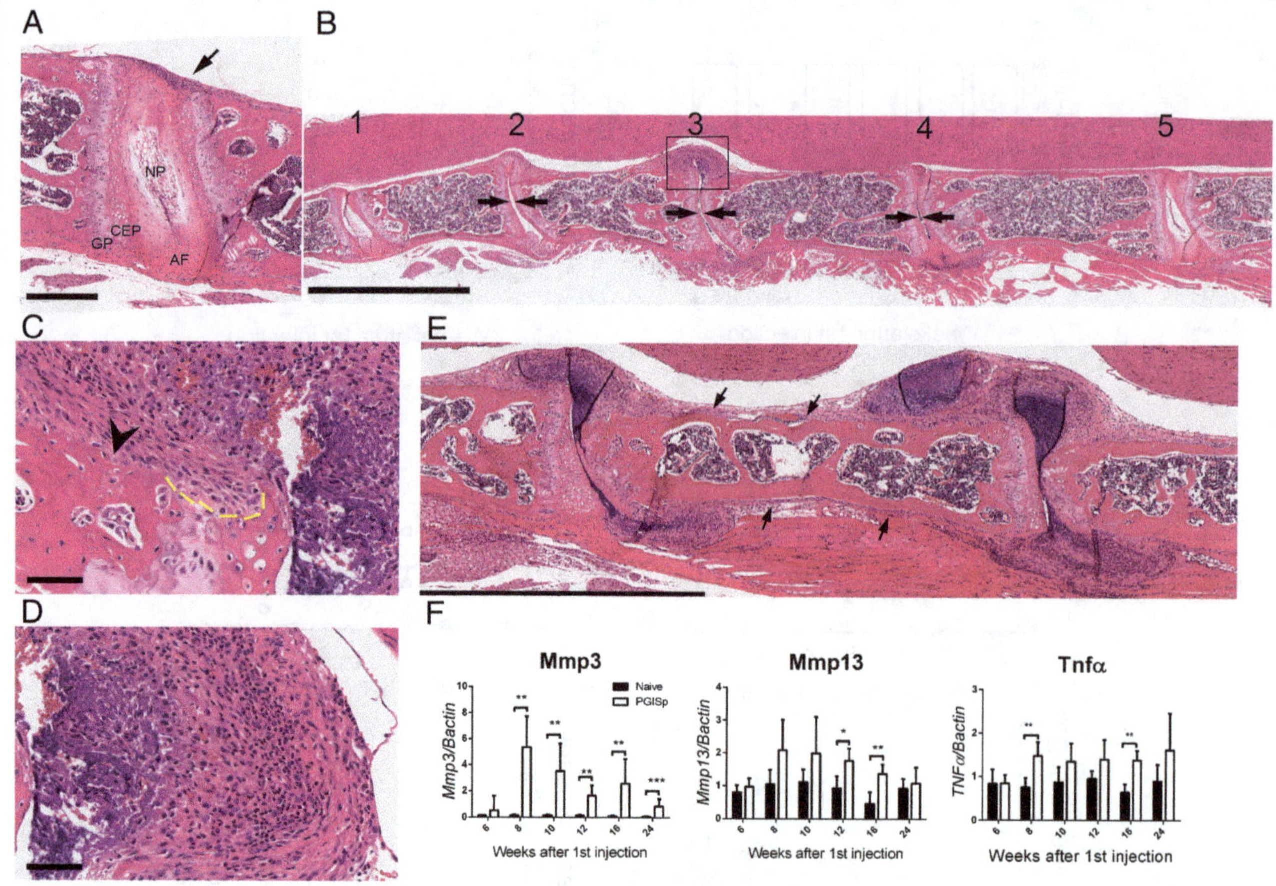

Fig. 2 Progression of spinal inflammation in PGISp mice. **a** Representative H&E stain of mild inflammation in an 8-week time point mouse. Inflammatory cells accumulate at the periphery of the disc (*arrow*), but the rest of the intervertebral disc appears normal. *AF* annulus fibrosus, *CEP* cartilaginous end plate, *GP* cartilaginous growth plate, *NP* nucleus pulposus. Scale bar = 300 μm. **b** Variable disease penetrance in an 8-week PGISp mouse: (1) and (5) unaffected intervertebral discs, (2) disc destruction combined with early chondrocyte formation, (3) severe inflammation and disc destruction, and (4) moderate inflammation with incomplete disc destruction. Scale bar = 2 mm. **c** Magnification of the boxed area in (b) shows bone erosion (*arrowhead*) and cartilage damage. The yellow dashed line indicates the eroded cartilage surface. Scale bar = 60 μm. **d** Magnification of the boxed area in (b) demonstrating large numbers of mononuclear cells presenting in the affected joints. Scale bar = 60 μm. **e** Inflammation expansion along the longitudinal ligament (*arrows*). **f** mRNA expression of *Mmp3*, *Mmp13* and *Tnf* in whole spine was analysed by qPCR and normalized to *β-actin*. Black bars represent naïve and open bars represent PGISp mice. Expression levels are presented as mean ± standard deviation. $^{***}P < 0.0001$, $^{**}P < 0.001$, $^{*}P < 0.01$ compared with naïve at the same time point, Mann-Whitney test. *MMP* matrix metalloproteinase, *TNFα* tumour necrosis factor-alpha

after priming, while all mice were affected, within any given PGISp mouse, both affected (Fig. 2b, joints 2 to 4) and unaffected (Fig. 2b, joints 1 and 5) vertebral joints were observed and there was a broad range of inflammation severity within a single spine (Fig. 2b, joints 2–4). Inflammatory pannus invading into the disc space was clearly associated with IVD destruction, resulting in joint space narrowing (Fig. 2b, space between arrows), and was often associated with bone erosion (Fig. 2c, arrowhead). Early hyaline cartilage damage, including eroded surfaces defined by excavated and empty chondrocyte lacunae, was confined to areas exposed to inflammatory infiltrate (Fig. 2c, yellow dash line represented eroded cartilage surface), similar to previous observation in vertebrae and sacroiliac joints in PGISp mice [7, 8].

Severe inflammation was characterised by marked infiltration of the AF by inflammatory cells, including polymorphonuclear cells, vascular structures and increased density of mixed morphology mesenchymal cells (Fig. 2c and d). In severely inflamed joints, periosteal expansion and inflammatory cell invasion frequently extended along the cortical surface of the vertebral body, possibly following the spinal ligaments, suggesting an entheseal or periosteal pathology or both (Fig. 2e, arrows). Overall the histopathology features suggest that the inflammatory process drives the IVD destruction, focal cartilage damage and focal bone erosion, particularly at the vertebral corners, all of which are reported features of AS axial pathology.

TNFα and matrix metalloproteinase-3 (MMP-3) and MMP-13 have been implicated in AS inflammatory processes and have been correlated with disease activity [11–13]. Therefore, mRNA expression of these genes in the whole spine was measured by qPCR (Fig. 2f). The basal level of *Mmp3* in unaffected mice was very low across the time course (Fig. 2f, black bars). PG immunisation induced a dramatic elevation of *Mmp3* at 8 weeks and expression levels of this transcript remained significantly higher in PGISp mice when compared with naive mice at all later time points (Fig. 2f). *Mmp13* was significantly elevated at weeks 12 and 16 in PGISp spines. *Tnf* expression was significantly increased in PGISp mice at 8 and 16 weeks (Fig. 2f). These data suggest that the inflammation-driven tissue remodelling molecular cascades are established by 8–10 weeks post-immunisation and decrease in parallel with inflammation during the later disease stages.

Disease-associated anabolic tissue formation

Expansion of mesenchymal cells, predominantly fibroblast-like (Fig. 3a i and ii, arrowheads) and chondrocyte-like (Fig. 3a i and ii, arrows), was noted in the bulging residual AF of affected vertebral joints and extending along the vertebral periosteal surface (Fig. 3a). The chondrocyte-like cell phenotype included rounded or polygonal morphology within a dense predominantly basophilic extracellular matrix (ECM) (Fig. 3a i and ii, arrows). In advanced

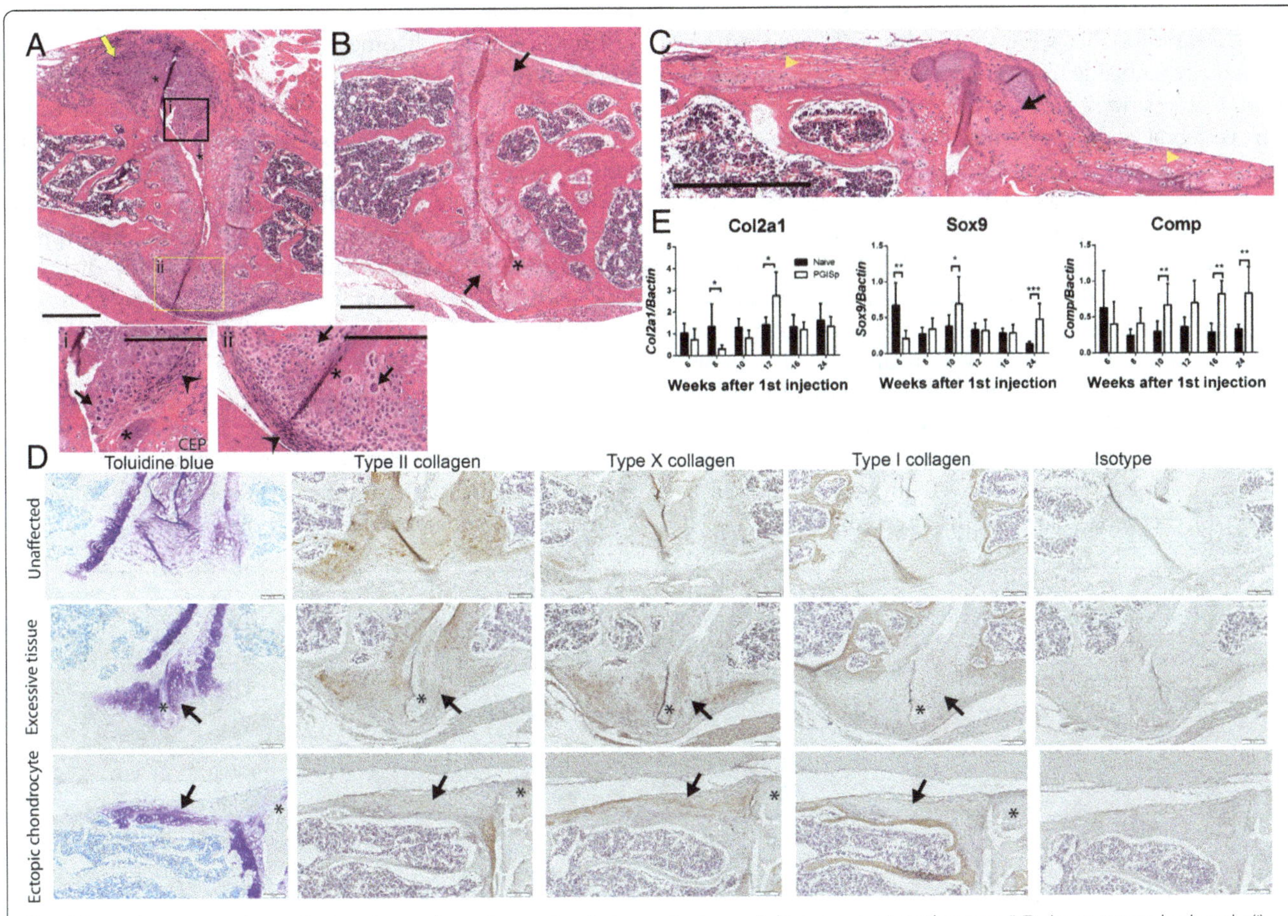

Fig. 3 Excessive tissue and ectopic chondrocyte formation are key features of advanced disease. **a** A 12-week mouse IVD demonstrates both early (i) and intermediate (ii) stages of excessive tissue formation using H&E stain. Scale bar = 300 μm. Inflammatory infiltrate (*yellow arrow*) surrounds the affected joint, while fibroblast-like cells (*arrowheads*) and chondrocyte-like cells (*arrows*) are located adjacently to the residual disc (*asterisks*). Scale bar = 200 μm in (i) and (ii). *CEP* cartilaginous end plate. **b** Excessive tissue at the periphery of the joint is greatly increased in more advanced disease (*arrows*). Representative image from a 24-week mouse. Scale bar = 400 μm. **c** In addition to excess tissue (*black arrow*), columnar chondrocytes expand ectopically along the cortical bone between affected joints (*yellow arrowheads*). Representative image from a 24-week mouse. Scale bar = 300 μm. **d** Representative images taken from 24-week mice show an unaffected IVD and affected joints with excessive or ectopic chondrocyte formation. Cartilaginous tissue (*arrows*) is positive for toluidine blue (proteoglycan content) and type II collagen. Type X collagen stains for hypertrophic chondrocytes while type I collagen delineates mature bone. Scale bar = 100 μm. **e** Spinal gene expression profiles of cartilage markers *Col2a1*, *Comp* and *Sox9* were analysed by qPCR reaction and normalized to β-actin. Black bars represent naïve and open bars represent PGISp mice. Expression levels are presented as mean ± standard deviation. $^{***}P < 0.0001$, $^{**}P < 0.001$, $^{*}P < 0.01$ compared with naïve at the same time point, Mann-Whitney test. *Col2a1* type II collagen, α 1, *COMP* cartilage oligomeric matrix protein, *Sox9* sex determining region Y- box 9

disease, ectopic cartilaginous tissue increased as the inflammatory cell infiltrate and density of fibroblast-like mesenchymal cells declined (Fig. 3b, arrows). Ectopic chondrogenesis/chondrophyte formation occurred only following disc destruction, and residual necrotic disk tissue was frequently evident (Fig. 3a, asterisks). Ectopic cartilage-like tissue containing embedded chondrocytes in columnar formation parallel to the vertebral periosteal cortical surface was also observed in some mice and was possibly associated with longitudinal ligament attachment points (Fig. 3c, yellow arrowheads). Interestingly, the cortical bone underlying the columnar cartilage-like tissues had evidence of erosive damage, including pitting of the periosteal surface (Fig. 2c). Inflammation was noted in similar regions of other mice (Fig. 2e, arrows), as were cells with chondroblast-like morphology embedded within dense ECM (Figs. 3aii and b). These features were not observed concomitantly on any given vertebral body, suggesting that while they occurred at a similar anatomical location, they were temporally staggered processes, although owing to cross-sectional experimental design, these observations are correlative.

The composition of the ectopic ECM present at sites of PGISp excess tissue formation was determined by assessing distribution of different types of collagen by immunohistochemistry (Fig. 3d). In unaffected vertebral joints (Fig. 3d, top row), the AF and endplate hyaline cartilage had high PG content (toluidine blue-positive) and predominantly contained type II collagen. Type I collagen was weakly present in AF but was a major component of the vertebral bone. In affected joints (Fig. 3d, middle and bottom row), the majority of the excessive tissue (Fig. 3d, arrows) had a high PG content and contained both type II and type X collagens, verifying pathologic chondroproliferation. Expression of type X collagen suggested that some chondrocytes were hypertrophic. Consistent with previous findings, weak collagen type I staining seen at the periphery of excessive tissue areas, potentially indicated progression towards formation of bone [8].

Spinal mRNA expression of cartilage matrix components and cartilage-forming regulatory proteins fluctuated during disease progression (Fig. 3e). Expression of cartilage components *col2a1* and *Sox9* was decreased at 8 and 6 weeks post-priming, respectively. From 10 weeks onwards, as inflammation peaked and excessive tissue formation increased, cartilage oligomeric matrix protein (*Comp*) was significantly elevated. *Col2a1* was upregulated at week 12 whereas *Sox9* increased at weeks 10 and 24. This trend suggests cartilaginous matrix expression was increased in PGISp mice after the peak of inflammation.

Mature osteophyte formation, defined as aberrant bone formation adjacent to cortical bone (Fig. 4a), was apparent. Osteophytes showed a variable collagen distribution with different areas containing collagen I-, II- or X-positive and osterix-positive cells (Fig. 4b). None of the PGISp mice at weeks 6 and 8 developed osteophytes, but 28.6 % of mice at week 10 had osteophytes, and the percentage increased to 71.4 %, 66.7 % and 75 % at weeks 12, 16 and 24, respectively. A noteworthy observation is that pathological tissue formation was observed only with vertebral joints that exhibited IVD destruction.

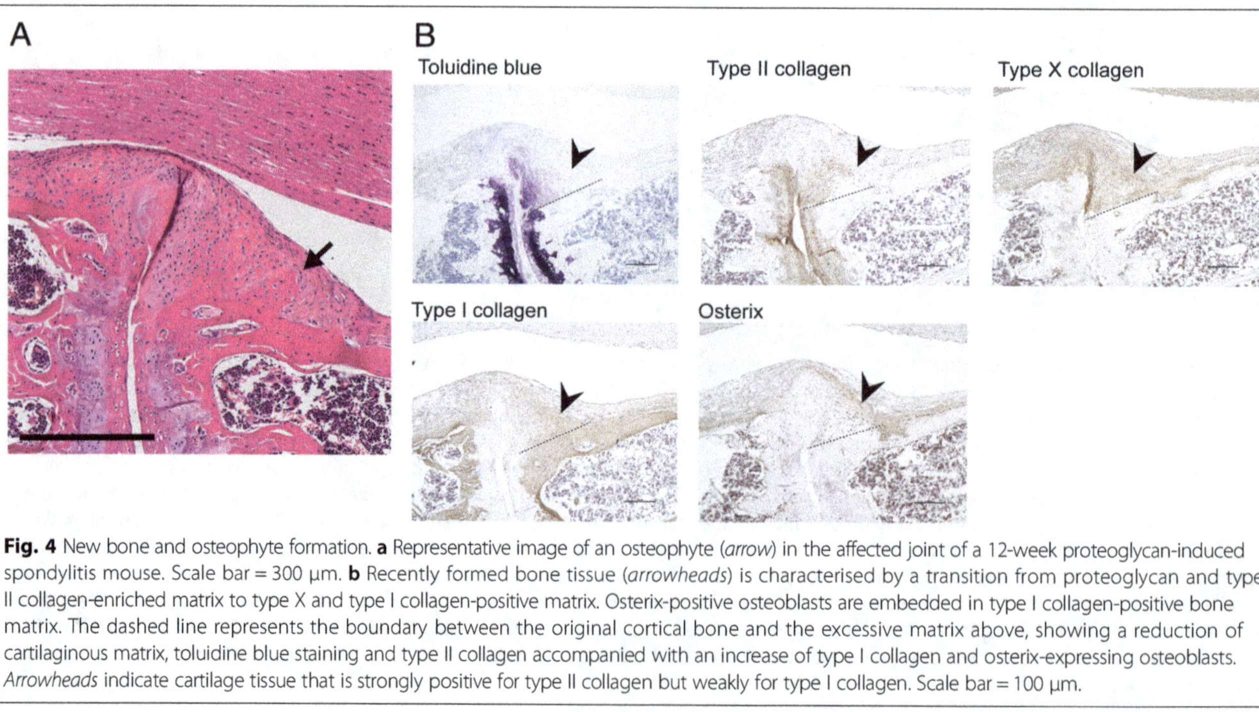

Fig. 4 New bone and osteophyte formation. **a** Representative image of an osteophyte (*arrow*) in the affected joint of a 12-week proteoglycan-induced spondylitis mouse. Scale bar = 300 μm. **b** Recently formed bone tissue (*arrowheads*) is characterised by a transition from proteoglycan and type II collagen-enriched matrix to type X and type I collagen-positive matrix. Osterix-positive osteoblasts are embedded in type I collagen-positive bone matrix. The dashed line represents the boundary between the original cortical bone and the excessive matrix above, showing a reduction of cartilaginous matrix, toluidine blue staining and type II collagen accompanied with an increase of type I collagen and osterix-expressing osteoblasts. *Arrowheads* indicate cartilage tissue that is strongly positive for type II collagen but weakly for type I collagen. Scale bar = 100 μm.

Modelling of disease

To unbiasedly model the interdependence of the different scoring criteria irrespectively of time post-PG priming, we developed an algorithm to define different disease stages. This algorithm used an unsupervised clustering approach based purely on average affected vertebral joint scores across all the criteria measured. This clustering defined three disease stages which interestingly corresponded broadly to the time point post-priming—stage 1: early (mainly week 6 to 8, Fig. 5a, left box); stage 2: intermediate (mainly weeks 10 to 12, Fig. 5a, middle box); and stage 3: advanced (mainly weeks 16–24, Fig. 5a, right box). Stage 3 could also be divided into two subgroups with a very late cluster consisting of almost entirely 24-week mice. We further dissected the data to identify the scoring metrics that best delineated each stage. The scores for inflammation (Fig. 5b), excessive tissue formation (Fig. 5c) and ectopic chondrocyte formation (Fig. 5d) strongly differentiated between these three groups. The early stage showed mild to moderate inflammation, low excessive tissue and low ectopic chondrocyte formation. The intermediate stage displayed severe inflammation and moderate excessive tissue and ectopic chondrocyte formation. The advanced stage showed decreased inflammation but pronounced excess tissue and ectopic chondrocyte formation.

Discussion

Inflammation and syndesmophyte formation are two defining hallmarks in AS. However, the relationships between these features, as well as the underlying controlling factors, are poorly understood. Key questions that remain to be answered are whether the enthesis is the site of disease initiation, whether inflammation is necessary for radiographic disease progression, and what is the nature of the pathological osseous tissue laid down. By detailed analysis of disease progression in the PGISp mouse model of AS, we have provided insights into these questions. Specifically we have demonstrated that osteoproliferation is seen only at sites where inflammation previously occurred, strongly suggesting that inflammation and IVD destruction are required for disease progression to bone formation.

The detailed histology analysis in the present study revealed that the inflammatory invasion started at the periphery of the AF. Association of inflammation with the AF has been previously noted in this model but was not identified as the inflammation initiating point within spine [7, 8]. Spinal enthesitis presenting as pannus formation outside of the AF was also reported in HLA-B27 transgenic rats [14] and curdlan-treated SKG mice [15]. We also showed that inflammatory infiltrate and ectopic chondroproliferation expanded along the adjacent vertebrae cortical bone surfaces. Although we do not show definitive proof of entheses in these regions, it is well established that the longitudinal spinal ligaments have frequent attachment points in this area [16, 17].

The limited effects of anti-TNF therapies on radiographic progression raised the question as to whether inflammation is required for osteoproliferation in AS. Our detailed histological examination suggests inflammation, excessive tissue formation and ectopic chondrocyte formation typify early, intermediate and late disease stages, respectively. We demonstrated that early mesenchymal expansion initiated before resolution of inflammation. Although averaging of histological scores suggests overlap between the disease stages, examination of individual vertebrae showed that severe inflammation was never found simultaneously with severe excessive tissue formation within the same joint, supporting sequential rather than parallel progression of these disease features. Therefore, our model predicts that inflammatory lesions are likely to have decreased, if not resolved, in the later disease stages typified by syndesmophyte formation. This prediction is supported by MRI studies in AS patients that have shown that (1) new syndesmophytes are seen more frequently in vertebral corners with resolved inflammation [18] and (2) 68 % of syndesmophytes developed from vertebral corners without active inflammation during the 2-year observation period [19]. However, some consideration needs to be given to the sensitivity limits of MRI for detecting mild inflammation [20].

Excessive tissue formation occurred only at vertebral joints in which the IVD itself had been destroyed, implying that disease initiates with inflammation which leads to disc destruction. As inflammation decreases, excessive tissue formation commences with ectopic chondrocyte formation occurring late. Such a progression concurs with the "TNF-brake hypothesis" proposed by Maksymowych *et al.* [18], who suggest that a high level of inflammatory TNF actually inhibits osteoproliferation and this inhibition is eased as TNF levels drop with resolution of inflammation. This also matches data from rheumatoid arthritis models in which osteoblast function is inhibited in the presence of inflammation [21] and induced after inflammation resolution [22]. However, we also see elevated TNF expression in the spines of the PGISp mice from inflammation throughout the excess tissue production phases, suggesting that TNF may play a role in the osteoproliferation as well as inflammation. Alternatively, these elevated levels might also reflect the disease heterogeneity within individual vertebrae and local TNF levels may result in site-specific impacts on osteoblast regulation.

Enthesitis and osteoproliferation have also been reported in DBA/1 mice [23], HLA-B27/hβ2m transgenic rats [24] and curdlan-treated SKG mice [15]. However, the relationship between the processes is not well defined. In the DBA/1 mouse model of ankylosing enthesitis, chondrocyte proliferation was the leading cause of

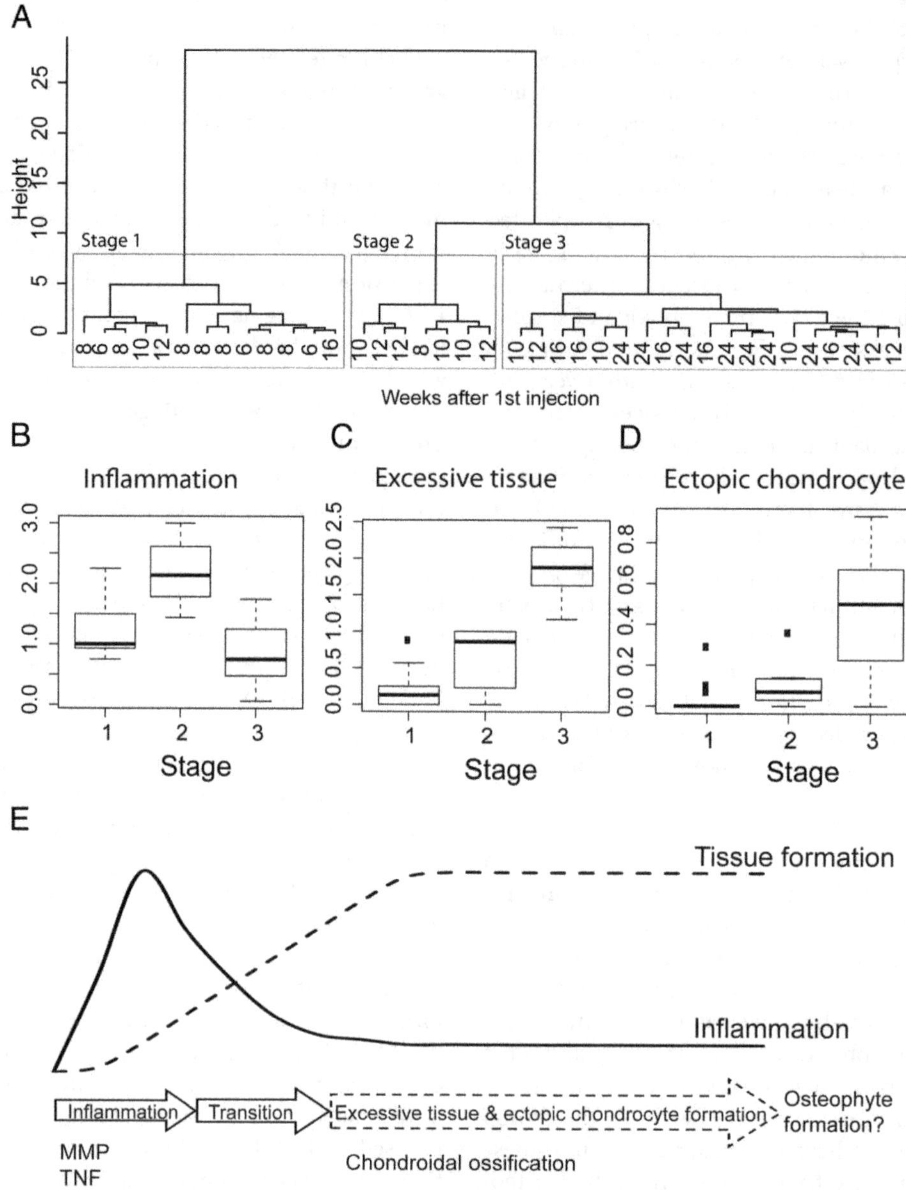

Fig. 5 Early, intermediate and late phases of disease progression are delineated by inflammation, excessive tissue and ectopic chondrocyte formation. **a** Unsupervised clustering differentiates the model into three stages corresponding with disease duration. The x-axis depicts the time points of the mice. The left box (stage 1), middle box (stage 2) and right box (stage 3) represent early, intermediate and late stages of disease development, respectively. Scores for (**b**) inflammation, (**c**) excessive tissue formation and (**d**) ectopic chondrocyte formation are distinct between these three groups. **e** Axial disease was initially characterised by transient inflammation that included vertebral joint infiltration by monocular cells, activation of tissue remodelling (matrix metalloproteinases, or MMPs) and pro-arthritic inflammatory pathways (tumour necrosis factor, or TNF). Vertebral joint inflammation culminated in destructive changes, including destruction of the intervertebral disc, the latter of which was irreparable and would have considerable impact on joint biomechanics. In advanced disease, inflammation is decreased; however, excessive tissue and ectopic chondrocyte formation driven by chondroidal ossification was the predominant feature and occurred only in joints in which the IVD had been severely compromised

ankle ankylosis [23, 25]. The entheseal proliferation and inflammatory infiltrate were minor in this model, and treatment with glucocorticoids [26], but not etanercept [27], did ameliorate inflammation but had no effect on the ankylosis. In a longitudinal study in HLA-B27/hβ2m transgenic rats, osteoproliferation was found external to the joint space separate to inflammatory infiltrates [24] but was present simultaneously, suggesting distinct but parallel processes. Interestingly, although blocking TNF signalling before or after onset prevented or reduced arthritis, respectively [28], chondroproliferation and its activation of relevant bone morphogenetic protein signalling were prevented only by early treatment. In the SKG mouse model, bone formation and erosion were shown to be adjacent to inflammation, although progressive association of these different features is unclear as a detailed longitudinal study was not undertaken [15]. So although evidence from other animal models is ambiguous, our extensive analysis in the PGISp model clearly supports a direct progression from inflammation to cartilage-bone formation.

Direct connection of the ectopic chondrocytes and cartilage to the vertebral end plate or growth plate cartilage was not a consistent histological feature in our model, indicating that these ectopic tissues were not due to expansion of existing cartilage structures. The AF [29], periosteum [30] and ligament [16] all contain potential chondrocyte progenitors. Therefore, it is possible the chondrogenesis is initiated using progenitors located within these disease-affected tissues without direct involvement of pre-existing cartilage. Several features of the excessive tissue in the advanced disease, such as cartilage formation and chondrocyte hypertrophy, resembled endochondral ossification. Hypertrophic chondrocytes have been shown to be able to transform directly into osteoblasts and osteocytes [31]. Bleil *et al.* recently demonstrated that zygapophyseal joint ankylosis was caused by direct transformation from cartilage to bone without chondrocyte hypertrophy [32]. The direct transformation/ossification from chondrocytes represents chondroidal ossification [2, 32] and might be the primary mechanism of excessive tissue formation in the PGISp model. Examples of mature syndesmophytes were rare in this study but more evident in later disease stages. This finding suggests that the transformation of cartilage to bone in PGISp mice is a slow process modelling the prolonged window between disease onset and radiographic change in patients with AS [33].

Our results suggest that if inflammation is not treated early enough to prevent irreparable structural damage, further osteoproliferation at that location will progress even if the inflammatory process is resolved/attenuated. The benefits of early intervention regarding both spondylitis and radiographic progression have been demonstrated with different treatments. After treatment with infliximab for 16 weeks, 61 % of patients with short disease duration (13.4 months) had 40 % improvement from baseline [34] whereas only 47 % of patients with long disease duration (7.7 years) reached the same criteria after 24 weeks of treatment [35]. Delaying TNF intervention therapy for 10 years was related to faster radiographic progression compared with those who started treatment within 10 years of disease onset [36]. The benefit of early intervention was also seen using NSAIDs. AS patients with short disease duration (<5 years) had less radiographic progression [37] compared with those with long disease duration (11.9 years) [38] following chronic high-dose NSAID treatment. These studies suggest that anti-inflammatory therapies exert better clinical outcomes in patients with early AS/spondyloarthritis compared with those whose disease is established.

Conclusions

In summary, our study indicates inflammation leads to IVD destruction in the PGISp mouse AS model. The latter is a prerequisite for induction of excessive tissue formation, and chondroidal ossification rather than endochondral or intramembranous ossification appears to be the most likely mechanism. Extrapolation of these findings to human disease suggests that early intervention with potent anti-inflammatory therapeutic regimens may prevent inflammation-induced destructive changes and consequently reduce the frequency of osteoproliferative events and joint fusion.

Abbreviations

AF: Annulus fibrosus; AS: Ankylosing spondylitis; Col2a1: Type II collagen, α 1; ECM: Extracellular matrix; EDTA: Ethylenediaminetetraacetic acid disodium salt dehydrate; H&E: Haematoxylin and eosin; HLA: Human leukocyte antigen; IVD: Intervertebral disc; MMP: Matrix metalloproteinase; MRI: Magnetic resonance imaging; NSAID: Non-steroidal anti-inflammatory drug; PCR: Polymerase chain reaction; PG: Proteoglycan; PGISp: Proteoglycan-induced spondylitis; qPCR: Quantitative real-time reverse transcription polymerase chain reaction; RT: Room temperature; Sox9: Sex determining region Y- box 9; TBS: Tris-buffered saline; TNF: Tumour necrosis factor.

Competing interests

The authors declare that they have no competing interests.

Authors' contributions

H-WT generated and analysed data and wrote the manuscript. MEP generated and analysed data. TTG provided reagents and helped conceive the project. AFM analysed data. TJK, ARP and GPT conceived the project and analysed data. MAB conceived the project. All authors contributed to writing the manuscript and approved the final version.

Acknowledgements

This study was supported by National Health and Medical Research Council (NHMRC) project grant APP1006450. The cartilage extract was kindly provided by TTG. H-WT was supported by a University of Queensland PhD Scholarship. ARP is supported by NHMRC Career Development Fellowship 519744 and the Mater Foundation. MAB is supported by NHMRC Senior Principal Research Fellowship APP1024879, and TTG by the National Institutes of Health/National Institute of Arthritis and Musculoskeletal and Skin Diseases (R01 AR062991).

Author details

[1]The University of Queensland Diamantina Institute, Translational Research Institute, 37 Kent Street, Woolloongabba, QLD 4102, Australia. [2]Section of Molecular Medicine, Department of Orthopedic Surgery, Rush University Medical Center, 1735 W. Harrison Street, Cohn Research Building, Chicago, IL 60612, USA. [3]The University of Queensland, Queensland Brain Institute, QBI Building, St Lucia, QLD 4072, Australia. [4]The University of Queensland-Mater Research Institute, Translational Research Institute, 37 Kent Street, Woolloongabba, QLD 4102, Australia.

References

1. Benjamin M, Toumi H, Suzuki D, Hayashi K, McGonagle D. Evidence for a distinctive pattern of bone formation in enthesophytes. Ann Rheum Dis. 2009;68:1003–10.
2. Francois RJ, Gardner DL, Degrave EJ, Bywaters EG. Histopathologic evidence that sacroiliitis in ankylosing spondylitis is not merely enthesitis. Arthritis Rheum. 2000;43:2011–24.
3. Appel H, Maier R, Wu P, Scheer R, Hempfing A, Kayser R, et al. Analysis of IL-17+ cells in facet joints of patients with spondyloarthritis suggests that the innate immune pathway might be of greater relevance than the Th17-mediated adaptive immune response. Arthritis Res Ther. 2011;13:R95.
4. Appel H, Kuhne M, Spiekermann S, Ebhardt H, Grozdanovic Z, Kohler D, et al. Immunohistologic analysis of zygapophyseal joints in patients with ankylosing spondylitis. Arthritis Rheum. 2006;54:2845–51.
5. Appel H, Kuhne M, Spiekermann S, Kohler D, Zacher J, Stein H, et al. Immunohistochemical analysis of hip arthritis in ankylosing spondylitis: evaluation of the bone-cartilage interface and subchondral bone marrow. Arthritis Rheum. 2006;54:1805–13.
6. Appel H, Maier R, Bleil J, Hempfing A, Loddenkemper C, Schlichting U, et al. In situ analysis of interleukin-23- and interleukin-12-positive cells in the spine of patients with ankylosing spondylitis. Arthritis Rheum. 2013;65:1522–9.
7. Bárdos T, Szabó Z, Czipri M, Vermes C, Tunyogi-Csapó M, Urban RM, et al. A longitudinal study on an autoimmune murine model of ankylosing spondylitis. Ann Rheum Dis. 2005;64:981–7.
8. Haynes KR, Pettit AR, Duan R, Tseng HW, Glant TT, Brown MA, et al. Excessive bone formation in a mouse model of ankylosing spondylitis is associated with decreases in Wnt pathway inhibitors. Arthritis Res Ther. 2012;14:R253.
9. Finnegan A, Grusby MJ, Kaplan CD, O'Neill SK, Eibel H, Koreny T, et al. IL-4 and IL-12 regulate proteoglycan-induced arthritis through Stat-dependent mechanisms. J Immunol. 2002;169:3345–52.
10. Calin A, Elswood J. The relationship between pelvic, spinal and hip involvement in ankylosing spondylitis–one disease process or several? Br J Rheumatol. 1988;27:393–5.
11. Yang C, Gu J, Rihl M, Baeten D, Huang F, Zhao M, et al. Serum levels of matrix metalloproteinase 3 and macrophage colony-stimulating factor 1 correlate with disease activity in ankylosing spondylitis. Arthritis Rheum. 2004;51:691–9.
12. Soliman E, Labib W, el-Tantawi G, Hamimy A, Alhadidy A, Aldawoudy A. Role of matrix metalloproteinase-3 (MMP-3) and magnetic resonance imaging of sacroiliitis in assessing disease activity in ankylosing spondylitis. Rheumatol Int. 2012;32:1711–20.
13. Arends S, van der Veer E, Groen H, Houtman PM, Jansen TL, Leijsma MK, et al. Serum MMP-3 level as a biomarker for monitoring and predicting response to etanercept treatment in ankylosing spondylitis. J Rheumatol. 2011;38:1644–50.
14. Hammer RE, Maika SD, Richardson JA, Tang JP, Taurog JD. Spontaneous inflammatory disease in transgenic rats expressing HLA-B27 and human beta 2 m: an animal model of HLA-B27-associated human disorders. Cell. 1990;63:1099–112.
15. Ruutu M, Thomas G, Steck R, Degli-Esposti MA, Zinkernagel MS, Alexander K, et al. beta-glucan triggers spondylarthritis and Crohn's disease-like ileitis in SKG mice. Arthritis Rheum. 2012;64:2211–22.
16. Cai HX, Yayama T, Uchida K, Nakajima H, Sugita D, Guerrero AR, et al. Cyclic tensile strain facilitates the ossification of ligamentum flavum through beta-catenin signaling pathway: in vitro analysis. Spine (Phila Pa 1976). 2012;37:E639–46.
17. Loughenbury PR, Wadhwani S, Soames RW. The posterior longitudinal ligament and peridural (epidural) membrane. Clin Anat. 2006;19:487–92.
18. Maksymowych WP, Chiowchanwisawakit P, Clare T, Pedersen SJ, Ostergaard M, Lambert RG. Inflammatory lesions of the spine on magnetic resonance imaging predict the development of new syndesmophytes in ankylosing spondylitis: evidence of a relationship between inflammation and new bone formation. Arthritis Rheum. 2009;60:93–102.
19. van der Heijde D, Machado P, Braun J, Hermann KG, Baraliakos X, Hsu B, et al. MRI inflammation at the vertebral unit only marginally predicts new syndesmophyte formation: a multilevel analysis in patients with ankylosing spondylitis. Ann Rheum Dis. 2012;71:369–73.
20. Appel H, Loddenkemper C, Grozdanovic Z, Ebhardt H, Dreimann M, Hempfing A, et al. Correlation of histopathological findings and magnetic resonance imaging in the spine of patients with ankylosing spondylitis. Arthritis Res Ther. 2006;8:R143.
21. Walsh NC, Reinwald S, Manning CA, Condon KW, Iwata K, Burr DB, et al. Osteoblast function is compromised at sites of focal bone erosion in inflammatory arthritis. J Bone Miner Res. 2009;24:1572–85.
22. Matzelle MM, Gallant MA, Condon KW, Walsh NC, Manning CA, Stein GS, et al. Resolution of inflammation induces osteoblast function and regulates the Wnt signaling pathway. Arthritis Rheum. 2012;64:1540–50.
23. Corthay A, Hansson AS, Holmdahl R. T lymphocytes are not required for the spontaneous development of entheseal ossification leading to marginal ankylosis in the DBA/1 mouse. Arthritis Rheum. 2000;43:844–51.
24. van Duivenvoorde LM, Dorris ML, Satumtira N, van Tok MN, Redlich K, Tak PP, et al. Relationship between inflammation, bone destruction, and osteoproliferation in the HLA-B27/human beta(2) -microglobulin-transgenic rat model of spondylarthritis. Arthritis Rheum. 2012;64:3210–9.
25. Lories RJ, Matthys P, de Vlam K, Derese I, Luyten FP. Ankylosing enthesitis, dactylitis, and onychoperiostitis in male DBA/1 mice: a model of psoriatic arthritis. Ann Rheum Dis. 2004;63:595–8.
26. Braem K, Deroose CM, Luyten FP, Lories RJ. Inhibition of inflammation but not ankylosis by glucocorticoids in mice: further evidence for the entheseal stress hypothesis. Arthritis Res Ther. 2012;14:R59.
27. Lories RJ, Derese I, de Bari C, Luyten FP. Evidence for uncoupling of inflammation and joint remodeling in a mouse model of spondylarthritis. Arthritis Rheum. 2007;56:489–97.
28. Milia AF, Ibba-Manneschi L, Manetti M, Benelli G, Generini S, Messerini L, et al. Evidence for the prevention of enthesitis in HLA-B27/hbeta(2)m transgenic rats treated with a monoclonal antibody against TNF-alpha. J Cell Mol Med. 2011;15:270–9.
29. Nosikova Y, Santerre JP, Grynpas MD, Kandel RA. Annulus fibrosus cells can induce mineralization: an in vitro study. Spine J. 2013;13:443–53.
30. Ito Y, Fitzsimmons JS, Sanyal A, Mello MA, Mukherjee N, O'Driscoll SW. Localization of chondrocyte precursors in periosteum. Osteoarthritis Cartilage. 2001;9:215–23.
31. Yang L, Tsang KY, Tang HC, Chan D, Cheah KS. Hypertrophic chondrocytes can become osteoblasts and osteocytes in endochondral bone formation. Proc Natl Acad Sci U S A. 2014;111:12097–102.
32. Bleil J, Maier R, Hempfing A, Schlichting U, Appel H, Sieper J, et al. Histomorphologic and histomorphometric characteristics of zygapophyseal joint remodeling in ankylosing spondylitis. Arthritis Rheumatol. 2014;66:1745–54.
33. van Tubergen A, Weber U. Diagnosis and classification in spondyloarthritis: identifying a chameleon. Nat Rev Rheumatol. 2012;8:253–61.
34. Barkham N, Keen HI, Coates LC, O'Connor P, Hensor E, Fraser AD, et al. Clinical and imaging efficacy of infliximab in HLA-B27-Positive patients with magnetic resonance imaging-determined early sacroiliitis. Arthritis Rheum. 2009;60:946–54.
35. van der Heijde D, Dijkmans B, Geusens P, Sieper J, DeWoody K, Williamson P, et al. Efficacy and safety of infliximab in patients with ankylosing spondylitis: results of a randomized, placebo-controlled trial (ASSERT). Arthritis Rheum. 2005;52:582–91.
36. Haroon N, Inman RD, Learch TJ, Weisman MH, Lee M, Rahbar MH, et al. The impact of tumor necrosis factor alpha inhibitors on radiographic progression in ankylosing spondylitis. Arthritis Rheum. 2013;65:2645–54.
37. Poddubnyy D, Haibel H, Listing J, Marker-Hermann E, Zeidler H, Braun J, et al. Baseline radiographic damage, elevated acute-phase reactant levels, and cigarette smoking status predict spinal radiographic progression in early axial spondylarthritis. Arthritis Rheum. 2012;64:1388–98.
38. Wanders A, Heijde D, Landewe R, Behier JM, Calin A, Olivieri I, et al. Nonsteroidal antiinflammatory drugs reduce radiographic progression in patients with ankylosing spondylitis: a randomized clinical trial. Arthritis Rheum. 2005;52:1756–65.

In vivo pre-activation of monocytes in patients with axial spondyloarthritis

Kristina Conrad[1], Peihua Wu[2], Joachim Sieper[1,2] and Uta Syrbe[1,2*]

Abstract

Introduction: Innate immune responses, including monocyte functions, seem to play an important role in the pathogenesis of axial spondyloarthritis (axSpA). Therefore, we characterized the phenotype and functional state of monocytes of patients with axSpA.

Methods: Fifty-seven patients with axSpA, 11 patients with rheumatoid arthritis (RA), and 29 healthy controls were included in the study. We determined the percentage of classic, intermediate, and non-classic monocytes according to CD14 and CD16 expression and the expression of Toll-like receptor (TLR) 1, 2, and 4 in whole blood by flow cytometry. The percentage of monocytes producing interleukin (IL)-1beta, IL-6, tumor necrosis factor alpha (TNFα), IL-12/23p40, and IL-1 receptor antagonist (IL-1ra) was detected by flow cytometry after stimulation of whole blood without and with different TLR and nucleotide-binding oligomerization domain ligands—i.e., lipopolysaccharide (LPS), fibroblast-stimulating lipopeptid-1, PAM_3CSK_4, and muramyl dipeptide (MDP)—for 5 h. IL-10 production was measured after 18 h of stimulation in supernatants by enzyme-linked immunosorbent assay.

Results: In patients with axSpA but not patients with RA, we found higher frequencies of classic monocytes than in controls (median of 90.4 % versus 80.4 %, $P < 0.05$), higher frequencies of monocytes spontaneously producing IL-1beta and IL-1ra ($P < 0.05$), and a higher percentage of monocytes producing IL-1beta after MDP stimulation ($P < 0.05$). Elevated cytokine production was confined to axSpA patients under conventional therapy (non-steroidal anti-inflammatory drugs) and not found in patients under TNFα inhibitor treatment. The LPS-induced production of IL-6 and IL-10 was lower in axSpA patients compared with controls ($P < 0.05$). Monocytic TLR expression was unaffected in patients with axSpA.

Conclusion: Enhanced spontaneous and MDP-induced cytokine secretion by monocytes suggests *in vivo* pre-activation of monocytes in axSpA patients under conventional therapy which is reverted under TNF inhibitor treatment.

Introduction

Axial spondyloarthritis (AxSpA) is the prototypic form of spondyloarthritis, a group of related diseases comprising AxSpA, reactive arthritis, arthritis related to inflammatory bowel disease, psoriasis, and uveitis [1]. AxSpA, nowadays subdivided into non-radiographic axSpA and ankylosing spondylitis (AS), is characterized by inflammation within the axial skeleton, predominately of the sacroiliac joints [1].

The pathogenesis and triggers of inflammation in axSpA are still unclear. AxSpA is strongly associated with the major histocompatibility complex (MHC) class I molecule HLA-B27; however, the involvement of CD8 T-cell responses could not be proven so far. In fact, in the HLA-B27 transgenic rat model, CD8 T cells are dispensable for disease induction [2]. Apart from presenting specific antigens to $CD8^+$ T cells, HLA-B27 has the capability to induce endoplasmic reticulum stress [3]. In innate immune cells, this can trigger cytokine responses or modify the responsiveness of these cells to other stimulants, suggesting that innate immune functions might play a role in the pathogenesis of axSpA.

Monocytes belong to the innate, first-line defence against infections. They recognize bacterial structures by pattern

* Correspondence: uta.syrbe@charite.de
[1]Charité-Universitätsmedizin Berlin, CBF, Medizinische Klinik für Gastroenterologie, Infektiologie und Rheumatologie, Hindenburgdamm 30, Berlin 12203, Germany
[2]Deutsches Rheumaforschungszentrum, Charitéplatz 1, Berlin 10117, Germany

recognition receptors, including Toll-like receptor (TLR) and nucleotide-binding oligomerization domain (NOD)-like-receptors. Ligation of TLR or NOD receptors rapidly triggers production of proinflammatory cytokines such as interleukin-1 (IL-1), IL-6, and tumor necrosis factor alpha (TNFα) in monocytes [4, 5]. Proinflammatory responses are tightly controlled by concomitant induction of anti-inflammatory mediators, such as IL-1ra, which competes with IL-1 for binding to the IL-1 receptor 1 [6], and IL-10, which is produced by monocytes at later time points after stimulation and downregulates TNFα production [7].

There are some reports that showed enhanced transcription and protein expression of inflammation-associated genes in blood monocytes of patients with AS, suggesting aberrant activation or disturbed responsiveness of monocytes in patients with axSpA [8, 9].

To further decipher potential involvement of monocytes in the pathogenesis of axSpA, we studied here the phenotype and function of monocytes from patients with axSpA. We performed a phenotypic analysis of monocytes and determined their spontaneous and TLR and NOD ligand-induced cytokine production.

Methods

Study subjects

Peripheral venous whole blood was collected in heparinised Vacutainer tubes (BD, Heidelberg, Germany) from 29 healthy donors (15/29 male, mean age of 35.3 ± 8.3 years) and from 57 patients with axSpA (39/57 male, mean age of 38.0 ± 10.6 years) meeting the Assessment of Spondyloarthritis International Society criteria for axSpA, of whom 39 patients (68.4 %) fulfilled the modified New York criteria for diagnosis of AS. Eleven patients (2/11 male, mean age of 59.7 ± 18.8 years) with rheumatoid arthritis (RA) were included as inflammatory controls. The number of patients and controls used for individual parts of the study (phenotypic analysis and cytokine analysis) is stated in each figure legend. Fifty-three (92.9 %) of the 57 patients with axSpA were HLA-B27-positive. Thirty-four patients with axSpA received conventional treatment with continuous or on-demand non-steroidal anti-inflammatory drugs (NSAIDs), and 23 patients received TNFα inhibitors. None of the patients with axSpA received disease-modifying anti-rheumatic drugs (DMARDs). Ten out of eleven patients with RA received prednisolone, eight out of 11 received synthetic DMARD therapy (four methotrexate, two hydroxychloroquine, one sulfasalacine, and one methotrexate plus sulfasalacine), and two patients received treatment with biologics (one TNFα inhibitor and one anti-IL-6 receptor antibody). Disease activity was determined according to the Bath ankylosing spondylitis disease activity index (BASDAI) [10]. C-reactive protein (CRP) was determined at the routine clinical laboratory of the Charité.

The study was approved by the local ethical commission of the Charité. All patients and control subjects gave consent to the study.

Phenotypic characterization of peripheral blood monocytes

To analyse the expression of phenotypic surface markers, 2 ml of heparinized whole blood was incubated with 8 ml of erythrocyte lysing buffer (Qiagen, Hilden, Germany) on ice to lyse erythrocytes. The remaining cells were stained with the respective antibodies against CD14 (clone M5E2 PerCPcy5.5; BD), CD16 (clone eBioCB16 APC; ebioscience, Frankfurt, Germany), HLA-DR (clone L243 fluorescein isothiocyanate (FITC); BD Heidelberg, Germany), CD64 (clone 10.1 PE; Dako, Glostrup, DK), CD80 (clone 2D10 PE; biolegend, San Diego, CA, USA), CD115 (clone 12-3A3-1B10 PE; ebioscience), and CD163 (clone GHI/61PE; BD). For analysis of TLR expression, 50 µl of heparinized whole blood was incubated at room temperature with the respective antibodies against TLR1, i.e., CD281 (clone GD2.F4 TLR-1), TLR2, i.e., CD282 (clone TL2.1 TLR-2), and TLR4, i.e., CD284 (clone HTA125 TLR-4; all PE; ebioscience) in the dark for 15 min. Afterwards, erythrocytes were lysed with fluorescence-activated cell sorting (FACS) lysing solution (BD) and leukocytes were analysed by flow cytometry by using a FACS Calibur from Becton Dickinson (San Jose, CA, USA) and FlowJo 7.6.4 Software.

In vitro stimulation of whole blood with Toll-like receptor and nucleotide-binding oligomerization domain ligands and intracellular cytokine detection

Heparinized peripheral blood (1 ml) was stimulated for 5 h without or with the TLR 1/2 ligand PAM_3CSK_4 (5 µg/ml), the TLR 2/6 ligand fibroblast-stimulating lipopeptid-1 (FSL-1; 1 µg/ml), the TLR 4 ligand lipopolysaccharide (LPS) (*Escherichia coli* O111:B4; 100 ng/ml), and the NOD2 ligand muramyl dipeptide (MDP) (2.5 µg/ml). All stimulants were purchased from invivoGen (San Diego, CA, USA).

To prevent cytokine secretion, 10 µg/ml brefeldin A (BFA) (Sigma-Aldrich, Steinheim, Germany) was added for the last 3 h of stimulation. After stimulation, erythrocytes were lysed with FACS lysing solution and the remaining cells were fixed by 2 % paraformaldehyde (Roth, Karlsruhe, Germany). Intracellular cytokines and CD68 were stained after permeabilization in 0.5 % saponin/phosphate-buffered saline buffer (Sigma-Aldrich, Steinheim, Germany) by using the following antibodies: anti-CD68-PerCPcy5.5 (clone Y1/82A; biolegend), anti-IL-12/23p40 (clone eBioHP40; e-bioscience, Frankfurt, Germany), anti-TNFα-FITC (clone Mab11; BD), anti-IL-1β-Alexa Fluor 647 (clone JK1B-1; biolegend), anti-IL-6-FITC (clone MQ2-13A5; BD), and anti-IL-1ra-PE (clone AS17; BD). Cytokine expression was detected on a cellular level by using flow cytometric analysis. CD68 was used for identification of monocytes after stimulation, which yielded better separation of monocytes than CD14 after stimulation.

In vitro stimulation of whole blood with Toll-like receptor and nucleotide-binding oligomerization domain ligands and detection of interleukin-10 production by enzyme-linked immunosorbent assay

To determine IL-10 production, heparinised whole blood was mixed 1:2 with RPMI supplemented with 10 % fetal calf serum and stimulated without and with the respective TLR and NOD ligands for 18 h. Supernatants were harvested by centrifugation, snap-frozen, and stored at −20 °C until measurement of IL-10 by enzyme-linked immunosorbent assay (ELISA) (BD OptEIA, Heidelberg, Germany).

Statistical analysis

Statistical analysis was performed by using GraphPad Prism 5 software (GraphPad Inc., La Jolla, CA, USA) and SPSS 19 software (IBM, Ehningen, Germany). Data are shown as individual measurements and medians. Non-parametric tests (Mann–Whitney *U* test and Kruskal-Wallis test and Dunn's post test) were used for comparisons between groups. For variance analysis, we log-transformed data with uneven distribution and used linear regression analysis for metric variables and analysis of variance (ANOVA) for categorical variables.

Results

Expansion of classic monocytes in the peripheral blood of patients with axial spondyloarthritis

To analyse the distribution of monocyte subsets (i.e., classic, intermediate, and non-classic monocytes) within the peripheral blood of axSpA patients in comparison with healthy controls and RA patients as an inflammatory control, monocytes were gated according to forward and side scatter and expression of HLA-DR (Fig. 1a). In patients with axSpA, the percentage of classic monocytes ($CD14^{++}CD16^{-}$) was significantly higher than in healthy controls (median of 90.5 % versus 80.4 %, $P < 0.05$; Fig. 1b) whereas intermediate ($CD14^{++}CD16^{+}$) and non-classic ($CD14^{+}CD16^{+}$) subsets were reduced in patients with axSpA (Fig. 1b). In patients with RA, non-classic monocytes were also reduced whereas differences in classic and intermediate monocyte subsets were not significantly different from controls. Subanalysis of axSpA patients grouped according to treatment into patients with conventional treatment (i.e., on demand or continuous NSAID treatment) or treatment with biologics showed significantly lower frequencies of intermediate $CD14^{++}CD16^{+}$ monocytes in patients under conventional as well as in patients treated with biologics compared with healthy controls, whereas the difference in frequencies of $CD14^{++}$ $CD16^{-}$ monocytes reached statistical significance only in patients under standard therapy compared with healthy patients ($P < 0.01$) but not in patients under biological treatment (Fig. 1c).

The expression of HLA-DR as an antigen-presenting molecule, CD80 as a co-stimulatory molecule, CD163 as a scavenger receptor, CD64 as the Fc receptor, or CD115 as an activation marker on monocytes showed no difference between axSpA patients and controls ($P > 0.05$; data not shown).

In vivo pre-activation of monocytes of axial spondyloarthritis patients according to proinflammatory cytokine production

To determine spontaneous as well as TLR and NOD ligand-induced production of cytokines by monocytes, we incubated whole blood of 42 patients with axSpA (32 male, 10 female; mean age of 37.2 ± 9.8 years), 8 patients with RA (2 male, 6 female; mean age of 59.7 ± 18.8 years; all patients on prednisolone and DMARD treatment, no treatment with biologics), and 26 controls (13 male; 13 female; mean age of 35.4 ± 7.1 years) without any stimulator or added 2.5 μg/ml MDP (NOD-2 ligand), 100 ng/ml LPS (TLR4 ligand), 1 μg/ml FSL-1 (TLR2/6 ligand), or 5 μg/ml PAM_3CSK_4 (TLR1/2 ligand). Cytokine expression was determined in monocytes which were identified according to CD68 expression (Fig. 2a).

The percentage of monocytes spontaneously producing IL-1β was significantly higher in axSpA patients compared with healthy controls (Fig. 2b). A similar non-significant trend toward higher production was observed for IL-6 and TNFα production in patients with axSpA, whereas the IL-12/23p40 production was not increased.

Stimulation with MDP and also stimulation with FSL-1 elicited a higher cytokine production by monocytes, particularly of IL-1β, but also to lesser extent of IL-6 and TNFα, in patients with axSpA (Fig. 2b). For instance, after MDP stimulation, 19.2 % (median) of the monocytes of patients with axSpA versus 8 % of monocytes of healthy controls ($P < 0.01$) produced IL-1β. In contrast, IL-12/23 p40 production by monocytes was low (i.e., below 5 %) after MDP and FSL stimulation and was without difference between axSpA patients and healthy controls. In contrast, patients with RA did not show an elevated spontaneous or MDP- or FSL-induced production of proinflammatory cytokines, despite a minimal but significant increase in the percentage of IL-12/23p40-producting monocytes in unstimulated cultures. In contrast, no difference was observed between axSpA patients and controls in IL-1β and TNFα production in response to LPS, which elicited the highest cytokine response in monocytes. In patients with axSpA, more than 80 % of blood monocytes produced IL-1β in response to LPS and about 60 % produced TNFα, which was not different from controls. Also, on a per-cell basis, LPS

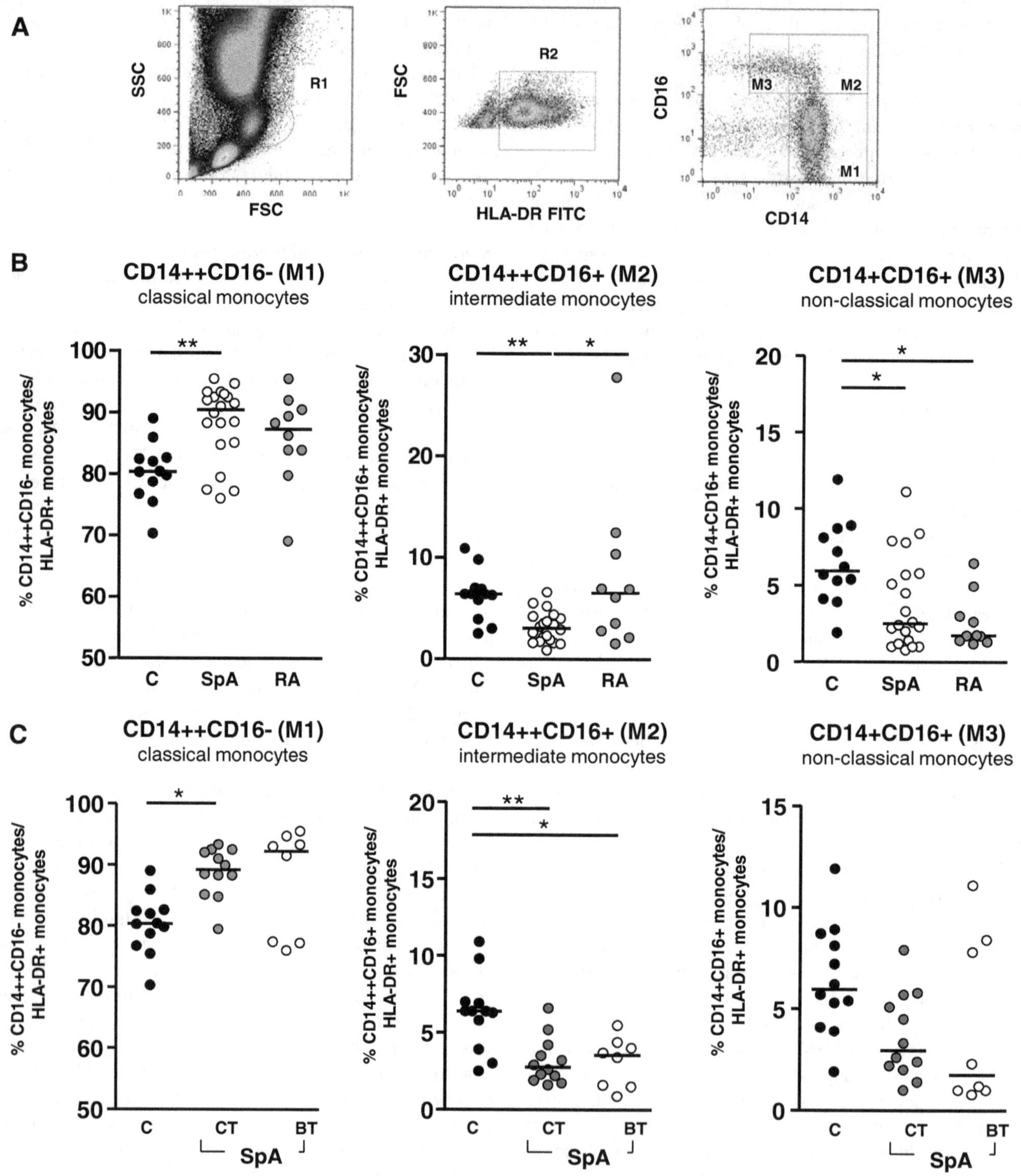

Fig. 1 (See legend on next page.)

(See figure on previous page.)
Fig. 1 Elevated percentage of classic monocytes in patients with axial spondyloarthritis (axSpA). **a** The percentage of classic $CD14^{++}CD16^{-}$ (M1), intermediate $CD14^{++}CD16^{+}$ (M2), and non-classic $CD14^{+}CD16^{+}$ (M3) monocytes was determined by fluorescence-activated cell sorting in whole blood of controls, patients with axSpA, and patients with rheumatoid arthritis (RA). The percentage of classic, intermediate, and non-classic monocytes was determined among monocytes which were gated according to forward (FSC) and side (SSC) scatter (R1) and HLA-DR expression (R2). **b** The percentage of classic, intermediate, and non-classic monocytes (individual measurements and median) is shown from measurements in 12 controls (C), 20 patients with axSpA (SpA), and 12 patients with RA (RA). $*P < 0.05$, $**P < 0.01$ (Kruskal-Wallis test and Dunn's post test). **c** The percentage of the respective populations in axSpA patients separated into patients under conventional treatment (SpA CT) ($n = 12$) and patients receiving biologics (i.e., tumor necrosis factor inhibitors) (SpA BT) ($n = 8$) compared with controls (c). $*P < 0.05$, $**P < 0.01$ (Kruskal-Wallis test and Dunn's post test). *FITC* fluorescein isothiocyanate

elicited higher responses than MDP, FSL-1, or PAM_3CSK_4 as indicated by the higher mean fluorescence intensity of the IL-1β staining (Fig. 2a).

However, LPS stimulation resulted in significantly less IL-6-producing monocytes in axSpA patients compared with controls (median of 63.2 % versus 72.1 %; $P < 0.01$; Fig. 2b). Also, in patients with RA, LPS-induced IL-6 and even TNFα production was reduced in comparison with healthy controls (Fig. 2b). No significant difference between axSpA patients and controls was found in monocytic cytokine production in response to PAM_3CSK_4 stimulation (Fig. 2b).

The elevated spontaneous and MDP, and FSL-1, induced proinflammatory cytokine production by monocytes of patients with axSpA suggests in vivo pre-activation of monocytes in these patients.

Elevated frequency of monocytes spontaneously producing interleukin-1 receptor antagonist in axial spondyloarthritis and rheumatoid arthritis patients

To determine whether the preactivation of monocytes in patients with axSpA is counterbalanced by an induction of anti-inflammatory mediators, we analysed the production of IL-1ra and IL-10. IL-1ra was detected by intracellular staining and FACS, whereas IL-10 which is induced at later time points after activation was measured by ELISA in the supernatant of whole blood stimulations performed in the absence of BFA. (Such cultures were performed only in axSpA patients and controls.)

The percentage of monocytes spontaneously producing IL-1ra was significantly elevated in axSpA patients but also RA patients compared with healthy controls (Fig. 3a). In contrast, no difference was found after stimulation with the different stimuli in the percentage of IL-1ra-producing monocytes between axSpA or RA patients and controls.

The IL-10 production induced by LPS was significantly lower in axSpA patients compared with controls (median of 1860 versus 3314 pg/ml; $P < 0.05$). In contrast, no difference was found in spontaneous or MDP-, FSL-1-, or PAM_3CSK_4-induced IL-10 production between axSpA patients and controls (Fig. 3).

Analysis of association of monocytic cytokine production with clinical parameters and treatment in patients with axial spondyloarthritis

To determine the association between cytokine production and the state of disease progression according to the presence of radiographic sacroiliitis or the treatment, we log-transformed the data of patients with axSpA and performed a univariate variance analysis. This analysis (ANOVA) revealed association of spontaneous cytokine production (IL-1β, $P = 0.009$; IL-6, $P = 0.03$; TNFα, $P = 0.012$) and FSL-1-induced IL-6 production ($P = 0.007$) with therapy—conventional treatment versus treatment with biologics (i.e., TNFα inhibitors)—but no association with disease state (i.e., presence of radiographic sacroiliitis).

Monocytic pre-activation is confined to axial spondyloarthritis patients under conventional treatment

As the previous analysis suggested an impact of the therapy on the cytokine responses by monocytes, we performed a subanalysis of the data by stratifying the axSpA patients according to therapy into patients receiving conventional treatment and patients receiving TNFα inhibitors. This subanalysis revealed that elevated spontaneous production of IL-1β, IL-6, and TNFα was confined to axSpA patients under conventional treatment (Fig. 4). In this group, the percentage of monocytes spontaneously producing IL-1β and TNFα was significantly higher than in patients under TNFα inhibitor (i.e., biological treatment) ($P < 0.05$).

Also, the enhanced production of proinflammatory cytokines in response to MDP and FSL-1 was restricted to the group of patients under conventional treatment (Fig. 4). In this group of patients, the percentage of monocytes producing IL-1β and IL-6 after MDP and FSL-1 stimulation was significantly higher than in controls even after subtraction of the percentage of monocytes spontaneously producing these cytokines (data not shown). In contrast, no difference was found between patients under conventional treatment and patients under TNFα inhibitor treatment in the percentage of monocytes producing IL-12/23p40 (spontaneous or MDP- or FSL-induced).

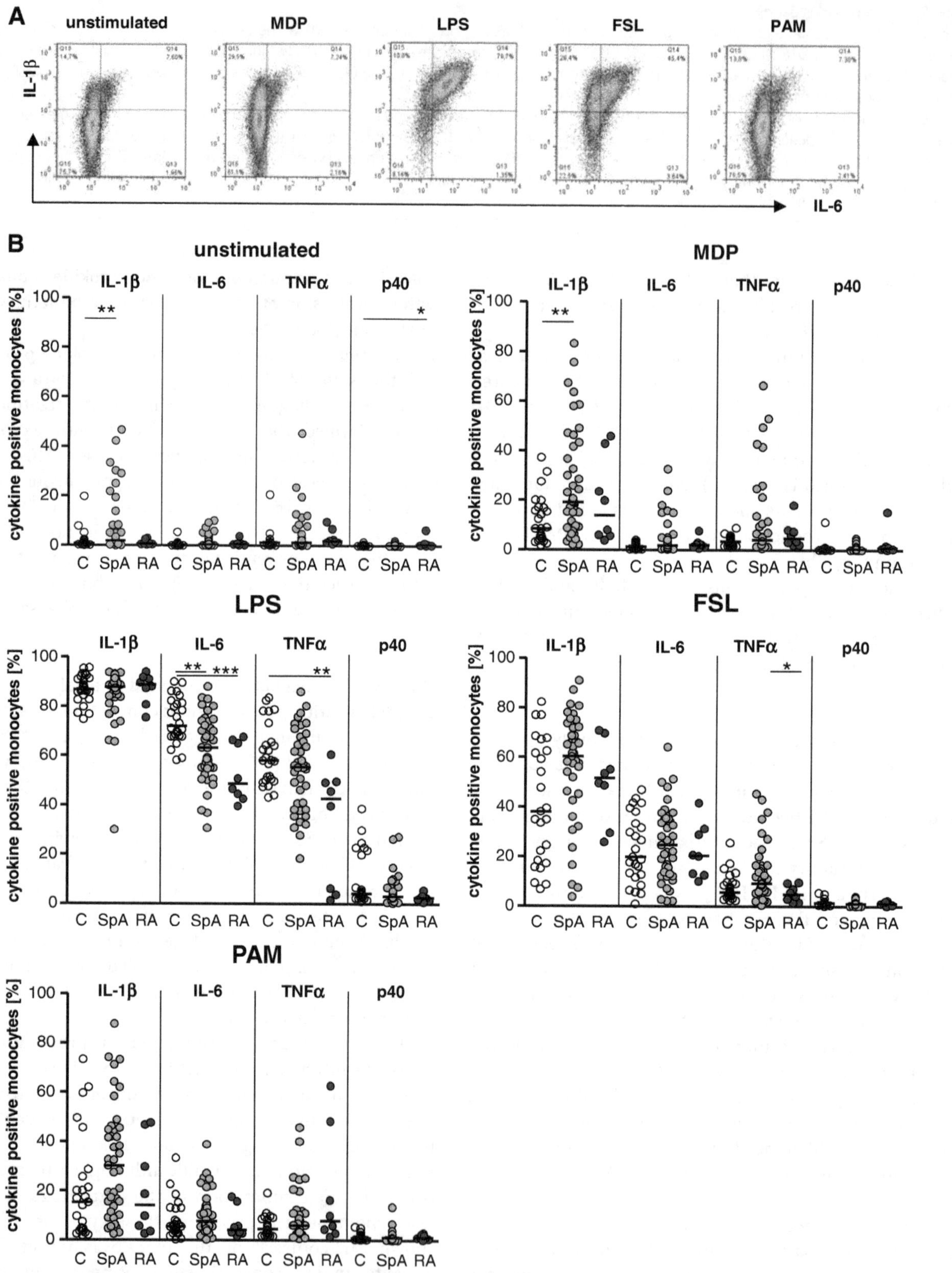

Fig. 2 (See legend on next page.)

(See figure on previous page.)

Fig. 2 Elevated spontaneous and muramyl dipeptide (MDP)-induced proinflammatory cytokine production by monocytes from patients with axial spondyloarthritis (axSpA). Cytokine production by monocytes after stimulation of whole blood without (unstimulated) or with MDP, lipopolysaccharide (LPS), fibroblast-stimulating lipopeptid-1 (FSL), and PAM_3CSK_4 (PAM) for 5 h with brefeldin A added for the last 3 h. Cytokine production was analysed after intracellular staining by fluorescence-activated cell sorting. Monocytes were identified according to CD68 expression. **a** A representative example of cytokine production of $CD68^+$ monocytes of a patient with axSpA in whole blood without stimulation and stimulation with the respective stimuli is shown. **b** The percentage of cytokine-positive cells among $CD68^+$ monocytes (individual measurement and median) in response to the different stimuli in controls (C) ($n = 26$), patients with axSpA (SpA) ($n = 42$), and patients with rheumatoid arthritis (RA) ($n = 8$) is given. $^*P < 0.05$; $^{**}P < 0.01$ (Kruskal-Wallis test and Dunn's post test). *IL* interleukin, *TNFα* tumour necrosis factor alpha

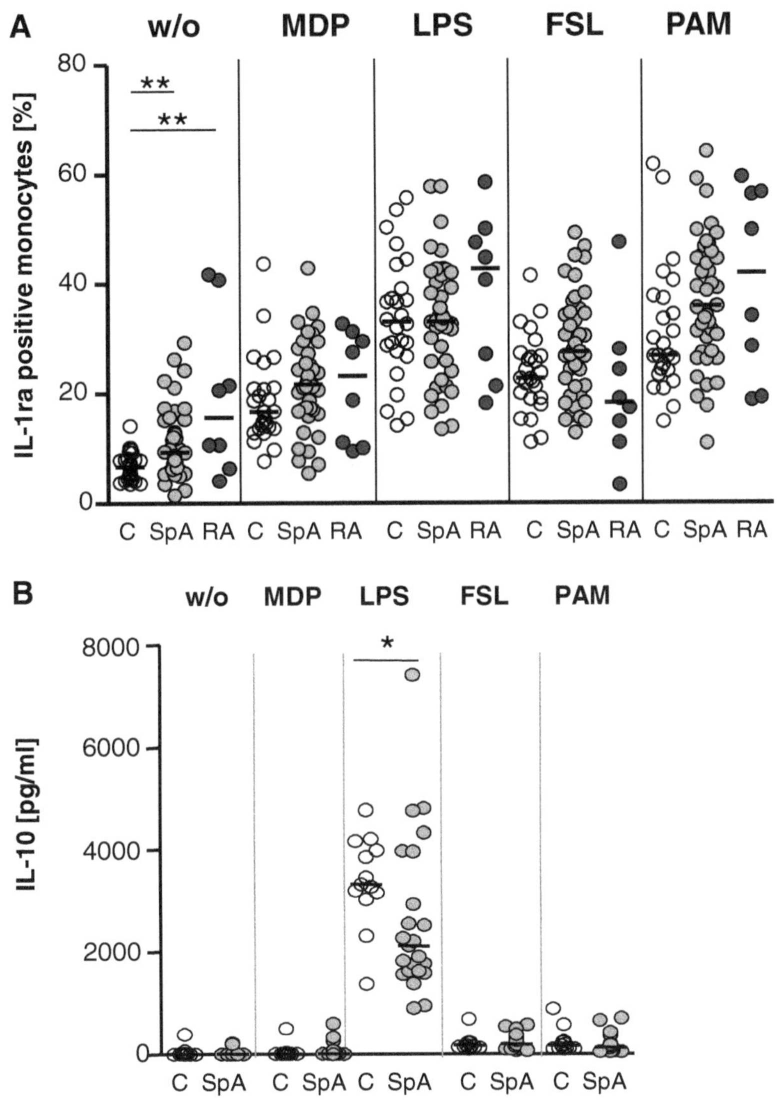

Fig. 3 a Elevated spontaneous production of interleukin-1 receptor antagonist (IL-1ra) by monocytes of patients with axial spondyloarthritis (axSpA) and rheumatoid arthritis (RA). The percentage of IL-1ra-producing monocytes among $CD68^+$ monocytes was determined as in Fig. 2. The percentage of cytokine-positive cells (individual measurement and median) in response to the different stimuli in controls (C) ($n = 26$), patients with axSpA (SpA) ($n = 42$), and patients with RA (RA) ($n = 8$) is given. $^{**}P < 0.01$ (Kruskal-Wallis test and Dunn's post test). Whole blood of patients with axSpA (SpA) ($n = 26$) and controls (C) ($n = 13$) was stimulated without or with indicated stimulators for 18 h. **b** IL-10 was measured in the supernatant by enzyme-linked immunosorbent assay. $^*P < 0.05$ (Mann–Whitney *U* test). *FSL* fibroblast-stimulating lipopeptid-1, *LPS* lipopolysaccharide, *MDP* muramyl dipeptide, *PAM* PAM_3CSK_4, *w/o* without

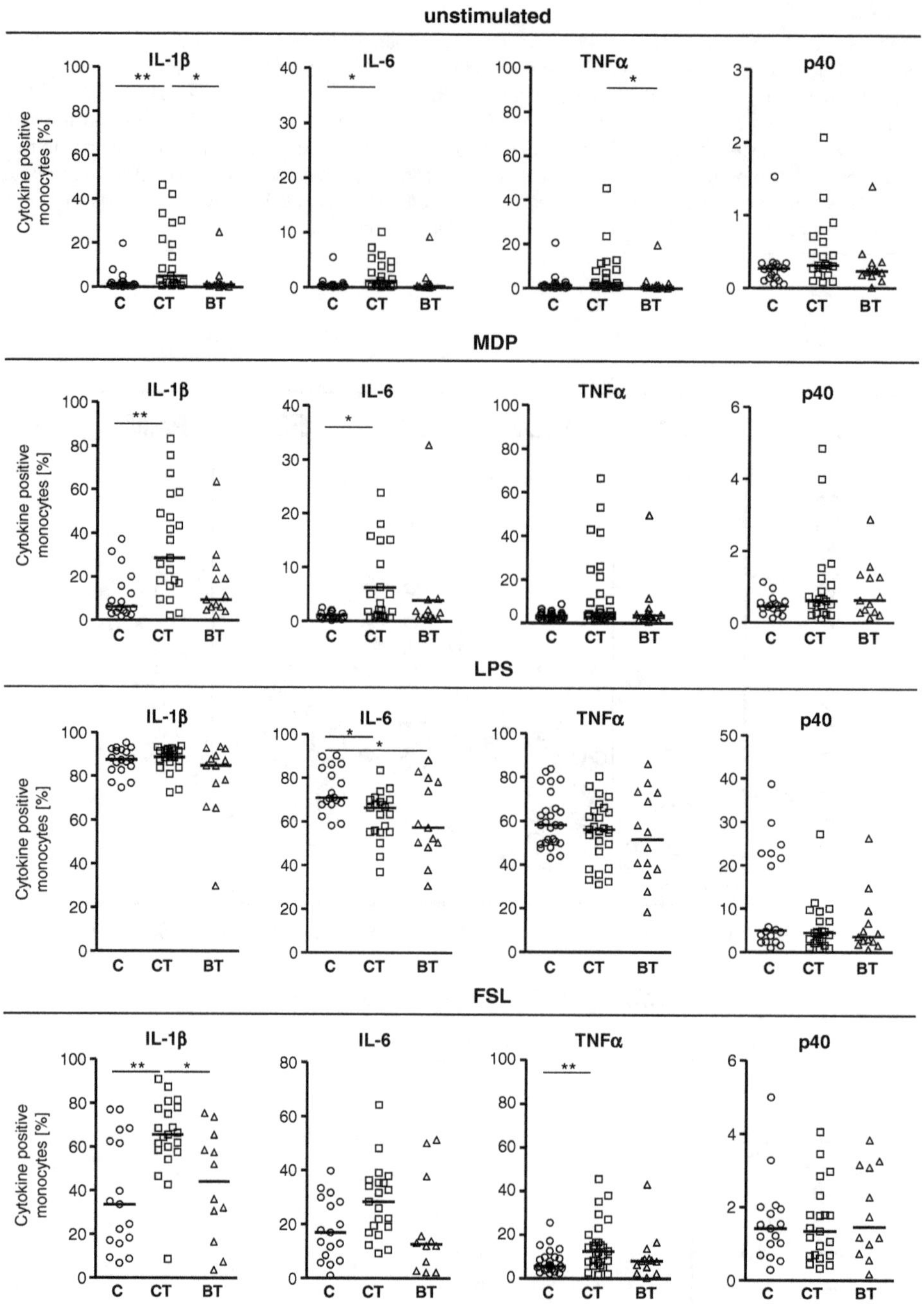

Fig. 4 Disturbed cytokine responses are found predominately in axial spondyloarthritis patients under conventional treatment. Subanalysis of monocytic cytokine production (Fig. 3) in patients stratified according to treatment into a group of patients receiving conventional treatment spondyloarthritis (CT) ($n = 20$) and patients receiving biological treatment (i.e., TNF inhibitor treatment) (BT) ($n = 12$) compared with healthy controls (C) ($n = 17$). *$P < 0.05$; **$P < 0.01$ (Kruskal-Wallis test and Dunn's post test). *FSL* fibroblast-stimulating lipopeptid-1, *IL* interleukin, *LPS* lipopolysaccharide, *MDP* muramyl dipeptide, *TNFα* tumour necrosis factor alpha

Interestingly, LPS-induced cytokine responses did not differ between both groups of patients; that is, IL-6 (Fig. 4) and IL-10 production (data not shown) was reduced in both groups of patients compared with controls ($P < 0.05$). Moreover, there was no difference in the percentage of IL-1ra-producing monocytes between patients under conventional treatment and patients under TNFα inhibitor treatment (data not shown).

To determine the association between monocytic cytokine production and clinical parameters such as inflammatory parameters, presence of radiographic sacroiliitis, and disease activity in patients with axSpA under conventional treatment, we performed an ANOVA and linear regression analysis. In this analysis, monocytic cytokine production (unstimulated and MDP-, LPS-, and FSL-1-stimulated) was not associated with CRP, but a strong association of monocytic cytokine production was observed with BASDAI (Table 1).

Difference in cytokine production by monocytes is not due to differences in Toll-like receptor expression in patients with axial spondyloarthritis

To determine whether differences in TLR ligand-induced monocytic cytokine production between axSpA patients and controls are due to differences in expression of TLR ligands, we analysed the expression of TLR 1, 2, and 4 on monocytes. No difference was found in surface expression of either of the receptors on monocytes in axSpA patients and RA patients compared with controls (Fig. 5).

Table 1 *P* values from univariate analysis of variance between clinical variables and cytokine responses in axial spondyloarthritis patients ($n = 20$) under standard treatment (*P* values, log-transformed data)

	Sacroiliitis	CRP	BASDAI
Unstimulated			
IL-1	0.980	0.539	0.011
IL-6	0.604	0.829	0.025
TNF	0.856	0.984	0.006
IL-1RA	0.299	0.449	0.181
IL-10	0.488	0.584	0.318
MDP			
IL-1	0.300	0.126	0.040
IL-6	0.693	0.698	0.034
TNF	0.439	0.963	0.007
IL-1RA	0.098	0.433	0.010
IL-10	0.634	0.812	0.177
LPS			
IL-1	0.888	0.584	0.005
IL-6	0.546	0.625	0.029
TNF	0.692	0.516	0.001
IL-1RA	0.543	0.744	0.048
IL-10	0.691	0.742	0.010
FSL			
IL-1	0.492	0.470	0.642
IL-6	0.389	0.483	0.669
TNF	0.861	0.918	0.669
IL-1RA	0.227	0.390	0.040
IL-10	0.714	0.199	0.037

CRP C-reactive protein, *BASDAI* Bath ankylosing spondylitis disease activity index, *IL* interleukin, *TNF* tumor necrosis factor, *MDP* muramyl dipeptide, *LPS* lipopolysaccharide, *FSL* fibroblast-stimulating lipopeptid

Discussion

In this study, we observed an elevated frequency of classic (i.e., $CD14^{++}CD16^{-}$) monocytes and a reduction in non-classic (i.e., $CD14^{+}CD16^{+}$) monocytes in peripheral blood of patients with axSpA and this is in accordance with a study by Surdacki et al. [11]. TNFα inhibitor treatment did not reverse these phenotypic differences. In patients with RA, we also observed a trend toward an increase of classic monocytes at the expense of non-classic monocytes. This is in line with data from Klimek et al. [12] but in contrast to other studies which reported an expansion of CD14/CD16 double-positive (i.e., non-classic) monocytes in RA [13, 14]. These discrepancies are most likely related to differences in therapy; in particular, glucocorticoid therapy has been described to deplete $CD14^{+}CD16^{+}$ monocytes [15]. In patients with Crohn's disease, an expansion of non-classic monocytes was described [16]. It was suggested that the imbalance between monocyte subsets in patients with Crohn's disease is due to recruitment of the classic monocytes, which are more migratory than the non-classic monocytes, to sites of inflammation [16]. Therefore, the difference between axSpA and Crohn's disease may be caused by differences in the extent of local inflammation which controls recruitment of monocytes. On the other hand, HLA-B27 could also affect the differentiation of monocyte subsets and promote the differentiation of classic monocytes.

Thiesen et al. analysed cytokine production of sorted human monocyte subsets and found that classic monocytes, though considered more phagocytic and less inflammatory, produced higher levels of proinflammatory cytokines than the non-classic monocytes [16]. Interestingly, we observed enhanced spontaneous as well as MDP- and FSL-1-induced production of proinflammatory cytokines in patients with axSpA and, according to the data by Thiesen et al., this could be related to the expansion of classic monocytes.

The enhanced cytokine production by monocytes of patients with axSpA in particular to suboptimal stimuli such as MDP and FSL-1, which require co-activating signals such as ineffective doses of LPS [17] or low levels of cytokines, suggests that monocytes of patients with axSpA are pre-activated in vivo. This is also suggested by mRNA expression profiles showing enhanced IL-1 receptor expression in blood cells of patients with axSpA [18] and by results of protein profiling of monocytes of axSpA patients that showed enhanced expression of proteins involved in TLR signaling, leukocyte extravasation, and other inflammatory pathways [8]. Genome association studies [19] and experimental [20] and clinical [21] data suggest an involvement of the IL-23-Th17 pathway

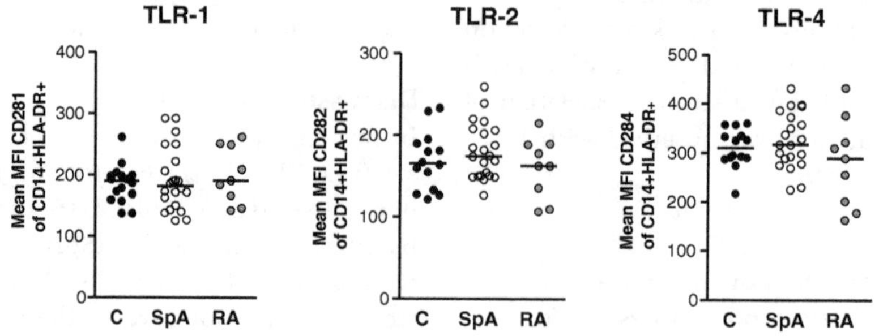

Fig. 5 No difference in Toll-like receptor (TLR) 1, 2, and 4 expression on CD14$^+$ monocytes between axial spondyloarthritis patients and controls. The expression of TLR-1, TLR-2, and TLR-4 on monocytes was determined in healthy controls (C) ($n = 16$), patients with axial spondyloarthritis (SpA) ($n = 22$), and patients with rheumatoid arthritis (RA) ($n = 9$) by surface staining and fluorescence-activated cell sorting and is given as the mean fluorescence intensity (MFI). Monocytes were identified according to CD14 expression

in axSpA. However, the production of IL-12/23p40 production was rather low in peripheral blood monocytes in our study and with no difference between axSpA patients and controls. Even after strong stimulation with LPS, only about 5 % of the monocytes produced IL-12/23p40, suggesting that monocytes are not a major source of this cytokine. In fact, our own analysis of the bone marrow of facet joints of patients with AS revealed myeloperoxidase-positive cells and, to a lesser extent, macrophages and dendritic cells as sources of IL-23 [22].

In contrast to the enhanced cytokine responses to MDP and FSL-1, cytokine production in response to LPS was, at least partially, reduced in patients with axSpA. Reduced LPS responses are observed in endotoxin tolerance which is induced by pre-exposure of monocytes to low doses of LPS. However, the suppression of proinflammatory cytokine responses by monocytes of patients with axSpA is rather minor and accompanied by a strong suppression of anti-inflammatory IL-10 production, whereas the state of endotoxin tolerance and monocyte paralysis, as for instance observed in patients with sepsis, is characterized by a strongly suppressed proinflammatory response and partly preserved IL-10 production [23]. Thus, the decent reduction of cytokine responses to LPS which is the strongest of the tested stimuli may indicate exhaustion of monocytes after pre-activation rather than tolerization.

The enhanced spontaneous production of cytokines was restricted to axSpA patients under conventional treatment and is not found in axSpA patients under TNFα inhibitor treatment or in RA patients. However, LPS-induced IL-6 and IL-10 production was also reduced in axSpA patients who received TNFα inhibitor. This could be attributable to the presence of TNFα inhibitors in the whole blood stimulation which may neutralize some autocrine effects of TNFα produced during early activation. In particular, IL-10 depends on autocrine production of TNFα [7]. Also, in patients with RA, LPS-induced production of IL-6 and TNFα was reduced and this may also be related to glucocorticoid therapy [24].

Differences in cytokine responses to TLR ligands may be caused by differential expression of TLRs. In fact, enhanced expression of TLR 4 on blood monocytes has been described in patients with SpA [25]. However, in our study, no differences were found in the expression of TLR 1, 2, and 4 in axSpA patients compared with controls and this might be due to technical differences as we analysed expression in whole blood as compared with isolated peripheral blood mononuclear cells and used a different gating strategy.

Interestingly, stimulation of bone marrow cells and splenocytes from HLA-B27/huβ2m transgenic rats with TNFα [26] or zymosan or *Mycobacterium tuberculosis* also resulted in elevated production of IL-1α and IL-1β compared with control rats, indicating that the enhanced responsiveness of axSpA patients to bacterial triggers may be related to HLA-B27. On the other hand, the expansion of classic monocytes and in vivo pre-activation of monocytes in patients with axSpA could also be the result of in vivo activation by cytokines released by local inflammation or by bacterial components such as LPS which may translocate during intestinal inflammation as mucosal inflammation is a common feature in axSpA. Thus, about 5 % of patients with AS also suffer from overt inflammatory bowel disease [27] and about 50 % show microscopic gut lesions in the absence of gastrointestinal discomfort [28].

Delineation of potential triggers of the spontaneous cytokine production is difficult since cellular responses of monocytes to LPS and cytokines such as TNFα are strongly overlapping [29]. Only some genes such as apoptosis-related genes are selectively induced in monocytes by LPS in vitro [29] and analysis of their expression might provide clues on the activating signal of monocytes in patients with axSpA.

TNFα inhibitor treatment of axSpA normalized the functional state of monocytes as elevated cytokine responses were confined to axSpA patients under conventional treatment. The fact that MDP- and FSL-1-induced cytokine production was unaffected under TNFα inhibitor treatment suggests that the effect of TNFα inhibitor treatment is an in vivo effect rather than an in vitro effect. Thus, the TNFα inhibitor treatment may interfere with the triggers of monocytic cytokine production such as local cytokine production or bacterial antigen translocation.

Interestingly, we found that spontaneous MDP- and LPS-induced production of cytokines correlated with disease activity. As CRP correlated neither with BASDAI nor with the monocytic cytokine production, monocyte activation might be a more sensitive indicator of inflammation than CRP. However, the monocytic pre-activation, particularly the spontaneous production of IL-1β as well as IL-6, does not seem to be directly pathogenic as blockade of IL-1 [30] as well as IL-6 [31] is of limited or no efficacy in reducing disease activity in AS. The enhanced IL-1β and IL-6 production by monocytes rather seems to be an indicator of systemic innate immune activation while other immune functions of monocytes or other cell types may exert the pathogenic effects.

Conclusions

This study reveals in vivo pre-activation of monocytes in axSpA patients indicated by enhanced spontaneous as well as MDP- and FSL-induced cytokine production by monocytes which correlates with BASDAI. This in vivo pre-activation is confined to patients under conventional therapy and reverted under TNFα inhibitor treatment. Further work should delineate the triggers of this systemic activation of innate cells.

Abbreviations

ANOVA: Analysis of variance; AS: Ankylosing spondylitis; axSpA: Axial spondyloarthritis; BASDAI: Bath ankylosing spondylitis disease activity index; BFA: Brefeldin A; CRP: C-reactive protein; DMARD: Disease-modifying anti-rheumatic drug; ELISA: Enzyme-linked immunosorbent assay; FACS: Fluorescence-activated cell sorting; FITC: Fluorescein isothiocyanate; FSL-1: Fibroblast-stimulating lipopeptid-1; IL: Interleukin; LPS: Lipopolysacchride; MDP: Muramyl dipeptide; NOD: Nucleotide oligomerization domain; NSAID: Non-steroidal anti-inflammatory drug; RA: Rheumatoid arthritis; TLR: Toll-like-receptor; TNFα: Tumour necrosis factor alpha.

Competing interests

The authors declare that they have no competing interests.

Authors' contributions

US and JS helped to design the study, draft the manuscript, and analyse the data. KC helped to perform the assays, collect the data, analyse the data, and draft the manuscript. PW helped to perform the assays, collect the data, and draft the manuscript. All authors read and approved the final manuscript.

Acknowledgements

This work was supported by the German Federal Ministry of Education and Research (Bundesministerium für Bildung und Forschung, or BMBF) through the ArthroMark project. We thank all patients for participation in the study and doctors and study nurses in the rheumatology department at the Charité, Campus Benjamin Franklin, for acquisition of samples.

References

1. Braun J, Sieper J. Ankylosing spondylitis. Lancet. 2007;369:1379–90. doi:10.1016/S0140-6736(07)60635-7.
2. May E, Dorris ML, Satumtira N, Iqbal I, Rehman MI, Lightfoot E, et al. CD8 alpha beta T cells are not essential to the pathogenesis of arthritis or colitis in HLA-B27 transgenic rats. J Immunol. 2003;170:1099–105.
3. Colbert RA, DeLay ML, Klenk EI, Layh-Schmitt G. From HLA-B27 to spondyloarthritis: a journey through the ER. Immunol Rev. 2010;233:181–202. doi:10.1111/j.0105-2896.2009.00865.x.
4. Freudenberg MA, Galanos C. Bacterial lipopolysaccharides: structure, metabolism and mechanisms of action. Int Rev Immunol. 1990;6:207–21.
5. Beutler B, Kruys V. Lipopolysaccharide signal transduction, regulation of tumor necrosis factor biosynthesis, and signaling by tumor necrosis factor itself. J Cardiovasc Pharmacol. 1995;25:S1–8.
6. Garlanda C, Dinarello CA, Mantovani A. The interleukin-1 family: back to the future. Immunity. 2013;39:1003–18. doi:10.1016/j.immuni.2013.11.010.
7. Platzer C, Meisel C, Vogt K, Platzer M, Volk HD. Up-regulation of monocytic IL-10 by tumor necrosis factor-alpha and cAMP elevating drugs. Int Immunol. 1995;7:517–23.
8. Wright C, Edelmann M, di Gleria K, Kollnberger S, Kramer H, McGowan S, et al. Ankylosing spondylitis monocytes show upregulation of proteins involved in inflammation and the ubiquitin proteasome pathway. Ann Rheum Dis. 2009;68:1626–32. doi:10.1136/ard.2008.097204.
9. Gu J, Marker-Hermann E, Baeten D, Tsai WC, Gladman D, Xiong M, et al. A 588-gene microarray analysis of the peripheral blood mononuclear cells of spondyloarthropathy patients. Rheumatology (Oxford). 2002;41:759–66.
10. Garrett S, Jenkinson T, Kennedy LG, Whitelock H, Gaisford P, Calin A. A new approach to defining disease status in ankylosing spondylitis: the Bath Ankylosing Spondylitis Disease Activity Index. J Rheumatol. 1994;21:2286–91.
11. Surdacki A, Sulicka J, Korkosz M, Mikolajczyk T, Telesinska-Jasiowka D, Klimek E, et al. Blood monocyte heterogeneity and markers of endothelial activation in ankylosing spondylitis. J Rheumatol. 2014;41:481–9. doi:10.3899/jrheum.130803.
12. Klimek E, Mikolajczyk T, Sulicka J, Kwasny-Krochin B, Korkosz M, Osmenda G, et al. Blood monocyte subsets and selected cardiovascular risk markers in rheumatoid arthritis of short duration in relation to disease activity. Biomed Res Int. 2014;2014:736853. doi:10.1155/2014/736853.
13. Kawanaka N, Yamamura M, Aita T, Morita Y, Okamoto A, Kawashima M, et al. CD14+, CD16+ blood monocytes and joint inflammation in rheumatoid arthritis. Arthritis Rheum. 2002;46:2578–86. doi:10.1002/art.10545.
14. Rossol M, Kraus S, Pierer M, Baerwald C, Wagner U. The CD14(bright) CD16+ monocyte subset is expanded in rheumatoid arthritis and promotes expansion of the Th17 cell population. Arthritis Rheum. 2012;64:671–7. doi:10.1002/art.33418.
15. Dayyani F, Belge KU, Frankenberger M, Mack M, Berki T, Ziegler-Heitbrock L. Mechanism of glucocorticoid-induced depletion of human CD14 + CD16+ monocytes. J Leukoc Biol. 2003;74:33–9.
16. Thiesen S, Janciauskiene S, Uronen-Hansson H, Agace W, Hogerkorp CM, Spee P, et al. CD14(hi)HLA-DR(dim) macrophages, with a resemblance to classic blood monocytes, dominate inflamed mucosa in Crohn's disease. J Leukoc Biol. 2014;95:531–41. doi:10.1189/jlb.0113021.
17. Fritz JH, Girardin SE, Fitting C, Werts C, Mengin-Lecreulx D, Caroff M, et al. Synergistic stimulation of human monocytes and dendritic cells by Toll-like receptor 4 and NOD1- and NOD2-activating agonists. Eur J Immunol. 2005;35:2459–70. doi:10.1002/eji.200526286.
18. Sharma SM, Choi D, Planck SR, Harrington CA, Austin CR, Lewis JA, et al. Insights in to the pathogenesis of axial spondyloarthropathy based on gene expression profiles. Arthritis Res Ther. 2009;11:R168. doi:10.1186/ar2855.
19. Cortes A, Hadler J, Pointon JP, Robinson PC, Karaderi T, Leo P, et al. Identification of multiple risk variants for ankylosing spondylitis through high-density genotyping of immune-related loci. Nat Genet. 2013;45:730–8. doi:10.1038/ng.2667.
20. Sherlock JP, Joyce-Shaikh B, Turner SP, Chao CC, Sathe M, Grein J, et al. IL-23 induces spondyloarthropathy by acting on ROR-gammat + CD3 + CD4-CD8- entheseal resident T cells. Nat Med. 2012;18:1069–76. doi:10.1038/nm.2817.
21. Poddubnyy D, Hermann KG, Callhoff J, Listing J, Sieper J. Ustekinumab for the treatment of patients with active ankylosing spondylitis: results of a 28-week, prospective, open-label, proof-of-concept study (TOPAS). Ann Rheum Dis. 2014;73:817–23. doi:10.1136/annrheumdis-2013-204248.
22. Appel H, Maier R, Bleil J, Hempfing A, Loddenkemper C, Schlichting U, et al. In situ analysis of interleukin-23- and interleukin-12-positive cells in the spine of patients with ankylosing spondylitis. Arthritis Rheum. 2013;65:1522–9. doi:10.1002/art.37937.

23. Randow F, Syrbe U, Meisel C, Krausch D, Zuckermann H, Platzer C, et al. Mechanism of endotoxin desensitization: involvement of interleukin 10 and transforming growth factor beta. J Exp Med. 1995;181:1887–92.
24. Boumpas DT, Paliogianni F, Anastassiou ED, Balow JE. Glucocorticosteroid action on the immune system: molecular and cellular aspects. Clin Exp Rheumatol. 1991;9:413–23.
25. De Rycke L, Vandooren B, Kruithof E, De Keyser F, Veys EM, Baeten D. Tumor necrosis factor alpha blockade treatment down-modulates the increased systemic and local expression of Toll-like receptor 2 and Toll-like receptor 4 in spondylarthropathy. Arthritis Rheum. 2005;52:2146–58. doi:10.1002/art.21155.
26. Layh-Schmitt G, Yang EY, Kwon G, Colbert RA. HLA-B27 alters the response to tumor necrosis factor alpha and promotes osteoclastogenesis in bone marrow monocytes from HLA-B27-transgenic rats. Arthritis Rheum. 2013;65:2123–31. doi:10.1002/art.38001.
27. Stolwijk C, van Tubergen A, Castillo-Ortiz JD, Boonen A. Prevalence of extra-articular manifestations in patients with ankylosing spondylitis: a systematic review and meta-analysis. Ann Rheum Dis. 2015;74:65–73. doi:10.1136/annrheumdis-2013-203582.
28. Van Praet L, Van den Bosch FE, Jacques P, Carron P, Jans L, Colman R, et al. Microscopic gut inflammation in axial spondyloarthritis: a multiparametric predictive model. Ann Rheum Dis. 2013;72:414–7. doi:10.1136/annrheumdis-2012-202135.
29. Smiljanovic B, Grun JR, Steinbrich-Zollner M, Stuhlmuller B, Haupl T, Burmester GR, et al. Defining TNF-alpha- and LPS-induced gene signatures in monocytes to unravel the complexity of peripheral blood transcriptomes in health and disease. J Mol Med (Berl). 2010;88:1065–79. doi:10.1007/s00109-010-0648-8.
30. Haibel H, Rudwaleit M, Listing J, Sieper J. Open label trial of anakinra in active ankylosing spondylitis over 24 weeks. Ann Rheum Dis. 2005;64:296–8. doi:10.1136/ard.2004.023176.
31. Sieper J, Braun J, Kay J, Badalamenti S, Radin AR, Jiao L, et al. Sarilumab for the treatment of ankylosing spondylitis: results of a Phase II, randomised, double-blind, placebo-controlled study (ALIGN). Ann Rheum Dis. 2015;74:1051–7. doi:10.1136/annrheumdis-2013-204963.

Permissions

All chapters in this book were first published in AR&T, by BioMed Central; hereby published with permission under the Creative Commons Attribution License or equivalent. Every chapter published in this book has been scrutinized by our experts. Their significance has been extensively debated. The topics covered herein carry significant findings which will fuel the growth of the discipline. They may even be implemented as practical applications or may be referred to as a beginning point for another development.

The contributors of this book come from diverse backgrounds, making this book a truly international effort. This book will bring forth new frontiers with its revolutionizing research information and detailed analysis of the nascent developments around the world.

We would like to thank all the contributing authors for lending their expertise to make the book truly unique. They have played a crucial role in the development of this book. Without their invaluable contributions this book wouldn't have been possible. They have made vital efforts to compile up to date information on the varied aspects of this subject to make this book a valuable addition to the collection of many professionals and students.

This book was conceptualized with the vision of imparting up-to-date information and advanced data in this field. To ensure the same, a matchless editorial board was set up. Every individual on the board went through rigorous rounds of assessment to prove their worth. After which they invested a large part of their time researching and compiling the most relevant data for our readers.

The editorial board has been involved in producing this book since its inception. They have spent rigorous hours researching and exploring the diverse topics which have resulted in the successful publishing of this book. They have passed on their knowledge of decades through this book. To expedite this challenging task, the publisher supported the team at every step. A small team of assistant editors was also appointed to further simplify the editing procedure and attain best results for the readers.

Apart from the editorial board, the designing team has also invested a significant amount of their time in understanding the subject and creating the most relevant covers. They scrutinized every image to scout for the most suitable representation of the subject and create an appropriate cover for the book.

The publishing team has been an ardent support to the editorial, designing and production team. Their endless efforts to recruit the best for this project, has resulted in the accomplishment of this book. They are a veteran in the field of academics and their pool of knowledge is as vast as their experience in printing. Their expertise and guidance has proved useful at every step. Their uncompromising quality standards have made this book an exceptional effort. Their encouragement from time to time has been an inspiration for everyone.

The publisher and the editorial board hope that this book will prove to be a valuable piece of knowledge for researchers, students, practitioners and scholars across the globe.

List of Contributors

Sofia Exarchou and Carl Turesson
Rheumatology, Department of Clinical Sciences, Malmö, Lund University, Inga Marie Nilssons gata 3,205 02 Malmö, Sweden

Lars Erik Kristensen
Rheumatology, Department of Clinical Sciences, Malmö, Lund University, Inga Marie Nilssons gata 3,205 02 Malmö, Sweden
The Parker Institute, Department of Rheumatology, Bispebjerg and Frederiksberg Hospital, the Capital Region of Copenhagen, Copenhagen, Denmark

Ulf Lindström, Helena Forsblad-d'Elia and Lennart TH Jacobsson
Department of Rheumatology and Inflammation Research, Sahlgrenska Academy at University of Gothenburg, Gothenburg, Sweden

Johan Askling
Clinical Epidemiology Unit & Rheumatology Unit, Department of Medicine Solna, Karolinska Institute, Stockholm, Sweden

Jonas K Eriksson and Martin Neovius
Clinical Epidemiology Unit, Department of Medicine Solna, Karolinska Institute, Stockholm, Sweden

Wei Wang
Department of Orthopedics, Chengdu Military General Hospital, Chengdu city, People's Republic of China

Gen-jin Yang
School of Pharmacy, Second Military Medical University, Shanghai city, People's Republic of China

Ju Zhang
Department of Rheumatology, Changhai Hospital, Shanghai city, People's Republic of China

Chen Chen
Physical Examination Center, Changhai Hospital, Shanghai city, People's Republic of China

Zhen-yu Jia, Jia Li and Wei-dong Xu
Department of Orthopedics, Changhai Hospital, Shanghai city, People's Republic of China

Manouk de Hooge, Roberta Ramonda, Mariagrazia Lorenzin, Paola Frallonardo, Leonardo Punzi, Augusta Ortolan and Andrea Doria
Rheumatology Unit, Department of Medicine – DIMED, University of Padova, Via Giustiniani,35128 Padova, Italy

Eva Klingberg, Anna Deminger and Hans Carlsten
Department of Rheumatology and Inflammation Research, Sahlgrenska Academy at the University of Gothenburg, Guldhedsgatan 10A, S-413 46 Gothenburg, Sweden

Helena Forsblad-d'Elia
Department of Rheumatology and Inflammation Research, Sahlgrenska Academy at the University of Gothenburg, Guldhedsgatan 10A, S-413 46 Gothenburg, Sweden
Rheumatology Unit, Department of Public Health and Clinical Medicine, Umeå University, Umeå, Sweden

Hans Strid
Department of Internal Medicine, Södra Älvsborgs Sjukhus, Borås, Sweden
Department of Internal Medicine and Clinical Nutrition, Sahlgrenska Academy at the University of Gothenburg, Gothenburg, Sweden

Arne Ståhl
Department of Microbiology and Immunology, Sahlgrenska Academy at the University of Gothenburg, Gothenburg, Sweden

Lena Öhman
Department of Microbiology and Immunology, Sahlgrenska Academy at the University of Gothenburg, Gothenburg, Sweden
Sweden School of Health and Education, University of Skövde, Skövde, Sweden

Fiona Maas, Elisabeth Brouwer and Hendrika Bootsma
Rheumatology and Clinical Immunology, University Medical Center Groningen, University of Groningen, RB Groningen, The Netherlands

Suzanne Arends and Anneke Spoorenberg
Rheumatology and Clinical Immunology, University Medical Center Groningen, University of Groningen, RB Groningen, The Netherlands
Rheumatology, Medical Center Leeuwarden, Leeuwarden, The Netherlands

Reinhard Bos and Freke R. Wink
Rheumatology, Medical Center Leeuwarden, Leeuwarden, The Netherlands

Junqing Zhu
Department of Rheumatology, Nanfang Hospital, Southern Medical University, Guangzhou, Guangdong 510515, China

Aiwu Li, Ertao Jia, Juan Xu, Shixian Chen and Yinger Huang
Department of Internal Medicine of Traditional Chinese Medicine, College of Traditional Chinese Medicine, Southern Medical University, Guangzhou, Guangdong 510510, China

Juan Li
Department of Internal Medicine of Traditional Chinese Medicine, College of Traditional Chinese Medicine, Southern Medical University, Guangzhou, Guangdong 510510, China
Department of Rheumatology, Nanfang Hospital, Southern Medical University, Guangzhou, Guangdong 510515, China

Yi Zhou
Department of Obstetrics, Guangdong Women and Children Hospital, Guangzhou, Guangdong 511400, China

Xiang Xiao
Department of Radiology, Nanfang Hospital, Southern Medical University, Guangzhou, Guangdong 510515, China

Walter P. Maksymowych and Stephanie Wichuk
Department of Medicine, University of Alberta, 568 Heritage Medical Research Building, Edmonton, AB T6G 2S,Canada

Maxime Dougados
Paris Descartes University; Department of Rheumatology - Hôpital Cochin, Assistance Publique - Hôpitaux de Paris; INSERM (U1153): Clinical Epidemiology and Biostatistics, PRES Sorbonne Paris-Cité, Paris, France

Heather Jones, Jack F. Bukowski and Lisa Marshall
Pfizer, Collegeville, PA, USA

Annette Szumski
inVentiv Health, Princeton, NJ, USA

Robert G. Lambert
Department of Radiology and Diagnostic Imaging, University of Alberta, Edmonton, AB, Canada

Ruben Burgos-Vargas
Department of Rheumatology, General Hospital of Mexico, Mexico City, Mexico

James Cheng-Chung Wei
Division of Allergy, Immunology and Rheumatology, Chung Shan Medical University Hospital, No. 110, Sec., Jianguo N. Road, South District, Taichung City 4020,Taiwan
Institute of Medicine, Chung Shan Medical University, Taichung City, Taiwan
Graduate Institute of Integrated Medicine, China Medical University, Taichung City, Taiwan

Mahboob U. Rahman
University of Pennsylvania, Philadelphia, PA, USA
Pfizer, Collegeville, PA, USA

Ehab Mahgoub, Ena Singh, Constance Hammond, Ron Pedersen, Qi Shen and Bonnie Vlahos
Pfizer, Collegeville, PA, USA

Nurullah Akkoc
Dokuz Eylül University, İzmir, Turkey

Syed Atiqul Haq
Bangabandhu Sheikh Mujib Medical University, Dhaka, Bangladesh

Mohammed Hammoudeh
Hamad Hospital, Doha, Qatar

Lyndon John Llamado
Pfizer Asia Pacific Region, Makati, Philippines

Khalid Shirazy
Pfizer Africa and Middle East Region, Dubai, UAE

Sameer Kotak
Pfizer, New York, NY, USA

Mikhail Protopopov, Joachim Sieper and Hildrun Haibel
Department of Gastroenterology, Infectiology and Rheumatology, Charité - Universitätsmedizin Berlin, Hindenburgdamm 30, 12203 Berlin, Germany

Denis Poddubnyy
Department of Gastroenterology, Infectiology and Rheumatology, Charité - Universitätsmedizin Berlin, Hindenburgdamm 30, 12203 Berlin, Germany
German Rheumatism Research Centre, Charitéplatz,10117 Berlin, Germany

Martin Rudwaleit
Department of Gastroenterology, Infectiology and Rheumatology, Charité - Universitätsmedizin Berlin, Hindenburgdamm 30, 12203 Berlin, Germany
Klinikum Bielefeld Rosenhöhe, An der Rosenhöhe 27, 33647 Bielefeld, Germany

Joachim Listing
German Rheumatism Research Centre, Charitéplatz, 10117 Berlin, Germany

Baek-Lok Oh
Department of Ophthalmology, Armed Forces Capital Hospital, Seongnam, Gyeonggi-do, South Korea

Jeong Seok Lee and Eun Young Lee
Division of Rheumatology, Department of Internal Medicine, Seoul National University College of Medicine, Seoul National University Hospital, Seoul, South Korea

Hee Young Lee
Center for Preventive Medicine and Public Health, Seoul National University Bundang Hospital, Seongnam, Gyeonggi-do, South Korea

Hyeong Gon Yu
Department of Ophthalmology, Seoul National University College of Medicine, Seoul National University Hospital, Seoul, South Korea

Janneke J. de Winter, Marleen G. van de Sande and Dominique L. Baeten
Department of Clinical Immunology and Rheumatology, Amsterdam Rheumatology and immunology Center, Academic Medical Center/ University of Amsterdam, Amsterdam, The Netherlands
Department of Immunology and Rheumatology, Medical University Hannover, Hannover, Germany

Torsten Witte
Department of Immunology and Rheumatology, Medical University Hannover, Hannover, Germany

Niklas Baerlecken
Department of Immunology and Rheumatology, Medical University Hannover, Hannover, Germany
Private Practice, Cologne, Germany

Inger Berg
Department of Rheumatology, Diakonhjemmet Hospital, Oslo, Norway

Roberta Ramonda
Rheumatology unit, Department of medicine, University of Padua, Padua, Italy

Désirée van der Heijde and Floris A. van Gaalen
Department of Rheumatology, Leiden University Medical Center, Leiden, The Netherlands

Natasha Miller and Stephen J. Duffield
Musculoskeletal biology I, Institute of Ageing and Chronic Disease, University of Liverpool, Liverpool, UK

Laura Chadwick, Nicola J. Goodson and Sizheng Zhao
Musculoskeletal biology I, Institute of Ageing and Chronic Disease, University of Liverpool, Liverpool, UK
Department of Academic Rheumatology, Aintree University Hospital, Liverpool, UK

Daniel Thong
Department of Academic Rheumatology, Aintree University Hospital, Liverpool, UK

David M. Hughes
Department of Biostatistics, Institute of Translational Medicine, University of Liverpool, Liverpool, UK

Oh Chan Kwon, Seokchan Hong, Chang-Keun Lee, Bin Yoo and Yong-Gil Kim
Division of Rheumatology, Department of Internal Medicine, University of Ulsan, College of Medicine, Asan Medical Center, 88 Olympic-ro 43-gil, Songpa-gu, Seoul 05505, South Korea

Sang-Won Lee and Yong-Beom Park
Division of Rheumatology, Department of Internal Medicine, Yonsei University College of Medicine, Seoul, South Korea

Ji Seon Oh
Clinical Research Center, University of Ulsan College of Medicine, Asan Medical Center, Seoul, South Korea

Sang Hoon Lee
Department of Radiology and Research Institute of Radiology, University of Ulsan College of Medicine, Asan Medical Center, Seoul, South Korea

Javier Rueda-Gotor, Fernanda Genre, Alfonso Corrales, Ricardo Blanco, Patricia Fuentevilla, Virginia Portilla and Trinitario Pina
Epidemiology, Genetics and Atherosclerosis Research Group on Systemic Inflammatory Diseases, Division of Rheumatology, Hospital Universitario Marqués de Valdecilla, IDIVAL, University of Cantabria, Avenida de Valdecilla,s/n, 39008 Santander, Spain

Miguel A. González-Gay
Epidemiology, Genetics and Atherosclerosis Research Group on Systemic Inflammatory Diseases, Division of Rheumatology, Hospital Universitario Marqués de Valdecilla, IDIVAL, University of Cantabria, Avenida de Valdecilla,s/n, 39008 Santander, Spain
Cardiovascular Pathophysiology and Genomics Research Unit, School of Physiology, Faculty of Health Sciences, University of the Witwatersrand, Johannesburg, South Africa

Rosa Expósito and Cristina Mata
Division of Rheumatology, Hospital Comarcal, Laredo, Cantabria, Spain

Carlos González-Juanatey
Division of Cardiology, Hospital Lucus Augusti, Lugo, Spain

Luis Rodriguez-Rodriguez
Division of Rheumatology, Instituto de Investigación Sanitaria del Hospital Clínico San Carlos (IDISSC), Hospital Clínico San Carlos, Madrid, Spain

Robert Landewé
Clinical Immunology and Rheumatology, Amsterdam Rheumatology & Immunology Center and Academic Medical Center, University of Amsterdam, Amsterdam, Netherlands

Tommi Nurminen
UCB Pharma, Monheim, Germany

Owen Davies
UCB Pharma, Slough, UK

Dominique Baeten
UCB Pharma, Brussels, Belgium

Hyemin Jeong and Chan Hong Jeon
Division of Rheumatology, Department of Internal Medicine, Soonchunhyang University Hospital, Bucheon, South Korea

Eun-Kyung Bae and Hunnyun Kim
Samsung Biomedical Research Institute, Seoul, South Korea

Yeong Hee Eun, In Young Kim, Hyungjin Kim, Jaejoon Lee, Eun-Mi Koh and Hoon-Suk Cha
Division of Rheumatology, Department of Internal Medicine, Samsung Medical Center, Sungkyunkwan University School of Medicine, 81 Irwon-Ro, Gangnam-gu, Seoul 0635, South Korea

Fernanda Manente Milanez, Carla G. S. Saad, Vilma T. Viana, Júlio C. B. Moraes, Percival Degrava Sampaio-Barros, Célio R. Goncalves and Eloísa Bonfá
Division of Rheumatology, Faculdade de Medicina da Universidade de São Paulo - Reumatologia, Av. Dr. Arnaldo, n° 455, 3° andar, sala 319,São Paulo, SP 05403-010, Brazil

Grégory Vinícius Périco
URC - Unidade Radiológica Criciúma, Rua Antonio de Lucca, 139 - Centro - Criciúma, Santa Catarina, SC 88811-50,Brazil

Ulf Lindström and Lennart Jacobsson
Department of Rheumatology and Inflammation Research, Institute of Medicine, Sahlgrenska Academy, University of Gothenburg, Guldhedsgatan 10A, 405 30 Gothenburg, Sweden

Elisabeth Lie
Department of Rheumatology and Inflammation Research, Institute of Medicine, Sahlgrenska Academy, University of Gothenburg, Guldhedsgatan 10A, 405 30 Gothenburg, Sweden
Department of Rheumatology, Diakonhjemmet Hospital, Diakonveien 1,Vinderen, 0319 Oslo, Norway

Helena Forsblad-d'Elia
Institution of Public Health and Clinical Medicine/ Rheumatology, Umeå University, Lasarettsgatan 7, 901 87 Umeå, Sweden

Johan Askling
Rheumatology Unit and Clinical Epidemiology Unit, Department of Medicine Solna, Karolinska Institutet, Nobels väg 5, Solna 171 76 Stockholm, Sweden

Lars Erik Kristensen
The Parker Institute, Department of Rheumatology, Frederiksberg and Bispebjerg Hospital, Nordre Fasanvej 57, 2000 Frederiksberg, Denmark

Sofia Exarchou
Section of Rheumatology, Department of Clinical Sciences, Lund University, Barngatan 2B, 221 85 Lund, Sweden

Adrian Ciurea and Beate Steininger
Department of Rheumatology, University Hospital Zurich, Gloriastrasse 25, CH-8091 Zurich, Switzerland

Pascale Exer
Private Rheumatology Practice, Basel, Switzerland

Ulrich Weber
King Christian 10th Hospital for Rheumatic Diseases, Gråsten, Denmark
South Jutland Hospital, Denmark Institute of Regional Health Research, University of Southern Denmark, Odense, Denmark

Giorgio Tamborrini
Department of Rheumatology, Bethesda Hospital, Basel, Switzerland

Rudolf O. Kissling
Department of Rheumatology, Balgrist University Hospital, Zurich, Switzerland

Jürg Bernhard
Department of Rheumatology and Rehabilitation, Bürgerspital, Solothurn, Switzerland

Almut Scherer
Swiss Clinical Quality Management Foundation, Zurich, Switzerland

Roberta Ramonda and Leonardo Punzi
Rheumatology Unit, Department of Medicine DIMED, University of Padova, Via Giustiniani,,Padova 35128, Italy

Antonio Marchesoni
Division of Rheumatology, Day Hospital Unit, Istituto Ortopedico G. Pini, Milano, Italy

Antonio Carletto
Rheumatology Unit, University of Verona, Verona, Italy

Gerolamo Bianchi
Department of Locomotor System, Division of Rheumatology, ASL3-Azienda Sanitaria Genovese, Arenzano, Genova, Italy

Maurizio Cutolo
Research Laboratory and Academic Division of Clinical Rheumatology, Department of Internal Medicine, IRCCS A.O.U. San Martino-IST, University of Genova, Genova, Italy

Raffaele Scarpa
Rheumatology Research Unit, Department of Clinical and Experimental Medicine, University Federico II, Napoli, Italy

Gianfilippo Bagnato
Department of Clinical and Experimental Medicine, University of Messina, Messina, Italy

Giovanni Triolo
Department of Internal Medicine, Rheumatology Unit, University of Palermo, Palermo, Italy

Guido Valesini
Rheumatology Unit, La Sapienza University of Roma, Roma, Italy

Ignazio Olivieri
Rheumatology Department, San Carlo Hospital, Potenza, Italy

Yang Cui, Jinping Zheng, Xiao Zhang and Riqiang Luo
Department of Rheumatism, Guangdong General Hospital, Guangdong Academy of Medical Sciences, No. 106, Zhongshaner Road, Guangzhou, China

Hui Zeng
Medical Imaging Centre, Guangdong General Hospital, Guangdong Academy of Medical Sciences, Guangzhou 510010, China

Eugenio de Miguel
Department of Rheumatology, IdiPaz, University Hospital La Paz, Madrid, Spain

Victoria Navarro-Compán
Department of Rheumatology, IdiPaz, University Hospital La Paz, Madrid, Spain
Department of Rheumatology, Leiden University Medical Center, Leiden, The Netherlands

Désirée van der Heijde
Department of Rheumatology, Leiden University Medical Center, Leiden, The Netherlands

Robert Landewé
Department of Clinical Immunology & Rheumatology, Academic Medical Center, University of Amsterdam, Amsterdam, The Netherlands
Department of Rheumatology, Atrium Medical Center Heerlen, Heerlen, The Netherlands

Raquel Almodóvar and Pedro Zarco
Department of Rheumatology, University Hospital Foundation Alcorcón, Madrid, Spain

Carlos Montilla
Department of Rheumatology, Hospital Clínico Universitario de Salamanca, Salamanca, Spain

Emma Beltrán
Department of Rheumatology, Hospital Universitario General de Valencia, Valencia, Spain

Hsu-Wen Tseng, Miranda E. Pitt, Tony J. Kenna, Matthew A. Brown and Gethin P. Thomas
The University of Queensland Diamantina Institute, Translational Research Institute, 37 Kent Street, Woolloongabba, QLD 410,Australia

Allan F. McRae
The University of Queensland Diamantina Institute, Translational Research Institute, 37 Kent Street, Woolloongabba, QLD 410,Australia
The University of Queensland, Queensland Brain Institute, QBI Building, St Lucia, QLD 407,Australia

Tibor T. Glant
Section of Molecular Medicine, Department of Orthopedic Surgery, Rush University Medical Center, 1735 W. Harrison Street, Cohn Research Building, Chicago, IL 6061,USA

Allison R. Pettit
The University of Queensland-Mater Research Institute, Translational Research Institute, 37 Kent Street, Woolloongabba, QLD 410,Australia

Kristina Conrad
Charité-Universitätsmedizin Berlin, CBF, Medizinische Klinik für Gastroenterologie, Infektiologie und Rheumatologie, Hindenburgdamm 30, Berlin 1220,Germany

Joachim Sieper and Uta Syrbe
Charité-Universitätsmedizin Berlin, CBF, Medizinische Klinik für Gastroenterologie, Infektiologie und Rheumatologie, Hindenburgdamm 30, Berlin 1220,Germany
Deutsches Rheumaforschungszentrum, Charitéplatz,Berlin 10117, Germany

Peihua Wu
Deutsches Rheumaforschungszentrum, Charitéplatz, Berlin 10117, Germany

Index

www.ingramcontent.com/pod-product-compliance
Lightning Source LLC
LaVergne TN
LVHW080656210926
848485LV00003B/383